Blood and Marrow Transplantation Long-Term Management

Prevention and Complications

Blood and Marrow Transplantation Long-Term Management

Prevention and Complications

EDITED BY

Bipin N Savani MD

Professor of Medicine
Director, Long Term Transplant Clinic
Hematology and Stem Cell Transplantation Section
Vanderbilt University Medical Center
Nashville, TN, USA

WILEY Blackwell

Registered office: John Wiley & Sons, Ltd, The Atrium, Southern Gate, Chichester, West Sussex, PO19 8SQ, UK

Editorial offices: 9600 Garsington Road, Oxford, OX4 2DQ, UK
The Atrium, Southern Gate, Chichester, West Sussex, PO19 8SQ, UK
111 River Street, Hoboken, NJ 07030-5774, USA

For details of our global editorial offices, for customer services and for information about how to apply for permission to reuse the copyright material in this book please see our website at www.wiley.com/wiley-blackwell

Library of Congress Cataloging-in-Publication Data
Blood and marrow transplantation long-term management : prevention and complications / edited by Bipin N Savani.
p. ; cm.
Includes bibliographical references and index.
ISBN 978-1-118-47340-5 (cloth)
I. Savani, Bipin N., editor of compilation.
[DNLM: 1. Hematopoietic Stem Cell Transplantation. 2. Disease-Free Survival. 3. Long-Term Care. 4. Survivors. 5. Transplantation, Homologous. WH 380]
RM171.4
616.02'774–dc23
2013018410

A catalogue record for this book is available from the British Library.

Wiley also publishes its books in a variety of electronic formats. Some content that appears in print may not be available in electronic books.

Cover image: iStockphoto.com

Set in 9/12 pt Minion by Toppan Best-set Premedia Limited
Printed and bound in Malaysia by Vivar Printing Sdn Bhd

1 2013

Contents

Foreword

by John Barrett

The science and clinical application of stem cell transplantation began soon after the Second World War, prompted by intensive research to find ways to treat radiation sickness. But substantial numbers of allogeneic stem cell transplants only began to be performed in the1970s. Decade by decade the number of transplant centers has increased, and the number of successful transplants has increased. Long-term survivors from transplant thus represent a new field of medicine born out of the success of a procedure that is every year becoming both increasingly applied and more successful in its outcome.

No reliable data exist as to how many long-term survivors are now living, but we can make some estimates: The World Blood and Marrow Transplantation Organization (WBMT) has assembled data from over 1400 stem cell transplant teams from 72 countries in 5 continents. In recent years the combined *reported* world output for stem cell transplants is in the order of 50 000 transplants a year. As a rough estimate, this represents about half a million transplants per decade, but this figure is conservative given a steady increase in the number of transplants being performed in all parts of the world every year. Assuming a conservative global 30% long-term survival for the 1 million transplants performed in the last 20 years, we can expect around 300 000 long-term transplant survivors. Allowing for underreporting and adding in survivors from all transplants since 1970, it is likely that there are substantially more than half a million long-term survivors from transplant world wide.

This book is therefore timely and at the same time unique: the first textbook on long-term survivorship after stem cell transplantation. It will be an invaluable source for all practitioners and caregivers responsible for the lifelong management of this burgeoning group of individuals. Bipin Savani, the editor, has assembled what must be the definitive text on this subject and has called upon 74 co-authors to put together this authoritative book. Section 1 sets the stage, with contributions from acknowledged experts in the field from Europe and the USA, covering the organizational aspects of long-term care of transplant patients. Section 2 is devoted to management of the major issues facing our survivors: second malignancies, graft-versus-host disease, infections, organ-specific complications, and the long-term screening systems needed to manage transplant recipients over the years. As risks of serious complications diminish, the quality of life of the survivors becomes a paramount and not-to-be forgotten consideration. It is appropriate that Section 3, in its entirety, deals with the supportive care and management of our survivors who have been changed in many ways by the transplant procedure. Finally, the list of appendices is a source of practical "go-to" information that caregivers of all types will find extremely helpful in the management of our population of valiant survivors.

In clinical medicine, which is often subject to vogues and trends with short-lived impact, the care of stem cell transplant recipients stands out as a critical area of medicine which will inevitably grow in importance and remain with us over the years ahead. *Blood and Marrow Transplantation Long Term Management: Prevention and Complications*, is a book well shaped to introduce the field and is likely to run into multiple editions in the decades to come. My congratulations go to Dr Savani and the world-class panel of authors for this timely and essential contribution to the practice of stem cell transplantation!

John Barrett
Stem Cell Allogeneic Transplantation Section
Hematology Branch
National Heart, Lung and Blood Institute
National Institutes of Health
Bethesda MD, USA

Foreword
by Stephanie J Lee

Survivors of hematopoietic cell transplantation have already faced myriad challenges to their health. The majority received treatment for their diseases before transplantation. Almost all have received supportive care and frequent monitoring. The transplant process itself may have been physically painful and debilitating, and the emotional journey can be exhausting. Afterwards, patients and their families face recovery, reintegration, and the rest of their lives.

This book is about that last concept: "the rest of their lives." Transplant survivors have higher rates of cancers, heart and kidney disease, diabetes, infections, and premature death than people who have not had the transplant experience. It is tragic that in the course of trying to cure one life-threatening disease we may be sowing the seeds of collateral suffering and deaths from other diseases. Some treating physicians may view late effects as the inevitable price to pay for cure. The premise of this book is that the goal of transplantation should not just be eradication of the underlying disease, but also the return to as much of a normal and healthy life as possible. We care providers have a responsibility to transplant survivors to improve our ability to address the physical and emotional sequelae of transplantation. I use the term "providers" because many survivors no longer receive care from oncologists or hematologists, but instead are treated by general pediatricians or internists. Increasingly, mid-level providers, pharmacists, and other health professionals will help care for transplant survivors and need this information too.

This book presents the most current knowledge about how to prevent, detect, and treat problems that arise after hematopoietic cell transplantation. In some cases, extensive epidemiologic studies and case series have defined the increased risks; for other complications, rare occurrences are known to happen but the true incidence is less certain. Our understanding of late effects prevention is still largely at the stage of identifying clinical risk factors. Genetic and environmental factors either are not examined or are poorly understood. Treatment approaches are primarily based on knowledge gained from other patient populations. High-quality studies designed to develop and test prevention and treatment strategies in transplant survivors are logistically daunting and rarely performed because of decentralized patient care, patient heterogeneity, lack of funding, or lack of effective interventions. Thus, another purpose of this book is to highlight gaps in our clinical knowledge and treatment armamentarium so that additional studies can be performed. It is my fervent hope that this book will soon be out of date and in need of another edition, since that would mean that much more information about late effects is accumulating and treatments have advanced.

Some say the true meaning of cure is being able to forget that you had a transplant. But your body and organs do not forget. Late effects of transplantation, the unintended adverse consequences of our aggressive attempts to eradicate hematologic cancers and other diseases, cause significant morbidity and mortality. We can decrease their impact by making sure that providers are prepared to diagnose them and provide the best treatments available. The message of this book is one of optimism: better information and proactive care can help people stay healthier "for the rest of their lives" despite having had a transplant.

Stephanie J Lee MD, MPH
Professor of Medicine
University of Washington School of Medicine
Member, Fred Hutchinson Cancer Research Center
Seattle, WA, USA

Foreword

by John Goldman

Though, sadly, there was been little progress in recent years in some areas of medicine, the clinical use of hematopoietic stem cell transplantation is not one of them. If 50 years ago one had suggested to an experienced hematologist that one could collect nucleated cells from the marrow or indeed from the blood of normal persons and infuse them in relatively small numbers into a suitably "prepared" patient with leukemia or another hematologic or immunologic disorder and thereby cure the disease, the suggestion would have been greeted with incredulity. In reality, the pioneering preclinical work of many laboratory scientists, the increased understanding of histocompatibility antigen, and the dedicated commitment of clinicians such as Georges Mathé, Robert Good, and Don Thomas laid the foundations for the first successful bone marrow transplants in the 1970s. It is difficult today to appreciate the scepticism or, indeed, formal opposition with which the initial work of these enthusiasts was met.

In the beginning of the 21st century, stem cell transplantation in some form or another is practised in 60 to 70 countries of the world and there is no aspiring hematologist who does not learn early that there are certain diseases for which allogeneic or autologous stem cell transplantation offers a real chance of cure or at worst just useful palliation. This means that the number of persons surviving and in many cases cured of a serious and usually life-threatening disease has increased enormously in recent years. This collection of papers written by experts in the field of stem cell transplantation could not have been contemplated by earlier researchers in the field for the simple reason that the number of patients who had survived long term would have been very few. Today, clinical data on transplant recipients are carefully collected and analysed by two very valuable organizations: on a global scale by the International Center for Blood and Marrow Transplant Research and by the European Group for Blood and Marrow Transplantation, which focuses mainly on Europe. Data collated by these two agencies and the multiplicity of individual publications covering many aspects of health in patients alive at 5, 10, or more years after a transplant procedure show clearly that some long-term survivors do still have specific problems associated with their original transplant procedures, but most of these are relatively minor and eminently treatable. The fact that there are so many "ex-patients" alive today is a truly impressive testament to the progress that has been made in this field since the 1960s.

Professor John Goldman DM, FRCP, FRCPath, FMedSci
Hammersmith Hospital
Imperial College London
Centre for Haematology
Du Cane Road
London, UK

List of Contributors

Imad Abboud MD
Attending Physician
Nephrology Department
Saint Louis Hospital
(Assistance Publique-Hôpitaux de Paris)
Paris, France

Sairah Ahmed MD
Assistant Professor
Department of Stem Cell
Transplantation and Cellular Therapy
University of Texas
MD Anderson Cancer Center
Houston, TX, USA

Joseph H Antin MD
Professor of Medicine
Division of Hematologic Malignancies
Dana-Farber Cancer Institute
Boston, MA, USA
Harvard Medical School
Boston, MA, USA

Andrea Bacigalupo MD
Head
Divisione di Ematologia e
Trapianto di Midollo Osseo
IRCCS AOU San Martino-IST
Genoa, Italy

Preet Bagi MD
Assistant Clinical Investigator
The National Institute of Diabetes and
Digestive and Kidney Diseases (NIDDK)
National Institutes of Health
Bethesda, MD, USA

Helen Baldomero BMS
Biomedical Scientist
Hematology Division
Basel University Hospital
Basel, Switzerland

Shichun Bao MD, PhD
Assistant Professor of Medicine
Division of Diabetes, Endocrinology
and Metabolism
Department of Medicine
Vanderbilt University Medical Center
Nashville, TN, USA

Margaret Bevans RN, PhD, AOCN
Clinical Nurse Scientist
LCDR, United States Public Health Service
National Institutes of Health, Clinical Center
Bethesda, MD, USA

Jeffrey B Boord MD, MPH
Assistant Professor of Medicine
Division of Cardiovascular Medicine
Vanderbilt Heart and Vascular Institute
Nashville, TN, USA

Michael W Brown
Registered Principal at LPL Financial
Private Wealth Management Group
LLC, Crossville, TN, USA

Paolo F Caimi MD
Assistant Professor
Department of Medicine
Division of Hematology and Oncology
Case Western Reserve University
Cleveland, OH, USA
Case Comprehensive Cancer Center
Cleveland, OH, USA

Anna Campanati
Clinica Determatologica
Dipartimento di Scienze Cliniche e Molecolari
Università Politecnica delle Marche
Ancona, Italy

Kristin Clay Chabarria MS
Medical Student
Louisiana State University Health
Science Center School of Medicine
New Orleans, LA, USA

James E Crowe Jr MD
Ingram Professor of Cancer Research
Department of Pediatrics
Vanderbilt University Medical Center
Nashville, TN, USA
Department of Pathology,
Microbiology, and Immunology
Vanderbilt University Medical Center
Nashville, TN, USA

Corey Cutler MD, MPH, FRCP(C)
Associate Professor of Medicine
Harvard Medical School
Division of Hematologic Malignancies
Dana-Farber Cancer Institute
Boston, MA, USA

Kathryn Dahir MD
Assistant Professor of Medicine
Division of Diabetes, Endocrinology,
and Metabolism
Department of Medicine
Vanderbilt University Medical Center
Nashville, TN, USA

Michael Dickenmann MD
Professor
Clinic for Transplantation Immunology
and Nephrology
University Hospital Basel
Basel, Switzerland

Stephen Dummer MD
Professor of Medicine and Surgery
Division of Infectious Diseases
Department of Medicine
Vanderbilt University School of Medicine
Nashville TN, USA

Dara L Eckerle Mize MD
Clinical Fellow
Division of Diabetes, Endocrinology
and Metabolism
Vanderbilt University Medical Center
Nashville, TN, USA

Sharon Elad DMD, MSc
Professor and Chair
Division of Oral Medicine
Eastman Institute for Oral Health
University of Rochester Medical Center
Rochester, NY, USA

Brian G Engelhardt MD, MSCI
Assistant Professor of Medicine
Division of Hematology and Oncology
Department of Medicine
Vanderbilt University Medical Center
Nashville, TN, USA

Cheryl A Fassler MD
Associate Professor of Medicine
University of Tennessee Health
Science Center
Baptist Hospital
Nashville, TN, USA

M Kathleen Figaro MD, MS
Clinical Fellow
Division of Diabetes, Endocrinology
and Metabolism
Vanderbilt University Medical Center
Nashville TN, USA

John P Galvin MD, MPH
Instructor
Division of Hematology/Oncology
Department of Medicine
Feinberg School of Medicine
Northwestern University
Chicago, IL, USA

Lee Gazourian MD
Instructor in Medicine
Division of Pulmonary Medicine
Brigham and Women's Hospital
Boston, MA, USA

Stacey A Goodman MD
Professor of Medicine
Hematology and Stem Cell Transplant
Vanderbilt University
Nashville, TN, USA

Joerg P Halter MD
Attending Physician
Hematology Department,
Basel University Hospital
Basel, Switzerland

Kristina K Hardy PhD
Assistant Professor
Department of Psychiatry and
Behavioral Science
George Washington University
Neuropsychology Division
Children's National Medical Center
Washington, DC, USA

Shahrukh Hashmi MD, MPH
Senior Associate Consultant
Division of Blood and Marrow Transplantation
William J. von Liebig Transplant Center
Mayo Clinic College of Medicine
Rochester, MN, USA

Darlene Haven BS
Senior Manager, Medical Marketing
National Marrow Donor Program®
/Be The Match®
Minneapolis, MN, USA

Theo Heller MD
Chief, Translational Hepatology Unit
Liver Disease Branch
The National Institute of Diabetes
and Digestive and Kidney Diseases (NIDDK)
National Institutes of Health
Bethesda, MD, USA

LaQuisa Hill MD
Internal Medicine Residency Program
Department of Medicine
Vanderbilt University
Nashville, TN, USA

Vincent T Ho MD
Associate Professor of Medicine
Division of Hematologic Malignancies
Dana-Farber Cancer Institute
Boston, MA, USA
Harvard Medical School
Boston, MA, USA

David A Jacobsohn MD, ScM
Chief
Division of Blood and Marrow Transplantation
Children's National Medical Center
Center for Cancer and Blood Disorders
Washington, DC, USA

Shubhada Jagasia MD, MMHC
Associate Professor of Medicine
Director-Vanderbilt Eskind Diabetes Clinics
Director-Inpatient Diabetes and Endocrinology
Division of Endocrinology, Diabetes and Metabolism
Vanderbilt University Medical Center
Nashville, TN, USA

Prathima Jasti MD
Clinical Fellow
Division of Diabetes, Endocrinology
and Metabolism
Department of Medicine
Vanderbilt University Medical Center
Nashville, TN, USA

Tajana Klepac Pulanic MD
Post-Doctoral Fellow
University of Zagreb
School of Medicine
Zagreb, Croatia
Community Health Center East
Zagreb, Croatia

Vipul T Lakhani MD
Assistant Professor of Medicine
Associate Program Director
Endocrinology Fellowship
Division of Diabetes, Endocrinology
and Metabolism
Vanderbilt University Medical Center
Nashville, TN, USA

Hillard M Lazarus MD, FACP
The George & Edith Richman
Professor and Distinguished
Scientist in Cancer Research Professor of Medicine
Case Western Reserve University
Director, Novel Cell Therapy
University Hospitals
Case Medical Center
Case Comprehensive Cancer Center
Cleveland, OH, USA

Helen Leather BPharm
Research Assistant Professor
Department of Medicine
Division of Hematology/Oncology
University of Florida
Gainesville, FL, USA

Mark R Litzow MD
Professor of Medicine
Division of Hematology
College of Medicine
Mayo Clinic
Rochester, MN, USA

Melissa Logue ANP-BC
Blood & Marrow Transplant Nurse Practitioner
Vanderbilt University Medical Center
Hematology and Stem Cell Transplantation Section
Division of Hematology/Oncology
Department of Medicine
Vanderbilt University Medical Center
Nashville, TN, USA

Catherine E Lucid ACNP-BC, MSN
Stem Cell Transplant Nurse Practitioner
Hematology and Stem Cell
Transplantation Section
Division of Hematology/Oncology
Vanderbilt University Medical Center
Nashville, TN, USA

Keith Luckett MD
Clinical Fellow
Division of Infectious Diseases
Department of Medicine
Vanderbilt University School of Medicine
Nashville, TN, USA

Navneet S Majhail MD, MS
Medical Director
National Marrow Donor Program
Adjunct Associate Professor of Medicine
University of Minnesota
Minneapolis, MN, USA

Daniela Massi MD
Professore associato
Servizio di Anatomia Patologica
Universita' di Firenze
Florence, Italy

Jayesh Mehta MD
Professor
Northwestern Memorial Hospital
Chicago, IL, USA

Melissa A Merideth MD
Obstetrician/Gynecologist
Geneticist
Medical Genetics Branch
National Human Genome Research Institute
National Institutes of Health
Bethesda, MD, USA

Yago Nieto MD, PhD
Professor of Medicine
University of Texas
MD Anderson Cancer Center
Houston, TX, USA

Attilio Olivieri MD
Head of Stem Cell Transplant Unit
Clinica di Ematologia
Dipartimento di Scienze
Cliniche e Molecolari
Università Politecnica delle Marche
Ancona, Italy

Jakob R Passweg MD
Professor of Hematology
Hematology Division
Basel University Hospital
Basel, Switzerland

Steven Pavletic MD
Head, Graft-versus-Host and Autoimmunity Unit
Center for Cancer Research
National Cancer Institute
Bethesda, MD, USA

Evelio Perez-Albuerne MD, PhD
Assistant Professor, Attending Physician
Division of Blood and Marrow Transplantation
Children's National Medical Center
Center for Cancer and Blood Disorders
Washington, DC, USA

Brandon Perry MD
Clinical Fellow
Division of Diabetes, Endocrinology
and Metabolism
Department of Medicine
Vanderbilt University Medical Center
Nashville, TN, USA

J Douglas Rizzo MD, MS
Professor of Medicine, Associate Director
Medical College of Wisconsin and
Center for International Blood and
Marrow Transplant Research
Milwaukee, WI, USA

Alicia Rovó MD
Assistant Professor
Hematology Department
Basel University Hospital
Basel, Switzerland

Nina Salooja FRCPath, MD
Honorary Clinical Senior Lecturer
Department of Medicine
Imperial College London
Hammersmith Hospital
London, UK

Niharika Samala MD
Clinical Fellow
Liver Disease Branch
The National Institute of Diabetes
and Digestive and Kidney Diseases (NIDDK)
National Institutes of Health
Bethesda, MD, USA

Bipin N Savani MD
Professor of Medicine
Director
Long Term Transplant Clinic (LTTC)
Hematology and Stem Cell
Transplantation Section
Division of Hematology/Oncology
Department of Medicine
Vanderbilt University Medical Center
Nashville, TN, USA

Carl P Schwarze MD
Professor
University Children's Hospital
Tübingen, Germany

Paul Shaughnessy MD
Clinical Director Adult BMT
Texas Transplant Physician Group
San Antonio, TX, USA

Gérard Socié MD, PhD
Head of the Hematology Transplantation
AP-HP Hospital Saint Louis
Professor of Hematology
University Paris VII Denis Diderot
Paris, France

Katrina M Stokes MSSW, LCSW
Stem Cell Transplant Social Worker
Department of Veterans Affairs
National Transplant Center
Tennessee Valley Healthcare System
Nashville, TN, USA

Pamela Stratton MD
Head, Gynecology Consult Service
Program in Reproductive and
Adult Endocrinology
Eunice Kennedy Shriver National
Institute of Child Health and Human Development
National Institutes of Health
Bethesda, MD, USA

Daniel R Thomas MS, RD, CNSC
Registered Dietician
Vanderbilt University Medical Center
Nashville, TN, USA

André Tichelli MD
Professor of Hematology
Hematology Department
Basel University Hospital
Basel, Switzerland

Nathaniel Treister DMD, DMSc
Assistant Professor of Oral Medicine
Harvard School of Dental Medicine
Division of Oral Medicine and Dentistry
Dana-Farber/Brigham and Women's
Cancer Center
Boston, MA, USA

Gaurav Trikha MD, MBBS
Assistant Professor of Medicine
Division of Infectious Diseases
Shands Hospital at University of Florida
Gainesville, FL, USA

Andrea L Utz MD, PhD
Assistant Professor of Medicine
Division of Diabetes, Endocrinology and Metabolism
Vanderbilt University Medical Center
Nashville, TN, USA

Gerald L Weinhouse MD
Assistant Professor of Medicine
Division of Pulmonary Medicine
Brigham and Women's Hospital
Boston, MA, USA

Lori Wiener PhD
Co-Director, Behavioral Science Core
Head, Psychosocial Support and
Research Program
Center for Cancer Research
Pediatric Oncology Branch
National Institutes of Health
Bethesda, MD, USA

John R Wingard MD
Price Eminent Scholar and
Professor of Medicine
Deputy Director for Research
University of Florida Shands Cancer Center
Director, Bone Marrow Transplant Program
Division of Hematology/Oncology
University of Florida College of Medicine
Gainesville, FL, USA

Angela M Woods MSN, APRN, ACNP-BC
Transplant Nurse Practitioner
National VA Transplant Program
Bone Marrow/ Stem Cell Transplant Service
Veterans Affairs Medical Center
Nashville, TN, USA

Elizabeth Wulff-Burchfield MD
Clinical Fellow
Division of Hematology/Oncology
Department of Medicine
Vanderbilt University Medical Center
Nashville, TN, USA

Lauren Zatarain MD
Hematolgy/Oncology Fellow
Division of Hematology/Oncology
Vanderbilt University
Nashville, TN, USA

1

SECTION 1

Late effects concepts

CHAPTER 1

Introduction

Bipin N Savani

Long Term Transplant Clinic (LTTC), Hematology and Stem Cell Transplantation Section, Division of Hematology/Oncology, Department of Medicine, Vanderbilt University Medical Center and Veterans Affairs Medical Center, Nashville, TN, USA

Background

Allogeneic hematopoietic cell transplantation (allo-HCT) provides curative therapy for a variety of diseases. Over the past several decades, significant advances have been made in the field of allo-HCT and now allo-HCT has become an integral part of treatment modality for a variety of hematological malignancies and nonmalignant diseases. Advances in transplantation technology and supportive care measures have resulted in significant decrease in early mortality, resulting in continued growth in the number of long-term HCT survivors.

These patients have increased risks for a variety of late complications (Figure 1.1), which can cause morbidity and mortality [1].

As HCT survivorship increases, the focus of care has shifted to the identification and treatment of long-term complications that may affect long-term survival and quality of life [2–7]. Preventive care and early detection and treatments are important aspects to reducing morbidity and mortality in long-term survivors after HCT. This book focuses on the essential knowledge about diagnosis, screening, treatment, and long-term surveillance of long-term survivors after HCT.

Long-term survivorship after hematopoietic cell transplantation

Since the first three cases of successful allo-HCT in 1968, the number of allo-HCTs performed annually has increased steadily over the past three decades [8–11]. It is estimated that by 2015 more than 100 000 patients will receive HCT (combined allogeneic and autologous) annually throughout the world, and numbers are increasing rapidly. Long-term survival after HCT has improved significantly since its inception over 40 years ago owing to improved supportive care and early recognition of long-term complications. With broadening indications, more options for HCT, and improvement in survival, there may be up to a million long-term survivors after HCT by 2020 worldwide [12].

The rapidly growing population of HCT survivors creates an obligation to educate patients and physicians about the late complications observed in patients after this therapy. Historically, limitation of allo-HCT has been transplant-related mortality (TRM). In order to offer the curative allo-HCT treatment option in most patients, safer regimens with acceptable graft-versus-host disease (GVHD)-associated morbidity and TRM are preferred. A recently published M.D. Anderson Cancer Center study showed an excellent overall survival and progression-free survival (85% and 83%, respectively, after median follow-up of 60 months) for relapsed follicular lymphoma after fludarabine, cyclophosphamide, and rituximab reduced-intensity conditioning (RIC) allo-HCT [13]. Similarly, many disease-specific transplant regimens are in development to improve transplant outcome after HCT.

In this era, a stem cell source can be found for virtually all patients who have an indication to receive allo-HCT. Since 2007, more allo-HCT procedures have been

Blood and Marrow Transplantation Long-Term Management: Prevention and Complications, First Edition. Edited by Bipin N Savani.

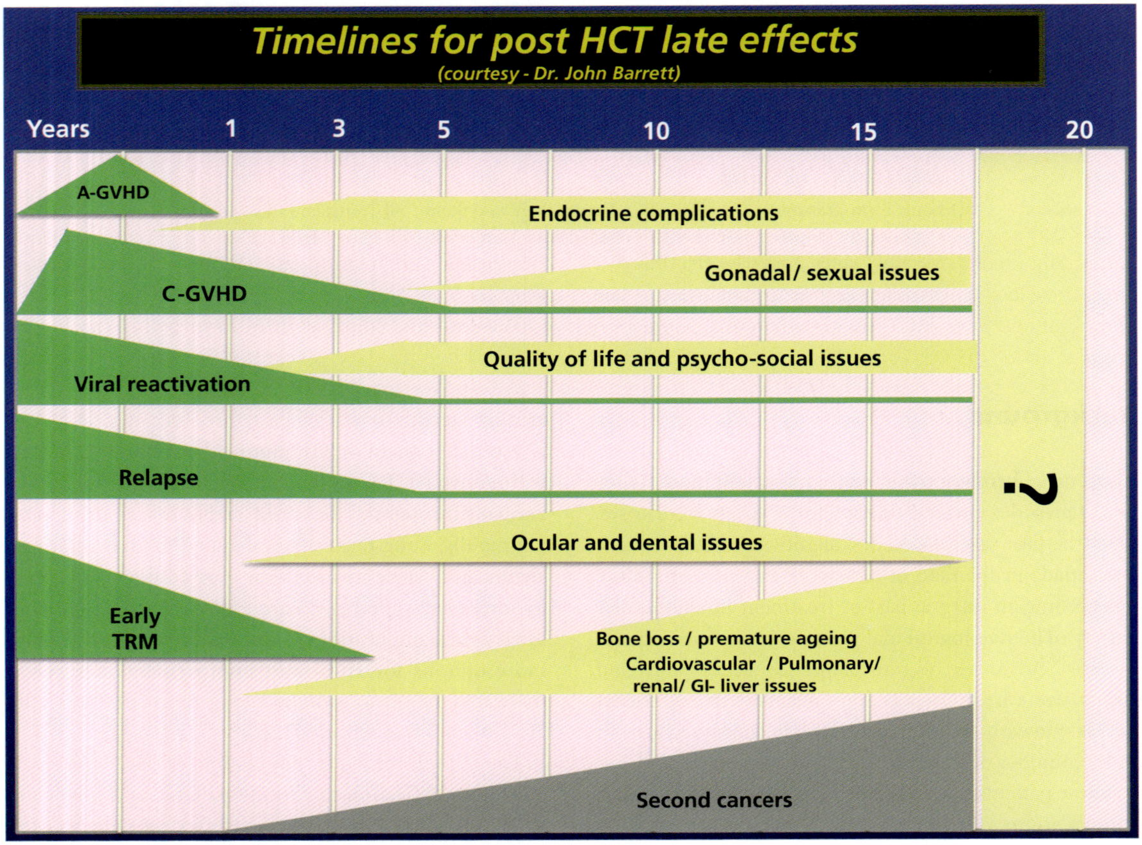

Figure 1.1 Timelines for post-HCT late effects. (Courtesy of Dr John Barrett.)

performed using alternative donor stem cell sources, such as volunteer unrelated donors or cord blood, than have been performed using related donors [9]. RIC haploidentical-related donor or cord blood transplantations have emerged as alternatives to fill the gap for those patients who do not have a matched related donor or unrelated donor, and the outcomes of these types of transplantations are expected to be better than chemotherapy alone or even better than auto-HCT for selected indications. The result of this is a steadily increasing number of long-term survivors after allo-HCT, creating an enlarging pool of children and young and mature adults who are at risk of long-term complications of allo-HCT.

Late effects after hematopoietic cell transplantation

Several studies have investigated the late effects of allo-HCT recipients, and the cumulative incidence of a late effect among long-term survivors has been reported to be 32–93.2% [7, 14–17]. Bresters et al. [15] reported that the cumulative incidence of late effects was 93.2% after a median follow-up time of 7.2 years after HCT, and Sun et al. [16] reported that survivors were twice as likely as their siblings to develop a chronic condition and 3.5 times as likely to develop severe conditions.

Among long-term survivors after allo-HCT, mortality rates are four- to nine-fold higher than observed in an age-adjusted general population for at least 30 years after HCT, yielding an estimated 30% lower life expectancy than someone who has not been transplanted [17]. Among long-term survivors, the most common causes of excess deaths other than recurrent malignancy are chronic GVHD, infections, second malignancies, respiratory diseases, and cardiovascular disease [10, 18–20]. Higher than average rates of second malignancies and cardiopulmonary, infectious, endocrine, and renal diseases, bone loss or avascular necrosis, and many other late complications after HCT suggest that this population requires more frequent screening and earlier interventions than the general population [21–24].

Chronic GVHD is a multisystem chronic alloimmune and autoimmune disorder that occurs later after allo-HCT. It is characterized by immunosuppression, immune dysregulation, decreased organ function, significant morbidity, and impaired survival. Approximately 10–30% of patients require continued immunosuppressive treatment beyond 5 years from the initial diagnosis of chronic GVHD. Therefore, it is not surprising that corticosteroid and other immunosuppressive therapies are major contributors of late complications after allo-HCT. Several factors impact on recovery from and late effects of allo-HCT, including prior therapy for the underlying disease, pre-transplant comorbidities and psychosocial status, intensity of the transplant conditioning regimen, and, most importantly, duration of chronic GVHD and immunosuppressive therapy [12, 25 26].

Developing resources and a guide for long-term survivors

Transplant society guidelines for screening and preventive practices for pediatric and adult survivors of auto- and allo-HCT were updated and published in 2012 [27]. Ongoing research is focused on better understanding of late-effect issues and prediction of posttransplant long-term complications, which allows transplant-eligible patients to incorporate this knowledge into more informative decision making. Therefore, significant resources should be focused on the better implementation of how patients and physicians use extensive data regarding post-transplant late complications in clinical care.

We also recommend early referral or discussion with a transplant center for enrollment of patient in available late-effect studies and for management guidelines. A better understanding of the pathogenesis of late effects will allow for more effective screening to identify patients at risk prior to the HCT procedure, and allow more effective monitoring to detect early evolution of the late effects after HCT. This may, in turn, allow for improved therapeutic decision making while evaluating patients for HCT, and early institution of treatments directed at preventing and treating late effects in patients at risk after HCT.

With survivorship, a shift in survivorship care occurs from large transplant centers to community health care providers. As a result, many hematologists/oncologists and primary care physicians are assuming the post-HCT late-effects care of long-term survivors. Long-term survivors should be assessed lifelong after HCT; all health care providers involved in the follow-up of these patients should be aware of the premature health threats of long-term complications after transplantation. This book offers practical advice and outlines late-effect experts personal approaches in managing long-term complications after HCT.

Declaration of commercial interest

None.

References

1. Savani BN. How can we improve life expectancy and quality of life in long-term survivors after allogeneic stem cell transplantation? Semin Hematol. 2012;49:1–3.
2. Syrjala KL, Martin PJ, Lee SJ. Delivering care to long-term adult survivors of hematopoietic cell transplantation. J Clin Oncol. 2012;30:3746–3751.
3. Khera N, Storer B, Flowers ME, et al. Nonmalignant late effects and compromised functional status in survivors of hematopoietic cell transplantation. J Clin Oncol. 2012;30: 71–77.
4. Socie G, Stone JV, Wingard JR, et al. Long-term survival and late deaths after allogeneic bone marrow transplantation. Late Effects Working Committee of the International Bone Marrow Transplant Registry. N Engl J Med. 1999;341: 14–21.
5. Socie G, Salooja N, Cohen A, et al. Nonmalignant late effects after allogeneic stem cell transplantation. Blood. 2003;101: 3373–3385.

6. Flowers MED, Deeg HJ. Delayed nonmalignant complications after hematopoietic cell transplantation. In: Appelbaum FR, Forman SJ, Negrin RS, Blume KG, (eds). Thomas' Hematopoietic Cell Transplantation. West Sussex, UK: Wiley-Blackwell, 2009; pp. 1620–1637.
7. Wingard JR, Majhail NS, Brazauskas R, et al. Long-term survival and late deaths after allogeneic hematopoietic cell transplantation. J Clin Oncol. 2011;29:2230–2239.
8. Thomas ED. A history of bone marrow transplantation. In: Appelbaum FR, Forman SJ, Negrin RS, Blume KG (eds). Thomas' Hematopoietic Cell Transplantation. West Sussex, UK: Wiley-Blackwell, 2009; pp. 3–7.
9. Pasquini MC, Wang Z. Current use and outcome of hematopoietic stem cell transplantation: CIBMTR Summary Slides. 2012. Available from: http://www.cibmtr.org/referencecenter/slidesreports/summaryslides/pages/index.aspx (accessed 29 April 2013).
10. Socie G, Rizzo JD. Second solid tumors: screening and management guidelines in long-term survivors after allogeneic stem cell transplantation. Semin Hematol. 2012;49:4–9.
11. Gratwohl A, Baldomero H, Aljurf M, et al. Hematopoietic stem cell transplantation: a global perspective. JAMA. 2010;303:1617–1624.
12. Savani BN, Griffith ML, Jagasia S, Lee SJ. How I treat late effects in adults after allogeneic stem cell transplantation. Blood. 2011;117:3002–3009.
13. Khouri IF, McLaughlin P, Saliba RM, et al. Eight-year experience with allogeneic stem cell transplantation for relapsed follicular lymphoma after nonmyeloablative conditioning with fludarabine, cyclophosphamide, and rituximab. Blood. 2008;111:5530–5536.
14. Mo XD, Xu LP, Liu DH, et al. Nonmalignant late effects in survivors of partially matched donor hematopoietic stem cell transplantation. Biol Blood Marrow Transplant. 2013; 19:777–783.
15. Bresters D, van Gils IC, Kollen WJ, et al. High burden of late effects after haematopoietic stem cell transplantation in childhood: a single-centre study. Bone Marrow Transplant. 2010;45:79–85.
16. Sun CL, Francisco L, Kawashima T, et al. Prevalence and predictors of chronic health conditions after hematopoietic cell transplantation: a report from the Bone Marrow Transplant Survivor Study. Blood. 2010;116:3129–3139.
17. Martin PJ, Counts GW Jr, Appelbaum FR, et al. Life expectancy in patients surviving more than 5 years after hematopoietic cell transplantation. J Clin Oncol. 2010;28: 1011–1016.
18. Bhatia S, Francisco L, Carter A, et al. Late mortality after allogeneic hematopoietic cell transplantation and functional status of long-term survivors: report from the Bone Marrow Transplant Survivor Study. Blood. 2007;110:3784–3792.
19. Bacigalupo A, Chien J, Barisione G, Pavletic S. Late pulmonary complications after allogeneic hematopoietic stem cell transplantation: diagnosis, monitoring, prevention, and treatment. Semin Hematol. 2012;49:15–24.
20. Rovo A, Tichelli A. Cardiovascular complications in long-term survivors after allogeneic hematopoietic stem cell transplantation. Semin Hematol. 2012;49:25–34.
21. Kida A, McDonald GB. Gastrointestinal, hepatobiliary, pancreatic, and iron-related diseases in long-term survivors of allogeneic hematopoietic cell transplantation. Semin Hematol. 2012;49:43–58.
22. McClune B, Majhail NS, Flowers ME. Bone loss and avascular necrosis of bone after hematopoietic cell transplantation. Semin Hematol. 2012;49:59–65.
23. Gunasekaran U, Agarwal N, Jagasia MH, Jagasia SM. Endocrine complications in long-term survivors after allogeneic stem cell transplant. Semin Hematol. 2012;49:66–72.
24. Abboud I, Peraldi MN, Hingorani S. Chronic kidney diseases in long-term survivors after allogeneic hematopoietic stem cell transplantation: monitoring and management guidelines. Semin Hematol. 2012;49:73–82.
25. Rizzo JD, Curtis RE, Socie G, et al. Solid cancers after allogeneic hematopoietic cell transplantation. Blood. 2009;113: 1175–1183.
26. Curtis RE, Metayer C, Rizzo JD, et al. Impact of chronic GVHD therapy on the development of squamous-cell cancers after hematopoietic stem-cell transplantation: an international case–control study. Blood. 2005;105:3802–3811.
27. Majhail NS, Rizzo JD, Lee SJ, et al. Recommended screening and preventive practices for long-term survivors after hematopoietic cell transplantation. Bone Marrow Transplant. 2012;47:337–341.

2

CHAPTER 2

Overview: transplant data and increasing numbers of long-term survivors

Jakob R Passweg and Helen Baldomero
Hematology Division, Basel University Hospital, Basel, Switzerland

Hematopoietic stem cell transplantation (HSCT) has evolved to become a standard of care for many patients with congenital or acquired disorders of the hematopoietic system and for a wide variety of chemosensitive, hematologic malignancies [1–3]. Fifty years have passed since the first reports of successful bone marrow transplants from human leukocyte antigen (HLA)-identical siblings for patients with immune deficiency disorders. After an initially slow evolution, HSCT has seen rapid expansion over the last two decades and major changes in technology use [4–7].

HSCT is a high-cost, highly specialized procedure. It requires significant infrastructure and a network of specialists from multiple fields of medicine. It is not available without preparative work by setting up a transplant center and organizing all the auxiliary services required to perform this procedure. Information on indication and trends is essential for healthcare agencies in order to prepare the necessary infrastructure. Given costs for HSCT, use of this technology is predominantly limited to high- and middle-income countries where the expansion in procedures performed has occurred [3]. In such a complex field, standardization is necessary and scientific societies have classified indications for HSCT by the degree by which they are supported by scientific evidence [8]. Furthermore, quality management systems have been created in order to support transplant centers to achieve the best possible outcomes [9].

The European Group for Blood and Marrow Transplantation (EBMT) introduced an annual activity survey in 1990 that provides data on HSCT use by indication, type of transplant, donor type, and stem cell source [10]. Using data from that survey, we will highlight in this chapter the current trends in technology use and in changes occurring. As this book is on long-term complications of HSCT, we will try to estimate the number of patients at risk for such long-term complications in Europe based on transplant numbers as provided by the EBMT activity survey and based on survival estimates as provided by the EBMT database. Through the Worldwide Bone Marrow Transplant Group (WBMT), data from Europe have been combined with reports from North, Middle and South America, the eastern Mediterranean and Africa, and from Asia–Pacific registries in order to provide a world view of transplant activity [3]. In 2006, 50 417 transplants were reported to the WBMT from these global registries.

The European experience can be largely extrapolated to areas with similarly highly developed medical systems. We will limit the data presented here to the European experience as we do have a long-term view over more than 20 years of annual surveys [4].

Teams participating in the annual survey are requested to report annually by indication, stem cell source, and donor type. Quality control measures include several independent systems: confirmation of validity of the

Blood and Marrow Transplantation Long-Term Management: Prevention and Complications, First Edition. Edited by Bipin N Savani.

entered data by the reporting team, selective comparison of the survey data with data sets in the EBMT registry database, crosschecking with the national registries and onsite visits of selected teams. A total of 654 centers were contacted for the 2010 survey, of which 634 teams reported their numbers. This corresponds to a 97% return rate. In all, 22 active teams failed to report in 2010. By tradition, some centers outside of Europe are EBMT members and report data. These comprise 7% of the total data set and are included in all analyses.

According to the EBMT 2010 annual survey 33 362 transplants were performed in 30 012 patients. Of these 33 362 transplants, 13 345 were allogeneic and 20 017 autologous (Table 2.1). The indications for autologous and allogeneic HSCT are shown in Table 2.1. Only first transplants are shown, corresponding to number of patients rather than number of transplants. It is well known that indications for allogeneic and autologous HSCT differ and that more leukemia patients receive allogeneic HSCT and more patients with lymphoid neoplasia and plasma cell neoplasia receive autologous HSCT. The number of transplants for bone marrow failure, autoimmune disorders, and congenital diseases is smaller than those for malignancy. Figure 2.1 shows the evolution of transplant numbers for autologous and allogeneic HSCT, with a continuous increase between 1990 and 2010. Two changes in clinical practice are mirrored in the curves displayed. The first is the introduction of imatinib (in 1999) for the treatment of chronic myeloid leukemia, resulting in a transient slowing of allogeneic transplant numbers in the early 2000s. The second is the discontinuation of autologous HSCT for breast cancer after the publication of negative data, resulting in a hump in the curve depicting numbers of autologous HSCT performed. Current increases in transplant numbers are due to higher rates of allogeneic HSCT for leukemia and more recently in myelodysplastic syndrome and chronic lymphocytic leukemia. Autologous HSCT increases are mainly due to transplants for lymphoid neoplasias and plasma cell disorders.

If the total of transplanted patients from 1990 to 2010 is cumulated, there is a total of 375 948 patients that have been reported to the survey, of which 135 179 had an allogeneic HSCT (36%) and 240 769 an autologous

Table 2.1 Indications for allogeneic and autologous HSCT in 2010 in Europe; over 30 000 patients were reported to have undergone HSCT

Indication	Allogeneic 1st HSCT	Autologous 1st HSCT	Total
Leukaemia	8685	670	9355
Lymphoma	1411	7550	8961
Plasma cell disorder	566	7835	8401
Solid tumor	81	1504	1585
Bone marrow failure	676	1	677
Non-malignant disorder	773	159	932
Other	84	17	101
Total	12 276	17 736	30 012

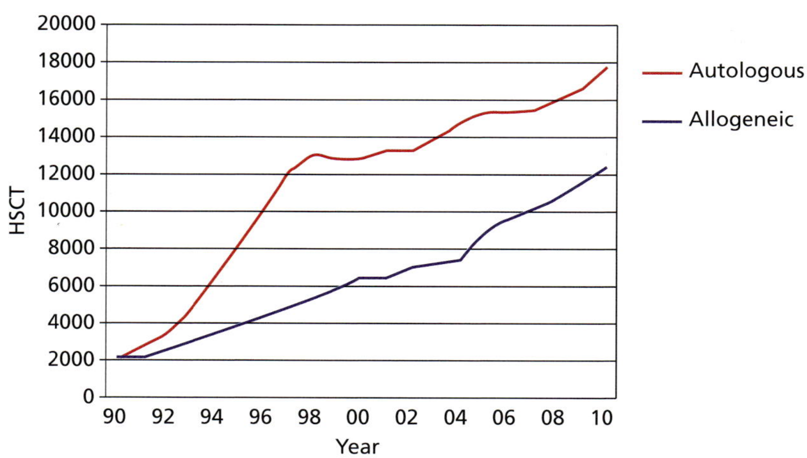

Figure 2.1 Development of autologous and allogeneic HSCT in Europe from 1990–2010 [4].

HSCT (64%). The main indications were leukemias with 125 139 patients (33% – 98 108 allogeneic (73%) and 27 031 autologous (22%)), lymphoid neoplasias with 189 299 patients (50% – 17 625 allogeneic (9%) and 171 674 autologous (91%)), solid tumors with 41 070 patients (11% – 1354 allogeneic (3%) and 39 716 autologous (97%)), and nonmalignant disorders with 17 953 patients (5% – 16 457 allogeneic (92%) and 1496 (8%) autologous). An additional 2487 patients (0.7% – 1635 allogeneic and 852 autologous), were listed as "other indications."

Trends over the last 20 years have included the shift from marrow as a stem cell source to using peripheral blood, first in autologous HSCT and later in allogeneic HSCT. The association of peripheral blood use for allogeneic HSCT with higher risks of chronic graft versus host disease has been recognized, and in nonmalignant disorders the trend towards increasing use of peripheral blood over marrow as a stem cell source has been halted. New sources of stem cells have been developed, such as cord blood, which is used in 7–8% of all allogeneic HSCT. A major shift in donor use for allogeneic HSCT is shown in Figure 2.2. Around the beginning of the last decade, the introduction of HLA high-resolution typing has resulted in better typed volunteer unrelated donors, resulting in better outcomes. As a consequence of this, and of the availability of high-resolution typing technology at a reasonable price, the unrelated donor registries have expanded and now include more than 20 million volunteer donors. Figure 2.2 shows that since 2007 and 2008 the number of unrelated donor transplants done in Europe has exceeded the number of transplants from sibling donors. The use of unrelated donors is in large part responsible for increasing transplant numbers, in addition to changes in transplant technology for allogeneic HSCT, in particular reduced-intensity conditioning transplants amounting to 30–60% of all allogeneic HSCT with variation between countries. Reduced-intensity conditioning HSCT has opened up the option of allogeneic HSCT in older patients, who are the majority of patients with hematologic malignancies, with median age of onset for most diseases being between 60 and 70 years of age.

Long-term survival after HSCT has increasingly become the center of attention in recent years [11–16]. It has been recognized that many of these patients suffer from late complications that need to be recognized, diagnosed, and treated appropriately. Furthermore, all patients, and in particular those treated many years ago as children having reached adult life, require medical care adapted to their prior medical experience, even though many of them lead an active life [15]. In addition, in the early years of HSCT, every patient treated was considered as a single medical achievement and patients were followed long term at their transplant center. With increasing numbers of transplants performed and with

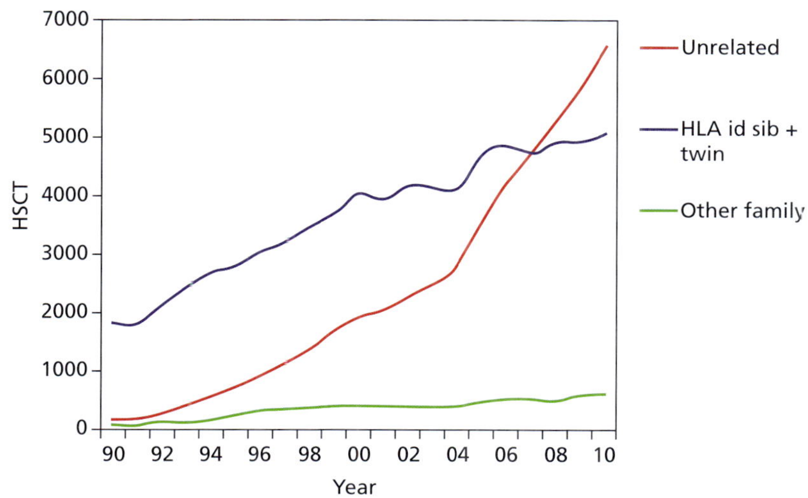

Figure 2.2 Allogeneic HSCT in Europe from 1990 to 2010 by donor type [4].

increasing numbers of long-term survivors, as shown above, organizing this care becomes increasingly difficult and some of this care may be delegated to referring physicians. Tools and guidelines have been developed to help with this care, and much of this will be discussed in the upcoming chapters.

A quantitative assessment of the magnitude of the issue of the number of patients requiring long-term care is difficult to provide, and modeling may be complex as transplant rates are increasing rapidly, as is the age of patients undergoing allogeneic and autologous HSCT. To estimate this number for Europe, we took the total cumulative number of patients transplanted in Europe during 1990–2010 that were reported to the EBMT activity survey and multiplied this number by survival estimates from the EBMT data registry, which indicate that, for 1990–2010, the overall survival at 5 years is approximately 53% and at 10 years this is 44%, including all diseases and all types of transplant. Extrapolating from this information, approximately 200 000 patients are expected to be alive in Europe having had an HSCT in the past. This estimate may be criticized as being imprecise, as there are patients included that are from non-European centers; all the patients transplanted before 1990 are not counted, and appropriate adjustments for patient age and from the recent increase in transplant activity are not made. Nonetheless, this number, however imprecise, provides a stimulus for the tasks ahead. These patients are at risk of late effects and are the focus of our attention.

References

1. Copelan EA. Hematopoietic stem-cell transplantation. N Engl J Med. 2006;354:1813–1826.
2. Appelbaum FR. Hematopoietic cell transplantation at 50. N Engl J Med. 2007;357:1472–1475.
3. Gratwohl A, Baldomero H, Aljurf M, et al. Hematopoietic stem cell transplantation: a global perspective. JAMA. 2010;303:1617–1624.
4. Passweg JR, Baldomero H, Gratwohl A, et al. The EBMT activity survey: 1990–2010. Bone Marrow Transplant. 2012;47:906–923. doi: 10.1038/bmt.2012.66.
5. Gratwohl A, Schwendener A, Baldomero H, et al. Changes in use of hematopoietic stem cell transplantation; a model for diffusion of medical technology. Haematologica. 2010; 95:637–643.
6. Gratwohl A, Baldomero H, Schwendener A, et al. The EBMT activity survey 2008 impact of team size, team density and new trends. Bone Marrow Transplant. 2011;46:174–191.
7. Gratwohl A, Baldomero H, Horisberger B, *et al.* Current trends in haematopoietic stem cell transplantation in Europe. Blood. 2002;100:2374–2386.
8. Ljungman P, Bregni M, Brune M, et al. Allogeneic and autologous transplantation for haematological diseases, solid tumours and immune disorders: current practice in Europe 2009. Bone Marrow Transplant. 2010;45(2):219–234. Epub 2009 Jul 6.
9. Gratwohl A, Brand R, Niederwieser D, et al. Introduction of a quality management system and outcome after hematopoietic stem-cell transplantation. J Clin Oncol. 2011; 29(15):1980–1986. Epub 2011 Apr 11.
10. Gratwohl A. Bone marrow transplantation activity in Europe 1990. European Group for Bone Marrow Transplantation (EBMT). Bone Marrow Transplant. 1991;8(3): 197–201.
11. Pulsipher MA, Skinner R, McDonald GB, et al. National Cancer Institute, National Heart, Lung and Blood Institute/ Pediatric Blood and Marrow Transplantation Consortium First International Consensus Conference on Late Effects after Pediatric Hematopoietic Cell Transplantation: The Need For Pediatric-Specific Long-Term Follow-Up Guidelines. Biol Blood Marrow Transplant. 2012;18(3):334–347. Epub 2012 Jan 14.
12. Armenian SH, Sun CL, Kawashima T, et al. Long-term health-related outcomes in survivors of childhood cancer treated with HSCT versus conventional therapy: a report from the Bone Marrow Transplant Survivor Study (BMTSS) and Childhood Cancer Survivor Study (CCSS). Blood. 2011;118(5):1413–1420. Epub 2011 Jun 7.
13. Majhail NS, Rizzo JD, Lee SJ, et al. Recommended screening and preventive practices for long-term survivors after hematopoietic cell transplantation. Bone Marrow Transplant. 2012;47(3):337–341.
14. Wingard JR, Majhail NS, Brazauskas R, et al. Long-term survival and late deaths after allogeneic hematopoietic cell transplantation. J Clin Oncol. 2011;29(16):2230–2239. Epub 2011 Apr 4.
15. Sanders JE, Woolfrey AE, Carpenter PA, et al. Late effects among pediatric patients followed for nearly 4 decades after transplantation for severe aplastic anemia. Blood. 2011;118(5):1421–1428. Epub 2011 Jun 7.
16. Socié G, Stone JV, Wingard JR, et al. Long-term survival and late deaths after allogeneic bone marrow transplantation. Late Effects Working Committee of the International Bone Marrow Transplant Registry. N Engl J Med. 1999;341(1): 14–21.

3

CHAPTER 3

Long-term transplant clinic setup

André Tichelli, Joerg P Halter, Jakob R Passweg, and Alicia Rovó
Hematology Division, Basel University Hospital, Basel, Switzerland

Introduction

With the increasing number of hematopoietic stem cell transplants (HSCTs) performed yearly worldwide, and the improvement of survival after transplantation, the number of patients surviving 2 years and longer after transplantation is continuously increasing. Between 1980 and 2010, the European Group for Blood and Marrow Transplantation (EBMT) registry included 339 402 patients who underwent either first autologous (211 543) or allogeneic (127 859) HSCT. From these 339 402 patients, 150 235 (44.3%) patients survived 2 years or longer since first HSCT: 97 531 autologous and 52 704 allogeneic HSCT (unpublished data from the EBMT registry). By 2020, there may be worldwide up to half a million long-term survivors after allogeneic HSCT [1]. Long-term recipients who have overcome the acute toxicity phase of HSCT and are in remission of their primary disease have completed their treatment and will no longer be considered as patients. Nevertheless, long-term HSCT recipients, similar to cancer patients, do not return to prediagnosis status [2] and, therefore, cannot be considered as healthy persons. Indeed, about two-thirds of the transplanted patients will experience at least one late effect that is not related to the primary disease, but the direct or indirect consequence of the cancer treatment or the transplant procedure [3]. Malignant and nonmalignant late complications after HSCT will interfere with the general health condition, the quality of life, family life, and the reinsertion in social life at school or at employment of the patient. During the transplantation period the focus of care has extended from the cure of the primary disease to the screening and management of late effects and improvement of quality of life. The transition from the acute phase of HSCT to post-treatment care is critical to maintain long-term health. At this phase, recipients of transplantation need specialized follow-up care. This involves not only the patient themselves and their family, but also the transplantation center and its organization.

In cancer medicine, the need of special attention to long-term cancer patients has been recognized for more than 50 years. The definition of long-term survivor and the concept of cancer survivorship were introduced by the Institute of Medicine by engaging a committee to examine medical and psychological issues of cancer survivors and to make recommendations to improve their health care and quality of life. According to the Institute of Medicine, cancer survivorship is the phase of care that follows primary treatment. However, this definition allows a wide range of interpretation, depending on the time of diagnosis, the completion of treatment, and the time interval between the diagnosis and the end of treatment of the cancer. A Cancer Survivorship Program is intended to provide a specialized follow-up care to long-term survivors who are in remission after having completed their cancer treatment, usually for at least 2 years or longer. Some of the controversial issues of a survivorship program concern the type and frequency of optimal follow-up care, the increased expenses caused, as well as the extra time and the physical space needed to run such a program. In many countries the costs of the follow-up care are no longer covered by the insurances that covered expenses of the cancer treatment. Cancer survivors are

Blood and Marrow Transplantation Long-Term Management. Prevention and Complications, First Edition. Edited by Bipin N Savani.

usually seen once a year in a follow-up program. However, this cancer survivorship program does not replace the regular primary health care of long-term survivors. Both, regular primary health care and long-term follow-up are complementary.

Compared with cancer survivorship care, posttransplant long-term follow-up programs emerged with some delay. The reason for this delay is obvious, since efficient cancer therapies have been available now for more than 60 years, whereas the first transplantation centers started about 30–35 years ago. The transplant survivorship programs have adopted much from the experience of the cancer survivorship programs and, therefore, they are roughly based on the models of cancer survivorship care. In analogy to cancer survivorship, the long-term survivors after HSCT are usually defined as patients currently in remission of their primary disease and surviving 2 years or longer since completion of transplantation. However, survivorship after HSCT has its own particularities owing to the type and intensity of the conditioning regimen, the prolonged immune incompetence, and, in patients treated with allogeneic HSCT, the late effects due to graft-versus-host disease (GVHD) and its treatment. Survivorship programs and long-term transplant clinics will therefore share many characteristics with cancer survivorship programs, but also present some features of their own.

Setting up a long-term transplant clinic is a challenging but rewarding experience for a transplantation center. When a center starts with a transplantation program, the whole team is initially confronted with the immediate survival and disease control. The major focus is placed on problems related to acute toxicity, relapse, GVHD, and infectious complications. Usually, there is not much time left for patients without acute medical issues. With advancing time, the number of long-term survivors of the new transplant center is increasing. Their needs and expectations become different. In general, they require less acute medical interventions and immediate care, but have increasing expectations of good physical and mental health and quality of life. For the long-term survivorship care, the focus is on careful screening, prevention, and early treatment of possible late effects that interfere with good health condition. Transition from acute care to long-term follow-up is a process rather than an event. Some particular aspects have to be considered when choosing a model of a long-term transplant clinic. A common outpatient HSCT clinic, where acute care and long-term follow-up are mixed, allows continuity in the care, but faces the risk that the particular needs of long-term survivors are left behind the daily care of the new posttransplant patients. In contrast, dedicated long-term follow-up clinics run into the danger of losing continuity of care from the acute phase to the follow-up care. Community-based models, where long-term survivors are followed by community healthcare providers, discharge the transplant centers from the ever-increasing of burden of long-term survivors. However, these primary care doctors are not necessarily experts in chemotherapy agents, specific transplantation problems, and in long-term effects after HSCT. Furthermore, they are not surrounded by a complete network of specialists needed for the care of long-term survivors.

In this chapter, the setup of a long-term transplant clinic and the essential functions and components of a survivorship care program will be outlined. Different models of survivorship programs and clinics will be considered, and the minimal requirements discussed. This chapter consists of two parts. In the first part we will present the lessons learned from the experience of cancer survivorship programs. In the second part we will concentrate on the particular aspects of transplant survivorship clinic programs.

What we have learned from cancer survivorship models

The concept of survivorship in cancer patients was created by the National Coalition for Cancer Survivorship (NCCS) in 1986. Accordingly, a cancer survivor is a person with a cancer diagnosis who has completed treatment. The Institute of Medicine and leaders in cancer survivorship have recommended cancer centers to examine and evaluate the setup of services for survivors. In a first step, general recommendations and the development of guidelines have been assessed for pediatric and adult cancer survivors [4, 5]. Today, the Institute of Medicine provides a template for the four essential elements of the survivorship care: prevention and detection of late effects, surveillance, interventions to manage side effects, and coordination of care and information [6]. Cancer survivors' needs vary depending on the type of disease and the treatments received. Long-term events may be different for survivors of a breast cancer, a prostate cancer, or a colon cancer [7]. Furthermore, the late effects and long-term needs are different for patients who received local radiation therapy, Doxorubicin-containing chemotherapy, hormonal treatment, or invalidating surgery. Nevertheless, some of the long-term issues are shared by most of the cancer survivors.

The Children's Oncology Group (COG) recently described survivorship services and, based on their findings, discussed the models of care that are in use for childhood cancer survivors and adult survivors of childhood cancer. Of the 220 COG institutions, 175 completed an Internet-based survey [8]. According to this survey, late effects services are available in 87% of the responding centers and 59% of these institutions provide a specialized care program for their pediatric population. The main barriers to care for pediatric cancer survivors were the lack of dedicated time for the program (29% of responses), not enough funding to support the program (20%), deficits in knowledge about cancer survivorship (17%), lack of health-care insurance or insurance limitations (12.7%), lack of survivor desire to be followed by the late effects team (7%), and no perceived need to support a late effects program (6.7%).

A variety of models have been proposed for the long-term follow-up cancer care and clinic setup [9]. A follow-up program can be built up on a cancer-center-based model, a community-based model, or a combined cancer center and community model [10]. Each of these models has its advantages and disadvantages, in respect of continuity of care, education of survivors, family and health care providers, resources and cost effectiveness, convenience for the survivor and their family, and opportunities for research on long-term survivorship and late effects. A combination of the cancer center and community model, where the role of each part has been predefined, appears to be the most ideal. An emerging concept in combining community and cancer center follow-up is to involve a virtual or Web-based follow-up program, which could be designed to bridge the two models of follow-up [4].

A survivor follow-up program aims to prevent and to detect late complications of cancer treatment that will interfere later with physical and mental health. This can be obtained by promoting healthy behaviors and introducing risk-adapted screening procedures to allow early detection. Special attention has to be brought to quality of life, including physical and psychological functioning, sexuality, and fertility issues of long-term survivors. The long-term follow-up program has also to be concerned about collateral damage caused by the cancer and cancer treatment, such as financial embarrassments, limitations in insurance coverage, and obstacles encountered at employment and at school. Today, in many countries, efforts are undertaken to build up a national system for cancer survivorship care. For instance, in the UK, based on the experience of 38 test communities, the Department of Health, Macmillan Cancer Support, and NHS Improvement worked out a document that provides an emerging vision for improved care and support for people living with and beyond cancer [11].

A study, including eight centers from the LIVESTRONG Survivorship Center of Excellence Network, evaluated survivorship models and aimed to identify barriers and facilitators influencing survivorship care [12]. Accordingly, there is not one single best model for survivorship care that could fit for all cancer centers; and for a given institution, changes often take place as a result of the increase of long-term survivors, the availability of resources and work space, the experience of the team, and changes in the organizational structure of the center. The development into a definitive model can be the result of different attempts until the optimal structure has been obtained. According to the above-mentioned study, the most important prerequisite for the development and the support of a survivorship care program included an organization and leadership commitment as well as the existence of a well-trained staff dedicated on survivorship. To succeed, the survivorship care model not only has to be supported from the top down, but also from bottom-up by the long-term follow-up team. Lack of dedicated work space and of personnel resources was often mentioned as the major barrier for a survivorship care center. The lack of financial support for salaries and research, as well as reimbursement for clinical services, remained a key issue for the centers. Last but not least, an appropriate clinical information system was in most centers either not existing or not adapted for the long-term follow-up care of cancer patients.

Transition from pediatric to adult long-term care

Survivors of childhood cancer have a high rate of illness due to chronic health conditions [13]. Long-term survivors treated during childhood for cancer will need lifelong health care. However, the best way to accomplish lifelong health care for adult survivors of childhood cancer is not clearly defined. Several modes of cancer survivor care are applied, mainly depending on the size of the pediatric oncology center and the center's preferences: cancer center-based model (I) without referral, where adult survivors are kept indefinitely at the treating institution; community referral model (II), where survivors are transitioned at adulthood to their primary care professionals; hybrid model (III), where the survivors are transitioned to community health-care providers who collaborate closely with the treating institution for all questions concerning long-term survivorship; adult hemato-oncology model (IV), where the survivors are transitioned definitively to an adult hemato-oncology department [8].

The transition from pediatric cancer care to adult-focused care is challenging and needs to overcome a number of barriers. Barriers of successful health care for these adult survivors included the survivor's psychological condition and knowledge about their primary disease, the attitude of pediatric and adult health-providers, and the health system itself. Unlike their adult counterparts, childhood cancer survivors have often limited access to information on the diagnosis and treatment of their malignancy, as well as on adverse effects that can occur later in life. They may have been too young to understand and their parents may have decided to shield them from details of their disease. In a cross-sectional survey on 635 consecutive adult survivors of childhood cancer, 72% accurately reported their diagnosis with precision. Most of the participants correctly reported on their treatment history for chemotherapy and radiation therapy. However, knowledge deficits existed about basic facts of their medical history, such as the use and dose of anthracycline and site of radiation [14].

Despite a significant risk of late effects after cancer treatment, the majority of adult survivors of childhood cancer do not receive regular medical care focused on their long-term risk. Only 17.8% of a large cohort of 8522 long-term survivors reported a specific medical follow-up visit within the previous 2 years. Medical care was not a barrier for most, since nearly 90% of the survivors had at least one medical visit during this period. Rather, the care that they received did not focus on their specific long-term risk and strategies to ameliorate them [15]. These results correspond to another large cohort from the Childhood Cancer Survivor Study: most of the survivors reported some contact with a medical system. The likelihood of a medical visit decreased as survivors aged and the interval from diagnosis increased. Less than 20% of survivors were seen in a cancer center, and a risk-based health care of adult survivors of childhood cancer was very uncommon [16].

The transition from childhood cancer treatment to adult long-term care is a long and difficult process. There is not one single way to proceed; however, there are some rules increasing the chances for a successful transition. An important step is to provide complete data on disease, treatment, and complications that occurred during the period before the transition, and to elaborate a personalized risk-based follow-up program. In a noncancer population, successful transfer was related to the existence of documented pediatric recommendations and patients' belief that the control should be performed in a highly specialized center [17]. The transition to adult care has to be planned and started well before the patient is transferred. During this transition phase, certain health professionals, such as social workers, psychologists, physical therapists, and nurses, could maintain the continuity of the care [18].

Long-term transplant clinic setup

Late mortality is increased in long-term survivors of allogeneic HSCT when compared with an age- and gender-matched general population. More than 25 years after transplantation there is still a twofold excess in death rate [19]. Some of the late complications, such secondary malignancies and vascular complications, are expected very late after transplantation. Even three decades after allogeneic HSCT, the cumulative incidence for secondary solid tumors or vascular complications continues to increase, with no indication of a plateau developing [20, 21]. Life expectancy among 5-year survivors after HCT is reduced by approximately 30% compared to the general population, regardless of current age or time from transplantation [22]. These data clearly demonstrate that individuals undergoing allogeneic HSCT, even when cured from their primary disease, will never become nonpatients. Therefore, there must be a lifelong commitment for post-transplant survivorship care.

When does survivorship care start? Most studies on late effects after HSCT include recipients surviving 2 years or longer after transplantation and in remission of their primary disease. However, in daily routine, the precise timing of survivorship care is not so stringent. In cancer patients, it is usually defined by the time the primary treatment ends. In many transplant centers the posttransplant survivorship begins when the patient no longer needs regular posttransplant care. At that time, annual survivorship visits are considered as a standard for long-term follow-up. However, transplant survivors with ongoing chronic GVHD and still on immunosuppressive treatment may need more regular controls at a specialized follow-up center. With growing numbers of long-term survivors after HSCT, many centers refer their patients back to the primary care provider or to the referring hemato-oncology center. However, there is often no clear plan and designated responsibilities between primary care clinicians and the survivorship clinic. This condition may result in fragmentation of care and poor communication between the different care providers. This obstacle could be overcome when promoting an integrated approach of long-term survivors involving all participants to work together as a team, and to define the responsibility of each part. The question is also when does survivorship care end? Cancer survivorship lasts until recurrence of primary disease, secondary cancer, or death of the patient. In the case of relapse or secondary cancer, survivors again become cancer patients reentering possibly in the acute phase of cancer treatment [6]. In analogy, this definition can also be applied for long-term survivors of HSCT.

Improvement in the overall quality of life of long-term survivors depends among other things on the education of health-care providers regarding the potential late effects that may occur after HSCT [23]. Educating health-care professionals on long-term follow-up may produce institutional changes and improve survivorship care and communication between the health-care providers involved. Within an National Cancer Institute funded educational program, 204 multidisciplinary teams from the USA participated in four annual courses on education for quality of survivorship cancer care. The course participants included administrators, social workers, nurse practitioners, physicians, and others and were followed up at 6, 12, and 18 months after the course for goal achievement and institutional evaluations. The institutional assessments increased significantly from baseline to 18 months. Psychological and emotional standards, which were deficient for most cancer survivors, improved over the time period. Also, the communication domain improved significantly [24].

There are no specific publications on survivorship clinic setup and long-term follow-up program for the transplant setting. A lot of information used for cancer survivorship is applicable to transplant survivorship care. There are, however, some basic differences between cancer and transplant survivorship care in the long term that affect the setup of a long-term transplant clinic and the posttransplant survivorship care program. The follow-up of cancer survivors is mainly concentrated on the cancer specificity and the treatment applied. In contrast, posttransplant long-term follow-up is much more focused on late effects due to the conditioning toxicity, the delayed immune reconstitution, and the consequences of chronic GVHD and its prolonged immunosuppressive treatment. The COG Late Effects Committee provided a comprehensive *Long-Term Follow-Up Resource Guide* describing the entire process required to establish the infrastructure for a long-term follow-up clinic [25]. The content of this resource guide is based on the expertise of individuals who have successfully established such centers at their institution. This resource guide addresses all issues needed to set up a long-term transplant clinic: various models of long-term follow-up care; transition issues; challenges and barriers; survivorship program development; multidisciplinary team composition; recommendations for the annual follow-up visit; billing and financial issues; integration of survivorship research.

Basis for long-term follow-up clinic setup

As for cancer survivors, there are a variety of models for long-term transplant clinics, all of them with distinct advantages and disadvantages. There is not one best model for all transplant centers, and for a given center the model may change over time. Some models of long-term follow-up clinics are shown in Table 3.1. Considerations for the choice of a model include factors such as available resources in personnel and work space, commitment of the head of the transplant center and the team to support a late effects program, the size and type of transplant center (allogeneic, autologous), the geographic area covered by the transplant center, the level of education of the primary care providers in survivorship after HSCT, and the national system of insurance covering long-term follow-up care. Independent of the chosen

Table 3.1 Different models of long term transplant clinics

Model	Advantages	Disadvantages
Outpatients long-term follow-up clinic integrated into outpatient clinic of the transplant center	Comfortable for patients and family Continuity of care ensured	Main attention brought to the acute medical problems of the posttransplant care Focus set on illness and not wellness Potential lack in interest or knowledge of late effects Research in late effects and long-term survivorship becomes of second rank
Independent specialized long-term follow-up clinic	Providers with expertise Emphasis on improving survivor knowledge after HSCT Risk-based screening and follow-up care Health education of the survivors Opportunity to train healthcare professionals Structured research of late effects	Requires multiples resources of personnel and work space Requires time In the case of an independent center, loss of expertise of the transplant center Continuity of care can get lost
Specialized long-term follow-up clinic integrated within the transplant center	Most advantages of the independent specialized long-term follow-up clinic, without loss of continuity	Requires multiples resources of personnel and work space
Community-based care	Convenience for the survivor and their family Promotes independence and reintegration into primary care	Limited provider knowledge and training regarding late effects Lack of time to devote to special physical and psychological needs of long-term survivors Lack of sub-specialist resources with survivorship expertise Difficult to coordinate research Difficult to update survivors regarding new information as it becomes available Difficult to update survivorship database
Combined approach between transplant center and community-based care	Combined advantages of specialized care and community-based care	Risk of insufficient predefined role of each part Risk of poor communication between each part

model, all survivors should maintain life-long regular contact with the care provider who has knowledge about the potential long-term effects and the causal relationship between transplantation and late effects.

The essential functions of a long-term transplant clinic are to take care of the health condition, prevent late effects, detect and treat as early as possible the late complications after HSCT, and assure quality of life of the long-term survivors after HSCT. Figure 3.1 presents the most relevant components of posttransplant survivorship care. Ideally, the posttransplant long-term clinic not only assures medical and psychological care, but also considers financial aspects, insurance issues, reinsertion in social life, and approaches problems related to school and employment. Long-term survivors are generally followed on an annual basis at the survivorship clinic. Therefore, the follow-up clinic needs space and personnel resources to meet the requirements of survivorship care. The minimum time required for initial and annual survivorship visits has been estimated to be approximately 120 min and 90 min, respectively [8]. The magnitude of risk and the time of appearance of late effects after transplantation for an individual patient depend on a multitude of factors. Accordingly, the follow-up program

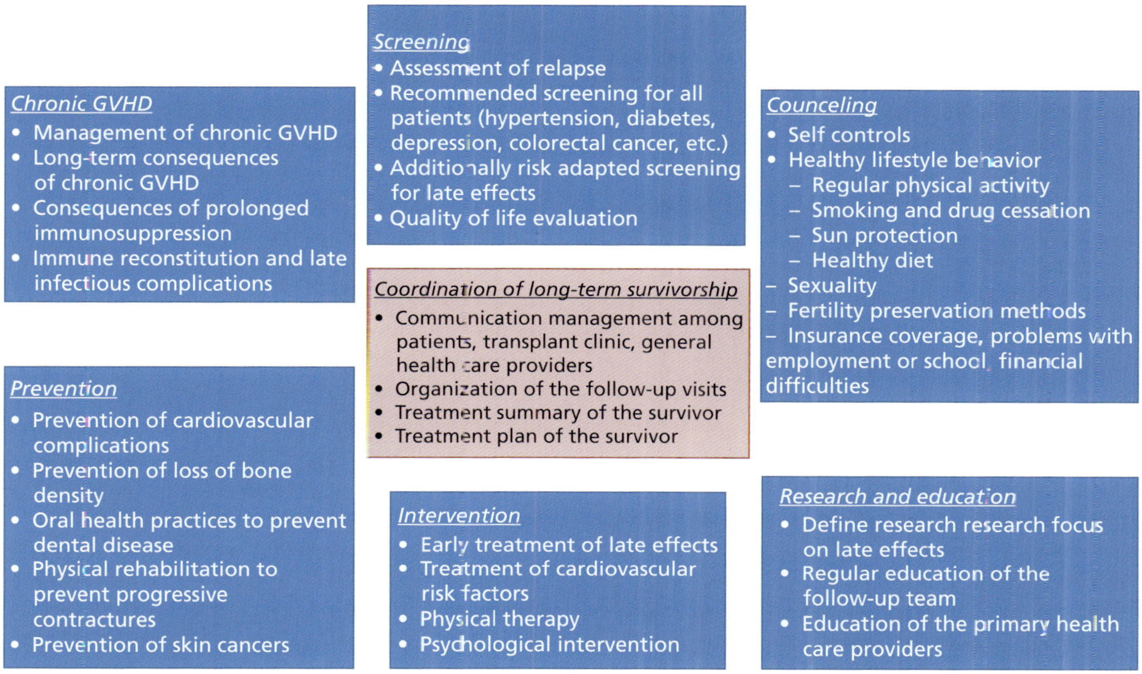

Figure 3.1 Components of post-transplant survivorship care.

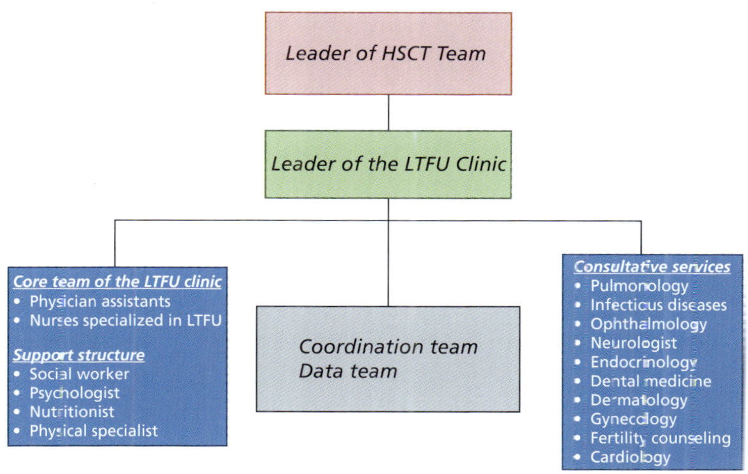

Figure 3.2 Building up a multidisciplinary team for a long-term follow-up (LTFU) transplant clinic.

should provide a risk-based survivor care and be customized to the patients.

The composition of the long-term transplant team is crucial. A well-functioning follow-up program requires a multidisciplinary approach (Figure 3.2). There is usually a core team, including physicians and nurses specialized in HSCT, GVHD, and long-term follow-up, coordinators of the program, medical social workers, nutritionists, physical therapists, and psychologists. This core team needs to be supported by a complex consultative network with specialists interested in the long-term follow-up of HSCT. The specialties involved may include pulmonology, infectious disease specialists, ophthalmology, neurology, endocrinology, dental medicine, dermatology, gynecology, fertility counseling, cardiology, and many others.

The annual visit has to be scheduled and prepared well in advance [25]. Prior to the visit, the team reviews the diagnosis, summarizes all relevant events of the post-transplant phase, and discusses the clinical and biological information obtained from the previous annual visit, taking into account the decisions drawn after the visit. Based on the treatment summary, the pre-ordered laboratory analysis, the radiologic evaluations, and other specific investigations can be determined and scheduled for the visit. Subspecialist referral has to be organized in advance as well. A preclinical team meeting can be helpful to disseminate information and to determine which team member will be involved during the visit. During the clinic visit, the family medical and psychosocial histories should be reviewed. A comprehensive physical exam has to be performed with focus on organs at risk, and a psychological assessment should be done by the social worker or psychologist. Health counseling is part of the annual visit, and includes general nutrition advice, directives on prohibition of active or passive smoke exposure and use of illegal drugs, and advice concerning alcohol use, sun exposure, healthy weight maintenance, and regular physical activities [26]. The post-clinic follow-up begins immediately after the clinic visit. A team meeting to summarize the patient status and the treatment consequences should be organized. During this meeting the various results and the impressions of the team members will be summarized in a systematic and written document. An automated mechanism should be in place to contact patients not arriving for the scheduled visit. Patients lost to follow-up should be traced and brought back into a health-care system. In order to improve adherence to follow-up health care, Internet-based survivorship care may be offered to long-term survivors of HSCT. It represents an important modality for augmenting onsite clinical services [27].

The "Recommended screening and preventive practices for long-term survivors after hematopoietic cell transplantation" represent the basis for the follow-up program. These recommendations, provided by an international group of transplantation experts, were published for the first time in 2006 [28, 29] and updated in 2012 [26, 30–32]. To assure an international applicability, the three transplant societies who initiated the project in 2006 (the Center for International Blood and Marrow Transplant Research, EBMT, and the American Society of Blood and Marrow Transplantation), invited transplant societies worldwide (the Asia–Pacific Blood and Marrow Transplantation Group, the Bone Marrow Transplant Society of Australia and New Zealand, the East Mediterranean Blood and Marrow Transplantation Group, and the Sociedada Brasileira de Transpante de Medula Ossea) to participate in the updated recommendations of 2012. In this multi-published paper, the working group recognized that the models and primary site for long-term follow-up will vary by country and available resources. Furthermore, some suggestions referring to the setup of a posttransplant survivorship clinic were made [26]:

- The HSCT recipient should be provided with a survivorship care plan that includes a treatment strategy summary and a follow-up plan to facilitate the transition from the immediate transplantation care to the long-term follow-up care.
- Primary health providers and hemato-oncologists that will take care of long-term survivors have to be educated on the unique exposures, risk factors, and medical issues of HSCT long-term survivors.
- Prevention, screening, and management of late complications of transplantation require a multidisciplinary approach. Therefore, the long-term follow-up program has to establish a multidisciplinary team.

The National Marrow Donor Program (NMDP), which is one of the leaders in providing hematopoietic stem cells to patients for unrelated HSCT, also supports patient care by elaborating material for medical education. The NMDP has recently developed guidelines in consultation with several leading transplant organizations for posttransplant care [33]. These guidelines, intended for health-care providers who have to follow up transplant survivors, provide recommendations on post-transplant screening, vaccination, and GVHD.

Table 3.2 shows the significant aspects that need to be considered when setting up a long-term transplant clinic. Before starting, the head of the transplant center and his team have to be convinced about the necessity of a follow-up transplant clinic and to decide which model is most appropriate for the present situation. Thereafter, the personnel and space resources available have to be

Table 3.2 Significant aspects to consider when building up a long-term follow-up transplant clinic

1. Commitment of the head of the HSCT center to have a long-term follow-up clinic
   a. Convince the core team of physicians and nurses that this needs to be done
   b. Define the resources required to start the program
2. Decision on the type of model to be chosen
   a. This model can change with time for a given center
   b. Define what will be the consequences on the transplant center
3. Define the team of the long-term clinic
   a. The core team composition
   b. The multidisciplinary network with the most important specialists involved in the long-term follow-up
4. Define the space needed for the long-term follow-up clinic
   a. Room for administrative work (preparation of the follow-up visit)
   b. Room for blood sample taking
   c. Room for clinic visit
   d. Room to isolate patients with communicable infectious diseases
5. Define the follow-up program for the survivor
   a. Define the process of a follow-up visit (preparation; clinic visit; post-clinic follow-up)
   b. Determining program parameters
   c. Organize post-clinic follow-up (tracking results; interpretation of the findings)
   d. Organize the documentation of the follow-up care
   e. Define how to assure all long-term follow-up and to deal with lost to follow-up
6. Define transition of survivors
   a. From regular posttransplant care to long-term survivorship care
   b. From pediatric to adult care
   c. From long-term follow-up clinic to primary health-care providers
7. Define reimbursement and financial issue
8. Define education and research issues on the long term
   a. Continuous education of the core team
   b. Education of the primary care providers and hemato-oncologists
   c. Links with patients/family organizations
   d. Research on long-term survivorship

assessed. Finally, the follow-up program has to be defined. The choice of a specific model and follow-up program does not need to be definitive. It can evolve with the changes affecting the transplant center, the survivorship needs, and the resources available to run a follow-up clinic. Nevertheless, whatever the decision of the transplant center is, the need for long-term survivorship care after HSCT will continuously increase in workload for the HSCT center and in importance for the health-care system.

Acknowledgment

We thank Carmen Ruiz de Elvira for the data provided on patients registered at the EBMT Central Registry Office.

References

1. Savani BN. How can we improve life expectancy and quality of life in long-term survivors after allogeneic stem cell transplantation? Semin Hematol. 2012;49(1):1–3.
2. Rowland JH. What are cancer survivors telling us? Cancer J. 2008;14(6):361–368.
3. Sun CL, Francisco L, Kawashima T, et al. Prevalence and predictors of chronic health conditions after hematopoietic cell transplantation: a report from the Bone Marrow Transplant Survivor Study. Blood. 2010;116(17):3129–3139.
4. Children's Oncology Group. Long-term follow-up guidelines for survivors of childhood, adolescent and young adult cancers. 2012.
5. Landier W, Bhatia S, Eshelman DA, et al. Development of risk-based guidelines for pediatric cancer survivors: the Children's Oncology Group Long-Term Follow-Up Guidelines from the Children's Oncology Group Late Effects Committee and Nursing Discipline. J Clin Oncol. 2004;22(24):4979–4990.
6. Hewitt M, Greenfield S, Stovall E (eds). From Cancer Patient to Cancer Survivor: Lost in Transition. Washington, DC: The National Academies Press, 2005.
7. NHS Improvement. Cancer Improvement. 2009. Available from: http://www.improvement.nhs.uk/cancer (accessed 9 May 2013).
8. Eshelman-Kent D, Kinahan KE, Hobbie W, et al. Cancer survivorship practices, services, and delivery: a report from the Children's Oncology Group (COG) Nursing Discipline, Adolescent/Young Adult, and Late Effects Committees. J Cancer Surviv. 2011;5(4):345–357.
9. McCabe SM, Baker SK, Huffman C, Miller K. Optimizing survivorship care: academic and community clinic models. In: Feuerstein M, Ganz PA (eds). Health Services for Cancer Survivors. Dordrecht: Springer Science+Business Media, 2011; pp. 223–238.
10. Friedman DL, Freyer DR, Levitt GA. Models of care for survivors of childhood cancer. Pediatr Blood Cancer. 2006;46(2):159–168.

11. Department of Health, Macmillan Cancer Support, NHS Improvement. The National Cancer Survivorship Initiative Vision. Department of Health, 2010. Available from: http://www.ncsi.org.uk/wp-content/uploads/NCSI-Vision-Document.pdf (accessed 9 May 2013)
12. Campbell MK, Tessaro I, Gellin M, et al. Adult cancer survivorship care: experiences from the LIVESTRONG centers of excellence network. J Cancer Surviv. 2011;5(3):271–282.
13. Oeffinger KC, Mertens AC, Sklar CA, et al. Chronic health conditions in adult survivors of childhood cancer. N Engl J Med. 2006;355(15):1572–1582.
14. Kadan-Lottick NS, Robison LL, Gurney JG, et al. Childhood cancer survivors' knowledge about their past diagnosis and treatment: Childhood Cancer Survivor Study. JAMA. 2002;287(14):1832–1839.
15. Nathan PC, Greenberg ML, Ness KK, et al. Medical care in long-term survivors of childhood cancer: a report from the childhood cancer survivor study. J Clin Oncol. 2008; 26(27):4401–4409.
16. Oeffinger KC, Mertens AC, Hudson MM, et al. Health care of young adult survivors of childhood cancer: a report from the Childhood Cancer Survivor Study. Ann Fam Med. 2004;2(1):61–70.
17. Reid GJ, Irvine MJ, McCrindle BW, et al. Prevalence and correlates of successful transfer from pediatric to adult health care among a cohort of young adults with complex congenital heart defects. Pediatrics. 2004;113(3 Pt 1):e197–e205.
18. Henderson TO, Friedman DL, Meadows AT. Childhood cancer survivors: transition to adult-focused risk-based care. Pediatrics. 2010;126(1):129–136.
19. Bhatia S, Francisco L, Carter A, et al. Late mortality after allogeneic hematopoietic cell transplantation and functional status of long-term survivors: report from the Bone Marrow Transplant Survivor Study. Blood. 2007;110(10): 3784–3792.
20. Rizzo JD, Curtis RE, Socie G, et al. Solid cancers after allogeneic hematopoietic cell transplantation. Blood. 2009; 113(5):1175–1183.
21. Tichelli A, Bucher C, Rovo A, et al. Premature cardiovascular disease after allogeneic hematopoietic stem-cell transplantation. Blood. 2007;110(9):3463–3471.
22. Martin PJ, Counts GW, Appelbaum FR, et al. Life expectancy in patients surviving more than 5 years after heamtopoietic cell transplantation. J Clin Oncol. 2010;28(10);1011–1016.
23. Bhatia S, Meadows AT. Long-term follow-up of childhood cancer survivors: future directions for clinical care and research. Pediatr Blood Cancer. 2006;46(2):143–148.
24. Grant M, Economou D, Ferrell B, Uman G. Educating health care professionals to provide institutional changes in cancer survivorship care. J Cancer Educ. 2012;27(2):226–232.
25. Children's Oncology Group Nursing Discipline Clinical Practice Subcommittee/Survivorship in collaboration with the Late Effects Committee. Establishing and Enhancing Services for Childhood Cancer Survivors: Long-Term Follow-Up Program Resource Guide. Children's Oncology Group, 2007. Available from: http://www.survivorshipguidelines.org/pdf/LTFUResourceGuide.pdf (accessed 9 May 2013).
26. Majhail NS, Rizzo JD, Lee SJ, et al. Recommended screening and preventive practices for long-term survivors after hematopoietic cell transplantation. Bone Marrow Transplant. 2012;47(3):337–341.
27. Syrjala KL, Stover AC, Yi JC, et al. Development and implementation of an Internet-based survivorship care program for cancer survivors treated with hematopoietic stem cell transplantation. J Cancer Surviv. 2011;5(3):292–304.
28. Rizzo JD, Wingard JR, Tichelli A, et al. Recommended screening and preventive practices for long-term survivors after hematopoietic cell transplantation: joint recommendations of the European Group for Blood and Marrow Transplantation, the Center for International Blood and Marrow Transplant Research, and the American Society of Blood and Marrow Transplantation. Biol Blood Marrow Transplant. 2006;12(2):138–151.
29. Rizzo JD, Wingard JR, Tichelli A, et al. Recommended screening and preventive practices for long-term survivors after hematopoietic cell transplantation: joint recommendations of the European Group for Blood and Marrow Transplantation, Center for International Blood and Marrow Transplant Research, and the American Society for Blood and Marrow Transplantation (EBMT/CIBMTR/ASBMT). Bone Marrow Transplant. 2006;37(3):249–261.
30. Majhail NS, Rizzo JD, Lee SJ, et al. Recommended screening and preventive practices for long-term survivors after hematopoietic cell transplantation. Rev Bras Hematol Hemoter. 2012;34(2):109–133.
31. Majhail NS, Rizzo JD, Lee SJ, et al. Recommended screening and preventive practices for long-term survivors after hematopoietic cell transplantation. Hematol Oncol Stem Cell Ther. 2012;5(1):1–30.
32. Majhail NS, Rizzo JD, Lee SJ, et al. Recommended screening and preventive practices for long-term survivors after hematopoietic cell transplantation. Biol Blood Marrow Transplant. 2012;18(3):348–371.
33. Medical Education, National Marrow Donor Program. Recommended Post-Transplant Care: Long-Term Survival Guidelines. 2012. Available from: http://marrow.org/Physicians/Post-Transplant_Care/11008_Recommended_Post-Transplant_Care_MAY2012_PDF.aspx (accessed 9 May 2013).

CHAPTER 4

Late effects after allogeneic hematopoietic stem cell transplantation

Shahrukh Hashmi[1] *and Mark R Litzow*[2]

[1]Division of Blood and Marrow Transplantation, William J. von Liebig Transplant Center, Mayo Clinic, Rochester, MN, USA

[2]Division of Hematology, College of Medicine, Mayo Clinic, Rochester, MN, USA

Introduction and concepts

Late effects have traditionally been defined as the complications arising at least 6 months after hematopoietic stem cell transplantation (HSCT) [1], and include both relapse and nonrelapse complications. Although the relapse incidence is highest early after HSCT, most recipients remain at risk for relapse up to a year after HSCT and support the use of an intense monitoring program for high-risk patients with disease-specific morphologic, radiologic, and/or molecular parameters. Since patients with relapsed disease are treated with intensive therapies, they are conventionally excluded from the general management model of a typical long-term follow-up, as discussed in detailed in Chapter 3. The general concepts of nonrelapse late effects, including chronic graft-versus-host disease (cGVHD), are discussed in detail in this chapter.

Most of the late effects can be categorized based on the organ or system-specific complications and usually arise due to a complex interaction of various factors which may include:

1 a direct effect of cGVHD (e.g., sclerosing skin cGVHD resulting in contractures);

2 complications of poor baseline health (e.g., increased risk of increased risk of pulmonary complications in smokers); and

3 chemotherapy/radiotherapy- or immunosuppressive therapy (IST)-related complications (e.g., increased risk of solid secondary cancers or increased risk of diabetes, respectively)

The complications arising from either of these variables may coalesce to decrease both the survival and the quality of life (QOL; see Figure 4.1), thus making the biologic plausibility of a particular outcome with causation very difficult. An example of such an interaction in post-HSCT patients is infertility, which is a well-known phenomenon in the survivors of HSCT [2] and is associated with total body irradiation (TBI) due to endocrine disruption (central or gonadal) [3, 4]. cGVHD may also lead to unsuccessful conception due to anatomic complications, especially when vaginal stenosis or strictures develop [5]. Among the baseline health parameters, smoking has an established relationship with infertility [6] (though data are lacking regarding this association within the HSCT literature). Thus, various factors combine to cause adverse outcomes in an allogeneic HSCT survivor.

Certain late effects of allogeneic HSCTs are likely underestimated owing to an extended median time of occurrence of these effects. Since the majority of the adult HSCT recipients do not survive for more than 10 years, the data for the incidence of *very late* complications

Blood and Marrow Transplantation Long-Term Management: Prevention and Complications, First Edition. Edited by Bipin N Savani.

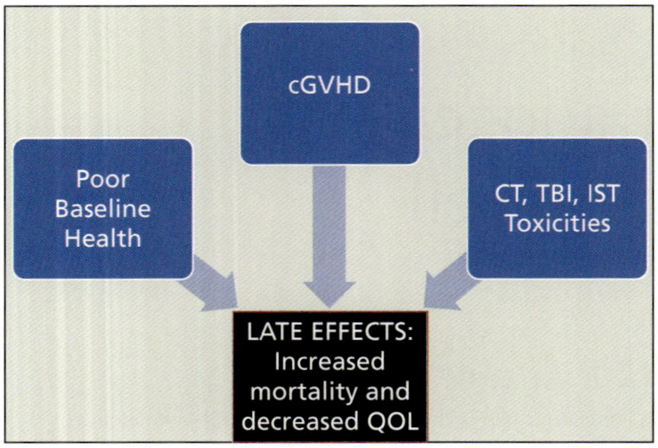

Figure 4.1 Dynamics of etiology of late effects in allogeneic HSCT survivors (cGVHD: chronic graft-versus-host disease; CT: chemotherapy; IST: immunosuppressive therapy; TBI: total body irradiation; QOL: quality of life).

Table 4.1 Nonrelapse late and very late effects of allogeneic HSCTs

1. Acute and chronic infections
2. Cutaneous complications
3. Oral cavity complications
4. Hepatic complications
5. Gastrointestinal (GI) complications
6. Genital complications
7. Renal complications
8. Ocular complications
9. Endocrine complications
10. Hypogonadism, infertility, pregnancy, and lactation issues
11. Dental complications
12. Musculoskeletal and bone complications
13. Pulmonary complications and obliterating bronchiolitis
14. Neurologic complications
15. Psychologic and social complications
16. Sexual dysfunction
17. Cardiovascular complications
18. Secondary solid malignancies
19. Secondary hematologic malignancies

(e.g., secondary solid cancers and cardiovascular effects) may not be appropriately captured and thus may lead to a biased estimate of the true incidence. A good example illustrating this notion is the pediatric lymphoma survivor study [7] in which the heart disease incidence of the treated patients was found to be five times higher than the general population, but the risk of myocardial infarction started to increase only after 10 years of treatment. This study had a median follow-up of approximately 19 years, which is hard to replicate in adult allogeneic HSCT studies. Therefore, it is likely that secondary solid cancers and cardiovascular complications may increase with longer follow-up in allogeneic HSCT cohorts.

The late effects of cGVHD occur in a nonsystematic fashion. Once cGVHD starts to manifest in a particular organ or system, quite frequently other organs/systems may also show signs of involvement with cGVHD, leading to the hypothesis of a uniform pathogenesis of cGVHD in which a series of immunologic events contribute to an autoimmune-like systemic syndrome [8]. However, histologic and immunologic studies indicate a wide variety of differences in pathologic manifestations among different organs involved with cGVHD; for example, in liver cGVHD, the biopsies have indicated the presence of lobular hepatitis and a reduction or absence of small bile ducts with cholestasis resembling primary biliary cirrhosis [9], whereas in cutaneous cGVHD, epidermal atrophy and dense focal dermal fibrosis are apparent without any significant inflammation [10]. Furthermore, specific organ late effects thought to occur only from cGVHD may have other etiologic factors playing a role. For example, some studies of obliterative bronchiolitis (OB) have indicated a strong association with the presence of cGVHD [11], but some OB cases in HSCT recipients have also been reported to occur in the absence of cGVHD [12]. In summary, the exact pathogenesis of the late effects manifested as organ-specific cGVHD are complex and a detailed discussion of this issue is beyond the scope of this chapter.

Identification of the effects

Various methods of identifying late effects can be utilized. Unfortunately, since many organs or organ systems can be involved simultaneously, a strict timeline for the preventive landmarks post-HSCT cannot be formulated. *Very late effects* can be defined as those occurring at least 5 years post-HSCT. A general guidance strategy for psychologic and organ-based aspects of late effects is delineated. The common nonrelapse late effects occurring after HSCTs are depicted in Table 4.1 and a brief description of each complication is given in the next section along with an introduction to the preventive and surveillance strategies.

Late effects

1. Acute and chronic infections

Infections occurring late in allogeneic-HSCT recipients typically have an onset within the first year of transplant, but HSCT recipients remain at risk for a long period of time, especially when being treated with IST for cGVHD. After an allogeneic-HSCT, it may take few months or up to a year for the immune system to completely reconstitute, thus justifying scheduled re-vaccinations at regular intervals late after transplant, as indicated per the current immunization guidelines unless treatment for GVHD is ongoing. Owing to both IST and cGVHD, immune recovery can be delayed and a functional immunodeficiency state can persist posttransplant beyond 1 year due to impairment of both humoral and cell-mediated immunity (mainly due to persistent lymphopenia), decreased opsonization, and hyposplenism in certain cases. The risks of acute infections are heightened by mucocutaneous damage, which occurs due to skin, oral, and gastrointestinal (GI) cGVHD, and due to iatrogenic reasons (e.g., intravenous catheters for extracorporeal photophoresis). Extra care should be taken to examine the catheter sites, and for surveillance of skin or oral mucosal tears due to cGVHD.

Among the late viral infections, Epstein–Barr virus is exceedingly common, but infrequently causes any permanent late sequelae (except posttransplant lymphoproliferative disorder, as discussed later in "17. Cardiovascular complications"). Varicella zoster virus (VZV) and cytomegalovirus (CMV) are the most common organisms causing complications. The VZV-mediated infections typically occur during the first 6–12 months post-HSCT (approximately 80% of cases) [13]; disseminated disease is much more common in allogeneic-HSCTs than in autologous HSCTs (45% versus 25%) and the lesions are likely to last longer and heal more slowly than in normal adults [14], necessitating the need for prophylactic therapy with anti-VZV drugs for a long period of time even in the absence of cGVHD. Herpes simplex encephalitis, JC/BK infections, hepatitis B and C virus infections and reactivations, and HIV infection are rare late effects and do not need long-term surveillance.

Although not unique to allogeneic-HSCT, human herpesvirus 6 (HHV-6) infections occurring late in HSCTs deserve special attention in these patients as significant morbidity and mortality can be associated with this infection. HHV-6 infection can lead to memory loss, insomnia, confusion, hyperintense signals of the hippocampi on brain magnetic resonance imaging, and temporal lobe seizure activity on electroencephalography [15]. Since similar symptoms may occur in acute meningitis and in some cases of calcineurin inhibitor (CNI)-associated encephalopathy, a high level of suspicion for HHV-6 encephalitis is required in order to send the appropriate diagnostic tests for this condition.

Late-onset fungal infections include candidal species, invasive aspergillosis, *Fusarium* species and the Zygomycetes. They are more common within a few months of allogeneic-HSCTs and do not require surveillance besides a heightened awareness and prompt diagnostic testing in symptomatic patients for urgent treatment, particularly in high-risk patients such as cGVHD patients on high-dose corticosteroids.

The usual suspects for late-onset bacterial infections include staphylococcus species, pseudomonas species, and the encapsulated bacteria [16–18]. The risk of pneumococcal infection is greatest among patients with IgG deficiencies [19] and with severe cGVHD [20], thereby re-enforcing the need for prophylactic antibiotics (e.g., oral penicillin therapy) and pneumococcal vaccinations (see Chapter 11 and Appendix A). Recently, *Clostridium difficile* (C.diff) colitis has been found to have a significantly increased incidence in HSCT recipients [21], which occurred more frequently in early HSCT periods. Interestingly, GI GVHD was found be strongly associated with an increased risk for recurrent C.diff colitis (OR 4.23, $P = 0.02$).

HSCT recipients residing in certain developing countries may be more susceptible to endemic conditions (e.g., tuberculosis, Chagas disease, schistosomiasis) which may manifest as late effects post allogeneic-HSCT. These endemic infections can have a detrimental effect on QOL of HSCT recipients who are already prone to organ dysfunction due to organ involvement; for example, ocular GVHD patients living in areas where *Chlamydia trachomatis* is endemic are at significantly higher risk of blindness compared with the trachoma-free geographic locations.

Post-HSCT hypoglobulinemias can be related to cGVHD and are found most commonly in the cases of chronic lymphocytic leukemia. Routine use of antibiotics in asymptomatic hypoglobulinemic patients without evidence of recurrent infections is not indicated.

2. Cutaneous complications

Among the late effects, cutaneous cGVHD (skin and oral mucosal) is the most common organ/system involved by GVHD [22]. It manifests in a variety of manifestations from chronic eczematous form [23], to lichen planus-like lesions [24]. The affected skin can become progressively indurated and fixed to the underlying fascia, resulting in prominent morphea and scleroderma, which can lead to joint contractures [25] and significant compromise in QOL of HSCT patients.

Although skin cGVHD is one of the leading causes of morbidity in HSCT recipients, a thorough evaluation for other causes of cutaneous complications pertinent to allogeneic-HSCTs is warranted in symptomatic patients. Invasive mold infections can affect the skin of HSCT recipients. Photosensitive rash may represent GVHD or may occur as an adverse effect of certain medications commonly utilized in HSCT recipients for treatment or prevention of infections particularly with voriconazole [26]. In some patients, pre-HSCT chemotherapy with busulfan, cyclophosphamide, or hydroxyurea may lead to permanent darkening and/or thickening of skin, which may masquerade initial stages of cGVHD. Skin cancers are the most common solid malignancies occurring post-HSCT. Routine surveillance with dermatologic exams at annual intervals is recommended [1, 27].

3. Oral cavity complications

The oral mucosal involvement with GVHD frequently leads to extreme xerostomia, often resulting in pain secondary to aphthous-like ulcers [28]. Erythema within lichenoid plaques of buccal mucosa is diagnostic of cGVHD; however, a biopsy is frequently required to exclude the presence of co-infections or oral cancers. Oral cGVHD along with skin cGVHD can result in difficulty in opening of the mouth (similar to the manifestations of oral scleroderma), which can lead to many complications, including malnutrition and poor dental health. Complete loss of taste can also happen in oral cGVHD, which may further decrease the QOL significantly. Prompt recognition of early oral cGVHD and referral to oral surgery for localized treatments (along with systemic therapy) may help in preventing the above-mentioned complications.

4. Hepatic complications

Late liver effects after allogeneic-HSCT include cGVHD, viral hepatitis, and drug-induced hepatitis. Liver biopsies obtained from cGVHD patients have indicated chronic persistent hepatitis, lobular hepatitis, and reduction of small bile ducts with cholestasis, which resembles the pathologic manifestations of primary biliary cirrhosis. Untreated hepatic GVHD may lead to liver failure, which carries a very high mortality. Periodic evaluation with liver function tests may help in early diagnosis. Hepatitis B and C reactivations post-HSCT are rare, but a diagnostic work-up must include the viral serology to exclude these conditions.

Some 7–64% of cancer patients utilize some form of complementary and alternative medicine (CAM) therapies, though a literature gap exists with regard to this issue in the field of HSCT. Many CAM therapies are known to be hepatotoxic and in some cases may lead to hepatic failure. Some of the more frequently reported hepatotoxic CAM therapies include the Chinese remedies [29], mistletoe [30], and kava kava [31]. Efforts should be made to obtain comprehensive CAM history and appropriate advice should be provided to those HSCT patients who are using hepatotoxic CAM therapies to potentially avoid the potentially fatal late effect of hepatic failure.

Approximately one-third of HSCT survivors have evidence of iron overload [32] due to chronic transfusions during the pre- and peri-HSCT time period that may lead to secondary hemochromatosis. It may be reasonable to evaluate serum ferritin levels at 6–12 months post-HSCT; and in patients in whom the evidence of iron overload is found, the general principles of secondary hemochromatosis should be applied for organ-specific screening for complications (e.g., surveillance with ultrasound for liver cancers). Patients with evidence of significant iron overload can be considered for therapeutic phlebotomy if there is adequate recovery of erythropoiesis or possibly for iron chelation therapy.

5. Gastrointestinal (GI) complications

Apart from the oral cavity complications (see "3. Oral cavity complications" earlier), GI involvement with cGVHD is not uncommon. Common manifestations include involvement of the esophagus, resulting in progressive dysphagia, painful ulcers, and gradual weight loss and esophageal webs. Since the incidence of secondary cancers is also increased in allogeneic-HSCT patients, endoscopies should be performed in patients with symptoms of dysphagia. Abdominal pain/cramping, nausea/vomiting, weight loss, diarrhea, and early satiety are also common in GI GVHD [33].

Apart from GI GVHD, late GI effects include GI cancers, medication adverse effects, which include steroid-induced gastritis/esophagitis, mycophenolate-induced colitis, and lastly infections particularly due to CMV colitis. Prompt recognition and treatment of these conditions is warranted to avoid complications.

6. Genital complications

In females, the most frequent late effect manifesting as a genital complaint is vaginal–vulvar GVHD. It typically occurs around the 10th month post-HSCT and presents with vaginal pain, discomfort, and vaginal scarring [34]. Since this late effect can be successfully treated with topical cyclosporine/steroids/estrogen therapies in early stages, vaginal exams at regular intervals (see Chapters 18 and 23) should be performed for early detection. Other late effects include cervical cancers, vaginal candidiasis, and herpes simplex infections.

In males, penile cGVHD is the most frequent genital late effect, which can result in Peyronie's disease or phimosis [35].

Annual comprehensive dermatologic evaluations in both men and women should include complete genital assessments for genital cancers and cGVHD screening.

7. Renal complications

The use of prior nephrotoxic chemotherapies (e.g., platinum based) and CNI therapy for prevention or treatment of GVHD predisposes to the development of chronic kidney disease [36] which can manifest as either glomerulonephritis or interstitial fibrosis. Among chronic infections, CMV and adenovirus are known offencers, and a search for these organisms is warranted if renal infections are suspected.

8. Ocular complications

Among allogeneic-HSCT recipients, blindness is perhaps the leading preventable cause contributing to the disability-adjusted life years.

Ocular cGVHD commonly results in decreased lacrimal gland function, resulting in chronic dry eye (keratoconjunctivitis sicca) as the main late effect and its incidence may be up to 40% among patients with cGVHD. Tear production can be measured with the Schirmer test. Non-cGVHD ocular complications include cataracts, ischemic retinopathy, and infections. Cumulative incidence of cataracts in children has been reported to be 36% at 15 years post-HSCT [37]. Although TBI has a strong association with cataracts [38], many patients remain at risk for cataract due to chronic corticosteroid therapy for cGVHD. Ischemic retinopathy is an uncommon complication but has been described in HSCT settings, particularly in the setting of systemic cyclosporin use.

Since complete vision loss impairs QOL of long-term HSCT survivors more than any other organ complication, it is imperative that the HSCT recipients have ophthalmologic examinations at regular intervals. Detailed management of ocular complications is given in Chapter 16.

9. Endocrine complications

Late endocrine effects of allogeneic-HSCT usually occur as a result of radiation, chemotherapy, or due to cGVHD treatments [39] Organs commonly involved include thyroid gland, gonads, and pancreatic islets. Despite frequent exposures to corticosteroid therapies, the HSCT recipients generally have a low incidence of hypoadrenalism. The major risk factor for hypothyroidism is TBI. The median time of occurrence of hypothyroidism is 4 years post-HSCT. Annual screening with biochemical markers is suggested. A 3.65 times higher incidence of diabetes mellitus (DM) compared with matched siblings has been reported in allogeneic-HSCT recipients [40]. At 2 years post-HSCT, up to one-third of patients may develop DM [41], thereby suggesting a role for screening for DM at annual intervals. Development of DM itself may accelerate the rate of other known complications, including cataracts and chronic kidney disease.

10. Hypogonadism, infertility, pregnancy, and lactation issues

Hypogonadism to varying degrees is common after allogeneic-HSCT, and myeloablative regimens quite frequently lead to permanent sterility [42]. TBI or busulfan-based therapies are major risk factors. Detailed fertility risk–benefit discussions pretransplantation in patients of child-bearing age are strongly suggested. Hormonal insufficiencies may manifest as loss of libido, erectile dysfunction, vaginal dryness, and dyspareunia. Hormonal assessment at 6 months post-HSCT and then annually with follicle-stimulating hormone (FSH), luteinizing hormone (LH), and estrogen in females and FSH, LH, and testosterone in symptomatic males is recommended.

For those patients who wish to conceive and do not have any evidence of hypogonadism, a general approach is to recommend conception planning after 2 years of HSCT since the majority of the primary disease relapses occur within that period of time. Since some allogeneic-HSCT patients are given maintenance chemotherapies, contraception may be utilized (if gonadal function normal) during that period of maintenance therapy to avoid pregnancy since the majority of the agents currently utilized for this purpose are teratogenic (e.g., hypomethylating agents). Similarly, those patients who are undergoing GVHD therapy may benefit from contraception, too, due to unknown teratogenic effects (e.g., CNI, sirolimus). Use of tyrosine kinase inhibitors for treatment of cGVHD or for post-HSCT maintenance therapy is a contraindication for pregnancy due to their known teratogenicity.

Besides the above-mentioned potential late pregnancy/fetal complications, caution must be exercised during lactation since most of the GVHD therapy drugs (CNI) are excreted in breast milk.

11. Dental complications

Late dental complications may arise as a result of TBI, chemotherapy, oral cGVHD, DM, or due to corticosteroid therapy [43]. Common effects include dental caries, endodontic disease, and periodontal disease. General principles of dental care of cancer patients should be adopted [44]. Detailed management options are given in Chapter 17.

12. Musculoskeletal and bone complications

Osteopenia and avascular necrosis (AVN) of the hip or other joints are well described late bone effects of HSCT which may occur as a result of corticosteroid therapy for GVHD [45]. AVN occurs frequently post-HSCT, and about 4–10% of the patients may be affected with at least one joint with AVN [46]. Vitamin D plus calcium supplementation and annual dual-energy X-ray absorptiometry scans for bone health are described in detail in Chapter 15.

Common late musculoskeletal effects include steroid-induced myopathy, fasciitis/scleroderma, and polymyositis, and up to a third of patients may report musculoskeletal symptoms even after 10 years of HSCT [47]. Sclerosis as a manifestation of cGVHD can affect the skin and subcutaneous tissues, including fasciae and joints. Prompt recognition of these complications by clinical exams, serology, and neurologic studies and early intervention may prevent permanent disability.

13. Pulmonary complications and obliterating bronchiolitis (OB)

Infections (particularly aspergillosis, HHV-6, CMV, respiratory syncytial virus, influenza and parainfluenza viruses), OB and pulmonary thromboembolism are the main pulmonary late effects of allogeneic-HSCT. OB occurs in 2–14% of allogeneic-HSCT recipients [48], and although classified as a manifestation of cGVHD, it can less commonly develop in patients with no other clinical manifestations of GVHD. Smoking, TBI, chemotherapy (particularly busulfan), preexisting lung disease, and early HSCT pulmonary complications are known risk factors. Surveillance strategies with history, exams and pulmonary function tests at regular intervals post-HSCT may help in avoidance of severe OB. This topic is further discussed in Chapter 14.

14. Neurologic complications

Late neurologic effects include neurocognitive defects, neuropathy, central nervous system (CNS) GVHD, and CNS infections. Neurocognitive impairment after allogeneic-HSCT is common, and up to 40% of the HSCT survivors may exhibit cognitive deficits even 5 years post-HSCT [49]. Neuropathy in HSCT survivors is highly prevalent and frequently is a result of pre-HSCT chemotherapies. CNS GVHD is an understudied area, but evidence indicating specific inflammatory GVHD changes in the brain is accumulating [50, 51], and its diagnosis requires an aggressive approach with brain biopsy since cerebrospinal fluid analysis and brain magnetic resonance images cannot differentiate CNS GVHD from other causes. CNS infections include HHV-6 and CMV encephalitis (see "1. Acute and chronic infections") besides the common microbial causes of meningitis.

Myasthenia gravis and demyelinating diseases, including Guillain–Barré syndrome, are rare complications. Progressive multifocal encephalopathy should also be considered in differential diagnosis of encephalopathies, if rituximab was given pre-HSCT, or for treatment of cGVHD.

15. Psychologic and social complications

The HSCT survivors and their caregivers are at significant risk of psychologic disorders [52]. Multiple factors may be responsible for this including pretransplant psychologic diagnosis or spiritual absence [53], GVHD, or disease relapse. Major depression, adjustment disorders, and anxiety disorders are the most common psychiatric diagnoses in these patients. Compared with their siblings, allogeneic-HSCT survivors are less likely to continue jobs or be married, and are more likely to report difficulty maintaining health insurance or acquiring life insurance [54, 55]. Late psychologic effects of HSCTs culminate when the psychologic health of spouses/partners is affected by the HSCT [56]. Thus, screening for the disorders affecting these psychologic and social domains at regular intervals is suggested and described in detail in Chapters 34–36.

16. Sexual dysfunction

Sexual late effects of allogeneic-HSCT occur in a significant number of survivors and are usually multifactorial in origin, with common etiologies being vulvar–vaginal GVHD, gonadal deficiencies, and depression, as discussed earlier. Detailed management is discussed in Chapter 18.

Very late effects

17. Cardiovascular complications

About one-third of HSCT patients are at increased risk of developing known cardiovascular risk factors (CVRFs) [57]. Acute GVHD and TBI have been reported to be risk factors specific to HSCT along with the well-recognized cardiotoxic chemotherapies (cyclophosphamide, anthracyclines, trastuzumab, etc.) and mediastinal radiation. Estimated prevalence of long-term cardiovascular complications has been reported to be approximately 5% at 5 years and 9% at 15 years [41, 58]; thus, this is categorized as a very late effect. cGVHD uniquely poses a significantly increased risk for development of CVRFs due to the toxicity of drugs. Corticosteroids and CNI increase the risk of both diabetes and hypertension, whereas sirolimus increases the risks of dyslipidemias CVRFs should be minimized with aggressive treatment strategies and with modification of preventable CVRFs (e.g., smoking, unhealthy diets). Routine post-HSCT care should incorporate measurements of blood pressure, nutritional counseling, obesity control, counseling for smoking cessation, and control of diabetes. Electrocardiogram/echocardiography performance at yearly intervals may be necessary in high-risk patients (e.g., those with CVRFs or anthracycline exposures).

18. Secondary solid malignancies

Allogeneic-HSCT recipients have a two- to threefold increased risk of developing this very late effect [59]. Solid malignancies are the fourth leading cause of mortality in patients surviving more than 2 years post-HSCT. The pattern of increase is linear over time: 1.2–1.6% at 5 years, 2.2–6.1% at 10 years, and 3.8–14.9% at 15 years [60–63]. Certain conditions significantly increase the risk, particularly Fanconi's anemia in which routine surveillance strategies for head/neck cancers should be utilized. Common solid cancers seen in allogeneic-HSCT survivors include thyroid, skin, oropharyngeal, and breast cancers.

Thyroid cancer is the fastest growing non-skin cancer in the USA [64], and its incidence is even higher in the HSCT recipients. A study from the EBMT Late-Effects Working Party suggested a threefold higher incidence of thyroid cancer in HSCT recipients than in the general population [65]. TBI, female gender, and cGVHD were found to be risk factors. A vigilant clinical exam of the thyroid gland and cervical nodes at yearly intervals is recommended.

Skin cancers are the most common solid malignancies post-HSCT. In a large series, the 20-year cumulative incidences of basal cell and squamous cell cancers were reported to be 6.5% and 3.4%, respectively [66]. TBI and GVHD were found to be risk factors. Annual dermatologic exam for skin cancer screening is recommended.

Breast cancer risk is elevated among HSCT recipients with a reported cumulative incidence of 11% at 25 years post-HSCT [67]. Risk factors include TBI and prior chemotherapies. Annual mammography is recommended.

19. Secondary hematologic malignancies

This late effect usually develops within a few years of allogeneic-HSCT, but it may occur after 5 years of HSCT. Donor-derived leukemia is a well-recognized entity [68, 69] along with posttransplant lymphoproliferative disease [70, 71]. An aggressive diagnostic approach is mandated when leukemia or posttransplant lymphoproliferative disease is suspected late in allogeneic-HSCTs.

Future directions

With the improvement in survival of allogeneic-HSCT patients [72], it is predicted that more late complications will be identified in the HSCT recipients. Evidence-based surveillance strategies for early recognition and prompt management of these late effects are best undertaken in multidisciplinary long-term follow-up. Future allogeneic HSCT studies should focus on assessing long-term outcomes by obtaining pretransplant risk factors for late effects and follow through of the late and very late complications in a prospective fashion.

References

1. Majhail NS, Rizzo JD, Lee SJ, et al. Recommended screening and preventive practices for long-term survivors after hematopoietic cell transplantation. Biol Blood Marrow Transplant. 2012;18(3):348–371.
2. Hammond C, Abrams JR, Syrjala KL. Fertility and risk factors for elevated infertility concern in 10-year hematopoietic cell transplant survivors and case-matched controls. J Clin Oncol. 2007;25(23):3511–3517.
3. Littley MD, Shalet SM, Morgenstern GR, Deakin DP. Endocrine and reproductive dysfunction following fractionated total body irradiation in adults. Q J Med. 1991;78(287): 265–274.
4. Cust MP, Whitehead MI, Powles R, et al. Consequences and treatment of ovarian failure after total body irradiation for leukaemia. BMJ. 1989;299(6714):1494–1497.
5. Corson SL, Sullivan K, Batzer F, et al. Gynecologic manifestations of chronic graft-versus-host disease. Obstet Gynecol. 1982;60(4):488–492.
6. Practice Committee of the American Society for Reproductive Medicine. Smoking and infertility. Fertil Steril. 2004; 81(4):1181–1186.
7. Aleman BM, van den Belt-Dusebout AW, De Bruin ML, et al. Late cardiotoxicity after treatment for Hodgkin lymphoma. Blood. 2007;109:1878–1886.
8. Blazar RB, Murphy WJ, Abedi M. Advances in graft-versus-host disease biology and therapy. Nat Rev Immunol. 2012;12:443–458.
9. Epstein O, Thomas HC, Sherlock S. Primary biliary cirrhosis is a dry gland syndrome with features of chronic graft-versus-host disease. Lancet. 1980;1(8179):1166–1168.
10. Wenzel J, Lucas S, Zahn S, Mikus S, et al. CXCR3<–>ligand-mediated skin inflammation in cutaneous lichenoid graft-versus-host disease. J Am Acad Dermatol. 2008;58(3): 437–442.
11. Epler GR. Bronchiolitis obliterans and airways obstruction associated with graft-versus-host disease. Clin Chest Med. 1988;9(4):551–556.
12. Holland HK, Wingard JR, Beschorner WE, et al. Bronchiolitis obliterans in bone marrow transplantation and its relationship to chronic graft-v-host disease and low serum IgG. Blood. 1988;72(2):621–627.
13. Kawasaki H, Takayama J, Ohira M. Herpes zoster infection after bone marrow transplantation in children. J Pediatr. 1996;128:353–356.
14. Atkinson K, Meyers JD, Storb R, et al. Varicella-zoster virus infection after marrow transplantation for aplastic anemia or leukemia. Transplantation. 1980;29:47–50.
15. Wainwright MS, Martin PL, Morse RP, et al. Human herpesvirus 6 limbic encephalitis after stem cell transplantation. Ann Neurol. 2001;50(5):612–619.
16. Ochs L, Shu XO, Miller J, et al. Late infections after allogeneic bone marrow transplantations: comparison of incidence in related and unrelated donor transplant recipients. Blood. 1995;86:3979–3986.
17. Youssef S, Rodriguez G, Rolston KV, et al. *Streptococcus pneumoniae* infections in 47 hematopoietic stem cell transplantation recipients: clinical characteristics of infections and vaccine-breakthrough infections, 1989–2005. Medicine (Baltimore). 2007;86:69–77.
18. Hoyle C, Goldman JM. Life-threatening infections occurring more than 3 months after BMT. 18 UK Bone Marrow Transplant Teams. Bone Marrow Transplant. 1994;14: 247–252.
19. Sheridan JF, Tutschka PJ, Sedmak DD, Copelan EA. Immunoglobulin G subclass deficiency and pneumococcal infection after allogeneic bone marrow transplantation. Blood. 1990;75:1583–1586.
20. Kulkarni S, Powles R, Treleaven J, et al. Chronic graft versus host disease is associated with long-term risk for pneumococcal infections in recipients of bone marrow transplants. Blood. 2000;95:3683–3686.

21. Alonso CD, Treadway SB, Hanna DB, et al. Epidemiology and outcomes of clostridium difficile infections in hematopoietic stem cell transplant recipients. Clin Infect Dis. 2012;54(8):1053–1063.
22. Joseph RW, Couriel DR, Komanduri KV. Chronic graft-versus-host disease after allogeneic stem cell transplantation: challenges in prevention, science, and supportive care. J Support Oncol. 2008;6:361–372.
23. Creamer D, Martyn-Simmons CL, Osborne G, et al. Eczematoid graft-vs-host disease: a novel form of chronic cutaneous graft-vs-host disease and its response to psoralen UV-A therapy. Arch Dermatol. 2007;143:1157–1162.
24. Sullivan KM, Shulman HM, Storb R, et al. Chronic graft-versus-host disease in 52 patients: adverse natural course and successful treatment with combination immunosuppression. Blood. 1981;57(2):267–276.
25. Jacobsohn DA, Kurland BF, Pidala J, et al. Correlation between NIH composite skin score, patient-reported skin score, and outcome: results from the Chronic GVHD Consortium. Blood. 2012;120:2545–2552.
26. Patel AR, Turner ML, Baird K, et al. Voriconazole induced phototoxicity masquerading as chronic graft-versus-host disease of the skin in allogeneic hematopoietic cell transplant recipients. Biol Blood Marrow Transplant. 2009; 15(3):370–376.
27. Rizzo JD, Wingard JR, Tichelli A, et al. Recommended screening and preventive practices for long-term survivors after hematopoietic cell transplantation: joint recommendations of the European Group for Blood and Marrow Transplantation, the Center for International Blood and Marrow Transplant Research, and the American Society of Blood and Marrow Transplantation. Biol Blood Marrow Transplant. 2006;12:138–151.
28. Schubert MM, Sullivan KM. Recognition, incidence, and management of oral graft-versus-host disease. NCI Monogr. 1990;(9):135–143.
29. Picciotto A, Campo N, Brizzolara R, et al. Chronic hepatitis induced by Jin Bu Huan. J Hepatol. 1998;28:165–167.
30. Harvey J, Colin-Jones DG. Mistletoe hepatitis. Br Med J (Clin Res Ed). 1981;282:186–187.
31. Centers for Disease Control and Prevention (CDC). Hepatic toxicity possibly associated with kava-containing products – United States, Germany, and Switzerland, 1999–2002. MMWR Morb Mortal Wkly Rep. 2002;51: 1065–1067.
32. Majhail NS, DeFor T, Lazarus HM, Burns LJ. High prevalence of iron overload in adult allogeneic hematopoietic cell transplant survivors. Biol Blood Marrow Transplant. 2008; 14:790–794.
33. Akpek G, Chinratanalab W, Lee LA, et al. Gastrointestinal involvement in chronic graft-versus-host disease: a clinicopathologic study. Biol Blood Marrow Transplant. 2003; 9(1):46–51.
34. Spiryda LB, Laufer MR, Soiffer RJ, Antin JA. Graft-versus-host disease of the vulva and/or vagina: diagnosis and treatment. Biol Blood Marrow Transplant. 2003;9(12): 760–765.
35. Grigg AP, Underhill C, Russell J, Sale G. Peyronie's disease as a complication of chronic graft versus host disease. Hematology. 2002;7(3):165–168.
36. Choi M, Sun CL, Kurian S, et al. Incidence and predictors of delayed chronic kidney disease in long-term survivors of hematopoietic cell transplantation. Cancer. 2008;113(7): 1580–1587.
37. Gurney JG, Ness KK, Rosenthal J, et al. Visual, auditory, sensory, and motor impairments in long-term survivors of hematopoietic stem cell transplantation performed in childhood: results from the Bone Marrow Transplant Survivor Study. Cancer. 2006;106:1402–1408.
38. Majhail NS, Ness KK, Burns LJ, et al. Late effects in survivors of Hodgkin and non-Hodgkin lymphoma treated with autologous hematopoietic cell transplantation: a report from the Bone Marrow Transplant Survivor Study. Biol Blood Marrow Transplant. 2007;13:1153–1159.
39. Brennan BM, Shalet SM. Endocrine late effects after bone marrow transplant. Br J Haematol. 2002;118:58–66.
40. Baker KS, Ness KK, Steinberger J, et al. Diabetes, hypertension, and cardiovascular events in survivors of hematopoietic cell transplantation: a report from the Bone Marrow Transplantation Survivor Study. Blood. 2007;109:1765–1772.
41. Majhail NS, Challa TR, Mulrooney DA, et al. Hypertension and diabetes mellitus in adult and pediatric survivors of allogeneic hematopoietic cell transplantation. Biol Blood Marrow Transplant. 2009;15:1100–1107.
42. Ranke MB, Schwarze CP, Dopfer R, et al. Late effects after stem cell transplantation (SCT) in children – growth and hormones. Bone Marrow Transplant. 2005;35(Suppl 1): S77–S81.
43. Sonis ST, Woods PD, White BA. Oral complications of cancer therapies. Pretreatment oral assessment. NCI Monogr. 1990;(9):29–32.
44. National Cancer Institute. Oral and Dental Management Before Cancer Therapy. 2013. Available from: http:// www.cancer.gov/cancertopics/pdq/supportivecare/ oralcomplications/HealthProfessional/page3 (accessed 11 May 2013).
45. Yao S, Smiley SL, West K, et al. Accelerated bone mineral density loss occurs with similar incidence and severity, but with different risk factors, after autologous versus allogeneic hematopoietic cell transplantation. Biol Blood Marrow Transplant. 2010;16:1130–1137.

46. Campbell S, Sun CL, Kurian S, et al. Predictors of avascular necrosis of bone in long-term survivors of hematopoietic cell transplantation. Cancer. 2009;115:4127–4135.
47. Syrjala KL, Langer SL, Abrams JR, et al. Late effects of hematopoietic cell transplantation among 10-year adult survivors compared with case-matched controls. J Clin Oncol. 2005;23:6596–6606.
48. Au BK, Au MA, Chien JW. Bronchiolitis obliterans syndrome epidemiology after allogeneic hematopoietic cell transplantation. Biol Blood Marrow Transplant. 2011;17:1072–1078.
49. Syrjala KL, Artherholt SB, Kurland BF, et al. Prospective neurocognitive function over 5 years after allogeneic hematopoietic cell transplantation for cancer survivors compared with matched controls at 5 years. J Clin Oncol. 2011;29:2397–2404.
50. Sostak P, Padovan CS, Eigenbrod S, et al. Cerebral angiitis in 4 patients with chronic GVHD. Bone Marrow Transplant. 2010;45:1181–1188.
51. Saad AG, Alyea E, Wen P, et al. Graft-versus-host disease of the CNS after allogeneic bone marrow transplantation. J Clin Oncol. 2009;27:e147–e149.
52. Rusiewicz A, DuHamel KN, Burkhalter J, et al. Psychological distress in long-term survivors of hematopoietic stem cell transplantation. Psychooncology. 2008;17:329–337.
53. Pereira DB, Christian LM, Patidar S, et al. Spiritual absence and 1-year mortality after hematopoietic stem cell transplant. Biol Blood Marrow Transplant. 2010;16(8):1171–1179.
54. Sun CL, Francisco L, Baker KS, et al. Adverse psychological outcomes in long-term survivors of hematopoietic cell transplantation: a report from the Bone Marrow Transplant Survivor Study (BMTSS). Blood. 2011;118:4723–4731.
55. Wong FL, Francisco L, Togawa K, et al. Long-term recovery after hematopoietic cell transplantation: predictors of quality-of-life concerns. Blood. 2010;115:2508–2519.
56. Bishop MM, Beaumont JL, Hahn EA, et al. Late effects of cancer and hematopoietic stem-cell transplantation on spouses or partners compared with survivors and survivor-matched controls. J Clin Oncol. 2007;25:1403–1411.
57. Armenian SH, Sun CL, Vase T, et al. Cardiovascular risk factors in hematopoietic cell transplantation (HCT) survivors: role in development of subsequent cardiovascular disease. Blood. 2012;120(23):4505–4512.
58. Tichelli A, Passweg J, Wójcik D, et al. Late cardiovascular events after allogeneic hematopoietic stem cell transplantation: a retrospective multicenter study of the Late Effects Working Party of the European Group for Blood and Marrow Transplantation. Haematologica. 2008;93:1203–1210.
59. Tichelli A, Rovo A, Passweg J, et al. Late complications after hematopoietic stem cell transplantation. Expert Rev Hematol. 2009;2:583–601.
60. Rizzo JD, Curtis RE, Socie G, et al. Solid cancers after allogeneic hematopoietic cell transplantation. Blood. 2009;113:1175–1183.
61. Kolb HJ, Socie G, Duell T, et al. Malignant neoplasms in long-term survivors of bone marrow transplantation (Late Effects Working Party of the European Cooperative Group for Blood and Marrow Transplantation and the European Late Effect Project Group). Ann Intern Med. 1999;131:738–744.
62. Bhatia S, Ramsay NK, Steinbuch M, et al. Malignant neoplasms following bone marrow transplantation. Blood. 1996;87:3633–3639.
63. Gallagher G, Forrest DL. Second solid cancers after allogeneic hematopoietic stem cell transplantation. Cancer. 2007;109:84–92.
64. Simard EP, Ward EM, Siegel R, Jemal A. Cancers with increasing incidence trends in the United States: 1999 through 2008. CA Cancer J Clin. 2012;62(2):118–128.
65. Cohen A, Rovelli A, Merlo DF, et al. Risk for secondary thyroid carcinoma after hematopoietic stem-cell transplantation: an EBMT Late Effects Working Party Study. J Clin Oncol. 2007;25:2449–2454.
66. Leisenring W, Friedman DL, Flowers ME, et al. Nonmelanoma skin and mucosal cancers after hematopoietic cell transplantation. J Clin Oncol. 2006;24:1119–1126.
67. Friedman DL, Rovo A, Leisenring W, et al. Increased risk of breast cancer among survivors of allogeneic hematopoietic cell transplantation: a report from the FHCRC and the EBMT-Late Effect Working Party. Blood. 2008;111:939–944.
68. Nakamizo A, Akagi Y, Amano T, et al. Donor-derived adult T-cell leukaemia. Lancet. 2011;377:1124.
69. Wiseman DH. Donor cell leukemia: a review. Biol Blood Marrow Transplant. 2011;17:771–789.
70. Krenauer A, Moll A, Pönisch W, et al. EBV-associated post-transplantation B-cell lymphoproliferative disorder following allogenic stem cell transplantation for acute lymphoblastic leukaemia: tumor regression after reduction of immunosuppression – a case report. Diagn Pathol. 2010;5:21.
71. Snyder MJ, Stenzel TT, Buckley PJ, et al. Posttransplant lymphoproliferative disorder following nonmyeloablative allogeneic stem cell transplantation. Am J Surg Pathol. 2004;28(6):794–800.
72. Gooley TA, Chien JW, Pergam SA, et al. Reduced mortality after allogeneic hematopoietic-cell transplantation. N Engl J Med. 2010;363:2091–2101.

CHAPTER 5

Late effects after autologous hematopoietic stem cell transplantation

Sairah Ahmed and Yago Nieto
University of Texas MD Anderson Cancer Center, Houston, TX, USA

Introduction

The first records of modern-day autologous hematopoietic cell transplantation (autoHCT) in humans was in 1958, when six patients with a variety of cancers were treated with wide-field intensive radiotherapy and then infused with autologous stem cells [1]. Autologous hematopoietic transplantation is now a well-established treatment for many malignant and nonmalignant disorders. Mobilization and collection of hematopoietic cells from peripheral blood with faster hematopoietic recovery has made this approach the treatment of choice for patients with relapsed lymphoma and standard of care for treatment of multiple myeloma [2]. Of 50 000–60 000 hematopoietic stem cell transplants performed worldwide annually, 35 000–40 000 are autologous [3]. With improvement in transplantation techniques, there are a growing number of autoHCT survivors as well as several late effects of transplantation that may account for a decrease in long-term survival for recipients of autologous transplants.

Bhatia et al. [4] published the results of a retrospective study examining late complications of autologous transplants in 2005 through the Bone Marrow Transplant Survivor Study. In that study of 854 patients with 2-year or longer survival, the probability of surviving 5 years was 80% and of surviving 10 years was 69% [4]. This cohort of patients was at a 13-fold increased risk for experiencing a late death compared with the general population, and 29% of patients in that study experienced a late death. Although 56% of these deaths were related to relapse of primary disease, the most frequent cause of nonrelapse death was subsequent malignancy [4]. This correlates to a 12-fold increased risk of malignant neoplasm when compared with the general population. Other studies have shown the increased risk of cancer incidence compared with the general population, and this is generally attributed to the use of radiation and chemotherapy [5–8]. Bhatia et al. also reported late death attributed to cardiac toxicity (2.4%), pulmonary complications (2%), and other treatment-related sequelae (15%) [4].

For malignant diseases, often patients are treated with cytotoxic chemotherapy prior to stem cell transplant. Some complications with significant late consequences can occur early in the posttransplant course; however, we will define late complications as all events occurring after 3 months post autologous hematopoietic stem cell transplantation. Potential long-term toxicities can occur from a number of agents (as seen in Table 5.1), and we will discuss some of the more common complications occurring from high-dose chemotherapy followed by autologous stem cell transplantation.

Blood and Marrow Transplantation Long-Term Management: Prevention and Complications, First Edition. Edited by Bipin N Savani.

Table 5.1 Main potential long-term toxicities of agents used at high doses

Drug	Nonhematologic complication
Busulfan	Pulmonary fibrosis
Carboplatin	Peripheral neuropathy
	Renal toxicity
Carmustine (BCNU)	Pulmonary fibrosis
	CNS toxicity
Cyclophosphamide	Cardiac toxicity
Ifosfamide	CNS toxicity
	Renal toxicity
Melphalan	Possible cardiac toxicity
Thiotepa	Neurotoxicity
	Pulmonary toxicity
	Cardiac toxicity
Total body irradiation (TBI)	Pulmonary toxicity
	Cardiac toxicity
	Endocrine side effects
	Growth retardation
Paclitaxel	CNS toxicity
	Peripheral neuropathy

CNS: central nervous system.

Pulmonary complications

Long-term pulmonary complications after autoHCT may rarely be related to opportunistic bacterial, viral, or fungal infections, but more often late complications are caused by treatment-related toxicity due to chemotherapy or radiation. Delayed onset pulmonary complications involving both airway and lung parenchyma are seen after transplant. Toxic pulmonary reactions, including chronic interstitial fibrosis and decrease in lung diffusing capacity, have been recognized in 16–64% of patients exposed to carmustine (bis-chloroethylnitrosourea, BCNU) in combination with a variety of other agents [9–12].

Idiopathic pneumonia syndrome (IPS), defined as lung injury following allogeneic or autologous hematopoietic stem cell transplantation for which an infectious etiology is not evident [13], has been reported in 4–28% of patients after an autoHCT [14–17]. The incidence of IPS appears to be higher after total body irradiation (TBI)-containing regimens compared with chemotherapeutic agents only [15]. Bilgrami et al. [18] retrospectively reviewed 271 patients receiving busulfan-containing myeloablative chemotherapy prior to an autoHCT without radiation and found a trend towards increased incidence of IPS, although not statistically significant. Wong et al. [77] also retrospectively reviewed the incidence of IPS in patients receiving cyclophosphamide, carmustine, and thiotepa followed by autoHCT for high-risk breast cancer and reported a 12% incidence, with median onset at 3 months posttransplant. BCNU-related IPS appears to be dose dependent, with doses greater than 1500 mg/m^2 leading to a profound increase in incidence of interstitial pneumonitis and pulmonary fibrosis [13, 19]. This dose-dependent relationship is expanded upon by Jones et al. [20], who retrospectively studied 38 patients who received an autoHCT using a conditioning regimen consisting of cyclophosphamide, cisplatin, and BCNU. Their analysis revealed that 20 (53%) of the 38 patients developed pulmonary injury following treatment and 12 (60%) of the 20 had values for area under the curve of BCNU concentration that exceeded 600 μg/(mL min), whereas only 2 (11%) of 18 without pulmonary injury had values above this level ($P < 0.03$). Both cyclophosphamide and BCNU have been implicated in causing pulmonary toxicity, but in this cohort of patients, 12 (86%) of 14 with BCNU area under the curve greater than 600 μg/(mL min) developed lung injury, which suggests a dose-dependent effect for toxicity mediated by BCNU.

Afessa et al. [21] retrospectively reviewed over 1200 patients who received autoHCTs and found more than 25% developed some type of pulmonary complication, the most common being infection (13.9%). Some 10% of pulmonary complications were non-infectious, with the most frequent being acute pulmonary edema (5%). Diffuse alveolar hemorrhage and peri-engraftment respiratory distress syndrome were both in the region of 2%, while IPS was diagnosed in 1% of patients. Independent factors associated with pulmonary complications included abnormal diffusing capacity of lung for carbon monoxide and transplant for acute myeloid leukemia (AML). Factors associated with mortality included female sex, history of pulmonary disease, advanced disease status at time of transplant, decreased forced vital capacity, decreased Karnofsky score, and underlying diagnosis of AML. The development of pulmonary complications posttransplant increased risk of death and adversely affected pulmonary function long term. Of the patients with an infectious pulmonary complication, 30.1% died within 1 year of infection, while patients with a noninfectious complication had 36.8% mortality within 1 year after diagnosis. This study indicates that the majority of pulmonary complications occur early during the post-transplant period, but their effects may be long lasting and predict for decreased overall survival.

Late cardiac and cardiovascular complications

In the setting of autologous transplantation, the majority of cardiac complications are due to myocardial injury as a consequence of chemotherapy [22]. Causes of late cardiotoxicity in cancer survivors include cardiomyopathy, overt congestive heart failure (CHF), valvular dysfunction, or arrhythmia [23]. Mediastinal radiation can lead to fibrosis and restrictive cardiomyopathy, as well as conduction pathway defects and subsequent arrhythmias [24]. Compared with the general population, women have a fourfold higher risk of late death due to cardiac complications after an autoHCT [25], while all long-term survivors have a threefold higher risk of cardiovascular complications when compared with age-matched controls [26, 27]. Known mediators of cardiac toxicity, including anthracyclines and radiation, have been well described; however, cardiotoxic exposures during transplant are more likely to be due to high-dose chemotherapy (including cyclophosphamide) and TBI [28]. TBI can lead to hypertension and diabetes mellitus, which are known to increase risk of cardiovascular complications [23, 29].

One of the most potentially cardiotoxic drugs used in autoHCT is cyclophosphamide. Nieto et al. [30] retrospectively evaluated 443 breast cancer patients treated with high-dose cyclophosphamide, cisplatin, and BCNU followed by autoHCT and found an overall 5.1% incidence of cardiac complications, both clinical and subclinical, while 2.4% developed cardiomyopathy and 2.2% developed cardiac arrhythmias. The median prior cumulative dose of anthracyclines in patients with clinical cardiomyopathy was 360 mg/m^2. Risk factors for cardiac toxicity included older age (≥55 years), and stage IV disease with prior radiation to the left chest wall. However, neither prior cumulative anthracyclines dose nor previous cyclophosphamide exposure correlated with risk. Numerous other studies [31–33] have shown a correlation between higher doses of cyclophosphamide and CHF and cardiac toxicity.

Melphalan is a different phosphoramide mustard with an apparently less cardiotoxic profile than that of cyclophosphamide. Bleeker et al. [34] retrospectively evaluated the frequency of cardiac dysfunction resulting from decreased left ventricular ejection fraction (LVEF) following high-dose melphalan and autoHCT for patients with multiple myeloma and systemic amyloidosis. Surveying a 20-year period, 1476 patients were evaluated and 2.8% of patients were found to have a decreased LVEF at 4 months posttransplant, which tended to correlate with higher doses of melphalan.

Armenian et al. [35] recently published a retrospective cohort analysis of 1327 patients who underwent an autoHCT at the City of Hope and found a cumulative incidence of CHF of 4.8% at 5 years, which increased to 9.1% at 15 years posttransplant. The cumulative incidence for female lymphoma survivors was 14.5% at 15 years. In their cohort they found a 4.5-fold increased risk of CHF compared with the general population. The median time to presentation was 2.3 years and the median age was 52.4 years, whereas median follow-up for the entire cohort was 5.3 years. They went on to match patients who developed CHF (88 cases) to autoHCT recipients who did not develop CHF (218 controls). Pretransplant exposure to anthracyclines, diagnosis of hypertension prior to and after transplant, and diagnosis of diabetes posttransplant were all statistically significant factors predicting for CHF on multivariate analysis. The pretransplant LVEF was comparable in both cases and controls [35]. In this analysis, heart failure accounted for 18.3% of the deaths in the cohort diagnosed with CHF after transplant.

Endocrine effects

Posttransplant complications are commonly seen in the endocrine system [36]. A review of the literature reveals that the relative risk of developing endocrine disorders is related to the number of previous chemotherapeutic treatments, use and type of radiation therapy as well as younger age at time of exposure [37, 38]. The most frequently seen abnormalities are persistent gonadal insufficiency, decreased bone density, and hypothyroidism [39].

Gonadal damage

Germ cell injury and damage to Leydig cells in men and follicular pattern ovarian damage in women have been well documented to be associated with alkylating agents and irradiation [38]. Tauchmanovà et al. examined late endocrine effects in patients who had undergone an autoHCT and revealed that some degree of gonadal damage was present in virtually all patients (97%). That study monitored endocrine dysfunction at 3 and 12 months posttransplant in 95 patients (47 men and 48 women) between ages of 16 and 55 [36] and found both hormonal abnormalities and follicular degeneration in women and impaired spermatogenesis in men. Women conditioned with busulfan/cyclophosphamide had lower estradiol levels than those conditioned with other regimens, such as high-dose melphalan or BCNU/etoposide/cytarabine/melphalan (BEAM), and men who received prior radiotherapy had significantly higher follicle-stimulating hormone levels, suggesting greater testicular injury.

Schimmer et al. retrospectively reviewed women after autoHCT and found that all women became menopausal after transplant, but 29% ultimately recovered their ovarian function. The median time to recovery was 24 months, and in their analysis an age younger than 20 (versus over 30 years) at time of transplant ($p = 0.03$) as well as regimens not containing TBI were predictive of recovery [40]. The 4- year actuarial likelihood of ovarian recovery was 35% for all female patients, 44% for women not receiving TBI, and 20% for women who received TBI-containing regimens. In that study, the predicted rate of recovery for women younger than 25 years of age at autoHCT, without exposure to TBI, was 79% [40]. These authors also prospectively examined male sexual function after an autoHCT. Seventy-five percent of men reported normal interest in sexual activities, with 87.5% reporting normal erectile function. Six of 16 male patients had decreased testosterone levels (38%), and decreased testosterone levels also correlated with erectile dysfunction in 2 of 16 men. No report of successful pregnancy after transplant was made in this study population, where median age was 39 years and median follow up was 3 years [41].

The Center for International Blood and Marrow Transplant Research (CIBMTR) recently reported on a large series of patients from 2002 to 2007, retrospectively evaluating pregnancy after transplant. Of the 178 pregnancies reported to CIBMTR, 33 pregnancies were after an autoHCT (20 women and 13 men). In 92% of these pregnancies there had been no TBI exposure, and age at autoHCT ranged from 10 to 49 years. For men who fathered a child after an autoHCT the median age at pregnancy was 32 years, the median time from autoHCT to pregnancy was 7 years, and 92% of pregnancies resulted in a live birth. For women who reported pregnancy after autoHCT, the median age at pregnancy was 28, the median time posttransplant was 6 years, and 90% of pregnancies resulted in a live birth. This study confirmed previous findings that fertility is most frequently preserved in patients receiving a transplant at a younger age (<30) and those who receive non-TBI-containing regimens.

Bone density

An extensive amount of research has been done regarding bone mineral density (BMD) loss after allogeneic HCT but much less is known about bone loss after an autoHCT. Schimmer et al. retrospectively examined 68 patients and observed that 54% had osteopenia or osteoporosis at the femur and 28% at the spine, at a median of 4.2 years after autoHCT [42]. Other prospective studies have shown conflicting reports of significant change in BMD at 3 and 12 months [43, 44]. Recently, Yao et al. prospectively assessed a large cohort of patients following allogeneic and autologous transplantation to identify risk factors and degree of BMD loss. Of the 206 patients that were assessed, 102 received an autoHCT. Median age was 57 years and 63% were male. Change of BMD was measured by dual-energy X-ray absorptiometry scan at the lumbar spine and dual femurs between baseline and day 100 after transplant. Accelerated BMD loss occurred after both autologous and allogeneic HCT with similar frequency; however, risk factors for BMD loss were different between transplant types: lymphoma was associated with greater bone loss after autoHCT than myeloma, whereas higher steroid dose was the most significant risk factor after allogeneic HCT. BMD loss was significantly accelerated following an autoHCT with a rate that was 27- to 37-fold higher than the expected loss rates in the general population associated with normal aging. On multivariate analysis, spinal BMD loss was associated with the diagnosis of lymphoma ($p = 0.005$), and for the femur the loss was associated with younger age at time of HCT and diagnosis of lymphoma ($p = 0.006$) [45].

Thyroid dysfunction

Thyroid dysfunction is one of the most frequent complications following autoHCT [46, 47]. Khera et al. retrospectively reviewed 492 patients and found an incidence of thyroid dysfunction of 7.5% pretransplant that increased to 14.2% posttransplant, with a median time to diagnosis of around 1 year after autoHCTs [46]. Tauchmanovà et al. [36] prospectively assessed 110 patients after an autoHCT and detected transient subclinical hyperthyroidism in 16% of patients, and transient "low T3" syndrome (also known as sick euthyroid syndrome) in 31% of patients. Subclinical hypothyroidism was observed in 12% of the cohort with increased frequency in patients previously exposed to neck or thoracic radiation. In total, thyroid abnormalities were seen in 66% of patients in their cohort, which appears higher than in previous studies, such as a prospective analysis of 111 autoHCT patients by Carlson et al. (18% incidence) [47]. Sanchez-Ortega et al. [48] described a 43% incidence of thyroid dysfunction in their study of 115 patients at a median post-autoHCT follow-up of 69 months. With findings closer in line with their Italian colleagues, they reported the rate of subclinical hypothyroidism at 38%, primary hypothyroidism 3%, and subclinical hyperthyroidism of 2%. Based on variability of time to diagnosis, all patients are recommended to undergo lifelong yearly thyroid evaluation, especially if there is a history of antecedent neck or thoracic radiation [36–38].

Secondary malignancies

The second most common cause of premature death due to late effects after an autoHCT, following disease relapse, is secondary malignancy. Reports for treatment-related myelodysplastic syndrome (t-MDS) or treatment-related AML (t-AML) are as high as 8–14% of patients who received high-dose chemotherapy with an autoHCT [49]. The majority of patients with t-MDS/t-AML have complex karyotypes, and the observed cytogenetic changes are often characteristic of known chemotherapy-induced damage by alkylating agents and topoisomerase II inhibitors [5, 49, 50]. Abnormalities of chromosomes 5 and/or 7 are the hallmark of t-MDS/t-AML following alkylating agent therapy [51], typically occurring a median of 5 years after exposure with antecedent cytopenias and a poor prognosis [52]. In contrast, patients developing t-AML after therapy with topoisomerase II inhibitors rarely present with MDS, occur after a shorter latency period (2–3 years), and have a more favorable response to induction chemotherapy, but continue to have a poorer prognosis than *de novo* AML [53]. Balanced translocations involving *MLL* at 11q23, *RUNX1* at 21q22, *CBFB* at 16q22, or *PML* (15q22) and *RARA* (17q12) are commonly found in t-AML following treatment with drugs targeting topoisomerase II [52].

Other known risk factors predicting increased risk of t-MDS/t-AML are older age at transplant [6, 7] and exposure to radiation treatment prior to or during transplant [5, 54, 55]. Although most deaths from secondary malignancy are from a hematologic origin, there is also a significant risk for solid tumors, especially with extended follow-up [4]. Tarella et al. [55] reviewed 1347 lymphoma patients after autoHCT and reported a cumulative incidence of solid tumors of 2.5% at 5 years and 6.7% at 10 years. Patients had a median survival of 3.8 years following the diagnosis of a solid tumor, the most frequently occurring malignancies being lung, gastrointestinal tract, skin, breast, head and neck, and bladder cancers. Seshadri et al. analyzed 372 patients who received an autoHCT for lymphoma and related an increase in relative risk 2.3 higher than the general population [56]. In their analysis there was no association of either prior radiation treatment or TBI with diagnosis of a secondary malignancy.

Table 5.2 summarizes the most recent evidence regarding treatment related malignancy after autologous transplantation.

Psychologic distress and quality of life after transplant

The diagnosis of cancer is stressful, and an autoHCT is one of the most aggressive forms of therapy that patients undergo. Most studies indicate a return to normal stress levels for the majority of patients, but there are still a minority who experience clinical or subclinical psychological distress [61]. Mosher et al. reviewed quality of life (QOL) after transplantation in 1434 survivors of whom 60% of their population had received an autoHCT; 15% of the autoHCT population met the criteria for moderate to severe depressive symptoms, and the most common problems that patients endorsed were fatigue (56%),

Table 5.2 Summary of recent evidence regarding treatment-related malignancy after autologous transplantation

Author	N	Conditioning	Incidence/risk	Predictive factors (adverse unless otherwise noted)
Micallef et al. [57], 2000	*N* = 230 NHL 1/1985 to 11/1996	Cyclophosphamide 60 mg/kg + fractionated TBI 12 Gy	*Incidence* at 6 yrs = 12% *Risk* 5 yrs = 14.2% 10 yrs = 36.5%	Prior fludarabine therapy Older age *No new cases of t-MDS/t-AML after TBI discontinued from conditioning
Krishnan et al. [6], 2000	*N* = 612 HL = 218 NHL = 394 1986 to 1998	TBI/VP-16/ cyclophosphamide Cyclophosphamide/BCNU/ vincristine	*Risk* 6 yrs = 8.6 ± 2.1% HL = 8.1% NHL = 9.1%	Priming with VP-16 for stem cell collection
Del Canizo et al. [58], 2000	*N* = 1411 AML = 557 NHL = 308 HL = 225 MM = 189 CML = 37 Solid tumors = 95	Variable including: TBI + cyclophosphamide BCNU, VP-16, ARA-C, melphalan Cyclophosphamide/BCNU/ vincristine	*Incidence* HL = 2.7% NHL = 1.6% MM = 0.5% AML = 0.2% Cumulative incidence at 5 yrs = 3.1%	
Hosing et al. [59], 2002	*N* = 493 NHL January 1990 to August 1999	TBI ± cyclophosphamide + VP-16 (TBI either 10.2 or 12 Gy)	*Risk* 5 yrs = 14.2%	TBI
Darrington et al. [54], 2003	*N* = 511 patients HL = 249 NHL = 262 4/1983 to 12/1991	HL: cyclophosphamide, etoposide, and carmustine NHL: TBI + alkylating agents (melphalan or cyclophosphamide)	*Incidence* HL, 5 yrs = 4%; 7 yrs = 10% NHL, 5 yrs = 4%; 7 yrs = 8% *Risk* at 5 yrs HL = 11% NHL = 12%	Age ≥40 yrs at transplant TBI-containing regimen
Metayer et al., 2003 [5]	*N* = 2739 NHL = 1784 HL = 955 1989–1995	Variable TBI + cyclophosphamide TBI + VP-16 ± cyclophosphamide VP-16 ± cyclophosphamide ± other drugs	*Incidence* 7 yrs = 3.7% NHL = 3.9% HL = 3.3% *Risk* at 7 yrs NHL = 8.9% HL = 7.1%	Intensity of pretransplant therapy TBI doses 13.2 Gy
Bhatia et al. [4], 2005 *data collected for pts surviving 2 yrs posttransplant	*N* = 854 AML = 158 ALL = 59 NHL = 392 HL = 245 1981 to 1998	TBI = 575 Cyclophosphamide = 828 Busulfan = 33 VP-16 = 635 BCNU = 234	*Incidence* 4.6% hematologic *Risk for second tumor* 12-fold higher than general population	

Table 5.2 (*Continued*)

Author	*N*	Conditioning	Incidence/risk	Predictive factors (adverse unless otherwise noted)
Kalaycio et al. [60], 2006	*N* = 526 NHL = 405 HL = 121 1/1993 to 12/2001	Oral busulfan 1 mg/kg × 14 doses Etoposide 50–60 mg/kg cyclophosphamide 60 mg/kg	*Incidence* 10 yrs = 6.8%	≥5 days apharesis Prior radiation ≥4 prior chemotherapy regimens
Seshadri et al. [56], 2009	*N* = 372 NHL 1/1987 to 12/2006	Etoposide + melphalan in 95% BEAM (BCNU, etoposide, cytarabine, melphalan) in 3% Other regimens in 2% Selected patients, TBI 12 Gy	*Incidence* 9% for second cancer (19 hematologic, 13 solid tumors) *Risk of 2nd cancer* at 3 yrs = 4.4% at 10 yrs = 12.9%	Salvage therapy using mini-BEAM
Tarella et al. [55], 2010	*N* = 1347 NHL = 1113 HL = 234 1985 to 2005	High-dose mitoxantrone/melphalan BEAM (BCNU, etoposide, cytarabine, melphalan) TBI = 79 patients Rituximab = 523	*Incidence for hematologic* 5 yrs = 3.09% 10 yrs = 4.52% 15 yrs = 6.80% *Incidence for solid tumors* 5 yrs = 2.54% 10 yrs = 6.79% 15 yrs = 9.14%	*Hematologic* Male sex Second harvest peripheral blood progenitor cells *Solid tumor* Advanced age Consolidation radiotherapy after transplant *Rituximab addition *protective**

ALL: acute lymphocytic leukemia; AML: acute myeloid leukemia; CML: chronic myelogenous leukemia; HL: Hodgkin's lymphoma; MM: multiple myeloma; NHL: non-Hodgkin's lymphoma.

worry that condition would worsen (36%), lack of sexual interest (31%), lack of sexual satisfaction (28%), and changes in appearance (30%) [61]. A higher level of education and autoHCT versus allogeneic HCT were correlated with fewer depressive symptoms. Wettergren et al. [62] prospectively evaluated 20 patients prior to and up to 12 months after an autoHCT and observed that the most frequent complaints were impaired function, fatigue, dyspnea, financial problems, and emotional distress. These issues had largely resolved at the 1 year mark. Frodin et al. [63] prospectively evaluated 111 patients for 3 years after an autoHCT for health-related QOL. They discovered patients recovered quickly and just 2 months after transplantation the baseline values for function, symptoms, and overall QOL were restored. At the 3-year follow-up, lymphoma patients indicated a better health-related QOL than MM patients. Recently, Braamse et al. [64] reviewed the literature for predictors of QOL in patients receiving allogeneic HCT or autoHCT. They reviewed 27 high-quality studies and 8 low-quality studies from 2002 to 2010. For patients undergoing autoHCT they identified the following predictors:

- *Predictors of global QOL.* Treatment with thalidomide in MM patients predicted worse functional well-being (weak evidence) [65].
- *Predictors of physical functioning.* Advanced disease risk status [66], pretransplant energy level, depression [67], previous delirium episode, and delirium severity [68] were studied as possible predictors for energy level, fatigue, and sleep quality (weak evidence).

• *Predictors of psychological functioning.* Evidence was inconsistent. Women were more likely to suffer from depression posttransplant in both allogeneic HCT and autoHCT [66] (strong evidence).
• *Predictors of social functioning.* Older age (≥65 years) predicted better social functioning posttransplant (strong evidence) [65].

The Bone Marrow Transplant Survivor Study [4] also reported on QOL for patients who survived 2 years or more after undergoing an autoHCT and found that survivors were more likely to report a health problem preventing them from holding a job or going to school when compared with siblings (15% versus 2%; $p < 0.001$). Older survivors (≥45 years) were 2.6-fold more likely to report difficulty in holding a job. Autologous stem cell transplant survivors were also more likely to report difficulty in obtaining or retaining health insurance (27% versus 5%; $p < 0.001$) or life insurance (33% versus 5%; $p < .001$).

Cognitive dysfunction

Cognitive difficulties have been reported by survivors of stem cell transplant in general and are associated with poorer physical and mental well-being [69]. The data about cognitive dysfunction reported on patients receiving autoHCTs is somewhat limited. There are two ways in which such impairments have been measured: objective neuropsychological assessment and self-reported measures of cognitive functioning. Ahles et al. [70] prospectively assessed 54 patients for neuropsychologic impact before and after autoHCT and found that cognitive functioning decreased posttransplant. They did not see an effect of prior history of intrathecal chemotherapy or cranial radiation. This study was limited by its short follow-up. Friedman et al. [71] conducted a longitudinal study in 117 transplant patients of which 59 were autoHCT recipients. Of the whole group, 39% were classified as impaired prior to transplant, and 47% of 33 with serial evaluations showed cognitive decline at 6 weeks, which improved to 33% at 28 weeks. On multivariate analysis they did not see an independent effect of the type of transplant (autoHCT versus allogeneic HCT). Jacobs et al. [72] used a sequential longitudinal design to assess 476 patients after transplant, with 79% of their cohort having received an autoHCT. Despite the fact that patients experienced cognitive deficits, including decreased motor speed, decreased attention, decreased executive functioning, and difficulty with memory prior to transplant and shortly after, they normalized their cognitive scoring within a year after transplant. The number of patients receiving allogeneic HCT performed worse and demonstrated less improvement over time of cognitive function compared with autoHCT patients. Van Dam et al. [73] prospectively studied 83 breast cancer patients who received either high-dose chemotherapy followed by autoHCT or standard-dose chemotherapy, and those patients were also measured against 50 early-stage patients treated definitively with surgery and radiation but without exposure to systemic chemotherapy. Their study revealed cognitive impairment in 32% of patients receiving an auto-HCT, 17% in patients treated at standard doses, and only 9% in control patients, with an 8.2-times higher risk of cognitive impairment in the first group and of 3.5 times in the second group, as compared with the control group [73]. In a follow-up evaluation [74], the authors found that at 4 years post therapy there was an improvement in cognitive function in all the chemotherapy groups, which may suggest that cognitive dysfunction may be transient in some patients.

Conclusions

The use of autoHCT has steadily increased since the mid 1980s, and with improvement in supportive care and transplant regimens there are a growing number of long-term survivors. As this population grows, they are also at a higher risk for long-term treatment-related complications that will affect not only their health but their overall sense of well-being. It is important not only to monitor patients posttransplant, but also to advise them of these potential long-term effects. Ultimately, the benefit from autologous transplant has to be weighed against the risk of disease as well as toxicity associated with treatment. There is evidence that patients are willing to risk substantial toxicity and increased risk of mortality for the chance of increased survival even with uncertain outcomes of treatment [75, 76]. With increasing knowledge about delayed effects of treatment, enhanced surveillance may improve outcomes of these late complications.

References

1. Kurnick NB, Montano A, Gerdes JC, Feder BH. Preliminary observations on the treatment of postirradiation hematopoietic depression in man by the infusion of stored autogenous bone marrow. Ann Intern Med. 1958;49(5):973–986. Epub 1958/11/01.
2. Blume KG, Forman SJ, Appelbaum FR (eds). Thomas' Hematopoietic Cell Transplantation, 3rd edition. Malden, MA: Blackwell, 2004.
3. Pasquini MC, Wang Z. Current use and outcome of hematopoietic stem cell transplantation: Part I CIBMTR summary slides, 2009. CIBMTR Newslett [serial online]. 2009;15(1): 7–11. Available from: http://www.cibmtr.org/Reference Center/Newsletters/Documents/Newsletter_Aug2009.pdf (accessed 12 May 2013).
4. Bhatia S, Robison LL, Francisco L, et al. Late mortality in survivors of autologous hematopoietic-cell transplantation: report from the Bone Marrow Transplant Survivor Study. Blood. 2005;105(11):4215–4222. Epub 2005/02/11.
5. Metayer C, Curtis RE, Vose J, et al. Myelodysplastic syndrome and acute myeloid leukemia after autotransplantation for lymphoma: a multicenter case-control study. Blood. 2003;101(5):2015–2023. Epub 2002/10/24.
6. Krishnan A, Bhatia S, Slovak ML, et al. Predictors of therapy-related leukemia and myelodysplasia following autologous transplantation for lymphoma: an assessment of risk factors. Blood. 2000;95(5):1588–1593. Epub 2000/02/26.
7. Bhatia S, Ramsay NK, Steinbuch M, et al. Malignant neoplasms following bone marrow transplantation. Blood. 1996;87(9):3633–3639. Epub 1996/05/01.
8. Bhatia S, Louie AD, Bhatia R, et al. Solid cancers after bone marrow transplantation. J Clin Oncol. 2001;19(2):464–471. Epub 2001/02/24.
9. Cagnoni PJ, Nieto Y, Shpall EJ, et al. High-dose chemotherapy with autologous hematopoietic progenitor-cell support as part of combined modality therapy in patients with inflammatory breast cancer. J Clin Oncol. 1998; 16(5):1661–1668. Epub 1998/05/20.
10. Kreisman H, Wolkove N. Pulmonary toxicity of antineoplastic therapy. Semin Oncol. 1992 19(5):508–520. Epub 1992/10/01.
11. Rubio C, Hill ME, Milan S, et al. Idiopathic pneumonia syndrome after high-dose chemotherapy for relapsed Hodgkin's disease. Br J Cancer. 1997;75(7):1044–1048. Epub 1997/01/01.
12. Ager S, Mahendra P, Richards EM, et al. High-dose carmustine, etoposide and melphalan ("BEM") with autologous stem cell transplantation: a dose–toxicity study. Bone Marrow Transplant. 1996;17(3):335–340. Epub 1996/03/01.
13. Clark JG, Hansen JA, Hertz MI, et al. NHLBI workshop summary. Idiopathic pneumonia syndrome after bone marrow transplantation. Am Rev Respir Dis. 1993;147(6 Pt 1):1601–1606. Epub 1993/06/01.
14. Ballester OF, Agaliotis DP, Hiemenz JW, et al. Phase I–II study of high-dose busulfan and cyclophosphamide followed by autologous peripheral blood stem cell transplantation for hematological malignancies: toxicities and hematopoietic recovery. Bone Marrow Transplant. 1996; 18(1):9–14. Epub 1996/07/01.
15. Carlson K, Backlund L, Smedmyr B, et al. Pulmonary function and complications subsequent to autologous bone marrow transplantation. Bone Marrow Transplant. 1994; 14(5):805–811. Epub 1994/11/01.
16. Wingard JR, Sostrin MB, Vriesendorp HM, et al. Interstitial pneumonitis following autologous bone marrow transplantation. Transplantation. 1988;46(1):61–65. Epub 1988/07/01.
17. Pecego R, Hill R, Appelbaum FR, et al. Interstitial pneumonitis following autologous bone marrow transplantation. Transplantation. 1986;42(5):515–517. Epub 1986/11/01.
18. Bilgrami SF, Metersky ML, McNally D, et al. Idiopathic pneumonia syndrome following myeloablative chemotherapy and autologous transplantation. Ann Pharmacother. 2001;35(2):196–201. Epub 2001/02/24.
19. Aronin PA, Mahaley MS Jr, Rudnick SA, et al. Prediction of BCNU pulmonary toxicity in patients with malignant gliomas: an assessment of risk factors. N Engl J Med. 1980;303(4):183–188. Epub 1980/07/24.
20. Jones RB, Matthes S, Shpall EJ, et al. Acute lung injury following treatment with high-dose cyclophosphamide, cisplatin, and carmustine: pharmacodynamic evaluation of carmustine. J Natl Cancer Inst. 1993;85(8):640–647. Epub 1993/04/21.
21. Afessa B, Tefferi A, Litzow MR, Peters SG. Outcome of diffuse alveolar hemorrhage in hematopoietic stem cell transplant recipients. Am J Respir Crit Care Med. 2002; 166(10):1364–1368. Epub 2002/10/31.
22. Majhail NS, Bajorunaite R, Lazarus HM, et al. Long-term survival and late relapse in 2-year survivors of autologous haematopoietic cell transplantation for Hodgkin and non-Hodgkin lymphoma. Br J Haematol. 2009;147(1):129–139. Epub 2009/07/04.
23. Armenian SH, Bhatia S. Cardiovascular disease after hematopoietic cell transplantation – lessons learned. Haematologica. 2008;93(8):1132–1136. Epub 2008/08/02.
24. Yahalom J, Portlock CS. Long-term cardiac and pulmonary complications of cancer therapy. Hematol Oncol Clin North Am. 2008;22(2):305–318, vii. Epub 2008/04/09.
25. Ruiz-Soto R, Sergent G, Gisselbrecht C, et al. Estimating late adverse events using competing risks after autologous stem-cell transplantation in aggressive non-Hodgkin

lymphoma patients. Cancer. 2005;104(12):2735–2742. Epub 2005/11/15.

26. Sun CL, Francisco L, Kawashima T, et al. Prevalence and predictors of chronic health conditions after hematopoietic cell transplantation: a report from the Bone Marrow Transplant Survivor Study. Blood. 2010;116(17):3129–3139; quiz 377. Epub 2010/07/27.
27. Syrjala KL, Langer SL, Abrams JR, et al. Late effects of hematopoietic cell transplantation among 10-year adult survivors compared with case-matched controls. J Clin Oncol. 2005;23(27):6596–6606. Epub 2005/09/20.
28. Tichelli A, Rovo A, Gratwohl A. Late pulmonary, cardiovascular, and renal complications after hematopoietic stem cell transplantation and recommended screening practices. Hematology Am Soc Hematol Educ Program. 2008;125-33:Epub 2008/12/17.
29. Baker KS, Ness KK, Steinberger J, et al. Diabetes, hypertension, and cardiovascular events in survivors of hematopoietic cell transplantation: a report from the bone marrow transplantation survivor study. Blood. 2007;109(4):1765–1772. Epub 2006/10/19.
30. Nieto Y, Cagnoni PJ, Bearman SI, et al. Cardiac toxicity following high-dose cyclophosphamide, cisplatin, and BCNU (STAMP-I) for breast cancer. Biol Blood Marrow Transplant. 2000;6(2A):198–203. Epub 2000/05/18.
31. Ayash LJ, Wright JE, Tretyakov O, et al. Cyclophosphamide pharmacokinetics: correlation with cardiac toxicity and tumor response. J Clin Oncol. 1992;10(6):995–1000. Epub 1992/06/01.
32. Goldberg MA, Antin JH, Guinan EC, Rappeport JM. Cyclophosphamide cardiotoxicity: an analysis of dosing as a risk factor. Blood. 1986;68(5):1114–1118. Epub 1986/11/01.
33. Braverman AC, Antin JH, Plappert MT, et al. Cyclophosphamide cardiotoxicity in bone marrow transplantation: a prospective evaluation of new dosing regimens. J Clin Oncol. 1991;9(7):1215–1223. Epub 1991/07/01.
34. Bleeker JS, Gertz MA, Pellikka PA, et al. Evaluation of pretransplant factors predicting cardiac dysfunction following high-dose melphalan conditioning and autologous peripheral blood stem cell transplantation. Eur J Haematol. 2012;89(3):228–235. Epub 2012/06/08.
35. Armenian SH, Sun CL, Shannon T, et al. Incidence and predictors of congestive heart failure after autologous hematopoietic cell transplantation. Blood. 2011;118(23):6023–6029. Epub 2011/10/07.
36. Tauchmanovà L, Selleri C, De Rosa G, et al. Endocrine disorders during the first year after autologous stem-cell transplant. Am J Med. 2005;118(6):664–670. Epub 2005/06/01.
37. Brennan BM, Shalet SM. Endocrine late effects after bone marrow transplant. Br J Haematol. 2002;118(1):58–66. Epub 2002/07/09.
38. Shalet SM, Didi M, Ogilvy-Stuart AL, et al. Growth and endocrine function after bone marrow transplantation. Clin Endocrinol (Oxf). 1995;42(4):333–339. Epub 1995/04/01.
39. Schimmer AD, Dranitsaris G, Ali V, et al. The autologous blood and marrow transplant long-term follow-up clinic: a model of care for following and treating survivors of autotransplant. Support Care Cancer. 2002;10(3):247–252. Epub 2002/03/21.
40. Schimmer AD, Quatermain M, Imrie K, et al. Ovarian function after autologous bone marrow transplantation. J Clin Oncol. 1998;16(7):2359–2363. Epub 1998/07/17.
41. Schimmer AD, Ali V, Stewart AK, et al. Male sexual function after autologous blood or marrow transplantation. Biol Blood Marrow Transplant. 2001;7(5):279–283. Epub 2001/06/13.
42. Schimmer AD, Mah K, Bordeleau L, et al. Decreased bone mineral density is common after autologous blood or marrow transplantation. Bone Marrow Transplant. 2001; 28(4):387–391. Epub 2001/09/26.
43. Ebeling PR, Thomas DM, Erbas B, et al. Mechanisms of bone loss following allogeneic and autologous hemopoietic stem cell transplantation. J Bone Miner Res. 1999;14(3):342–350. Epub 1999/02/23.
44. Gandhi MK, Lekamwasam S, Inman I, et al. Significant and persistent loss of bone mineral density in the femoral neck after haematopoietic stem cell transplantation: long-term follow-up of a prospective study. Br J Haematol. 2003; 121(3):462–468. Epub 2003/04/29.
45. Yao S, Smiley SL, West K, et al. Accelerated bone mineral density loss occurs with similar incidence and severity, but with different risk factors, after autologous versus allogeneic hematopoietic cell transplantation. Biol Blood Marrow Transplant. 2010;16(8):1130–1137. Epub 2010/03/02.
46. Khera N, Storer B, Flowers ME, et al. Nonmalignant late effects and compromised functional status in survivors of hematopoietic cell transplantation. J Clin Oncol. 2012; 30(1):71–77. Epub 2011/12/08.
47. Carlson K, Lonnerholm G, Smedmyr B, et al. Thyroid function after autologous bone marrow transplantation. Bone Marrow Transplant. 1992;10(2):123–127. Epub 1992/08/01.
48. Sanchez-Ortega I, Canals C, Peralta T, et al. Thyroid dysfunction in adult patients late after autologous and allogeneic blood and marrow transplantation. Bone Marrow Transplant. 2012;47(2):296–298. Epub 2011/03/23.
49. Armitage JO, Carbone PP, Connors JM, et al. Treatment-related myelodysplasia and acute leukemia in non-Hodgkin's lymphoma patients. J Clin Oncol. 2003;21(5):897–906. Epub 2003/03/01.
50. Borthakur G, Estey AE. Therapy-related acute myelogenous leukemia and myelodysplastic syndrome. Curr Oncol Rep. 2007;9(5):373–377. Epub 2007/08/21.

51. Smith SM, Le Beau MM, Huo D, et al. Clinical-cytogenetic associations in 306 patients with therapy-related myelodysplasia and myeloid leukemia: the University of Chicago series. Blood. 2003;102(1):43–52. Epub 2003/03/08.
52. Qian Z, Joslin JM, Tennant TR, et al. Cytogenetic and genetic pathways in therapy-related acute myeloid leukemia. Chem Biol Interact. 2010;184(1–2):50–57. Epub 2009/12/05.
53. Pedersen-Bjergaard J, Philip P. Balanced translocations involving chromosome bands 11q23 and 21q22 are highly characteristic of myelodysplasia and leukemia following therapy with cytostatic agents targeting at DNA-topoisomerase II. Blood. 1991;78(4):1147–1148. Epub 1991/08/15.
54. Darrington DL, Vose JM, Anderson JR, et al. Incidence and characterization of secondary myelodysplastic syndrome and acute myelogenous leukemia following high-dose chemoradiotherapy and autologous stem-cell transplantation for lymphoid malignancies. J Clin Oncol. 1994;12(12):2527–2534. Epub 1994/12/01.
55. Tarella C, Passera R, Magni M, et al. Risk factors for the development of secondary malignancy after high-dose chemotherapy and autograft, with or without rituximab: a 20-year retrospective follow-up study in patients with lymphoma. J Clin Oncol. 2011;29(7):814–824. Epub 2010/12/30.
56. Seshadri T, Pintilie M, Kuruvilla J, et al. Incidence and risk factors for second cancers after autologous hematopoietic cell transplantation for aggressive non-Hodgkin lymphoma. Leuk Lymphoma. 2009;50(3):380–386. Epub 2009/04/07.
57. Micallef IN, Lillington DM, Apostolidis J, et al. Therapy-related myelodysplasia and secondary acute myelogenous leukemia after high-dose therapy with autologous hematopoietic progenitor-cell support for lymphoid malignancies. J Clin Oncol. 2000;18(5):947–955. Epub 2000/03/01.
58. Del Canizo M, Amigo M, Hernandez JM, et al. Incidence and characterization of secondary myelodysplastic syndromes following autologous transplantation Haematologica. 2000;85(4):403–409. Epub 2000/04/11.
59. Hosing C, Munsell M, Yazji S, et al. Risk of therapy-related myelodysplastic syndrome/acute leukemia following high-dose therapy and autologous bone marrow transplantation for non-Hodgkin's lymphoma. Ann Oncol. 2002;13(3):450–459. Epub 2002/05/09.
60. Kalaycio M, Rybicki L, Pohlman B, et al. Risk factors before autologous stem-cell transplantation for lymphoma predict for secondary myelodysplasia and acute myelogenous leukemia. J Clin Oncol. 2006;24(22):3604–3610. Epub 2006/08/01.
61. Mosher CE, DuHamel KN, Rini C, et al. Quality of life concerns and depression among hematopoietic stem cell transplant survivors. Support Care Cancer. 2011;19(9):1357–1365. Epub 2010/07/28.
62. Wettergren L, Langius A, Bjorkholm M, Bjorvell H. Physical and psychosocial functioning in patients undergoing autologous bone marrow transplantation – a prospective study. Bone Marrow Transplant. 1997;20(6):497–502. Epub 1997/10/06.
63. Frodin U, Borjeson S, Lyth J, Lotfi K. A prospective evaluation of patients' health-related quality of life during auto-SCT: a 3-year follow-up. Bone Marrow Transplant. 2011; 46(10):1345–1352. Epub 2010/11/30.
64. Braamse AM, Gerrits MM, van Meijel B et al. Predictors of health-related quality of life in patients treated with auto- and allo-SCT for hematological malignancies. Bone Marrow Transplant. 2012;47(6):757–769. Epub 2011/07/05.
65. Sherman AC, Simonton S, Latif U, et al. Changes in quality-of-life and psychosocial adjustment among multiple myeloma patients treated with high-dose melphalan and autologous stem cell transplantation. Biol Blood Marrow Transplant. 2009;15(1):12–20. Epub 2009/01/13.
66. Prieto JM, Atala J, Blanch J, et al. Patient-rated emotional and physical functioning among hematologic cancer patients during hospitalization for stem-cell transplantation. Bone Marrow Transplant. 2005;35(3):307–314. Epub 2004/12/08.
67. Prieto JM, Blanch J, Atala J, et al. Clinical factors associated with fatigue in haematologic cancer patients receiving stem-cell transplantation. Eur J Cancer. 2006;42(12) 1749–1755. Epub 2005/11/30.
68. Fann JR, Roth-Roemer S, Burington BE, et al. Delirium in patients undergoing hematopoietic stem cell transplantation. Cancer. 2002;95(9):1971–1981. Epub 2002/10/31.
69. Andrykowski MA, Bishop MM, Hahn EA, et al. Long-term health-related quality of life, growth, and spiritual well-being after hematopoietic stem-cell transplantation. J Clin Oncol. 2005;23(3):599–608. Epub 2005/01/22.
70. Ahles TA, Tope DM, Furstenberg C, et al. Psychologic and neuropsychologic impact of autologous bone marrow transplantation. J Clin Oncol. 1996;14(5):1457–1462. Epub 1996/05/01.
71. Friedman MA, Fernandez M, Wefel JS, et al. Course of cognitive decline in hematopoietic stem cell transplantation: a within-subjects design. Arch Clin Neuropsychol. 2009;24(7): 689–698. Epub 2009/09/22.
72. Jacobs SR, Small BJ, Booth-Jones M, et al. Changes in cognitive functioning in the year after hematopoietic stem cell transplantation. Cancer. 2007;110(7):1560–1567. Epub 2007/08/10.
73. van Dam FS, Schagen SB, Muller MJ, et al. Impairment of cognitive function in women receiving adjuvant treatment for high-risk breast cancer: high-dose versus standard-dose chemotherapy. J Natl Cancer Inst. 1998;90(3):210–218. Epub 1998/02/14.

74. Schagen SB, Muller MJ, Boogerd W, et al. Late effects of adjuvant chemotherapy on cognitive function: a follow-up study in breast cancer patients. Ann Oncol. 2002;13(9):1387–1397. Epub 2002/08/28.
75. McQuellon RP, Muss HB, Hoffman SL, et al. Patient preferences for treatment of metastatic breast cancer: a study of women with early-stage breast cancer. J Clin Oncol. 1995;13(4):858–868. Epub 1995/04/01.
76. Mehta P, Rodrigue J, Nejame C, et al. Acquiescence to adjunctive experimental therapies may relate to psychological distress: pilot data from a bone marrow transplant center. Bone Marrow Transplant. 2000;25(6):673–676. Epub 2000/03/29.
77. Wong R, Rondon G, Saliba RM, et al. Idiopathic pneumonia syndrome after high-dose chemotherapy and autologous hematopoietic stem cell transplantation for high-risk breast cancer. Bone Marrow Transplant. 2003;31(12):1157–1163. Epub 2003/06/11.

CHAPTER 6

Graft-versus-host disease and late effects after hematopoetic stem cell transplantation

Gérard Socié
University Paris VII, Haematology/Transplantation, Hôpital Saint Louis, Paris, France

Introduction

Large numbers of patients now survive long term following hematopoietic stem cell transplantation (HSCT), and late clinical effects of stem cell transplantation (SCT) are, thus, of major concern. Chronic graft-versus-host disease (cGvHD) and the associated immunodeficiency are the primary causes of transplant-related mortality late after allogeneic SCT and contribute directly or indirectly to most late complications. Despite the advent of new treatment modalities, the incidence of cGvHD has remained high, related to several changes in clinical SCT practice: (i) the expanded use of human leukocyte antigen (HLA) matched unrelated and HLA nonidentical related donors; (ii) the increasing use of SCT in older patients; (iii) the increasing use of viable donor lymphocyte infusions after SCT to treat relapsed disease or to achieve full donor chimerism after nonmyeloablative transplantation; (iv) the increasing use of peripheral blood stem cells instead of bone marrow as a source of stem cells. In addition to cGvHD and its therapy, the major risk factor for late complications after SCT is the use of irradiation in the pretransplant conditioning regimen.

cGvHD – which was originally defined as occurring after the first 100 days post-HSCT – is now known to have a characteristic clinical presentation, which resembles autoimmune vascular diseases and is distinct from that of acute GvHD [1–3]. cGvHD occurs in 30–65% of allogeneic HSCT recipients, can be highly debilitating in its extensive form, and has a 5-year mortality rate of 30–50% that is mainly due to immune dysregulation and opportunistic infections. The pathophysiology of cGvHD mainly depends on the polarization of $CD4^+$ T cells into T helper 2 (TH2) cells, but there are six hallmarks that are unique to this syndrome (reviewed by Blazar et al. [4]). The first feature is damage to the thymus (a), which can be caused by the conditioning regimen or, more importantly, by prior occurrence of acute GvHD. This damage results in decreased negative selection of alloreactive $CD4^+$ T cells (b). There is immune deviation to a TH2-type cytokine response (c), which includes the production of interleukin (IL)-4, -5, and -11. This response leads to the release of fibrogenic cytokines – such as IL-2, IL-10, and transforming growth factor-β1 (TGFβ1) – and the activation of macrophages that produce platelet-derived growth factor and TGFβ1 (d). These molecules induce the proliferation and activation of tissue fibroblasts. Low numbers of regulatory T (TReg) cells are the fifth hallmark (e); and finally there is B cell dysregulation (f), which leads to the emergence of autoreactive B cells and the production of autoreactive antibodies. It has been suggested that autoreactive B cell activation may be

Blood and Marrow Transplantation Long-Term Management: Prevention and Complications, First Edition. Edited by Bipin N Savani.

due to the presence of high levels of B cell-activating factor (BAFF) in the lymphoid microenvironment. All these events contribute to an autoimmune-like systemic syndrome that is associated with fibroproliferative changes. These changes can occur in almost any organ of the body but mainly affect oral and ocular mucosal surfaces and the skin, lungs, kidneys, liver, and gut.

Immune reconstitution occurs gradually over time (generally 12–18 months) and is slower for allogeneic recipients, particularly those receiving umbilical cord blood, HLA-mismatched or T-cell-depleted grafts, and in survivors with graft-versus-host disease (GvHD) or those who have received prolonged immunosuppression [5]. T-helper lymphocyte (CD4) counts and CD4/CD8 ratios are good markers of immune reconstitution and some experts use these assessments as surrogate markers of the completeness of immune reconstitution to guide duration of viral or other infection prophylaxis after HSCT. Immune reconstitution has a pivotal role in the long-term issue of allogeneic SCT. cGvHD is the major factor affecting immune reconstitution of B cells and CD4- and CD8-T cells [6, 7]. Donor source (marrow versus peripheral blood), unrelated versus sibling transplant, and the degree of HLA compatibility between donor and recipient also affect the pace of immune reconstitution. Low B-cell count, inverted CD4/CD8 ratio, and a decreased immunoglobulin A level are all risk factors associated with late infections (reviewed by Fuji et al. [8]). Susceptibility to encapsulated bacteria (*Streptococcus pneumoniae*, *Haemophilus influenzae*, and *Neisseria meningitis*) has been well documented, especially in patients with current or previous cGvHD. Late (>2 years) fungal or cytomegalovirus infections are rare, and almost invariably occur in patients with ongoing immune suppression for GvHD. Varicella zoster, in contrast, is extremely frequent even in patients without GvHD, but usually occurs within several months of SCT after acyclovir prophylaxis has been discontinued. Finally, late *Pneumocystis carinii* (PCP) infections are more common in patients receiving active treatment for cGvHD. Since PCP prophylaxis with trimethoprim–sulfamethoxazole is highly active this regimen should be given to all patients receiving treatment for cGvHD and/or those with CD4-positive cells $<0.2 \times 10^9$/L. Probably, PCP prophylaxis should be continued for several weeks after the cessation of immunosuppressive therapy given the long-lasting T-cell defects characteristic of patients who have developed cGvHD. Finally, as described later, cGvHD is the main risk factor of squamous cell cancer occurring after SCT.

Extensive reviews with references have been published [9, 10]; thus, only selected references are included in this chapter. Since most chapters in this book also refer to the relationship between cGvHD and late effect, only the main concepts will be reviewed in two different sections:

- *nonmalignant late effects*, which are heterogeneous and, although often not life threatening, significantly impair the quality of life of long-term survivors [11];
- *secondary malignant diseases*, which are of particular clinical concern as more patients survive the early phase after SCT and remain free of their original disease [9, 10].

cGvHD and nonmalignant late effects

Ocular effects

Kerato-conjunctivitis sicca and cataracts are the two most common late complications affecting the anterior segment of the eye.

Cataract formation, particularly posterior subcapsular cataracts, has long been recognized in recipients of HSCT [12, 13]. The two main risk factors for cataract development are exposure to total body irradiation (TBI) and steroids therapy for cGvHD [12–14]. After single-dose TBI almost all patients developed cataracts within 3–4 years, and most if not all need surgical repair. The probability of developing cataracts after fractionated TBI is in the range of 30% at 3 years, but may be as high as 80% at 6–10 years after SCT. In a multivariate analysis, the use of TBI, single as compared with fractionated dose TBI, and the use of steroid treatment for longer than 3 months were associated with a significantly increased risk of cataract development [14]. The radiation effect was dose rate dependent [15, 16]. The largest series to date included a cohort of 1064 patients and identified factors independently associated with an increased risk of cataracts as older age (>23 years), higher radiation exposure rate (>4 cGy/min), allogeneic rather than autologous SCT, and steroid administration [15, 16]. Finally, in prospective studies comparing the incidence of cataracts and predisposing risk factors, patients who received cyclophosphamide and TBI had a higher incidence of cataracts than patients treated with busulfan and cyclophosphamide [17].

Kerato-conjunctivitis sicca of the eyes is usually part of a more general syndrome that also includes xerostomia, dryness of the skin, and, in women, vaginitis. All these manifestations are closely related to cGvHD [18–21]. In its most extensive form the clinical picture may be that of a Sjögren-like syndrome, as described in detail in other chapters of this book.

Pulmonary effects

Pulmonary effects were recently reviewed by Bacigalupo et al. [22].

Significant late toxicity involving both the airways and the lung parenchyma is observed in at least 15–40% of patients after SCT [11, 23–26]. Most studies have been performed in adult patients and results are still conflicting, owing to differences in patient selection and evaluation criteria, limited sample size, and short follow-up. Moreover, the various pulmonary syndromes are not well defined or definable because of overlapping mechanisms and because they represent a continuous spectrum rather than distinct disorders. Sensitivity to cytotoxic agents and irradiation, infections, and immune-mediated lung injury associated with GvHD are the most prominent factors that contribute to late respiratory complications. Impaired growth of both lungs and chest wall can be additional factors in patients who are transplanted as young children.

Restrictive lung disease

Restrictive lung disease is frequently observed 3–6 months after SCT in patients conditioned with TBI and receiving an allogeneic SCT, but in most cases it is not symptomatic. Restrictive disease is often stable and, in fact, may resolve, partially or completely, within 2 years of SCT. However, some patients do develop severe late restrictive defects and may eventually die from respiratory failure [25, 26].

Chronic obstructive lung disease

Chronic obstructive pulmonary disease with reduced FEV_1/FVC and FEV_1 develops in up to 20% of long-term survivors after SCT. The pathogenesis is not well understood, but cGvHD, TBI, hypo-gammaglobulinemia, GvHD prophylaxis with methotrexate, and infections have been described as risk factors [11].

Complications of bones and joints

This subject has recently been reviewed by McClune et al. [27].

Avascular necrosis of bone

The incidence of avascular necrosis (AVN) of bone has been reported at 4% to more than 10%. The mean time from transplant to the diagnosis of AVN is 18 months, and joint pain is usually the first sign [28–31]. The hip joint is affected in more than 80% of cases, with bilateral involvement occurring in more than 60% of cases. Other locations described include the knee (10% of patients with AVN), wrist, and ankle. Symptomatic relief of pain and orthopedic measures to decrease the pressure on the affected joints are of value, but most adult patients with advanced damage will require surgery. By 5 years about 80% of patients will have undergone total hip replacement. Short-term results of joint replacement are excellent in more than 85%, but further long-term follow-up is required, particularly in young patients, to determine outcome over an extended life span [32]. Steroid use (both total dose and duration) is the strongest risk factor for AVN [28–31].

Osteoporosis

HSCT can induce bone loss and osteoporosis via the toxic effects of TBI, chemotherapy, and iatrogenic hypogonadism and may be compounded by prolonged inactivity of patients after SCT (reviewed by Weilbaecher [33] and Schimmer et al. [34]). Osteopenia and osteoporosis are characterized by a reduced bone mass and increased susceptibility to bone fracture. These conditions are distinguished by the degree of reduction in bone mass and can be quantified on dual-energy X-ray absorptiometry. The cumulative dose and number of days of glucocorticoid therapy and the number of days of cyclosporine (CSP) or tacrolimus therapy showed significant associations with loss of bone mass. Nontraumatic fractures occurred in 10% of patients. Using World Health Organization criteria, nearly 50% of patients after SCT have low bone density, a third have osteopenia, and approximately 10% have osteoporosis by 12–18 months after SCT.

Few studies on the safety and efficacy of bisphosphonate for prevention of bone loss after HCT have been reported. Results of a randomized study in adult allogeneic HCT recipients showed less bone loss in patients receiving additional pamidronate (60 mg before and 1, 2,

3, 6, and 9 months after HCT) compared with patients receiving 1000 mg calcium carbonate and 800 IU vitamin D daily, and estrogen (women) or testosterone (men) alone. In a retrospective study of pediatric HCT recipients, treatment with bisphosphonates was well tolerated and was associated with improvement in bone mineral density [35]. Preventive measures of bone loss after HCT are indicated. Many experts recommend the use of antiresorptive treatments (gonadal hormonal replacement or bisphosphonates) in patients with gonadal failure and with cGvHD requiring treatment with glucocorticoid [36]. Hormone replacement after HCT should be individualized, with the pros and cons discussed carefully with each patient *before initiation of replacement, and reassessed at least yearly* if treatment is continued beyond 1–3 years after HCT. Increased risk of breast cancer, coronary heart disease, stroke, and venous thromboembolism was reported in the Women's Health Initiative study (nontransplanted women older than 50 years) with continuous combined estrogen–progestin replacement versus placebo, for an average of 5.2 years. Nonetheless, the study also showed a significantly reduced risk of bone fractures and colon cancer [37].

Late cardiovascular complications

This subject was recently reviewed by Rovó and Tichelli [38].

Cardiovascular disease is caused by disorders of blood vessels and is closely related to atherosclerosis. Atherosclerosis is now considered an inflammatory process, where endothelial lesions occur decades before clinical manifestations such as stroke, coronary heart disease, or peripheral arterial disease become manifest. Based on such concepts, cardiovascular disease might be expected decades after an endothelial damage occurs. Risk factors for arteriosclerosis in the general population are well established, and include smoking, arterial hypertension, obesity, diabetes, dyslipidemia, and physical inactivity. After SCT, endothelial damage is induced by the conditioning regimen, and endothelial cells have been documented as a target of GvHD. In addition, a higher incidence and degree of cardiovascular risk factors might be the result of posttransplant endocrine dysfunction, prolonged treatment with immunosuppressive drugs, or sedentary lifestyle. The increased incidence of cardiovascular events after allogeneic HCT supports the hypothesis that GvHD could be involved in the process. This is in line with the data on rarefaction of microvessels in patients with cGvHD. This loss of microvessels in the skin in cGvHD takes place independently of the epidermal injury. Patients with cGvHD have a significantly lower microvessel density in the subcutaneous compartment, compared with healthy controls. The correlation between GvHD and endothelial injury is also suggested in a study where donor-derived cells contributed to the endothelial repair of GvHD-induced lesions. Endothelial injury, due to a persistent vascular inflammation and endothelial cell death provoked by GvHD, could therefore be responsible for atherosclerosis and lead to premature cardiovascular accidents in long-term survivors after allogeneic SCT. Because of the long latency between an initial vascular injury and the appearance of a cardiovascular event, symptomatic cardiovascular disease might appear only decades after transplantation.

Secondary malignancies

Secondary malignancies are a known complication of conventional chemotherapy and radiation treatment for patients with a variety of primary cancers. Secondary cancers are now being increasingly recognized as a complication among SCT recipients. The magnitude of risk of secondary malignancies after SCT has been found to be increased fourfold to 11-fold compared with the general population. The estimated actuarial incidence is reported to be about 3–4% at 10 years, increasing to 10–12% at 15 years after allogeneic SCT [9, 10, 39–43].

Risk factors for the development of secondary malignancies include exposure to chemotherapy and radiation before transplantation, use of TBI and high-dose chemotherapy used in preparation for SCT, infection with viruses such as Epstein–Barr virus (EBV) and hepatitis B and C viruses, immunodeficiency after transplant, aggravated by the use of immunosuppressive drugs for prophylaxis and treatment of GvHD, including the use of monoclonal and polyclonal antibodies, HLA nonidentity, and T-cell depletion, the type of transplant (autologous versus allogeneic), the source of hematopoietic stem cells used, and the primary malignancy. However, assessment of risk factors for all secondary malignancies in aggregate is somewhat artificial because of the heterogeneous nature of the secondary malignancies, with differing clinico-pathological features, distinct pathogenesis, and hence very distinct risk factors associated with their development (reviewed by Socié and coworkers [9, 10]).

Currently, secondary malignancies after SCT are categorized into three distinct groups: (1) myelodysplasia and acute myeloid leukemia, (2) lymphoma, including lymphoproliferative disorders, and (3) solid tumors.

Secondary leukemia after allogeneic SCT

Secondary leukemia in the setting of allogeneic SCT refers to leukemia of donor cell origin or a *new* leukemia developing in surviving patient cells. Both are extremely rare complications, raising important questions on leukemogenesis. Recently, the Seattle team has suggested that transfer with the donor graft of otherwise silent malignant cells could also be responsible for leukemias arising from donor cells. However, no clear evidence links these secondary leukemias to cGvHD. Nevertheless, with increasing use of older donors (especially for patients receiving reduced-intensity conditioning) special attention must be given to the search for hematological abnormalities in the donor and of clear need for donor surveillance.

The development of new leukemias in patient cells is most likely related to cytotoxic conditioning therapy; there is no evidence to support a role of cGvHD.

Lymphomas

Posttransplant lymphoproliferative disorders (PTLDs) are the most common secondary malignancy in the *first year* after allogeneic SCT. Most of these cases are related to compromised immune function and EBV reactivation. The large majority of the PTLDs have a B-cell origin, although some T-cell PTLDs have been described [44, 45].

Nevertheless, several cases of late-occurring lymphomas have been reported in the literature. It is believed that these late-occurring lymphomas represent an entity that is distinct from the early-occurring B-cell PTLDs [46–49].

"Secondary" Hodgkin disease (HD) has also been observed among SCT recipients. SCT recipients followed as part of a large cohort study were at a sixfold increased risk of developing HD when compared with the general population [50]. Most of the reported cases were of the mixed cellularity subtype, and most of these cases contained the EBV genome. These cases differed from the EBV-associated PTLD by the absence of risk factors commonly associated with EBV-associated PTLD, by a later onset (>2.5 years), and relatively good prognosis. The increased incidence of HD among SCT recipients could possibly be explained by exposure to EBV and overstimulation of cell-mediated immunity, but no clear evidence for a link with cGvHD has been established.

Solid tumors

Solid tumors (recently reviewed by Socié and Rizzo [40]) have been described after syngeneic, allogeneic, and autologous SCT. The increase in the risk of solid tumors has ranged from 2.1-fold to 2.7-fold when compared with an age- and sex-matched general population [51, 52]. The risk increased with increasing follow-up, and, among those who survived 10 years or more after transplantation, was reported to be 8.3 times as high as expected in the general population. The types of solid tumors reported in excess among SCT recipients were those typically associated with exposure to radiation therapy, including melanoma, squamous cell carcinomas (SCCs) of the oral cavity and salivary glands, and cancers of the brain, liver, uterine cervix, thyroid, and breast as well as sarcomas of the bone and connective tissues.

Pathogenesis

Little is known about the pathogenesis of solid tumors. An interaction of cytotoxic therapy, genetic predisposition, viral infection, and GvHD with the resulting antigenic stimulation, and the use of immunosuppressive therapy all appear to play a role in the development of new solid tumors [53, 54].

Radiation-related cancers generally have a long latency period, and the risk of such cancers is particularly high among patients undergoing irradiation at a young age. A large series reported an increased risk of brain and thyroid cancers after TBI given as part of myeloablative conditioning, although most of these patients had also received cranial irradiation prior to SCT. Both thyroid cancer and brain tumors have been reported after exposure to radiation to the craniospinal axis and the neck when given as part of the conventional therapy for childhood acute lymphoblastic leukemia, HD, and *primary* brain tumors. Similarly, osteogenic sarcoma and other connective tissue tumors have been recognized as secondary malignancies developing after radiation therapy in nontransplanted patients. Those studies indicated a strong dose–response relationship for radiation exposure, in addition to an increased risk with increasing exposure to alkylating chemotherapy agents. The increased risk of thyroid, breast, brain, bone, and soft tissue malignancies seen after SCT appear to be related, at least in part, to cumulative doses of radiation exposure, both as a result of the pretransplant treatment regimens and the conditioning regimen used for transplantation.

Immunologic impairment may predispose patients to the development of SCC of the oral cavity and skin, particularly in the context of cGvHD. These tumors have been observed particularly in patients with aplastic anemia conditioned with limited field irradiation or treated with azathioprine for cGvHD [55]. In immune suppressed patients, oncogenic viruses, such as human papillomaviruses, may contribute to squamous-cell cancers of the skin and buccal mucosa. The observed excess risk of squamous-cell cancers of the buccal cavity and skin in males is unexplained, but may be indicative of an interaction between ionizing radiation, immunodeficiency, and, conceivably, factors such as smoking habits or alcohol consumption.

Patients with a family history of early-onset (<40 years of age) cancers are at an increased risk for developing secondary cancers, and genetic predisposition is likely to have a substantial impact on the risk of secondary cancers. Studies exploring genetic predisposition and gene–environment interactions have focused thus far on patients exposed to nontransplant conventional therapy for cancer. Future studies are needed in the transplant population to understand how genetic predisposition interacts with myeloablative chemotherapy, TBI, and the attendant posttransplant immunosuppression, thereby leading to secondary solid tumors.

Skin and mucosal carcinoma and cGVHD

As already implied, transplant recipients with cGvHD have an especially high risk of developing SCC of the oral cavity and skin, with rather aggressive behavior being noted for some of these tumors. Among solid organ transplant recipients the frequency of rejection episodes (requiring intensified immunosuppression) and the duration of immunosuppressive therapy strongly correlate with the occurrence of skin cancer. Patients undergoing SCT, in contrast to solid organ recipients, generally receive immunosuppressive therapy only for limited periods of time, unless they develop cGvHD. Thus, prolonged immunosuppression and (persistent) cGvHD are usually linked. A case–control analysis in SCT recipients was designed to quantify the association of GvHD and its therapy with the development of secondary SCC (including those of the oral mucosa) [55]. This case–control study included 183 patients with posttransplant solid cancers (58 SCC, 125 non-SCC) and 501 matched control patients within a cohort of 24 011 patients who received HCT at 215 centers worldwide. Results showed that cGvHD and its therapy were strongly related to the risk of SCC, whereas no such increase in risk was found for non-SCCs. Long duration of cGvHD therapy ($p = 0.0001$), the use of azathioprine, particularly when combined with CSP and steroids ($p = 0.0002$), and the severity of cGvHD ($p = 0.004$) were identified as major risk factors for the development of SCC. Since azathioprine was used mostly in patients who received prolonged immunosuppressive therapy and had severe cGvHD, the independent effects of these factors could not be evaluated. Consistent with a previous cohort study, there was no evidence that cGvHD or duration of therapy were related to the development of non-SCC solid cancers.

In a separate study the Seattle group evaluated the incidence of and risk factors for basal cell carcinoma (BCC) and SCC in survivors of SCT [56]. Patient-, disease-, treatment-, and toxicity-related factors were analyzed in regard to the risk of BCC and SCC in a retrospective cohort study of 4810 patients who received allogeneic SCT and who survived for at least 100 days. Among allogeneic SCT recipients, 237 developed at least one skin or mucosal cancer (BCC, $n = 158$; SCC, $n = 95$). Among the 95 SCCs, 24 occurred on internal mucosal surfaces, such as the tongue, tonsil, vocal cord, esophagus, and genitourinary tract (cervix, vagina, and vulva). The 20-year cumulative incidence rates of BCC and SCC were 6.5% and 3.4%, respectively. TBI was a significant risk factor for BCC (but not for SCC), most strongly among patients who were younger than 18 years at SCT. Light-skinned patients had an increased risk of BCC. Acute GvHD was associated with increased risk of SCC, and cGvHD with both BCC and SCC. Thus, this analysis suggested that immutable factors, such as age and complexion, have a significant impact on the development of BCC and SCC. However, specific treatment modalities (radiotherapy) and transplant-related complications (GvHD) may modify the risk. These additional risk factors suggest a contribution of immunologic mechanism and DNA and tissue repair in the development of BCC and SCC. Overall, these data confirmed previous reports which showed that exposure to ionizing radiation increased the risk of BCC but not SCC.

The major predisposing factor for cGvHD is preceding acute GvHD; that is, a syndrome characterized by alloreactivity and immunodeficiency. The immunodeficiency is further aggravated by the treatment of cGvHD, which may continue over several years. However, cGvHD, which most frequently affects the skin, liver, mouth, and eyes, also shows features of autoimmunity and inflammation. Both aspects are relevant since patients with autoimmune disorders develop malignant tumors more frequently than individuals with apparently normal immunity. Chronic inflammation and scar formation have also been associated with an increased risk of cancer. The interactions between inflammation and immunosuppression are not fully understood, but one might speculate that immunosuppression administered in a milieu of inflammation, as occurs with cGvHD, would interfere with tissue repair and thereby enhance the risk of tumor evolution. The risk would be further heightened when immunosuppressive therapies are given for prolonged periods, as observed in previous investigations in solid organ transplant recipients. If immunosuppression consisted of compounds which are known carcinogens then one would also expect new malignancies in recipients of SCT, which in fact has been reported in patients with severe aplastic anemia. In addition, it suggests that other components, in particular interactions with agents such as CSP, and the duration of treatment and severity of cGvHD are contributing factors. Reports from the early 1980s suggested that CSP, in many instances given at doses much higher than in use today, contributed to the development of malignancies, in particular PTLDs. More recent work suggests that CSP may induce phenotypic changes and enhance invasiveness of nontransformed cells via a TGF β-dependent mechanism. Finally, it should be noted that mycophenolate mofetil (which has largely replaced azathioprine in the treatment of cGvHD) has a mechanism of action similar to azathioprine and could, thus, represent a potent risk factor in the future!

Thyroid carcinoma and cGVHD

While thyroid carcinoma is generally considered a prototype of radiation-induced carcinoma, data from the European group strongly suggest that cGvHD may play a role in the genesis of this cancer. We performed a retrospective analysis comparing data obtained by means of a two-step questionnaire from the 166 centers who replied and data reported to the European Group for Blood and Marrow Transplantation (EBMT) registry on their transplantation activity [57]. During the follow-up period (1985 to 2003), 32 instances of thyroid carcinoma were found within the EBMT cohort of 68 936 patients who received SCT. The standardized incidence ratio of thyroid carcinoma in the transplant population was 3.26, in comparison with the general European population. Multivariate analysis revealed that young age at SCT was the strongest risk factor (relative risk RR = 24.61 for ages 0–10 years; RR = 4.80 for ages 11–20 years). Other risk factors were irradiation (RR = 3.44), female sex (RR = 2.79), and cGVHD (RR = 2.94). Nine patients showed no clinical signs of thyroid disease at diagnosis. Total thyroidectomy and iodine ablation was the standard treatment for the majority of patients, and only one patient died due to cancer progression.

References

1. Filipovich AH, Weisdorf D, Pavletic S, et al. National Institutes of Health consensus development project on criteria for clinical trials in chronic graft-versus-host disease: I. Diagnosis and staging working group report. Biol Blood Marrow Transplant. 2005;11(12):945–956.
2. Greinix HT, Loddenkemper C, Pavletic SZ, et al. Diagnosis and staging of chronic graft-versus-host disease in the clinical practice. Biol Blood Marrow Transplant. 2012;17(2): 167–175.
3. Wolff D, Gerbitz A, Ayuk F, et al. Consensus conference on clinical practice in chronic graft-versus-host disease (GVHD): first-line and topical treatment of chronic GVHD. Biol Blood Marrow Transplant. 2012;16(12):1611–1628.
4. Blazar BR, Murphy WJ, Abedi M. Advances in graft-versus-host disease biology and therapy. Nat Rev Immunol. 2012; 12(6):443–458.
5. Welniak LA, Blazar BR, Murphy WJ. Immunobiology of allogeneic hematopoietic stem cell transplantation. Annu Rev Immunol. 2007;25:139–170.
6. Vogelsang GB. How I treat chronic graft-versus-host disease. Blood. 2001;97(5):1196–1201.
7. Lee SJ, Vogelsang G, Flowers ME. Chronic graft-versus-host disease. Biol Blood Marrow Transplant. 2003;9(4):215–233.
8. Fuji S, Kapp M, Einsele H. Challenges to preventing infectious complications, decreasing re-hospitalizations, and

reducing cost burden in long-term survivors after allogeneic hematopoietic stem cell transplantation. Semin Hematol. 2012;49(1):10–14.

9. Deeg HJ, Socié G. Malignancies after hematopoietic stem cell transplantation: many questions, some answers. Blood. 1998;91(6):1833–1844.
10. Ades L, Guardiola P, Socié G. Second malignancies after allogeneic hematopoietic stem cell transplantation: new insight and current problems. Blood Rev. 2002;16(2):135–146.
11. Socié G, Salooja N, Cohen A, et al. Nonmalignant late effects after allogeneic stem cell transplantation. Blood. 2003; 101(9):3373–3385.
12. Tichelli A, Gratwohl A, Egger T, et al. Cataract formation after bone marrow transplantation. Ann Intern Med. 1993;119(12):1175–1180.
13. Deeg HJ, Flournoy N, Sullivan KM, et al. Cataracts after total body irradiation and marrow transplantation: a sparing effect of dose fractionation. Int J Radiat Oncol Biol Phys. 1984;10(7):957–964.
14. Benyunes MC, Sullivan KM, Deeg HJ, et al. Cataracts after bone marrow transplantation: long-term follow-up of adults treated with fractionated total body irradiation. Int J Radiat Oncol Biol Phys. 1995;32(3):661–670.
15. Belkacemi Y, Labopin M, Vernant JP, et al. Cataracts after total body irradiation and bone marrow transplantation in patients with acute leukemia in complete remission: a study of the European Group for Blood and Marrow Transplantation. Int J Radiat Oncol Biol Phys. 1998;41(3):659–668.
16. Belkacemi Y, Ozsahin M, Pene F, et al. Cataractogenesis after total body irradiation. Int J Radiat Oncol Biol Phys. 1996;35(1):53–60.
17. Socié G, Clift RA, Blaise D, et al. Busulfan plus cyclophosphamide compared with total-body irradiation plus cyclophosphamide before marrow transplantation for myeloid leukemia: long-term follow-up of 4 randomized studies. Blood. 2001;98(13):3569–3574.
18. Janin-Mercier A, Devergie A, Arrago JP, et al. Systemic evaluation of Sjögren-like syndrome after bone marrow transplantation in man. Transplantation. 1987;43(5):677–679.
19. Jabs DA, Wingard J, Green WR, et al. The eye in bone marrow transplantation. III. Conjunctival graft-vs-host disease. Arch Ophthalmol. 1989;107(9):1343–1348.
20. Gratwohl AA, Moutsopoulos HM, Chused TM, et al. Sjögren-type syndrome after allogeneic bone-marrow transplantation. Ann Intern Med. 1977;87(6):703–706.
21. Tichelli A, Duell T, Weiss M, et al. Late-onset keratoconjunctivitis sicca syndrome after bone marrow transplantation: incidence and risk factors. European Group or Blood and Marrow Transplantation (EBMT) Working Party on Late Effects. Bone Marrow Transplant. 1996;17(6): 1105–1111.
22. Bacigalupo A, Chien J, Barisione G, Pavletic S. Late pulmonary complications after allogeneic hematopoietic stem cell transplantation: diagnosis, monitoring, prevention, and treatment. Semin Hematol. 2012;49(1):15–24.
23. Soubani AO, Miller KB, Hassoun PM. Pulmonary complications of bone marrow transplantation. Chest. 1996; 109(4):1066–1077.
24. Cerveri I, Fulgoni P, Giorgiani G, et al. Lung function abnormalities after bone marrow transplantation in children: has the trend recently changed? Chest. 2001;120(6):1900–1906.
25. Crawford SW, Fisher L. Predictive value of pulmonary function tests before marrow transplantation. Chest. 1992; 101(5):1257–1264.
26. Crawford SW, Pepe M, Lin D, et al. Abnormalities of pulmonary function tests after marrow transplantation predict nonrelapse mortality. Am J Respir Crit Care Med. 1995; 152(2):690–695.
27. McClune B, Majhail NS, Flowers ME. Bone loss and avascular necrosis of bone after hematopoietic cell transplantation. Semin Hematol. 2012;49(1):59–65.
28. Enright H, Haake R, Weisdorf D. Avascular necrosis of bone: a common serious complication of allogeneic bone marrow transplantation. Am J Med. 1990;89(6):733–738.
29. Socié G, Cahn JY, Carmelo J, et al. Avascular necrosis of bone after allogeneic bone marrow transplantation: analysis of risk factors for 4388 patients by the Société Française de Greffe de Moëlle (SFGM). Br J Haematol. 1997;97(4): 865–870.
30. Socié G, Selimi F, Sedel L, et al. Avascular necrosis of bone after allogeneic bone marrow transplantation: clinical findings, incidence and risk factors. Br J Haematol. 1994; 86(3):624–628.
31. Fink JC, Leisenring WM, Sullivan KM, et al. Avascular necrosis following bone marrow transplantation: a case–control study. Bone. 1998;22(1):67–71.
32. Bizot P, Nizard R, Socié G, et al. Femoral head osteonecrosis after bone marrow transplantation. Clin Orthop Relat Res. 1998;357:127–134.
33. Weilbaecher KN. Mechanisms of osteoporosis after hematopoietic cell transplantation. Biol Blood Marrow Transplant. 2000;6(2A):165–174.
34. Schimmer AD, Minden MD, Keating A. Osteoporosis after blood and marrow transplantation: clinical aspects. Biol Blood Marrow Transplant. 2000;6(2A):175–181.
35. Carpenter PA, Hoffmeister P, Chesnut CH III,et al. Bisphosphonate therapy for reduced bone mineral density in children with chronic graft-versus-host disease. Biol Blood Marrow Transplant. 2007;13(6):683–690.
36. Couriel D, Carpenter PA, Cutler C, et al. Ancillary therapy and supportive care of chronic graft-versus-host disease: national institutes of health consensus development project

on criteria for clinical trials in chronic graft-versus-host disease: V. Ancillary Therapy and Supportive Care Working Group Report. Biol Blood Marrow Transplant. 2006;12(4): 375–396.

37. Rossouw JE, Anderson GL, Prentice RL, et al. Risks and benefits of estrogen plus progestin in healthy postmenopausal women: principal results from the Women's Health Initiative randomized controlled trial. JAMA. 2002;288(3): 321–333.
38. Rovó A, Tichelli A. Cardiovascular complications in long-term survivors after allogeneic hematopoietic stem cell transplantation. Semin Hematol. 2012;49(1):25–34.
39. Socié G. Secondary malignancies. Curr Opin Hematol. 1996;3(6):466–470.
40. Socié G, Rizzo JD. Second solid tumors screening and management guidelines in long-term survivors after allogeneic stem cell transplantation. Semin Hematol. 2012;49(1):4–9.
41. Witherspoon RP, Deeg HJ, Storb R. Secondary malignancies after marrow transplantation for leukemia or aplastic anemia. Transplantation. 1994;57(10):1413–1418.
42. Witherspoon RP, Fisher LD, Schoch G, et al. Secondary cancers after bone marrow transplantation for leukemia or aplastic anemia. N Engl J Med. 1989;321(12):784–789.
43. Deeg HJ, Witherspoon RP. Risk factors for the development of secondary malignancies after marrow transplantation. Hematol Oncol Clin North Am. 1993;7(2):417–429.
44. Cohen JI. Epstein–Barr virus lymphoproliferative disease associated with acquired immunodeficiency. Medicine (Baltimore). 1991;70(2):137–160.
45. Curtis RE, Travis LB, Rowlings PA, et al. Risk of lymphoproliferative disorders after bone marrow transplantation: a multi-institutional study. Blood. 1999;94(7):2208–2216.
46. Zutter MM, Durnam DM, Hackman RC, et al. Secondary T-cell lymphoproliferation after marrow transplantation. Am J Clin Pathol. 1990;94(6):714–721.
47. Meignin V, Devergie A, Brice P, et al. Hodgkin's disease of donor origin after allogeneic bone marrow transplantation for myelogeneous chronic leukemia. Transplantation. 1998; 65(4):595–597.
48. Rivet J, Moreau D, Daneshpouy M, et al. T-cell lymphoma with eosinophilia of donor origin occurring 12 years after allogeneic bone marrow transplantation for myeloma. Transplantation. 2001;72(5):965.
49. Schouten HC, Hopman AH, Haesevoets AM, Arends JW. Large-cell anaplastic non-Hodgkin's lymphoma originating in donor cells after allogenic bone marrow transplantation. Br J Haematol. 1995;91(1):162–166.
50. Rowlings PA, Curtis RE, Passweg JR, et al. Increased incidence of Hodgkin's disease after allogeneic bone marrow transplantation. J Clin Oncol. 1999;17(10):3122–3127.
51. Bhatia S, Louie AD, Bhatia R, et al. Solid cancers after bone marrow transplantation. J Clin Oncol. 2001;19(2):464–471.
52. Curtis RE, Rowlings PA, Deeg HJ, et al. Solid cancers after bone marrow transplantation. N Engl J Med. 1997; 336(13):897–904.
53. Daneshpouy M, Socie G, Clavel C, et al. Human papillomavirus infection and anogenital condyloma in bone marrow transplant recipients. Transplantation. 2001;71(1):167–169.
54. Socié G, Scieux C, Gluckman E, et al. Squamous cell carcinomas after allogeneic bone marrow transplantation for aplastic anemia: further evidence of a multistep process. Transplantation. 1998;66(5):667–670.
55. Curtis RE, Metayer C, Rizzo JD, et al. Impact of chronic GVHD therapy on the development of squamous-cell cancers after hematopoietic stem-cell transplantation: an international case-control study. Blood. 2005;105(10): 3802–3811.
56. Leisenring W, Friedman DL, Flowers ME, et al. Nonmelanoma skin and mucosal cancers after hematopoietic cell transplantation. J Clin Oncol. 2006;24(7):1119–1126.
57. Cohen A, Rovelli A, Merlo DF, et al. Risk for secondary thyroid carcinoma after hematopoietic stem-cell transplantation: an EBMT Late Effects Working Party Study. J Clin Oncol. 2007;25(17):2449–2454.

7

CHAPTER 7

Prominent role of allied health professionals (nurse practitioners, physician assistants, others) in long-term follow-up after hematopoietic stem cell transplantation

Catherine E Lucid

Hematology and Stem Cell Transplantation Section, Division of Hematology/Oncology, Vanderbilt University Medical Center, Nashville, TN, USA

Historically, the role of the allied health professional has been used in primary care clinics, walk-in clinics, or pediatrician offices. Training has and still does focus on these types of settings for the provider. There is a unique role for the allied health professional in the realm of transplantation, specifically stem cell transplantation (SCT). This embodies acute, critical, and primary outpatient care in its daily functioning. The nuts and bolts of the type of care that is provided are not typically taught in an educational setting other than brief lectures or electives. This lends itself to primarily preceptorship-type training in order to gain the skills necessary to take care of this patient population. The provider discussed here plays a large role in not only the physician extender position, but also in education and health maintenance for the long term.

The significant change in long-term care for the SCT patient is just that, that it is becoming more long term. Many years ago, the goal was a cure, and at that we were done. Now, we are focusing also just as much on the long-term issues related to this patient population. Once they arrive in a long-term setting, following the acute first 100 days, we have many more issues that we are wrestling with. The provider is focusing not only on the graft-versus-host disease (GHVD) prevention and maintenance as well as disease control, but now added to the mix is quality of life, impotency, hypogonadism, metabolic syndrome, vitamin deficiencies, secondary malignancies, and thyroid dysfunction to name a few. There is a great role for the other medical providers who are brought in to this multidisciplinary team, but the initial screening and triage starts with the allied health provider. Their specific recommendations, treatments, and protocols are described in detail in a number of other chapters in this book.

In order to explore this further, the following will outline the current process used by the allied health provider. The first component to the transition is the education that must be performed [1]. This is largely as important for the caregiver as it is for the patient. This

Blood and Marrow Transplantation Long-Term Management: Prevention and Complications, First Edition. Edited by Bipin N Savani.

includes topics such as GVHD, disease restaging, immunizations, routine maintenance, quality of life at home, as well as day-to-day contact information. Often times, this encourages the patient and caregiver to begin to explore issues with the transition home that they had yet to contemplate. Patients, but mostly caregivers, are often quite apprehensive about the transition home, and this allows them to begin to process this.

General outlines are given as to the timeline for upcoming treatments and testing. There is often great concern by patients as to how often routine scans or biopsies will be performed, and this allows for discussion to occur and plans to be made. One of the largest issues facing the provider is to encourage the patient and caregiver to begin to live "normal life" again and not to focus as much on their disease. This is extremely difficult owing to the fact that, at a minimum, the last 4 months has been consumed with their disease. Many times, the outline that the provider gives is very fluid in nature and does not follow completely with each patient. The important component is that the patient and caregiver trust that the team taking care of them, including the provider, has their best interest at the focus of their care.

Immunizations are another large component of education and maintenance provided by the allied health professional. Often, encouraging the patient that there is a schedule of immunizations and that we as a team follow these is very reassuring. Many patients question the re-immunization process and it is important that a significant amount of education be given to reiterate the importance of their role in getting back to normal life.

Empowerment of the patient and caregiver is critical in the transition to home. Events will occur in their routine, and patients need to be aware of who to call and when to be seen either locally or at the transplant center where they are being monitored. Transition to a local oncologist or primary care provider is a key point in the success of a long-term clinic. Patients often feel as though every issue, no matter how small or how large, needs to addressed by their long-term transplant team, whereas in fact this only inhibits returning to normal life. The process needs to be in place to have this care provided locally, especially for the many patients who live hours from their transplant center.

The routine of the provider includes seeing this patient population for routine visits, including every 4–6 weeks for the first year, then every 2 months till 18 months, and then every 6 months after that. At these visits, standard labs are ordered, including complete blood count, electrolytes, liver panel, immunosuppression drug levels if indicated, immunoglobulin G, viral testing, donor percentage. The very first visit includes a more in-depth list of labs, including thyroid-stimulating hormone, vitamin D, urine microalbumin, c-reactive protein, and free and total testosterone (male patients). These routine visits are mainly centered around monitoring for GVHD and infection prevention. Based on findings on exam and review of symptoms, it is typical to adjust medications at visits to treat GVHD or taper immunosuppression.

The following is an outline of the schedule followed by the allied health professional in the care of the long-term transplant patient in detail.

First visit. The first visit is typically around day+100, but will depend on the current health status of the patient. The first visit includes reviewing all of the day+100 data, including disease testing, pulmonary function testing, bone density, and extensive lab work. The lab work includes vitamin D, thyroid-stimulating hormone, free and total testosterone (male patient), urine microalbumin, c-reactive protein, and fasting lipids. Education plays a large role in the first long-term clinic visit and is given by the allied health professional [1]. A written teaching guide can also be very helpful at this visit to aid in remembering all that is said for the patient and caregiver support. A detailed review is done at this visit, and then at each subsequent visit the points are reiterated.

Subsequent first-year visits. These visits tend to focus primarily around chronic GVHD prevention and maintenance, infection prevention, and disease recurrence prevention. Each visit consists of a thorough review of systems and exam focused on primarily the various forms of GVHD. Medications are often titrated at these visits, and if no GVHD is present then standard tapering of immunosuppression occurs. There are many factors that impact tapering of immunosuppression, including GVHD presence, infection, disease type, and current status.

Annual visits. Annual visits tend to focus primarily on organ function and disease status. Testing is ordered based on history of disease, whether it be bone marrow biopsies, scans, or specific blood testing. Pulmonary function testing is also ordered annually to monitor for pulmonary changes following chemotherapy and stem cell transplant and for the possibility of pulmonary GVHD. Bone density scan testing is ordered every 2 years [2].

Immunizations include polio, tetanus, hepatitis B, and haemophilus influenza type B. These are given in three sets, each 2 months apart. Prevnar 13 is given at 6 months from transplant in three sets, 2 months apart. Titers for pneumococcal, hepatitis B, and heamophilus influenza B are drawn 2 years following transplant and boosters given when indicated.

It is clear to see that the role of the allied health provider in the clinical setting described above encompasses many forms. It is important that the provider understands the large role they play in continued education and health maintenance. Following an outline for labs, testing, and visits helps to give the program structure and a timeline. The ultimate goal is for the long-term survivor to be followed in a clinic where their transplant needs are met and health maintenance is achieved.

References

1. Cooke L, Grant M, Gemmil R. Discharge needs of allogeneic transplantation recipients. J Clin Oncol Nurs. 2012;16(4): 142–148.
2. Majhail NS, Rizzo JD, Lee SJ, et al. Recommended screening and preventive practices for long-term survivors after hematopoietic cell transplantation. Biol Blood Marrow Transplant. 2012;18:348–371.

2

SECTION 2
Management

8

CHAPTER 8

Screening and prevention guidelines for hematopoietic cell transplant survivors

Navneet S Majhail[1] *and J Douglas Rizzo*[2]

[1]National Marrow Donor Program and Center for International Blood and Marrow Transplant Research, Minneapolis, MN, USA

[2]Medical College of Wisconsin and Center for International Blood and Marrow Transplant Research, Milwaukee, WI, USA

Introduction

Several advances in transplantation techniques and supportive care practices over the last four decades have improved long-term survival of patients undergoing autologous or allogeneic hematopoietic cell transplantation (HCT). As patients survive longer, there is an increasing recognition that pre-, peri- and posttransplant exposures have the potential to compromise life expectancy and can contribute to development of late complications. These complications can cause substantial morbidity and mortality and can impair quality of life among HCT survivors. Many complications can be prevented or detected early and treated. This chapter reviews guidelines for preventive practices for autologous and allogeneic HCT survivors [1–3].

Guidelines for long-term follow-up of HCT recipients

Recognizing the need for appropriate systematic long-term follow-up of autologous and allogeneic HCT survivors, consensus recommendations for screening and preventive practices were developed and published in 2006 [4, 5]. An international group of experts was reconvened in 2011 to review and incorporate the best evidence available on late complications of HCT and update the long-term follow-up guidelines. The updated guidelines were published in March 2012 [1–3], and can be accessed at www.BeTheMatch.org/md-guidelines (print version and app version for smart phones). A patient-friendly version of the guidelines has also been developed by the National Marrow Donor Program and is available at www.BeTheMatch.org/Patient.

The guidelines take a pragmatic approach to the long-term followup of HCT survivors and describe the minimum set of evaluations that should be considered for screening and prevention of late complications. Recommendations are organized by organ system and important follow-up issues (e.g., psychosocial issues, fertility, general health maintenance, secondary cancers). The working group recognized the lack of high-quality studies to guide recommendations. Where literature was lacking, recommendations were based on the general supposition that early diagnosis of complications may lead to early interventions and treatment which ameliorate severity.

The guidelines were established using expertise from an international group of experts to increase their global

Blood and Marrow Transplantation Long-Term Management: Prevention and Complications, First Edition. Edited by Bipin N Savani.

applicability. Emphasis has been placed on identifying exposures that mediate specific late complications. On the same note, "special populations" that may need greater surveillance for selected late complications have been called out; these include pediatric HCT recipients, patients with graft-versus-host disease (GVHD), patients who received prolonged pre- or posttransplant corticosteroid exposure, and patients who received total body irradiation as part of conditioning. Recommendations for posttransplant vaccinations are included (adapted from the 2009 guidelines for preventing infectious complications among HCT recipients) [6, 7].

Table 8.1 highlights selected common late complications that can occur in HCT survivors and a summary of the long-term follow-up recommendations from the 2012 screening and prevention guidelines.

Utilizing guidelines to care for HCT survivors

The use of follow-up guidelines has the potential to overcome some barriers to long-term follow-up of HCT survivors. First, they can serve to increase patient awareness of their exposures, risks, and risk factors for specific late complications and appreciation of the importance and need for continued surveillance for late effects. The guidelines can facilitate a systematic approach to HCT survivor care at the level of transplant centers and community healthcare providers (e.g., primary care physicians and hematologists–oncologists). A survivorship care plan that includes a treatment summary and a follow-up care plan may be used to facilitate transition of HCT recipients from the early posttransplant phase to the survivor phase and enhance communication between transplant centers, community providers, and patients. This planning tool can serve as an instrument for reminding providers about appropriate surveillance for late complications based on an individual patient's risk factors and exposures. Although a survivor care plan template specific for HCT survivors is not available, transplant centers can use the guidelines as a template to provide this document to patients and their referring providers. This would greatly enhance survivor care as they transition from the transplant center back to their community healthcare providers and is especially relevant for patients who are not able to return to the transplant center for follow-up care (e.g., insufficient resources or live remote from the transplant center).

Areas for future research

A number of areas pertaining to the use of long-term follow-up guidelines warrant further investigation. More research is needed to understand the best models of long-term care for HCT survivors and their transition from transplant centers to the community. With the increasing demand for HCT, transplant centers frequently have to divert their limited resources towards extending HCT to a larger number of recipients and providing immediate care for recipients in the peri-transplant time period. They may lack the interest and resources for caring for long-term HCT survivors (especially patients without GVHD), and may consider this less important than making more transplants available to those who can benefit. Research can inform optimal care models that involve community healthcare providers, including non-physician providers (e.g., nurse practitioners, physician assistants), in the care of HCT survivors. Studies need to address whether the incorporation of guidelines-based survivor care plans into these care models can reduce morbidity from late complications and improve overall survival. The economic impact of using such care plans also needs to be investigated. Research is also needed on the implementation, dissemination, and utilization of follow-up guidelines among patients and their providers. This will also facilitate future revisions to the guidelines and will prevent underscreening or overscreening for late complications. Of note, no randomized controlled trial has been conducted to demonstrate that increased surveillance and early detection of late complications leads to improved outcomes. Access to long-term follow-up care may be limited for particular populations with limited resources and insurance coverage, and better evidence regarding averted complications may also be useful to close these access gaps.

The Institute of Medicine (IOM) published a report in 2005 suggesting the importance of integrating the patient into their survivorship care through treatment summaries and care plans [8]. Several specific recommendations were made: to raise awareness among patients and providers; to develop and use systematic evidence-based tools and guidelines for screening;

Table 8.1 Summary recommendations for screening and prevention of late complications in long-term HCT survivors

Tissues/organs	Late complications	General risk factors	Monitoring tests	Monitoring tests and preventive measures in all HCT recipients	Monitoring tests and preventive measures in special populations
Immune system	Infections	• Donor source • HLA disparity • T-cell depletion • GVHD • Prolonged immuno-suppression • Venous access devices	• CMV antigen or PCR in patients at high risk for CMV reactivation	• PCP prophylaxis for initial 6 months after HCT • Immunizations posttransplant according to published guidelines • Administration of antibiotics for endocarditis prophylaxis according to American Heart Association guidelines	• Patients with cGVHD: antimicrobial prophylaxis targeting encapsulated organisms and PCP for the duration of immunosuppressive therapy • Patients with cGVHD: screening for CMV reactivation should be based on risk factors, including intensity of immunosuppression.
Ocular	• Cataracts • Sicca syndrome • Microvascular retinopathy	• TBI/radiation exposure to head and neck • Corticosteroids • GVHD	• Ophthalmologic exam	• Routine clinical evaluation at 6 months and 1 year after HCT and at least yearly thereafter • Ophthalmologic examination with measurement of visual acuity and fundus examination at 1 year after HCT; subsequent evaluation based on findings and risk factors • Prompt ophthalmologic examination in patients with visual symptoms	• Patients with cGVHD: routine clinical evaluation and, if indicated, ophthalmologic examination more frequently
Oral	• Sicca syndrome • Caries	• GVHD • TBI/radiation exposure to head and neck	• Dental assessment	• Education about preventive oral health practices • Clinical oral assessment at 6 months and 1 year after HCT and at least yearly thereafter with particular attention to intra-oral malignancy evaluation • Dental assessment at 1 year after HCT and then at least yearly thereafter	• Pediatric recipients: yearly assessment of teeth development • Patients with cGVHD: consider more frequent oral and dental assesments with particular attention to intra-oral malignancy evaluation
Respiratory	• Idiopathic pneumonia syndrome • Bronchiolitis obliterans syndrome • Cryptogenic organizing pneumonia • Sino-pulmonary infections	• TBI/radiation exposure to chest • GVHD • Infectious agents • Allogeneic HCT • Busulfan exposure	• PFTs • Radiologic studies (e.g., chest X ray, CT scan)	• Routine clinical evaluation at 6 months and 1 year after HCT and at least yearly thereafter • Assessment of tobacco use and couselling against smoking • PFTs and focused radiologic assessment for allogeneic HCT recipients with symptoms or signs of lung compromise	• Patients with cGVHD: some experts recommend earlier and more frequent clinical evaluation and PFTs

(Continued)

Table 8.1 *(Continued)*

Tissues/organs	Late complications	General risk factors	Monitoring tests	Monitoring tests and preventive measures in all HCT recipients	Monitoring tests and preventive measures in special populations
Cardiac and vascular	• Cardiomyopathy • Congestive heart failure • Arrhythmias • Valvular anomaly • Coronary artery disease • Cerebrovascular disease • Peripheral arterial disease	• Anthracycline exposure • TBI/radiation exposure to neck or chest • Older age at HCT • Allogeneic HCT • Cardiovascular risk factors before/after HCT • Chronic kidney disease • Metabolic syndrome	• Cumulative dose of anthracyclines • Echocardiogram with ventricular function, ECG in patients at risk and in symptomatic patients • Fasting lipid profile (including HDL-C, LDL-C and triglycerides) • Fasting blood sugar	• Routine clinical assessment of cardiovascular risk factors as per general health maintenance at 1 year and at least yearly thereafter • Education and counseling on "heart" healthy lifestyle (regular exercise, healthy weight, no smoking, dietary counseling) • Early treatment of cardiovascular risk factors such as diabetes, hypertension, and dyslipidemia • Administration of antibiotics for endocarditis prophylaxis according to American Heart Association guidelines	
Liver	• GVHD • Hepatitis B • Hepatitis C • Iron overload	• Cumulative transfusion exposure • Risk factors for viral hepatitis transmission	• LFTs • Liver biopsy • Serum ferritin • Imaging for iron overload (MRI or SQUID)	• LFTs every 3–6 months in the first year, then individualized, but at least yearly thereafter • Monitor viral load by PCR for patients with known hepatitis B or C, with liver and infectious disease specialist consultation • Consider liver biopsy at 8–10 years after HCT to assess cirrhosis in patients with chronic HCV infection • Serum ferritin at 1 year after HCT in patients who have received RBC transfusions; consider liver biopsy or imaging study for abnormal results based on magnitude of elevation and clinical context; subsequent monitoring is suggested for patients with elevated LFTs, continued RBC transfusions, or presence of HCV infection	

Renal and genitourinary	• Chronic kidney disease • Bladder dysfunction • Urinary tract infections	• TBI • Drug exposure (e.g., calcineurin inhibitors, amphotericin, aminoglycosides) • CMV • Hemorrhagic cystitis	• Urine protein • Serum creatinine • BUN	• Blood pressure assessment at every clinic visit, with aggressive hypertension management • Assess renal function with BUN, creatinine and urine protein at 6 months, 1 year, and at least yearly thereafter • Consider further workup (kidney biopsy or renal ultrasound) for further workup of renal dysfunction as clinically indicated	
Muscle and connective tissue	• Myopathy • Fascitis/scleroderma • Polymyositis	• Corticosteroids • GVHD	• Evaluate ability to stand from a sitting position • Clinical evaluation of joint range of motion	• Follow general population guidelines for physical activity • Frequent clinical evaluation for myopathy in patients on corticosteroids	• Patients with cGVHD: physical therapy consultation in patients with prolonged corticosteroid exposure, fascitis, or scleroderma • Patients with cGVHD: frequent clinical evaluation by manual muscle tests or by assessing ability to go from sitting to standing position for patients on prolonged corticosteroids
Skeletal	• Osteopenia/ osteoporosis • Avascular necrosis	• Inactivity • TBI • Corticosteroids • GVHD • Hypogonadism • Allogeneic HCT	• Dual-photon densitometry • MRI to evaluate patients with joint symptoms	• Dual-photon densitometry at 1 year for adult women, all allogeneic HCT recipients, and patients who are at high risk for bone loss; subsequent testing determined by defects or to assess response to therapy • Physical activity, vitamin D, and calcium supplementation to prevent loss of bone density	• Patients with cGVHD: consider dual-photon densitometry at an earlier date in patients with prolonged corticosteroid or calcineurin inhibitor exposure
Nervous system	• Leukoencephalopathy • Late infections • Neuropsychological and cognitive deficits • Calcineurin neurotoxicity • Peripheral neuropathy	• TBI/radiation exposure to head • GVHD • Exposure to fludarabine • Intrathecal chemotherapy		• Clinical evaluation for symptoms and signs of neurologic dysfunction at 1 year and yearly thereafter • Diagnostic testing (e.g., radiographs, nerve conduction studies) for those with symptoms or signs	• Pediatric recipients: annual assessment for congnitive development milestones

(*Continued*)

Table 8.1 (*Continued*)

Tissues/organs	Late complications	General risk factors	Monitoring tests	Monitoring tests and preventive measures in all HCT recipients	Monitoring tests and preventive measures in special populations
Endocrine	• Hypothyroidism • Hypoadrenalism • Hypogonadism • Growth retardation	• TBI/radiation exposure (e.g., head and neck, CNS) • Corticosteroids • Young age at HCT • Chemotherapy exposure	• Thyroid function tests • FSH, LH, testosterone • Growth velocity in children	• Thyroid function testing yearly post-HCT, or if relevant symptoms develop • Clinical and endocrinologic gonadal assessment for post-pubertal women at 1 year, subsequent follow-up based on menopausal status • Gonadal function in men, including FSH, LH, and testosterone, should be assessed as warranted by symptoms	• Pediatric recipients: clinical and endocrinologic gonadal assessment for pre-pubertal boys and girls within 1 year of transplant, with further follow-up as determined in consultation with a pediatric endocrinologist • Pediatric recipients: monitor growth velocity in children annually; assessment of thyroid, and growth hormone function if clinically indicated • Patients with cGVHD: slow terminal tapering of corticosteroids for those with prolonged exposure • Patients with cGVHD: Consider stress doses of corticosteroids during acute illness for patients who have received chronic corticosteroids
Mucocutaneous	• Cutaneous sclerosis • Genital GVHD	• GVHD • TBI/radiation exposure to pelvis	• Pelvic exam	• Counsel patients to perform routine self-exam of skin and avoid excessive exposure to sunlight without adequate protection • Annual gynecologic exam in women to detect early involvement of vaginal mucosa by GVHD	• Patients with cGVHD and TBI recipients: consider more frequent gynecologic evaluation based on clinical symptoms
Second cancers	• Solid tumors • Hematologic malignancies • PTLD	• GVHD • TBI/radiation exposure • T-cell depletion • Exposure to alkylating agents or etoposide	• Mammogram • Screening for colon cancer (e.g., colonscopy, sigmoidoscopy, fecal occult blood testing) • Pap smear	• Counsel patients about risks of secondary malignancies annually and encourage them to perform self-exam (e.g., skin, testicles/genitalia) • Counsel patients to avoid high-risk behaviors (e.g., smoking) • Follow general population recommendations for cancer screening	• Patients with cGVHD: clinical and dental evaluation with particular attention towards oral and pharyngeal cancer • TBI and chest irradiation recipients: screening mammography in women starting at age 25 or 8 years after radiation exposure, whichever occurs later but no later than age 40

Psychosocial and sexual	• Depression • Anxiety • Fatigue • Sexual dysfunction	• Prior psychiatric morbidity • Hypogonadism	• Psychological evaluation	• Clinical assessment throughout recovery period, at 6 months, 1 year, and annually thereafter, with mental health professional counseling recommended for those with recognized deficits • Encouragement of robust support networks • Regularly assess level of spousal/caregiver psychological adjustment and family functioning • Query adults about sexual function at 6 months, 1 year, and at least annually thereafter
Fertility	• Infertility	• TBI/radiation exposure • Chemotherapy exposure	• FSH, LH levels	• Consider referral to appropriate specialists for patients who are contemplating a pregnancy or are having difficulty conceiving • Counsel sexually active patients in the reproductive age group about birth control post-HCT
General health				• Recommended screening as per general population

Reprinted from *Biology of Blood and Marrow Transplantation*, Volume 18 (3), NS Majhail et al., "Recommended screening and preventive practices for long-term survivors after hematopoietic cell transplantation", pp. 348–371, Copyright 2012, with permission from Elsevier.

BUN: blood urea nitrogen; cGVHD: chronic graft-versus-host disease; CMV: cytomegalovirus; CNS: central nervous system; CT: computed tomography; ECG: electrocardiogram; FSH: follicle-stimulating hormone; HCT: hematopoietic cell transplantation; HCV: hepatitis C virus; HDL-C: high-density lipoprotein cholesterol; LDL-C: low-density lipoprotein cholesterol; LFTs: liver function tests; LH: luteinizing hormone; MRI: magnetic resonance imaging; PCP: *Pneumocystis pneumonia*; PCR: polymerase chain reaction; PFTs: pulmonary function tests; PTLD: posttransplant lymphoproliferative disorder; RBC: red blood cell; SQUID: superconducting quantum interference device; TBI: total body irradiation.

develop quality measures for survivorship; to support and develop new models of care coordination for survivors; to educate health care providers; to ensure access to affordable care and recognize survivorship care as an essential benefit in payment policies; and to expand research. Despite these recommendations in a high-profile report, implementation of many of the recommendations has been very slow or nonexistent. Conclusively demonstrating, through well-defined studies, that recommendations such as those made by the IOM substantially improve outcomes for cancer patients and HCT recipients is likely to improve their uptake and implementation.

The working group that updated and published the 2012 guidelines for screening and prevention of HCT late effects recognized that many recommendations were based on expert consensus opinion. In fact, there has been little increase in high-level evidence to support screening practices since the initial publication in 2006. A need for more prospective studies and randomized clinical trials to guide development of evidence-based guidelines in the future was identified. A better understanding of barriers and facilitators to implementation of the guidelines in routine clinical practice is needed. Research is needed to increase awareness of the guidelines and to guide methods that can facilitate their utilization by transplant centers, community healthcare providers, and patients.

Notwithstanding these limitations, the long-term follow-up guidelines provide a framework for systematic care of pediatric and adult survivors of autologous and allogeneic HCT.

References

1. Majhail NS, Rizzo JD, Lee SJ, et al. Recommended screening and preventive practices for long-term survivors after hematopoietic cell transplantation. Bone Marrow Transplant. 2012;47(3):337–341.
2. Majhail NS, Rizzo JD, Lee SJ, et al. Recommended screening and preventive practices for long-term survivors after hematopoietic cell transplantation. Biol Blood Marrow Transplant. 2012;18(3):348–371.
3. Majhail NS, Rizzo JD, Lee SJ, et al. Recommended screening and preventive practices for long-term survivors after hematopoietic cell transplantation. Hematol/Oncol Stem Cell Ther. 2012;5(1):1–30.
4. Rizzo JD, Wingard JR, Tichelli A, et al. Recommended screening and preventive practices for long-term survivors after hematopoietic cell transplantation: joint recommendations of the European Group for Blood and Marrow Transplantation, Center for International Blood and Marrow Transplant Research, and the American Society for Blood and Marrow Transplantation (EBMT/CIBMTR/ASBMT). Bone Marrow Transplant. 2006;37(3):249–261.
5. Rizzo JD, Wingard JR, Tichelli A, et al. Recommended screening and preventive practices for long-term survivors after hematopoietic cell transplantation: joint recommendations of the European Group for Blood and Marrow Transplantation, the Center for International Blood and Marrow Transplant Research, and the American Society of Blood and Marrow Transplantation. Biol Blood Marrow Transplant. 2006;12(2):138–151.
6. Tomblyn M, Chiller T, Einsele H, et al. Guidelines for preventing infectious complications among hematopoietic cell transplant recipients: a global perspective. Bone Marrow Transplant. 2009;44(8):453–558.
7. Tomblyn M, Chiller T, Einsele H, et al. Guidelines for preventing infectious complications among hematopoietic cell transplantation recipients: a global perspective. Biol Blood Marrow Transplant. 2009;15(10):1143–1238.
8. Hewitt M, Greenfield S, Stovall E, (eds). From Cancer Patient to Cancer Survivor: Lost in Transition. Washington, DC: The National Academies Press, 2005.

9

CHAPTER 9

Secondary malignancies: prevalence, screening, prevention, and management guidelines

Paolo F Caimi[1,2] *and Hillard M Lazarus*[1,2]

[1]Department of Medicine, Division of Hematology and Oncology, Case Western Reserve University, Cleveland, OH, USA

[2]Division of Hematology and Oncology, Case Western Reserve University, Case Comprehensive Cancer Center, Cleveland, OH, USA

Introduction

High-dose chemotherapy with autologous hematopoietic progenitor cell transplant (HPCT) and allogeneic HPCT are treatment modalities that have allowed clinicians to provide curative intent therapies to a variety of hematologic malignancies and nonmalignant hematologic, metabolic, and immune disorders. Despite the potential for cure, survivors of HPCT have a significantly elevated risk of secondary neoplasms when compared with the general population. These secondary malignancies result in significant morbidity, mortality, and distress in patients, caregivers, and physicians and emphasize the need for lifelong surveillance and monitoring of HPCT recipients.

The risk factors and causes for development of secondary neoplasms after HPCT have not been fully elucidated, but it is likely that a multitude of variables influence the likelihood of each individual patient developing this problem. It is imperative that clinicians stay familiar with the patterns of presentation, surveillance methods, preventive measures, and treatment options of secondary neoplasms for our current HPCT survivors. At the same time, research must continue to elucidate the causes of these malignancies and to clarify the measures needed to decrease their incidence in future HPCT survivors.

Models

Secondary malignancies after HPCT follow three patterns: posttransplant lymphoproliferative disorders (PLTDs), myeloid malignancies, and solid tumors (Table 9.1).

Posttransplant lymphoproliferative disorders

These occur primarily in recipients of solid organ transplants and allogeneic HPCT, although rare cases have been reported in series of patients undergoing autologous HPCT [1, 2]. In contrast with solid organ transplant recipients, in whom PTLDs originate from host tissues, the majority of HPCT-associated PTLDs are of donor origin. The association of PTLD with EBV infection and intensive immunosupression has been clearly established [1–4].

The clinical presentation of PTLD is variable. B symptoms, including fever, weight loss, fatigue, and night sweats, are common. New lymphadenopathy should raise suspicion of PTLD after infection has been ruled out. Extranodal presentation is common, with gastrointestinal involvement being the most common, followed by primary central nervous system disease. PTLD represents the most common secondary malignancy in the first year

Blood and Marrow Transplantation Long-Term Management: Prevention and Complications, First Edition. Edited by Bipin N Savani.

Table 9.1 Models of secondary neoplasms after HPCT

	PTLDs	Secondary myeloid neoplasms	Secondary solid tumors
Type of HPCT	Allogeneic	Autologous	Allogeneic
Peak time of presentation	0–24 months	12–40 months	3.8–6.8 years
Risk factors	• EBV-negative recipient/ EBV-positive donor • Prior splenectomy • T-cell depletion, use of ATG or alemtuzumab • HLA mismatch • GVHD and immunosuppression • Early or advanced age	• Underlying diagnosis of lymphoma • TBI in conditioning • Peripheral blood mobilization with etoposide • Extensive prior exposure to chemotherapy, especially alkylating agents	• Men have higher risk of SCC of skin and oral cavity • Women have higher risk of thyroid neoplasms • HPV infection before transplant increases risk of SCC • TBI in conditioning regimen of children and young adults (<30 years) • GVHD and immunosuppression increases risk of secondary SCC

Compiled from Refs [4–6, 15].
ATG: antithymocyte globulin; EBV: Epstein–Barr virus; GVHD: graft-versus-host disease; HLA: human leukocyte antigen; HPV: human papillomavirus; SCC: squamous-cell carcinoma; TBI: total body irradiation.

after transplant, with HPCT recipients having earlier presentation than solid organ transplant recipients [4–7]. The onset of late lymphoid malignancies continues well into the first decade after transplantation.

The World Health Organization (WHO) classification of PTLD identifies three separate types of PTLDs [2–4, 7–9]: early lesions; polymorphic PTLD; monomorphic PTLD and Hodgkin lymphoma/Hodgkin lymphoma-like PTLD (see Table 9.2). Early lesions can develop at any time after transplantation but represent the first histologic changes of PTLD, characterized primarily by extensive lymphoid proliferation with limited disruption of normal lymph node architecture; they are not clonal, but chromosomal changes have been reported [10]. They are more common in younger patients and those who have not had previous EBV infections [9]. Polymorphic lesions present clonality and show tissue architecture effacement with cytologic variability and atypia. This entity is the most common type of PTLD in children and is related to initial EBV infection [11]. Monomorphic PTLDs are composed of a uniform cell population that follows the histologic patterns of B and T cell non-Hodgkin lymphoma, with the former being much more frequent. Histology compatible with Hodgkin lymphoma rarely also has been reported in cases of monomorphic PTLD [12, 13]. Detection of the EBV genome as well as immunoglobulin or T cell receptor gene rearrangement can be found in the majority of cases. Cytogenetic abnormalities are common in the majority of cases of monomorphic PTLD [2, 4, 8, 14]. A late form of EBV-negative monomorphic PTLD has been more recently characterized, with poor prognosis and response to therapy [7, 14, 15].

Myeloid malignancies

Secondary acute myeloid leukemia and myelodysplastic syndromes are designated by the WHO as therapy-related myeloid neoplasms. These disorders occur with much higher frequency among patients treated with high-dose chemotherapy and autologous HPCT than recipients of allogeneic HCT. Secondary myeloid malignancies tend to occur later than PTLD, reported median time of presentation ranges between 12 and 40 months [1, 4–6, 16]. The risk of therapy-related myeloid neoplasms is also elevated in allogeneic HPCT recipients, albeit to a lesser degree than after autologous HPCT [1, 16].

The mechanisms underlying the development of secondary myeloid malignancies are not completely understood, but they appear to be different between recipients of autologous HPCT versus allogeneic HPCT. In autologous HPCT, the factors contributing to secondary myeloid neoplasms include advanced age, extensive exposure to antineoplastic agents for treatment of the

Table 9.2 WHO classification of PTLD and characteristics of subtypes

	Morphologic characteristics	EBV association	
Early lesions	Involved tissue architecture preserved to some degree	• EBV genome positive • Recipient usually seronegative	• No clonality, but chromosomal changes can be found • More common in younger patients and those without previous EBV infection • Usually limited stage
Reactive plasmacytic hyperplasia	Abundant plasma cells, rare immunoblasts		
Infectious mononucleosis-like	Paracortical expansion and numerous immunoblasts		
Polymorphic PTLD	Effacement of involved tissue architecture with full range of B cell maturation stages in the tissue, giving it a pleomorphic aspect	• EBV genome positive • Recipient usually seronegative	• Can be either polyclonal or monoclonal • More commonly localized
Monomorphic PTLD B cell PTLD Diffuse large B cell lymphoma Burkitt lymphoma Plasma cell myeloma Plasmacytoma-like lesions T cell PTLD PTCL-NOS Other types	Effacement of architecture commonly with invasive tumor growth. Can be classified as lymphoma by morphology alone	• EBV genome positive or negative (majority of B cell are EBV positive; 25% of T cell are EBV positive) • Recipient usually seropositive	• Clonality with Ig gene or TCR gene rearrangement
Hodgkin lymphoma and Hodgkin-like PTLD	Effacement of architecture, compatible with classic Hodgkin lymphoma	• EBV genome positive	• Can be nodal or extranodal

Compiled from Refs [7, 9].
Ig: immunoglobulin; PTCL-NOS: peripheral T-cell lymphoma not otherwise specified; TCR: T cell receptor.

underlying disease [1, 3], hematopoietic progenitor cell mobilization and subsequent transplant conditioning, as well as the proliferative stress imposed on hematopoietic progenitor cells during engraftment and reconstitution of hematopoiesis [17]. It appears that patients who receive an autologous HPCT for relapsed lymphoma are at higher risk than patients transplanted for other malignancies. The survival benefit that results from the autologous HPCT, more pronounced in the transplantation of lymphoid malignancies, may underlie the development of secondary acute myeloid leukemia (AML)/myelodysplastic syndrome (MDS), as patients have enough survival time to develop these secondary malignancies [3, 4, 8]. Moreover, current conditioning regimens used for lymphomas are intense but not truly myeloablative, leaving the possibility of survival of hematopoietic progenitor cells exposed to the genotoxic effects of high-dose chemotherapy [17]. In addition, pharmacogenetic factors suggest there may be an inherited susceptibility to the development of secondary AML and MDS, which have been associated with polymorphisms of genes involved in the drug metabolism – in particular of alkylating agents – as well as genes involved in DNA repair [17, 18].

Allogeneic HPCT recipients have a much lower incidence of secondary AML/MDS. When these malignancies occur, they are more commonly of donor cell origin, and the underlying pathogenetic mechanisms are not clear. It has been proposed that leukemic transformation occurs through antigenic stimulation of donor cells from host tissues, through effects mediated by the recipient hematopoietic environment that developed the leukemia in the first place, or fusion of normal donor cells with leukemic cells that persist in the recipient [2, 14, 15].

Solid tumors

Secondary solid neoplasms can occur both after autologous and allogeneic HPCT, with a higher incidence in the latter population. The mechanisms appear to be multifactorial and are most likely an interaction between pretransplant risk factors (discussed below) with risks inherent to immunosuppression. Further, the exposure to chemotherapies and the development of chronic inflammation in the context of GVHD may foster this condition. Solid malignancies have a much longer latency period than PTLD or myeloid neoplasms, with a median time from transplant to diagnosis of 3.8–6.8 years [6, 7, 15]. While the incidence of both PTLD and myeloid malignancies tends to decline before the end of the first decade after HPCT, the incidence of solid malignancies never reaches a plateau and persists through several decades after HPCT [4–6, 16].

Epidemiology

Incidence

The most appropriate measure to estimate the increase in risk of secondary malignancies in HPCT recipients is the standardized incidence ratio (SIR), which represents the ratio between observed and expected cases, according to age and gender. The SIR for any secondary malignancy (excluding nonmelanoma skin cancers) has been reported to range between 4 and 11 [1, 4, 6, 16]. Using data from several retrospective series, the cumulative, long-term incidence of secondary neoplasms ranges from 6.9% 20 years post-HPCT [16] to as high as 12% 11 years post-HPCT [19]. The epidemiology of each specific model of secondary malignancy is as follows.

1 *PTLD.* As discussed above, PTLD presents typically in recipients of allogeneic HPCT, with a reported incidence between 1 and 2%, although rates in patients with multiple risk factors may be as high as 8–10% [20]. Compared with the general population, the risk of lymphoid malignancy is significantly elevated in recipients of allogeneic HPCT, with SIR ranging from 29.7 to 182 [20].

2 *AML/MDS.* Most secondary myeloid malignancies develop in recipients of autologous HPCT. The actuarial incidence has been reported to be in excess of 10% after 5–6 years [5] with a cumulative incidence reported between 1.4 and 8.9%; the SIR can be as high as 300 [5, 16, 21].

3 *Solid tumors.* The risk of secondary solid neoplasms appears to continue throughout the survival time of HPCT recipients, never reaching a plateau. In several large retrospective series, the cumulative incidence for solid tumors ranged from 3.8% at 20 years (SIR of 2.8; 95% confidence interval (CI) 2.0–3.7) as reported by investigators from the University of Minnesota [16] to 6.1% after 10 years (±1.6%) observed by investigators from the City of Hope Medical Center [15]. Curtis et al. reviewed the observational databases from the International Bone Marrow Transplant Registry and the Fred Hutchinson Cancer Research Center Registry [22] that included 20 000 HPCT survivors. The SIR for all solid neoplasms was 2.7. Solid tumors which were noted at a significantly increased rate include cancers of the buccal cavity (SIR 11.1), melanoma (SIR 5.0), thyroid (SIR 13.4), liver (SIR 7.5), brain (SIR 7.6), and connective tissue (SIR 8.0), cumulative incidences after 5, 10, and 15 years of 0.7% (95% CI 0.4–0.9%), 2.2% (95% CI 1.5–3.0%), and 6.7% (95% CI 3.7–9.6%). Long-term follow of survivors for 10 years or more after HPCT observed an elevation in the risk of breast cancer [23, 24]. In a recent report by Majhail [20], the risk of lung cancer was also observed to be elevated in patients who received allogeneic HPCT with busulfan and cyclophosphamide conditioning. Other common solid tumors, such as colon and prostate cancer, have not yet been observed to have an elevated incidence after HPCT.

Mortality from these secondary tumors represents 5–10% of all deaths after allogeneic HPCT and is the fourth cause of nonrelapse mortality in patients who survive more than 2 years after transplant [25, 26].

Risk factors for secondary malignancies after HPCT

The risk factors for development of secondary neoplasms after HPCT can be divided according to the specific type of malignancy they cause. However, a more encompassing classification takes into account the period of exposure to such predisposing factors (Table 9.3):

1 pretransplant risk factors
2 transplant risk factors
3 posttransplant risk factors.

Table 9.3 Risk factors for secondary neoplasms after HPCT

Pre-transplant factors	Transplant factors	Posttransplant factors
• Age • Gender • Underlying malignancy • Lifestyle (smoking) • HPV exposure • EBV exposure • Prior therapies and exposure to alkylating agents • Peripheral blood hematopoietic progenitor cell mobilization method (etoposide confers risk)	• Use of TBI in conditioning regimen • T cell depletion (PTLD)	• Acute and chronic GVHD (PTLD and solid neoplasms) • Immunosuppression, in particular the combination of cyclosporine, azathioprine, and corticosteroids

Pretransplant risk factors

In addition to age, gender, primary malignancy diagnosis, prior chemotherapy exposure, and cell mobilization method, other underlying risk factors associated with lifestyle, as well as genetic predisposition, may continue to affect the development of secondary malignancies through the survival of HPCT recipients.

Age

Younger recipients of HPCT are at increased risk of developing secondary solid malignancies [22], in particular when they receive radiation as part of the conditioning regimen [1, 24]. Younger age at transplant is a strong risk factor for thyroid carcinoma (relative risk (RR) 24.61 for age 0–10 years; RR 4.8 for age 11–20 years) [27]. Patients transplanted before age 18 years have an increased risk of breast cancer (hazard ratio: 9.5) and children who are EBV negative are at a higher risk of PTLD [28].

Gallagher and Forrest studied 926 consecutive allogeneic HPCT recipients and found that the absolute risk for a second solid malignancy increased with advancing age at transplant [29]. However, when compared with age and gender-specific cancer rates in British Columbia, patients younger than 40 years of age had a higher RR of second solid tumor (RR 3.42, 95% CI 1.37–7.05, $p = 0.005$), while the RR for patients older than 40 years of age was not statistically different (RR 1.32, 95% CI 0.57–2.61, $p = 0.26$). Patients older than 50 years of age appear to be at increased risk of developing PTLD.

Gender

Large cohort studies have identified male gender as a risk factor for development of SCC of the skin and oral cavity [22, 24]. Male gender has also been associated with higher risk of secondary AML/MDS after transplantation for lymphomas. Women are at higher risk for thyroid carcinoma after HPCT [27].

Previous antineoplastic therapies

The majority of HPCT survivors previously have received multiple antineoplastic agents, with many receiving more than one line of chemotherapy before their transplant. In autologous HPCT recipients, exposure to alkylating agents (mechlorethamine for treatment of Hodgkin lymphoma or cyclophosphamide for non-Hodgkin lymphoma) conferred increased risk of secondary AML/MDS [5]. The risk of secondary myeloid malignancies increases with the number of previous lines of chemotherapy before transplant.

Previous exposures

EBV seronegative patients are at greatest risk for development of PTLD.

Underlying diagnosis

The risk of AML/MDS is also increased in patients who undergo autologous HPCT for nonlymphoma diagnoses, including plasma cell myeloma [30], breast cancer [31, 32], and germ cell tumors [33]. However, the risk is significantly lower than that of transplanted lymphoma patients. Several factors have been proposed to cause this difference [17], including differences in the chemotherapy regimens and more prolonged survival of lymphoma patients, resulting in increased number of patients exposed to developing leukemia over time. Additional proposed factors are shared genetic factors that predispose both the AML/MDS and lymphoma and specific biological changes in lymphoma patients that increase the susceptibility of developing secondary AML/MDS.

Autologous cell mobilization method

Patients who received an autologous HPCT after peripheral blood hematopoietic cell mobilization with etoposide had a 4.7-fold increase in risk of developing secondary AML/MDS [21].

Transplant factors

Conditioning regimen

As expected, the characteristics of the conditioning regimen play an important role in the risk of development of secondary malignancies. TBI is an important risk factor for development of secondary solid tumors after allogeneic HPCT [23].

Exposure to radiation as part of the conditioning regimen appears to double the risk of secondary solid malignancies after allogeneic HPCT (SIR 2.7 versus 1.3 in HPCT recipients who did not get radiation). There has not been a consistent correlation between TBI dose and risk of second malignancies [22, 24]. TBI increases the risk of nonsquamous-cell cancers, in particular in patients surviving beyond 5 years after transplant. Children younger than 10 years of age appear to be at the highest risk of radiation-induced secondary malignancies, but the risk remains elevated in patients younger than 30 years of age [24].

Use of TBI in the conditioning regimen of autologous HPCT also appears to increase the risk of secondary AML/MDS, in particular for patients who receive etoposide for peripheral blood hematopoietic progenitor cell mobilization [21, 34].

It is not clear whether non-TBI-containing regimens used for conditioning both autologous and allogeneic HPCT result directly in an increased risk of secondary neoplasms [17]. Majhail et al. reported on the outcomes of 4318 patients who received an allogeneic HPCT for treatment of AML and chronic myeloid leukemia [35]. The risk of solid tumors continued to be higher than that expected for the general population (SIR 1.4, 95% CI 1.08–1.79, $p = 0.01$), albeit at a lower magnitude than patients receiving TBI-containing regimens.

Graft characteristics

Recipients of an *ex vivo* T-cell-depleted graft as well as those who receive *in vivo* T cell depletion with antithymocyte globulin or alemtuzumab are at significantly increased risk for PTLD [16, 20, 22, 25, 36]. Of note, selective T-cell-depletion methods appear to confer a higher risk of PTLD than methods that remove both B and T cells, possibly because the latter decrease the number of EBV-infected B cells in the graft [20, 36].

Posttransplant factors

GVHD and immunosuppressive therapy

An important posttransplant factor affecting development of secondary malignancies is the presence of chronic GVHD and the attendant use of prolonged immunosuppression. Solid neoplasms, including oral and cutaneous squamous-cell neoplasms, may develop early and late posttransplant [20, 22, 24]. The risk is increased further with more severe GVHD and prolonged exposure to immunosuppressants; patients requiring immunosuppression for more than 24 months had a significant increase in their risk of squamous neoplasms [37]. The risk associated with chronic GVHD is higher in patients who had preceding acute GVHD, a condition variably associated with SCC [37, 38]. A single study by Socié et al. found an inverse relationship between solid malignancies and GVHD, although nonmelanoma skin cancers were not included in the analysis [25].

Among the immunosuppressive therapies, the combination of azathioprine, cyclosporine, and corticosteroids had a highly significant correlation with SCC, with an 18-fold increase in risk. Use of other therapies, such as psoralen combined with ultraviolet A or limited field radiation, added to chronic GVHD treatment, further increase risk [37].

Chronic GVHD and its treatment may increase the risk of secondary neoplasms through several mechanisms, including chronic persistent inflammation [29, 39, 40] with genetic changes in epithelial cells, including telomere shortening. Immunosuppression may lead to decreased immune surveillance of abnormal epithelial cells, leading to pre-neoplastic lesions and subsequently to overt neoplasia. Immune suppression, in particular interference with T cell function, may also facilitate viral infection [15].

Viral infection

Epstein–Barr virus

As noted earlier in the chapter, EBV is implicated in the majority of PTLD cases, in particular with those that occur early after HPCT. EBV is capable of promoting B cell proliferation, leading to premalignant lesions characterized by lymphoid hyperplasia and subsequently to overt lymphoid malignancy [20, 28]. In contrast to what occurs in solid organ transplant recipients, EBV PTLD in HPCT recipients arises from donor lymphocytes [41].

Human papillomavirus and gynecologic surveillance

HPV is associated with SCCs of the female genital tract, oral cavity, and skin in both the general population and in immunosuppressed patients, including patients infected with HIV and solid organ transplant recipients. Savani et al. [42] reported that more than 40% of long-term female survivors of HPCT had abnormal cervical cytology and 20% had squamous intraepithelial neoplasia. Patients receiving immunosuppression for chronic GVHD had the highest risk for squamous intraepithelial neoplasia of the cervix. HPV exposure usually occurs in the pretransplant period, and the risk of developing a squamous malignancy is higher in older patients; however, its reactivation is a result of posttransplant immunosuppression. In pediatric recipients of HPCT, HPV exposure will occur in the posttransplantation period. The role of posttransplant vaccination against HPV will be discussed in the "Surveillance and prevention" section . The association of HPV infection and certain oral squamous-cell neoplasms has been well established in the general population [43]. De Araujo et al. [44] observed that Fanconi anemia and severe aplastic anemia patients treated with HPCT have a high prevalence of oral HPV infection, indicating a possible correlation with oral squamous neoplasms in this population.

Surveillance and prevention

The risk of secondary malignancies increases early after HPCT, with an elevated risk of PTLDs starting in the first year, while the incidence of secondary MDS and AML peaks during the first decade; solid tumors present a persistently elevated risk, continuing well beyond the first decade after HPCT. The care of HPCT survivors should include a focus on education regarding these increased risks, as well as the need for vigilance, screening, and adoption of preventive health behaviors. Contrary to expectation, the population of HPCT survivors has not been observed to have higher rates of preventive health practices than controls [45]. Surveillance guidelines are available for the long-term care of HPCT recipients [46]. Such specific measures for surveillance and prevention of secondary malignancies include the following:

- *Self-examination.* HPCT recipients should be encouraged to perform routine self examination of breasts as well as skin.
- *Mammogram.* Obtaining routine yearly mammograms beginning after age 40 years should be standard for all female HPCT recipients. Earlier initiation of screening and use of breast magnetic resonance imaging should be considered in young patients if 10 years or more have elapsed after HPCT.

Women who received chest irradiation between age 10 and 30 years as part of their pretransplant treatment have a significant increase in their risk of breast cancer. Screening should start at age 30 and include breast magnetic resonance imaging [47].

- *EBV viral load monitoring and treatment of EBV reactivation.* An increase in serum EBV viral load, measured by blood quantitative real-time polymerase chain reaction (RT-PCR), is associated with development of PTLD [48]. Patients at high risk of PTLD (Table 9.4) should have weekly monitoring of EBV viral load, starting from the day of transplant [49]. The duration of this monitoring schedule has not been established, with studies reporting that investigators monitor patients who do not have active GVHD for periods ranging from 3 to 6 months

Table 9.4 High risk of PTLD [15]

1. T-cell-depleted grafts
2. Use of ATG or alemtuzumab
3. EBV-positive donor and EBV-negative recipient
4. HLA mismatch
5. GVHD
6. Splenectomy

after HPCT [50, 51]. Patients with active GVHD should continue monitoring beyond the first 6 months.

There is no standard method of detection of EBV viral load; quantitative RT-PCR in whole blood is the preferred method used by many centers [49]. Commonly, 100 genome equivalents (geq) per milliliter is the threshold for diagnosis of EBV viremia. Data are limited for prophylactic antiviral therapy for HPCT with EBV viremia. Antiviral therapy can decrease replication of EBV, but has not shown to prevent PTLD and, therefore, is not recommended for prevention of EBV reactivation.

Preemptive therapy should be implemented for patients with EBV viral loads of 1000 geq/mL [52, 53] to 20 000 geq/mL [50]. The most commonly available treatment is the monoclonal antibody rituximab, aimed at decreasing the pool of B cells infected with EBV. Rituximab is given weekly at a dose of 375 mg/m^2 until there is a decrease in viremia by at least 1 log. Rituximab therapy will result in depletion of normal B cells lasting more than 6 months in HPCT recipients [54, 55], increasing the risk of viral infections. Moreover, rituximab does not result in persistent cellular immune response to EBV, allowing potentially for later reactivation and PTLD, especially if persistent immunosuppression is required [55, 56]. Other preemptive treatment strategies include infusion of donor-derived EBV-specific cytotoxic T lymphocytes [49, 55]. Because early after HPCT patients have profound immunosuppression with no immune regeneration, reduction of immunosuppression is unlikely to yield a response against EBV. Infusion of donor-derived, EBV-specific cytotoxic T lymphocytes should be considered in addition to rituximab primarily in patients who present with EBV reactivation several months after HPCT [57].

• *HPV vaccination.* Genital HPV disease, including anogenital condylomata and HPV-related genital dysplasia, has a high incidence in HPCT survivors [58, 59], in particular for those who receive long-term immunosuppression [42, 60]. Rather than reinfection, HPV reactivates from dormant virus, which correlates with the progressive disappearance of anti-HPV antibodies [42]. Reestablishing immunity against oncogenic HPV subtypes may decrease the rate of HPV reactivation, providing the rationale for vaccination with the HPV quadrivalent vaccine in women [61]. There are increasing data on the association between HPV and oral squamous neoplasms as well as the potential of HPV vaccines to prevent non-cervical cancers in both sexes [43]. Ongoing studies are investigating the rates of spontaneous seroconversion against HPV as well as the immunogenicity of the HPV quadrivalent vaccine in allogeneic HPCT recipients of both sexes older than 12 years of age [62]. Vaccination is done 1 year after HPCT or as soon as immunosuppression is discontinued. Three doses are given (0, 2, and 6 months) and repeated every 6 months in subjects who do not present seroconversion.

Therapeutic strategies

The treatment of HPCT survivors who develop secondary malignancies presents several challenges, most of them the result of the extensive previous therapy, the active or unresolved complications of the transplant, and the aggressive nature of the secondary neoplasms. To manage and avoid further complications, it is necessary to provide a comprehensive multidisciplinary approach to the care of these patients, including the involvement of the transplant team, surgical and medical oncologist, and supportive care specialists.

The treatment of secondary AML/MDS and solid neoplasms should follow the currently available therapies. A detailed discussion of these therapies is beyond the scope of this chapter. Specific attention must be given to squamous-cell neoplasms, which tend to be more aggressive in HPCT survivors, with early metastatic potential.

Chemotherapy may result in unexpected complications, either severe hematologic toxicity in patients with labile hematopoiesis or worsened mucocutaneous toxicity in patients with active or resolved chronic GVHD. Long-term complications of HPCT and previous therapies resulting in end organ damage, along with cumulative doses of chemotherapy and radiation, may present additional challenges. Surgical interventions such as tumor resections, while feasible, will have increased risk of complications in patients with long-standing immunosuppression or GVHD.

Treatment of posttransplant lymphoproliferative disorders

The treatment goals include the cure of the PTLD while maintaining integrity of the graft [7]. The therapeutic strategies for treatment of PTLD include restoration of the immune response against EBV and direct elimination of the neoplastic cells. The use of local treatment modalities, such as surgery or radiation, can be considered in patients with very localized disease and always in combination with reduction of immunosuppression or the monoclonal antibody rituximab.

Restoration of immunity against EBV

Reduction or withdrawal of immunotherapy may be an effective treatment approach in PTLD, in particular for patients with low tumor burden and "early" pathological lesions of PTLD [20, 55, 63]. After HPCT, reduction of immunotherapy may not be feasible in patients with severe acute or chronic GVHD. Additionally, this approach may not be effective in the early stages after HPCT because of the severe immunosuppression and incomplete immune reconstitution [2, 20, 55]. Patients with high tumor burden manifested multifocal extranodal disease, elevated serum lactate dehydrogenase, and B symptoms.

Unmanipulated donor lymphocyte infusions [55] or EBV-specific donor-derived cytotoxic T lymphocyte infusions may result in generating an immune response against the tumor and can control PTLD [7, 64], but infusion of unmanipulated lymphocytes carries the risk of development or worsening of GVHD. Haque et al. reported the results of a phase II trial of infusion of allogeneic EBV-specific cytotoxic T lymphocytes for treatment of PTLD developing after HPCT and solid organ transplants [65]. The overall response was 64% after 5 weeks and 52% after 6 months with no significant adverse events reported after infusion.

Elimination of neoplastic cells

The efficacy of rituximab in the treatment of PTLD in solid organ transplants has been well validated [66, 67]. Trappe et al. reported the results of a phase II study from the German PTLD Study Group and the European PTLD Network [68]. Sequential treatment with four weekly rituximab doses and the addition of CHOP chemotherapy in patients who did not have a complete response to rituximab resulted in overall response rates of 90%. Rituximab has been used in PTLD developing after HPCT, but the majority of reports were limited to case series [51, 55, 69–72]. The response rates range between 55 and 100%. Patients with multiple extranodal sites of disease, late onset after HPCT, and EBV-negative disease have a poor response to rituximab, and treatment with cytotoxic chemotherapy should be considered [20]. In PTLD secondary to solid organ transplants, use of regimens such as CHOP, ACVBP, and ProMACE-Cyta-BOM were associated with increased overall survival but also with an elevated rate of toxicity and treatment-related mortality [7, 73–76]. It can be expected that HPCT recipients will be at an equal or higher risk of toxicities from further treatment with chemotherapy and will require intensive supportive care.

Conclusion

Hematopoietic progenitor cell transplantation has become an accepted therapeutic approach for multiple hematologic and nonhematologic diseases. The safety of this procedure has improved significantly over the last two decades, and control of the acute and subacute complications of HPCT has led to longer survival of HPCT recipients. This has led to identification of a significantly elevated risk of secondary malignancies after autologous and allogeneic HPCT, resulting in significant mortality, morbidity, and distress in the transplant recipients, their families, and physicians.

It is fundamental for clinicians caring for HPCT recipients to remain aware of this elevated risk and to continue lifelong surveillance for malignancies in this patient population. Early detection and aggressive treatment of pre-neoplastic and cancerous lesions remains the cornerstone for improving outcomes in otherwise aggressive malignancies.

Future research should clarify the long-term effects of newer strategies introduced in HPCT such as reduced-intensity conditioning regimens, umbilical cord blood, and haploidentical transplants, and determine their effect on the risk of secondary neoplasms.

References

1. Friedman DL, Leisenring W, Schwartz JL, et al. Second malignant neoplasms following hematopoietic stem cell transplantation. Int J Hematol. 2004;79(3):229–234.
2. Adès L. Second malignancies after allogeneic hematopoietic stem cell transplantation: new insight and current problems. Blood Rev. 2002;16(2):135–146.

3. Bishop MR. The risk of secondary leukemias following autologous stem cell transplantation. Leuk Res. 1999; 23(3):281–282.
4. Ortega JJ, Olivé T, de Heredia CD, et al. Secondary malignancies and quality of life after stem cell transplantation. Bone Marrow Transplant. 2005;35:S83–S87.
5. Howe R, Micallef INM, Inwards DJ, et al. Secondary myelodysplastic syndrome and acute myelogenous leukemia are significant complications following autologous stem cell transplantation for lymphoma. Bone Marrow Transplant. 2003;32(3):317–324.
6. Bhatia S, Ramsay NK, Steinbuch M, et al. Malignant neoplasms following bone marrow transplantation. Blood. 1996;87(9):3633–3639.
7. Jagadeesh D, Woda BA, Draper J, et al. Post transplant lymphoproliferative disorders: risk, classification, and therapeutic recommendations. Curr Treat Options Oncol. 2012; 13(1):122–136.
8. Djokic M, Le Beau MM, Swinnen LJ, et al. Post-transplant lymphoproliferative disorder subtypes correlate with different recurring chromosomal abnormalities. Genes Chromosomes Cancer. 2005;45(3):313–318.
9. Swerdlow SH, Webber SA, Chadburn A, et al. Post transplant lymphoproliferative disorders. In: Swerdlow SH, (ed.). WHO Classification of Tumours of Haematopoietic and Lymphoid Tissues. Lyon, France: IARC, 2008; pp. 343–349.
10. Vakiani E, Nandula SV, Subramaniyam S, et al. Cytogenetic analysis of B-cell posttransplant lymphoproliferations validates the World Health Organization classification and suggests inclusion of florid follicular hyperplasia as a precursor lesion. Hum Pathol. 2007; 38(2):315–325.
11. Végso G, Hajdu M, Sebestyén A. Lymphoproliferative disorders after solid organ transplantation – classification, incidence, risk factors, early detection and treatment options. Pathol Oncol Res. 2011;17(3):443–454.
12. Okuno K, Horie Y, Kanai K, et al. Epstein–Barr virus associated post-transplant Hodgkin lymphoma in an adult patient after cord blood stem cell transplantation for acute lymphoblastic leukemia. J Clin Exp Hematop. 2009;49(1): 45–51.
13. Pitman SD, Huang Q, Zuppan CW, et al. Hodgkin lymphoma-like posttransplant lymphoproliferative disorder (HL-like PTLD) simulates monomorphic B-cell PTLD both clinically and pathologically. Am J Surg Pathol. 2006; 30(4):470–476.
14. Nelson BP, Nalesnik MA, Bahler DW, et al. Epstein–Barr virus-negative post-transplant lymphoproliferative disorders: a distinct entity? Am J Surg Pathol. 2000;24(3): 375–385.
15. Lowe T, Bhatia S, Somlo G. Second malignancies after allogeneic hematopoietic cell transplantation. Biol Blood Marrow Transplant. 2007;13(10):1121–1134.
16. Baker KS. New malignancies after blood or marrow stem-cell transplantation in children and adults: incidence and risk factors. J Clin Oncol. 2003;21(7):1352–1358.
17. Hake CR, Graubert TA, Fenske TS. Does autologous transplantation directly increase the risk of secondary leukemia in lymphoma patients? Bone Marrow Transplant. 2006; 39(2):59–70.
18. Knoche E, McLeod HL, Graubert TA. Pharmacogenetics of alkylator-associated acute myeloid leukemia. Pharmacogenomics. 2006;7(5):719–729.
19. Lowsky R, Lipton J, Fyles G, et al. Secondary malignancies after bone marrow transplantation in adults. J Clin Oncol. 1994;12(10):2187–2192.
20. Majhail NS. Secondary cancers following allogeneic haematopoietic cell transplantation in adults. Br J Haematol. 2011;154(3):301–310.
21. Krishnan A, Bhatia S, Slovak ML, et al. Predictors of therapy-related leukemia and myelodysplasia following autologous transplantation for lymphoma: an assessment of risk factors. Blood. 2000;95(5):1588–1593.
22. Curtis RE, Rowlings PA, Deeg HJ, et al. Solid cancers after bone marrow transplantation. N Engl J Med. 1997; 336(13):897–904.
23. Socié G, Rizzo JD. Second solid tumors: screening and management guidelines in long-term survivors after allogeneic stem cell transplantation. Semin Hematol. 2012;49(1):4–9.
24. Rizzo JD, Curtis RE, Socié G, et al. Solid cancers after allogeneic hematopoietic cell transplantation. Blood. 2009;113(5):1175–1183.
25. Socié G, Stone JV, Wingard JR, et al. Long-term survival and late deaths after allogeneic bone marrow transplantation. Late Effects Working Committee of the International Bone Marrow Transplant Registry. N Engl J Med. 1999; 341(1):14–21.
26. Wingard JR, Majhail NS, Brazauskas R, et al. Long-term survival and late deaths after allogeneic hematopoietic cell transplantation. J Clin Oncol. 2011;29(16):2230–2239.
27. Cohen A, Rovelli A, Merlo DF, et al. Risk for secondary thyroid carcinoma after hematopoietic stem-cell transplantation: an EBMT late effects working party study. J Clin Oncol. 2007;25(17):2449–2454.
28. Nourse JP, Jones K, Gandhi MK. Epstein–Barr virus-related post-transplant lymphoproliferative disorders: pathogenetic insights for targeted therapy. Am J Transplant. 2011; 11(5):888–895.
29. Gallagher G, Forrest DL. Second solid cancers after allogeneic hematopoietic stem cell transplantation. Cancer. 2007; 109(1):84–92.

30. Govindarajan R, Jagannath S, Flick JT, et al. Preceding standard therapy is the likely cause of MDS after autotransplants for multiple myeloma. Br J Haematol. 1996;95(2):349–353.
31. Kroger N, Damon L, Zander AR, et al. Secondary acute leukemia following mitoxantrone-based high-dose chemotherapy for primary breast cancer patients. Bone Marrow Transplant. 2003;32(12):1153–1157.
32. Rodenhuis S, Bontenbal M, Beex LVAM, et al. High-dose chemotherapy with hematopoietic stem-cell rescue for high-risk breast cancer. N Engl J Med. 2003;349(1):7–16.
33. Kollmannsberger C, Hartmann JT, Kanz L, et al. Therapy-related malignancies following treatment of germ cell cancer. Int J Cancer. 1999;83(6):860–863.
34. Travis LB, Weeks J, Curtis RE, et al. Leukemia following low-dose total body irradiation and chemotherapy for non-Hodgkin's lymphoma. J Clin Oncol. 1996;14(2):565–571.
35. Majhail NS, Brazauskas R, Rizzo JD, et al. Secondary solid cancers after allogeneic hematopoietic cell transplantation using busulfan–cyclophosphamide conditioning. Blood. 2011;117(1):316–322.
36. Landgren O, Gilbert ES, Rizzo JD, et al. Risk factors for lymphoproliferative disorders after allogeneic hematopoietic cell transplantation. Blood. 2009;113(20):4992–5001.
37. Curtis RE, Metayer C, Rizzo JD, et al. Impact of chronic GVHD therapy on the development of squamous-cell cancers after hematopoietic stem-cell transplantation: an international case–control study. Blood. 2005;105(10):3802–3811.
38. Leisenring W, Friedman DL, Flowers MED, et al. Nonmelanoma skin and mucosal cancers after hematopoietic cell transplantation. J Clin Oncol. 2006;1119–1126.
39. Bhatia S, Louie AD, Bhatia R, et al. Solid cancers after bone marrow transplantation. J Clin Oncol. 2001;19(2):464–471.
40. Demarosi F, Lodi G, Carrassi A, et al. Oral malignancies following HSCT: graft versus host disease and other risk factors. Oral Oncol. 2005;41(9):865–877.
41. Shapiro RS, McClain K, Frizzera G, et al. Epstein–Barr virus associated B cell lymphoproliferative disorders following bone marrow transplantation. Blood. 1988;71(5):1234–1243.
42. Savani BN, Stratton P, Shenoy A, et al. Increased risk of cervical dysplasia in long-term survivors of allogeneic stem cell transplantation – implications for screening and HPV vaccination. Biol Blood Marrow Transplant. 2008;14(9):1072–1075.
43. Gillison ML, Chaturvedi AK, Lowy DR. HPV prophylactic vaccines and the potential prevention of noncervical cancers in both men and women. Cancer. 2008;113(10 Suppl):3036–3046.
44. de Araujo MR, Rubira-Bullen I, Santos CF, et al. High prevalence of oral human papillomavirus infection in Fanconi's anemia patients. Oral Dis. 2011;17(6):572–576.
45. Bishop MM, Lee SJ, Beaumont JL, et al. The preventive health behaviors of long-term survivors of cancer and hematopoietic stem cell transplantation compared with matched controls. Biol Blood Marrow Transplant. 2010;16(2):207–214.
46. Rizzo JD, Wingard JR, Tichelli A, et al. Recommended screening and preventive practices for long-term survivors after hematopoietic cell transplantation: joint recommendations of the European Group for Blood and Marrow Transplantation, Center for International Blood and Marrow Transplant Research, and the American Society for Blood and Marrow Transplantation (EBMT/CIBMTR/ASBMT). Bone Marrow Transplant. 2006;37(3):249–261.
47. Saslow D, Boetes C, Burke W, et al. American Cancer Society guidelines for breast screening with MRI as an adjunct to mammography. CA Cancer J Clin. 2007;57(2):75–89.
48. Gärtner BC, Schäfer H, Marggraff K, et al. Evaluation of use of Epstein–Barr viral load in patients after allogeneic stem cell transplantation to diagnose and monitor posttransplant lymphoproliferative disease. J Clin Microbiol. 2002;40(2):351–358.
49. Styczynski J, Reusser P, Einsele H, et al. Management of HSV, VZV and EBV infections in patients with hematological malignancies and after SCT: guidelines from the Second European Conference on Infections in Leukemia. Bone Marrow Transplant. 2009;43(10):757–770.
50. Omar H, Hägglund H, Gustafsson-Jernberg A, et al. Targeted monitoring of patients at high risk of post-transplant lymphoproliferative disease by quantitative Epstein–Barr virus polymerase chain reaction. Transpl Infect Dis. 2009;11(5):393–399.
51. van Esser JWJ, Niesters HGM, van der Holt B, et al. Prevention of Epstein–Barr virus-lymphoproliferative disease by molecular monitoring and preemptive rituximab in high-risk patients after allogeneic stem cell transplantation. Blood. 2002;99(12):4364–4369.
52. Faraci M, Caviglia I, Morreale G, et al. Viral-load and B-lymphocyte monitoring of EBV reactivation after allogeneic hemopoietic SCT in children. Bone Marrow Transplant 2010;45(6):1052–1055.
53. van Esser JW, van der Holt B, Meijer E, et al. Epstein–Barr virus (EBV) reactivation is a frequent event after allogeneic stem cell transplantation (SCT) and quantitatively predicts EBV-lymphoproliferative disease following T-cell-depleted SCT. Blood. 2001;98(4):972–978.
54. Reddy N, Rezvani K, Barrett AJ, Savani BN. Strategies to prevent EBV reactivation and posttransplant lymphoproliferative disorders (PTLD) after allogeneic stem cell

transplantation in high-risk patients. Biol Blood Marrow Transplant. 2011;17(5):591–597.

55. Heslop HE. How I treat EBV lymphoproliferation. Blood. 2009;114(19):4002–4008.
56. Savoldo B, Rooney CM, Quiros-Tejeira RE, et al. Cellular immunity to Epstein–Barr virus in liver transplant recipients treated with rituximab for post-transplant lymphoproliferative disease. Am J Transplant. 2005;5(3):566–572.
57. Cesaro S, Murrone A, Mengoli C, et al. The real-time polymerase chain reaction-guided modulation of immunosuppression enables the pre-emptive management of Epstein–Barr virus reactivation after allogeneic haematopoietic stem cell transplantation. Br J Haematol. 2005; 128(2):224–233.
58. Sasadeusz J, Kelly H, Szer J, et al. Abnormal cervical cytology in bone marrow transplant recipients. Bone Marrow Transplant. 2001;28(4):393–397.
59. Daneshpouy M, Socié G, Clavel C, et al. Human papillomavirus infection and anogenital condyloma in bone marrow transplant recipients. Transplantation. 2001;71(1): 167–169.
60. Wang Y, Brinch L, Jebsen P, et al. A clinical study of cervical dysplasia in long-term survivors of allogeneic stem cell transplantation. Biol Blood Marrow Transplant. 2012; 18(5):747–753.
61. Tedeschi SK, Savani BN, Jagasia M, et al. Time to consider HPV vaccination after allogeneic stem cell transplantation. Biol Blood Marrow Transplant. 2010;16(8):1033–1036.
62. Savani BN, Goodman S, Barrett AJ. Can routine posttransplant HPV vaccination prevent commonly occurring epithelial cancers after allogeneic stem cell transplantation? Clin Cancer Res. 2009;15(7):2219–2221.
63. Heslop HE, Li C, Krance RA, et al. Epstein–Barr infection after bone marrow transplantation. Blood. 1994;83(6): 1706–1708.
64. Rooney CM, Smith CA, Ng CY, et al. Infusion of cytotoxic T cells for the prevention and treatment of Epstein–Barr virus-induced lymphoma in allogeneic transplant recipients. Blood. 1998;92(5):1549–1555.
65. Haque T, Wilkie GM, Jones MM, et al. Allogeneic cytotoxic T-cell therapy for EBV-positive posttransplantation lymphoproliferative disease: results of a phase 2 multicenter clinical trial. Blood. 2007;110(4):1123–1131.
66. Choquet S, Leblond V, Herbrecht R, et al. Efficacy and safety of rituximab in B-cell post-transplantation lymphoproliferative disorders: results of a prospective multicenter phase 2 study. Blood. 2006;107(8):3053–3057.
67. González-Barca E, Domingo-Domenech E, Capote FJ, et al. Prospective phase II trial of extended treatment with rituximab in patients with B-cell post-transplant lymphoproliferative disease. Haematologica. 2007;92(11):1489–1494.
68. Trappe R, Oertel S, Leblond V, et al. Sequential treatment with rituximab followed by CHOP chemotherapy in adult B-cell post-transplant lymphoproliferative disorder (PTLD): the prospective international multicentre phase 2 PTLD-1 trial. Lancet Oncol. 2012;13(2):196–206.
69. Kuehnle I, Huls MH, Liu Z, et al. CD20 monoclonal antibody (rituximab) for therapy of Epstein–Barr virus lymphoma after hemopoietic stem-cell transplantation. Blood. 2000;95(4):1502–1505.
70. Brunstein CG, Weisdorf DJ, DeFor T, et al. Marked increased risk of Epstein–Barr virus-related complications with the addition of antithymocyte globulin to a nonmyeloablative conditioning prior to unrelated umbilical cord blood transplantation. Blood. 2006;108(8):2874–2880.
71. Blaes AH, Cao Q, Wagner JE, et al. Monitoring and preemptive rituximab therapy for Epstein–Barr virus reactivation after antithymocyte globulin containing nonmyeloablative conditioning for umbilical cord blood transplantation. Biol Blood Marrow Transplant. 2010;16(2):287–291.
72. Wagner H-J, Cheng YC, Huls MH, et al. Prompt versus preemptive intervention for EBV lymphoproliferative disease. Blood. 2004;103(10):3979–3981.
73. Fohrer C, Caillard S, Koumarianou A, et al. Long-term survival in post-transplant lymphoproliferative disorders with a dose-adjusted ACVBP regimen. Br J Haematol. 2006;134(6):602–612.
74. Choquet S, Trappe R, Leblond V, et al. CHOP-21 for the treatment of post-transplant lymphoproliferative disorders (PTLD) following solid organ transplantation. Haematologica. 2007;92(2):273–274.
75. Elstrom RL, Andreadis C, Aqui NA, et al. Treatment of PTLD with rituximab or chemotherapy. Am J Transplant. 2006; 6(3):569–576.
76. Swinnen LJ, Mullen GM, Carr TJ, et al. Aggressive treatment for postcardiac transplant lymphoproliferation. Blood. 1995;86(9):3333–3340.

10

CHAPTER 10
Cutaneous chronic graft-versus-host disease

Attilio Olivieri[1], *Daniela Massi*[2], *Andrea Bacigalupo*[3], *and Anna Campanati*[4]

[1]Clinica di Ematologia, Dipartimento di Scienze Cliniche e Molecolari, Università Politecnica delle Marche, Ancona, Italy
[2]Servizio di Anatomia Patologica, Università di Firenze, Florence, Italy
[3]Divisione di Ematologia e Trapianto di Midollo Osseo, IRCCS AOU San Martino-IST, Genoa, Italy
[4]Clinica Dermatologica, Dipartimento di Scienze, Cliniche e Molecolari, Università Politecnica delle Marche, Ancona, Italy

Introduction

Cutaneous involvement is the most frequent manifestation of chronic graft-versus-host disease (cGVHD), occurring in about 75% of subjects. It is associated with significant morbidity, functional impairment, inferior quality of life, and requires prolonged immune suppressive therapy, which increases potentially lethal infectious complications [1, 2].

Cutaneous cGHVD is reminiscent of scleroderma (SSc) and may, or may not, be accompanied by involvement of other organs (liver, lung, gut, salivary glands). Several autoantibodies can be present in cGVHD patients, but their significance still remains unknown.

In spite of similarities with cutaneous fibrosis, the clinical presentation of skin cGVHD differs from SSc in several ways, including a general lack of the ischemic changes in distal extremities, characteristic autoantibody profile of SSc and internal organ disease as is seen in diffuse SSc (Table 10.1).

The new diagnostic criteria for cGVHD, proposed by the National Institutes of Health (NIH) in a dedicated Consensus Development Project, are based on different clinical manifestations, rather than on the cut-off of 100 days after transplantation, as discriminant between acute GVHD and cGVHD [3].

According to the NIH consensus criteria, some skin manifestations are diagnostic of cGVHD and do not require histopathological confirmation, that is, poikiloderma, lichen-like lesions, morphea-like sclerosis, and deep sclerosis/fasciitis.

Cutaneous cGVHD is characterized by a wide variety of clinical features (Table 10.2), but schematically the skin cGVHD manifestations can be classified into sclerotic and nonsclerotic lesions.

Sclerotic-type cGVHD (ScGVHD) of the skin encompasses several presentations, all sharing both inflammation and progressive fibrosis of the dermis and subcutaneous tissues and resembling morphea, systemic sclerosis, or eosinophilic fasciitis [4].

ScGVHD is generally a late manifestation of cGVHD, with a mean onset of 12–15 months after transplantation [5–7]. Since many studies do not differentiate between sclerotic and nonsclerotic disease, an accurate estimation of the burden of sclerotic variant (ScGVHD) is unknown [8, 9]. Skert et al. [10] estimated a 5-year cumulative incidence of 15% of ScGVHD among patients who developed cGVHD. Although ScGVHD has long been

Blood and Marrow Transplantation Long-Term Management: Prevention and Complications, First Edition. Edited by Bipin N Savani.

Table 10.1 Main distinctive characteristics between ScGVHD and systemic sclerosis

	Sclerotic-type chronic GVHD	Systemic sclerosis
Natural history	Patchy involvement, variable course	Symmetric, acral to proximal progression
Facial involvement	Rare, usually patchy involvement	Common, diffuse skin thickening (scleroderma facies)
Skin manifestations	Pleomorphic (sclerotic and lichenoid lesions)	Uniform (scleroderma; melanosis; ulcers)
Fibrosis	Dermis, hypodermis, and/or fascia	Dermis
Sclerodactily	Rare	Common
Raynaud phenomenon	Rare	Frequent
Autoantibodies	Variable, nonspecific (ANA, AMA, ASMA, ANCA, ACLA, anti-thyroid, anti-DNA (Patriarca Exp hematol2006)	Associated with specific subtypes (anti-centromeric; anti-Scl70)
Naifold videocapillaroscopic pattern	Aspecific pattern	"Scleroderma pattern": combination of giant capillaries, microhemorrhages, and avascular areas

ACLA: anti-cardiolipin antibody; AMA: anti-mitochondrial antibody; ANA: antinuclear antibody; ANCA: anti-neutrophil cytoplasmatic antibody; ASMA: anti-smooth muscle antibody.

recognized, little is known about pathophysiology, risk factors, and serological markers for this clinical variant; ScGVHD has been associated with higher platelet count and serum C3 complement level, and reduced forced vital capacity. These patients had significant impairments of joint range of motion, permanent contractures, and decreased grip strength; trunk involvement may also be associated with limited thoracic expansion. Total body irradiation (TBI) was associated with the development of ScGVHD, especially when used in reduced intensity conditioning regimens and higher body surface area (BSA) involvement was associated with poorer survival [4]. Compared with systemic sclerosis, cutaneous fibrotic involvement of the face, fingers, and toes and Raynaud phenomenon is less common.

Nonsclerotic cutaneous cGVHD lesions are heterogeneous and often preceded by unspecific symptoms, such as pain, pruritus, or photosensitivity [11]. In the past, these lesions have been generally defined as "lichenoid manifestations," but today the term "lichenoid" is no longer recommended because it should be referred to a histologic feature only [12]. The term "erythematous rash" is now used in the NIH guidelines to encompass several nonsclerotic manifestations of cGVHD; however, more specific descriptions of cutaneous lesions should be preferred, including lichen planus-like, ichthyosiform, poikilodermatous, papulosquamous, psoriasiform, eczematous, or exfoliative lesions [13–16].

Clinical manifestations and evolution of skin cGVHD

The assessment of the extent and severity of skin involvement is critical for defining prognosis and treatment of many cGVHD patients; recent data suggest that the evaluation of the NIH composite skin score has a good correlation with severity of symptoms [17, 18].

Onset of ScGvHD

At the onset, some cutaneous cGVHD manifestations may mimic autoimmune disease, facial lesions may be crusted, lichen planus-like, or poikilodermatous and often associated with atrophy, dyschromia, and telangiectasia (Figure 10.1). The evolution of skin lesions may be insidious and characterized by skin dryness, follicular prominence and ichthyosis (Figure 10.2).

The papular and desquamative lesions can be considered as "a great mimicker," able to resemble keratosis pilaris (Figure 10.3), pityriasis (Figure 10.4), eczema (Figure 10.5), or psoriasis (Figure 10.6).

Table 10.2 Clinical features and main characteristics of the different kinds of cutaneous involvement in cGVHD (by Dr Anna Campanati, Clinica Dermatologica, Dipartimento di Scienze Cliniche e Molecolari, Università Politecnica delle Marche)

Clinical features	Description
Xerosis/ichthyosis (Figure 10.2)	Generalized dry skin covered by "fish-like" scales and "dry dandruff"
Keratosis pilaris-like (Figure 10.3)	Presence of perifollicular erythema and keratinous plugs in follicular orifices
Lichen planus-like (Figure 10.7)	Purple, hyperpigmented papules arranged in annular, reticulated, arciform configuration; distribution pattern may be follicular, linear, or dermatomal; papular lesion can often coalesce to form extensive plaques. Vesicles may also be present
Lichen sclerosus-like (Figure 10.15)	Whitish, angular, flat, well-defined, indurated papules with an erythematous halo coalescing in shiny, whitish, and atrophic patches
Pityriasis-like (Figure 10.4)	Multiple macular patches of all sizes and shapes, and varying in pigmentation from fawn-colored to brown
Papulo-squamous-like Psoriasiform-like Eczematous-like (Figure 10.5, Figure 10.6, Figure 10.7, Figure 10.10, Figure 10.11, Figure 10.12)	Discrete guttate, annular, erythematous, infiltrated and scaly patches involving any part of the body including scalp, face, hands and feet, sometimes coalescing in extensive plaques.
Poikiloderma (Figure 10.1)	Presence of erythema, hypo- and hyperpigmentation, associated with extensive dermo-epidermal atrophy, and prominent blood vessels on the skin
Dyschromia (Figure 10.8, Figure 10.9)	Punctate or "confetti-like" spontaneous depigmentation resembling vitiligo or post-inflammatory hypopigmentation
Acral erythema (Figure 10.13, Figure 10.14)	Diffuse or patchy erythema of palms and soles associated with edema, variable hyperkeratosis and painful fissures; early forms may resemble hand and foot eczema
Vitiligo-like (Figure 10.8)	Sharply demarcated depigmented lesions with milky appearance and variable size and shape
Morphea-like (Figure 10.10, Figure 10.15, Figure 10.16)	Linear areas of induration, generally single and unilateral, although with hemiplegic distribution involving half the body
Sclerodermatous GVHD (Figure 10.17)	Skin appears shiny, taut, and thickened, tightly adhering to the underlying cutis. Skin thickening is frequently accompanied by hyperpigmentation, giving a salt-and-pepper appearance
Cellulitis (Figure 10.19)	Dermal fibrosis with the overlying epidermis relatively normal or with "peau d'orange" appearance, resembling eosinophilic fasciitis

Lichen planus

The lichen-planus-like lesions of cGVHD are often indistinguishable from those of classic lichen planus, with a focal or confluent pattern of distribution along the flexures (Figure 10.7). Moreover, an overlap *between* lichen-planus-like lesions and lichen-sclerosus-like lesions has also been reported [13]. Lichen-planus-like cGVHD may show vesicles reminiscent of those of herpes simplex or varicella-zoster virus infection [19].

Dyscromial lesions

Both hypo- and hyperpigmentations are commonly observed (Figure 10.8, Figure 10.9, Figure 10.10) [20]. These patients may show polymorphic skin lesions, which are sometimes difficult to distinguish from drug eruptions (Figure 10.11); however, the persistence of cutaneous manifestations despite drug withdrawal and the positive history of systemic cGVHD suggest the diagnosis of cutaneous cGVHD.

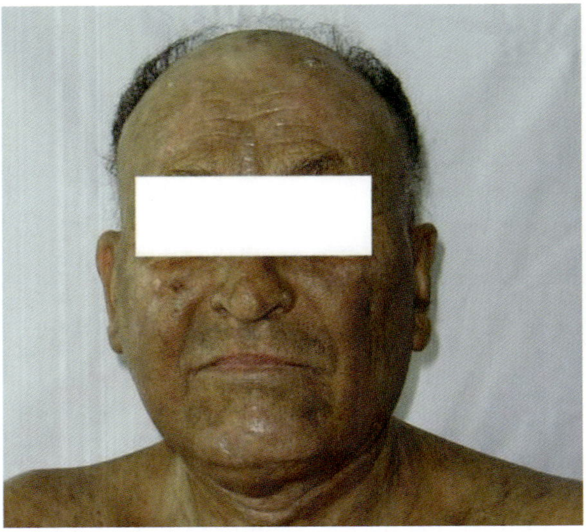

Figure 10.1 Epidermal GVHD characterized by face poikiloderma with hypo/hyperpigmentation, atrophic skin, and telangectasia.

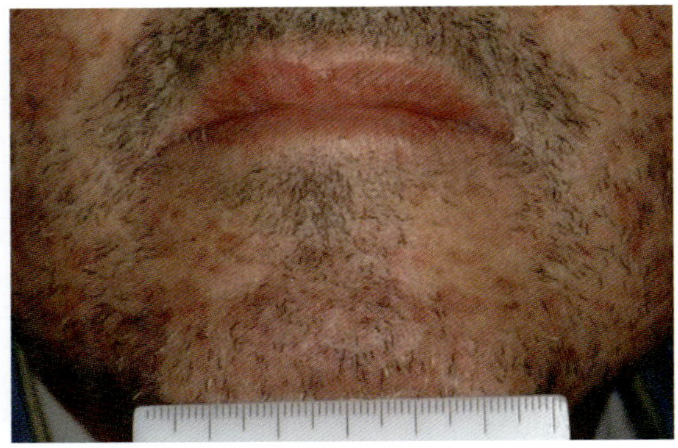

Figure 10.3 Epidermal GVHD characterized by keratosis pilaris-like eruption.

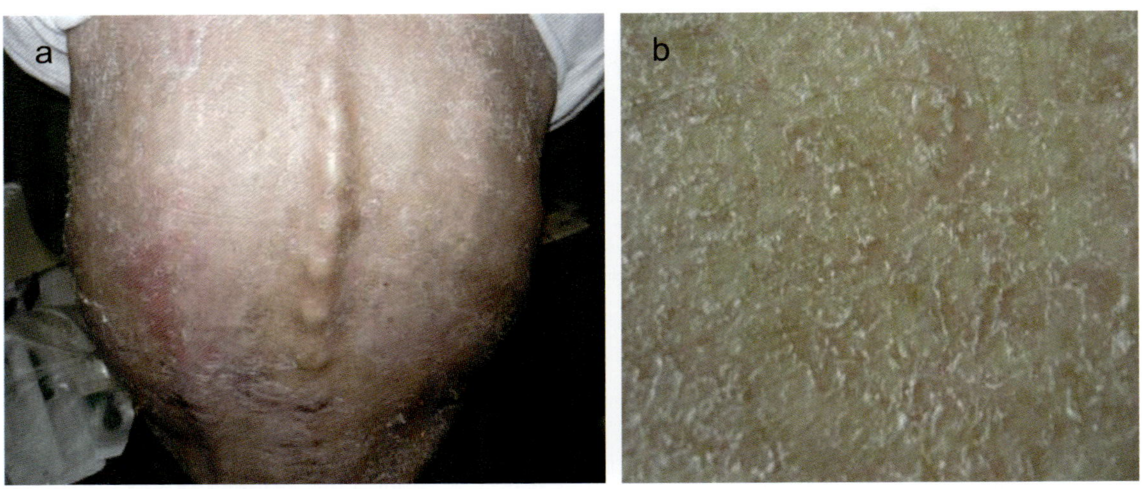

Figure 10.2 (a) Epidermal GVHD characterized by diffuse ichthyosiform xerosis on the back; (b) a particular of lamellar desquamation at strong magnification.

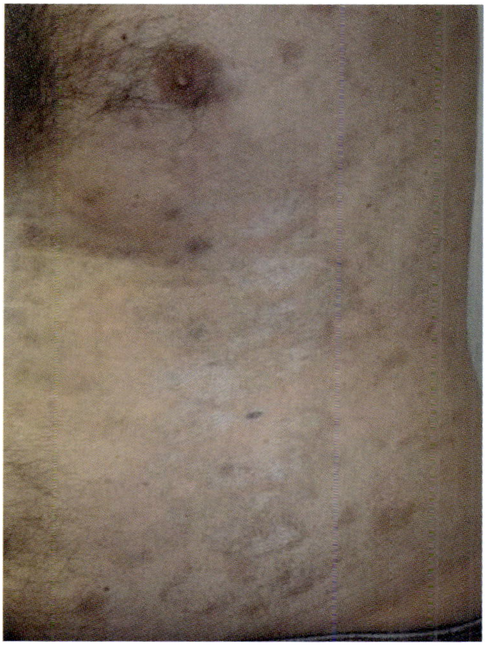

Figure 10.4 Epidermal GVHD characterized by desquamative and brownish patches of the trunk resembling pityriasis.

Figure 10.5 Epidermal GVHD characterized by eczematous features with diffuse, erythematous, and desquamative lesions on the back.

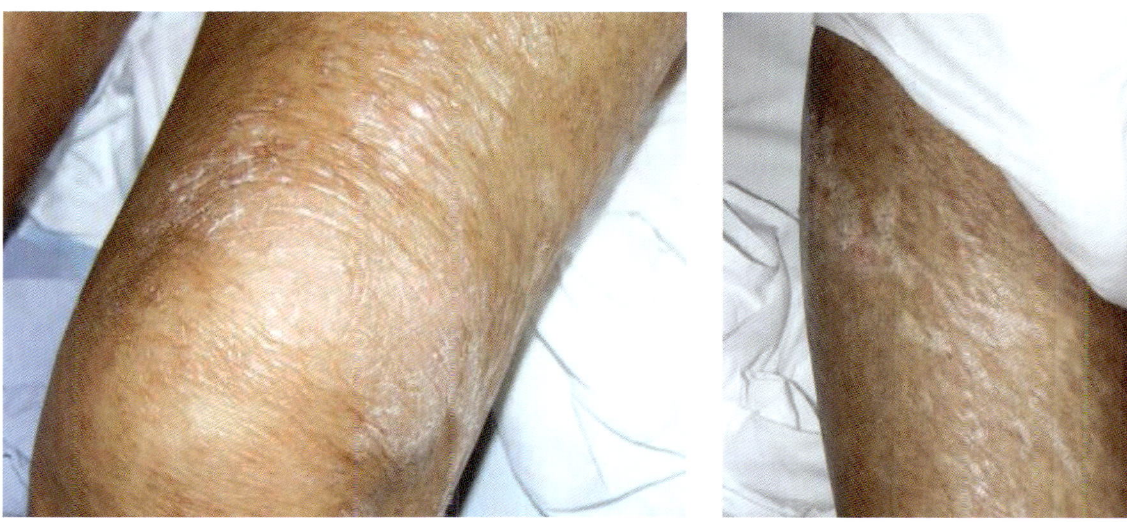

Figure 10.6 Epidermal GVHD characterized by psoriasiform changes with scaly plaques on the extensor surface of the lower limb.

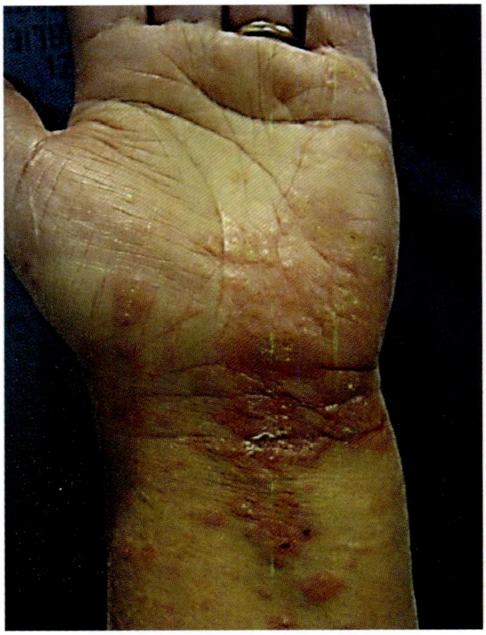

Figure 10.7 Epidermal GVHD may be indistinguishable from classical lichen planus.

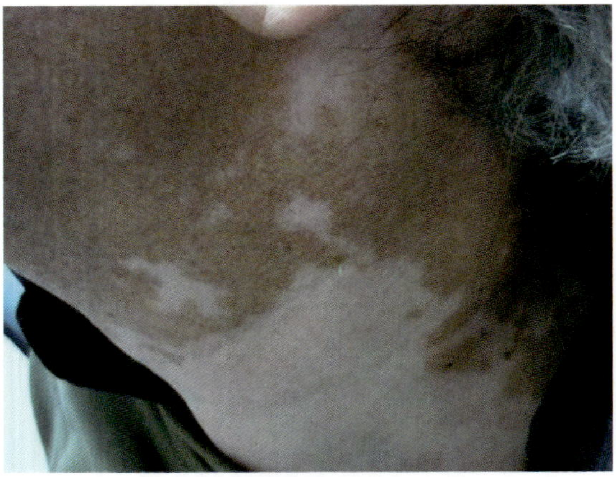

Figure 10.8 Epidermal GVHD characterized by a hypopigmented macula of the neck resembling vitiligo.

Erythrodermic cGVHD is typically preceded by papulosquamous, morbilliform, or annular eruptions.

Acral involvement is often observed in patients with cGVHD, with eczema-like lesions of the hands and/or feet (Figure 10.12), sometimes associated with erythema-

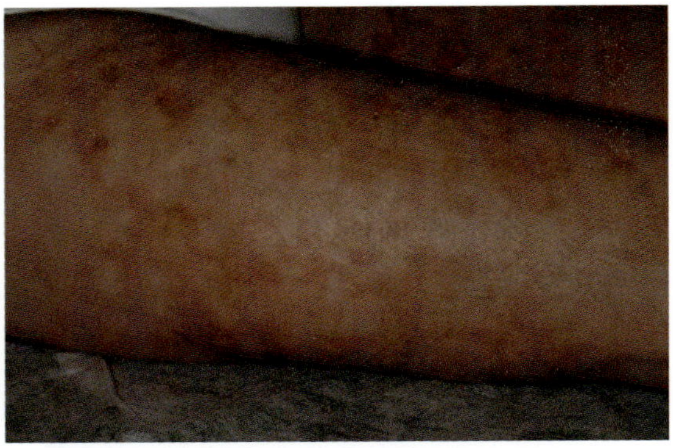

Figure 10.9 Epidermal GVHDcharacterized by diffuse hyperpigmentations of the lower limb with livedoid pattern of distribution.

multiforme-like lesions characterized by erosive features and fissures (Figure 10.13) and plantar hyperkeratosis (Figure 10.14) [21].

Sclerosis

Sclerotic manifestations are commonly observed during the late phase of cGVHD and may lead to a wide spectrum of clinical presentations. At the beginning the fibrotic lesions are limited to the papillary dermis, resulting in small gray–white papules and plaques, reminiscent of lichen sclerosus (Figure 10.15) [22]. The localized dermal fibrosis (commonly termed morphea) may present as nummular or irregular plaques and linear bundles associated with hypo- or hyperpigmentation (Figure 10.16).

cGVHD with morphea-like features is typically localized on previously damaged skin (Figure 10.10) sites (e.g., areas affected by varicella zoster, surgical intervention, or treated with radiotherapy) [23, 24]. Later diffuse dermal and subcutaneous sclerosis leads to hidebound induration of the skin reminiscent of systemic sclerosis (Figure 10.17).

Scarring alopecia and loss of skin appendages are frequently observed in the advanced phase of sclerotic involvement; also, nail dystrophy with thickening, ridging, onycholysis, pterygium, or complete nail loss is a common finding during the late phase of disease (Figure 10.18).

Sclerotic involvement of subcutaneous fat and fascia may be insidious, and the diagnosis may be delayed until the onset of contractures with significant motion

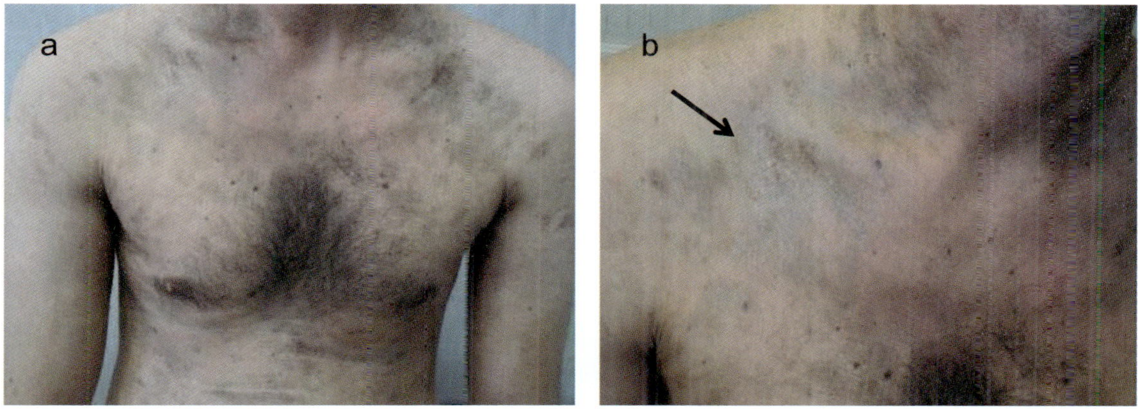

Figure 10.10 (a) Epidermal GVHD characterized by diffuse hyperpigmentation of the trunk; (b) a morphea-like plaque is located at the site of a previous indwelling venous port (black arrow).

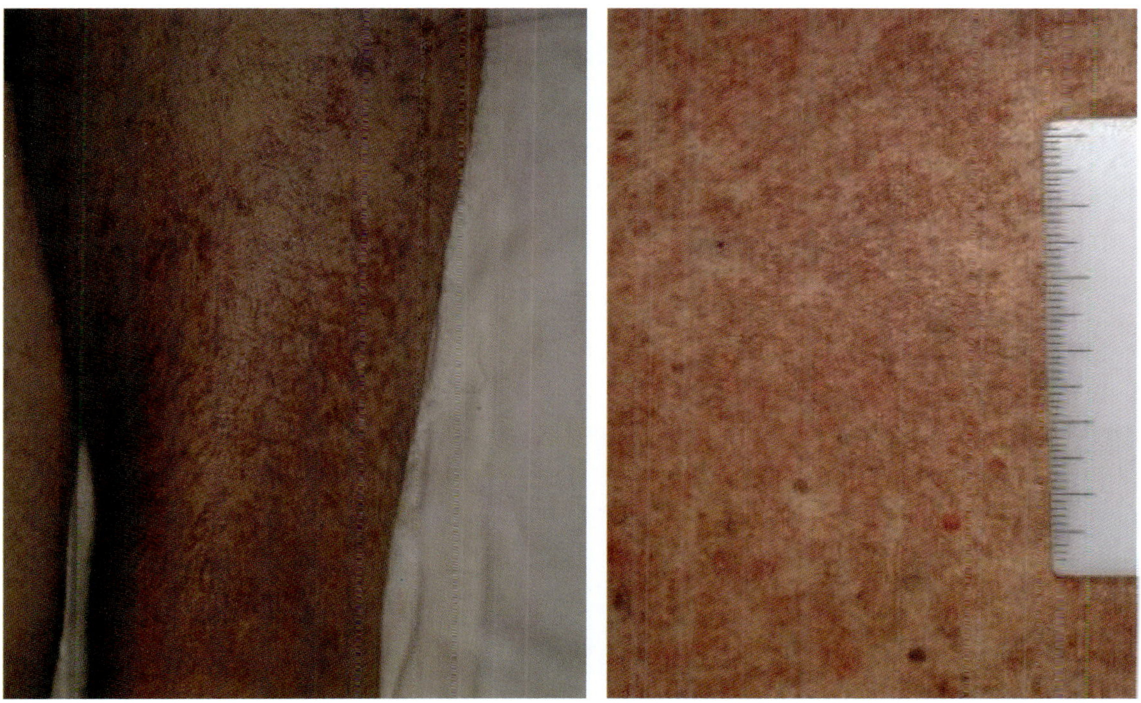

Figure 10.11 Epidermal GVHD characterized by diffuse purpuric macule of the lower limb resembling eczematous drug eruption.

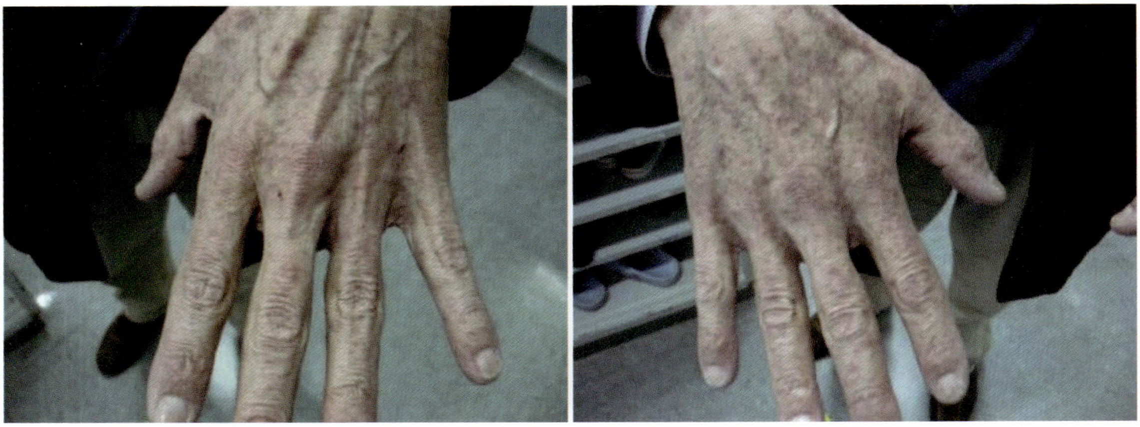

Figure 10.12 Epidermal GVHD characterized by an eczema-like eruption with papular and erythematous lesions diffused on the dorsum of the hand.

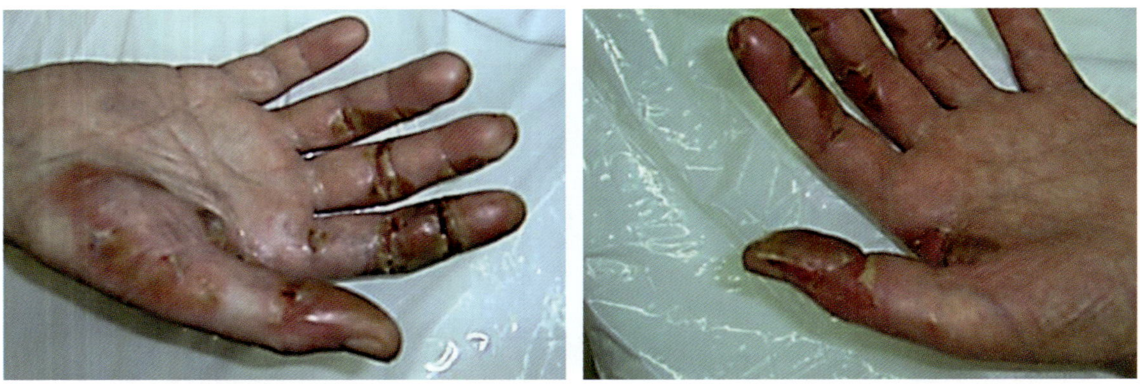

Figure 10.13 Epidermal GVHD characterized by erosive lesions and fissures of the palms.

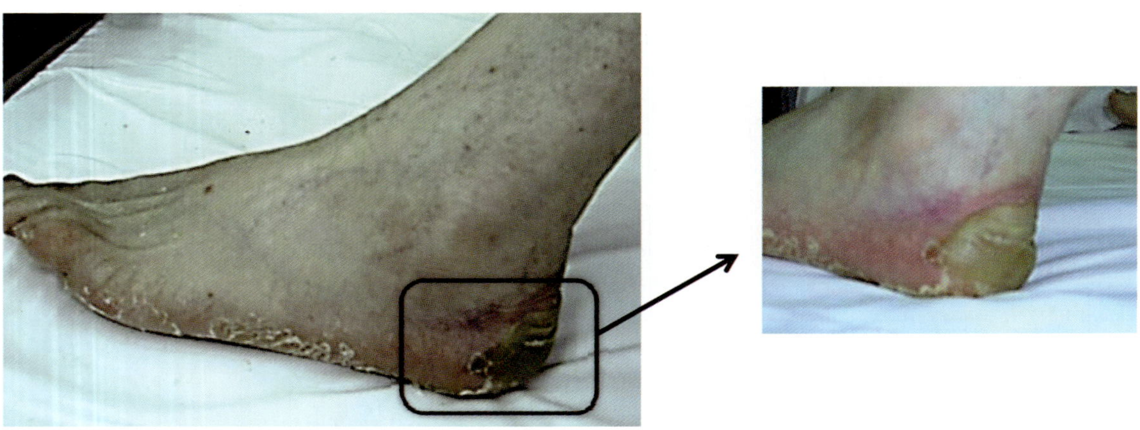

Figure 10.14 Epidermal GVHD characterized by erythema, desquamation, and plantar hyperkeratosis.

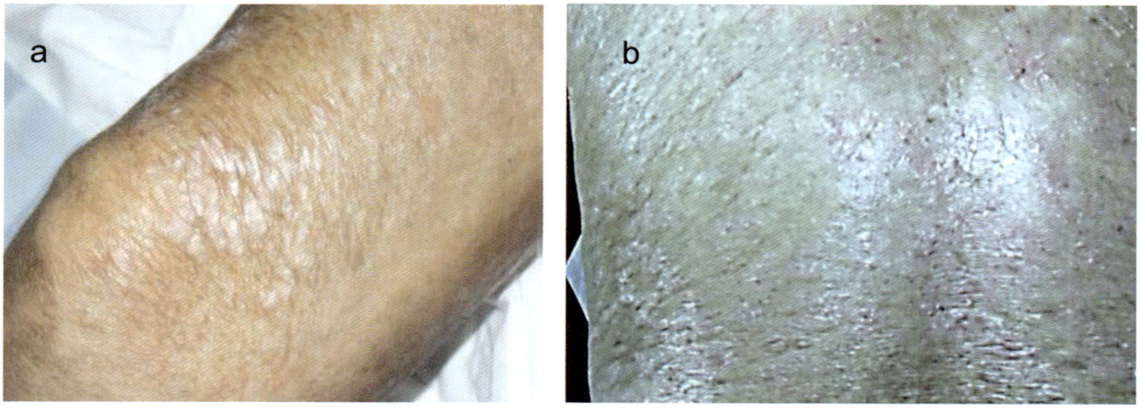

Figure 10.15 Epidermal GVHD characterized by (a) whitish papules or (b) diffuse hypopigmented and scaly plaques reminiscent of lichen sclerosus.

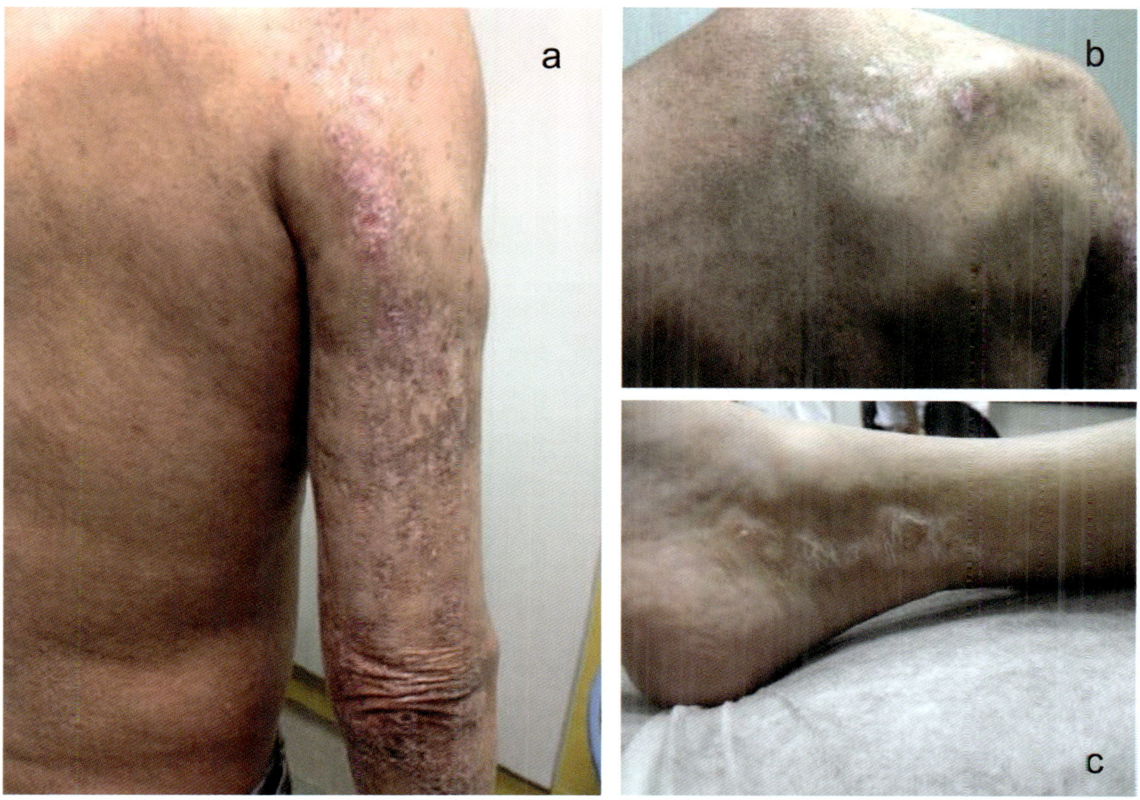

Figure 10.16 Epidermal GVHD characterized by band-like deep dermal sclerosis presenting in a linear pattern of distribution along upper limbs, shoulders, and legs.

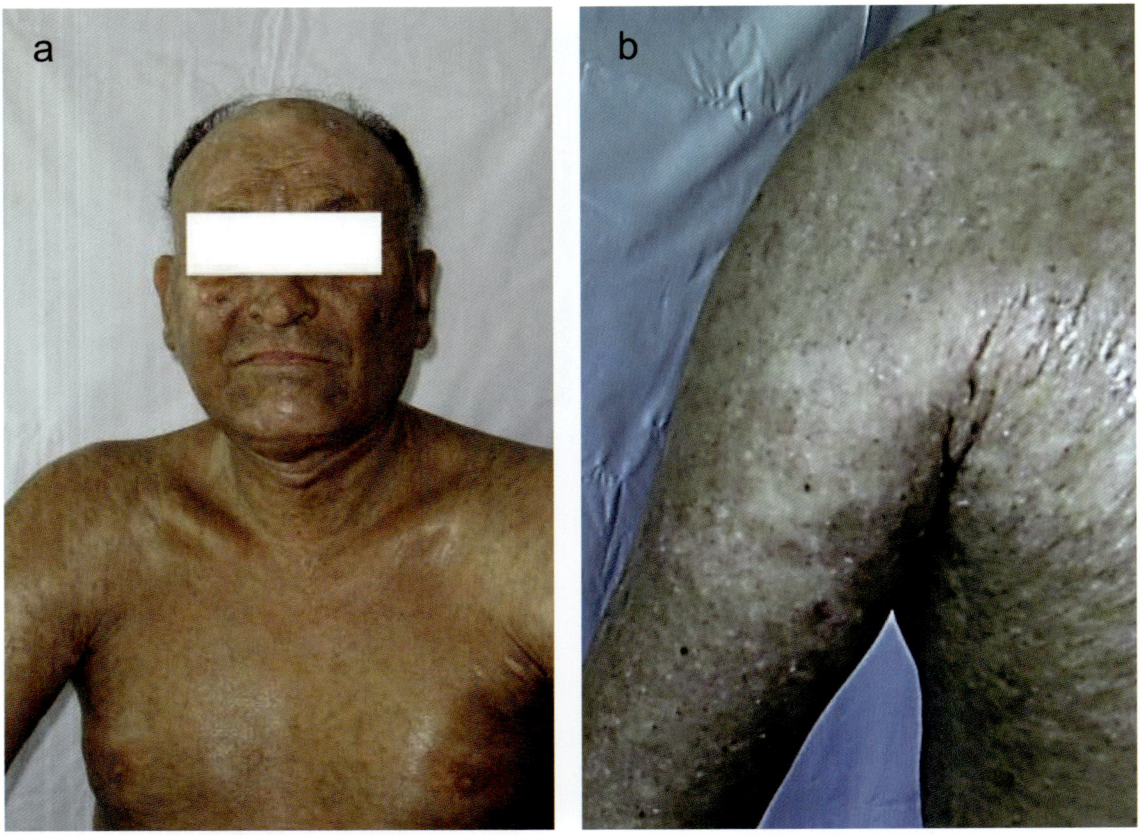

Figure 10.17 (a) Epidermal GVHD characterized by diffuse dermal and subcutaneous sclerosis leading to induration of the skin reminiscent of systemic sclerosis; (b) skin of the axillary folds appears translucent and inelastic.

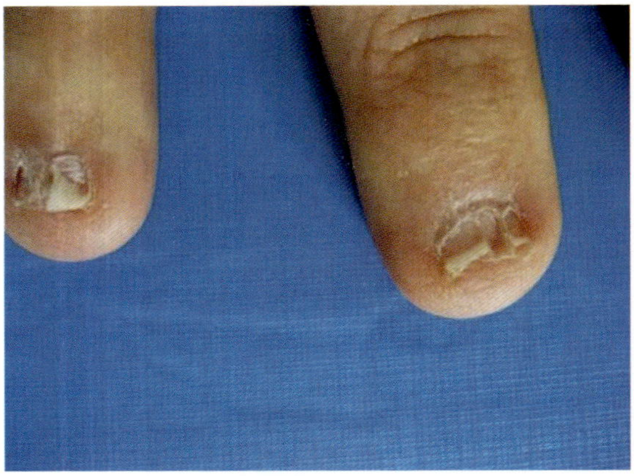

Figure 10.18 Epidermal GVHD characterized by dystrophy of the nail plate and focal pterygium.

limitations. Involvement of subcutaneous tissue typically shows as subcutaneous nodular texture, appreciable with deep palpation. Overlying hyperpigmentation with or without dermal fibrosis is common, or the overlying epidermis may appear relatively normal or with "peau d'orange" appearance, resembling eosinophilic fasciitis (Figure 10.19) [22, 25]. Chronic skin ulceration may occur in patients with long-standing sclerosis, especially in those receiving corticosteroids. Bullous lesions developing on sclerotic skin and epidermal atrophy are often complicated by local infections.

Additional signs and symptoms of evolving sclerotic disease include widespread calcinosis [26], acral edema, muscle weakness, and cramping [27].

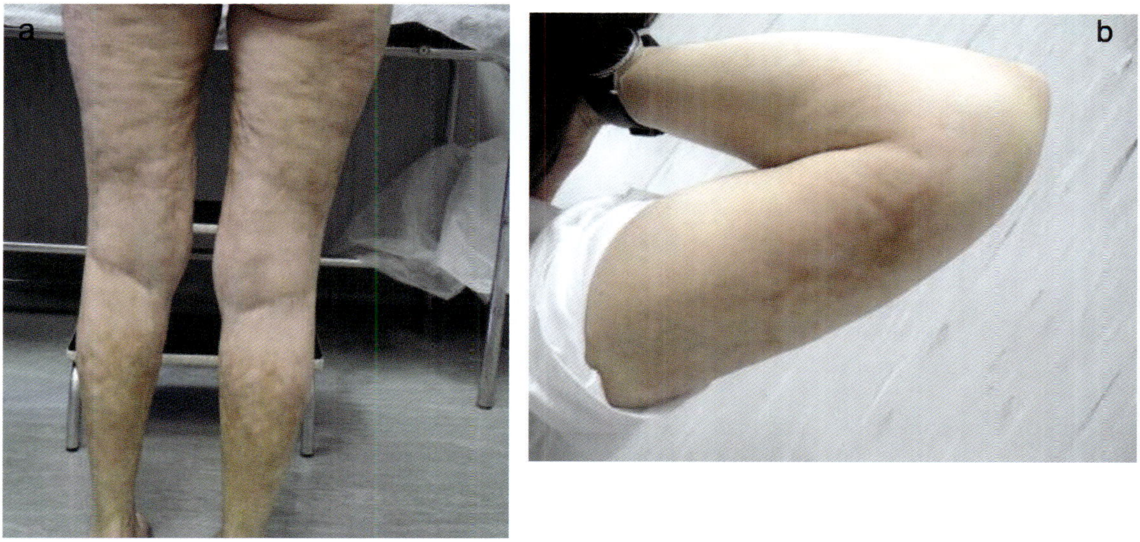

Figure 10.19 (a) Epidermal GVHD characterized by diffuse dermal fibrosis and the overlying epidermis with "peau d'orange" appearance, resembling eosinophilic fasciitis; (b) rippling and "cellulite" appearance in the axillae produced by subcutaneous septal fibrosis.

Sometimes it may be clinically difficult to differentiate edema associated with sclerotic skin involvement from drug-induced edema (e.g., sirolimus or imatinib). In these patients the limited motion ability is common and may be consequent to several causes, not mutually exclusive: weakness or muscle pain may be associated with myositis or myasthenia gravis (sometimes observed in cGVHD); a decreased range of motion may be secondary to pain, due to avascular necrosis, or chronic neuropathy.

In some situations, such as the absence of overt signs of dermal or fascial involvement, magnetic resonance imaging may be helpful [8, 9].

In a relevant proportion of patients with skin cGVHD, a concomitant visceral involvement (especially lung or esophagus), myalgias, and eosinophilia have been reported [28].

Mucous membranes are affected in most patients with cutaneous cGVHD [29], resulting in mucosal thickening (Figure 10.20) or punctate erosions, oral pain, and sicca syndrome, greatly interfering with nutrition and quality of life.

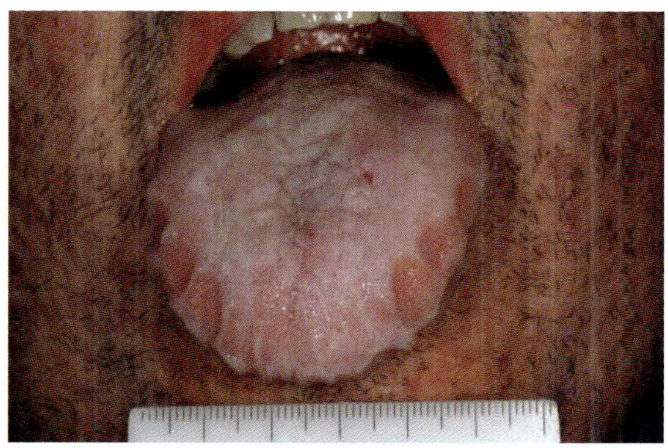

Figure 10.20 Epidermal GVHD characterized by thickening of the mucosa of the tongue.

The involvement of genital mucosa affects sexuality and the overall quality of life [30]. Vaginal GVHD develops later, with dryness, erosions, ulcerated or thickened mucosa, frequent vaginal infections, and symptoms of dyspareunia [31]. Similarly, phimosis may occur in males.

Pathogenesis

At least four different hypotheses regarding the pathogenesis of cGVHD have emerged:

• Hypothesis 1 postulates that cGVHD results from thymic damage, caused by acute GVHD, resulting in failure to delete T cells, recognizing antigens on donor or recipient cells [32].

• Hypothesis 2 implicates a central role for fibrogenic cytokines, such as transforming growth factor beta (TGF-β) and platelet-derived growth factor (PDGF), especially in the pathogenesis of fibrotic damage in the course of cGVHD.

• Hypothesis 3 implicates B cells and antibody-mediated mechanisms.

• Hypothesis 4 has recently invoked deficiency in the numbers or function of regulatory T (Treg) cells.

These four hypotheses are not mutually exclusive.

Animal models of cGVHD

Mouse models of cGVHD are generated by grafting donor bone marrow cells into a recipient that has the same major histocompatibility complex haplotype but comes from a different strain [33, 34]. Several current mouse models of cGVHD are characterized by a sclerodermatous phenotype [32, 35]. However, only specific combinations of donor/recipient strain result in this particular form of cGVHD; notably, simply swapping donor/recipient strain or minimally altering this combination may lead to a different model of murine cGVHD (i.e., lupus-like, antibody-mediated cGVHD) or even acute GVHD. Thus, the antigens and the kind of immune response are likely to participate to determine the clinical phenotype as well [35, 36]. These mouse models have contributed to elucidate several pathophysiological aspects of human cGVHD, but differences exist: in humans, cGVHD usually develops slowly and in patients pretreated with immunosuppressive agents as prophylaxis and/or therapy for acute GVHD; therefore, we cannot exclude the impact of either GVHD prophylaxis and/or subclinical acute GVHD on the subsequent development of cGVHD in humans [37]. As an example, early prophylactic use of corticosteroids in humans has been associated with increased risk of cGVHD.

In a classic model of sclerodermatous cGVHD, BALB/c (H-2d) mice are lethally irradiated and grafted with B10. D2 (H-2d) bone marrow and spleen cells across minor histocompatibility loci. In this model, skin and lung fibrosis is prominent and rapidly progressive; cytotoxic injury to epithelia is minimal and there is no evidence for vascular injury or autoantibodies at early time points. At the molecular level, fibrosis may be driven by infiltrating, TGF-β-producing mononuclear cells, preceding the upregulation of collagen mRNA and protein synthesis [38].

Pathogenetic pathways involved in cGVHD

Three pivotal actors have been studied in the development of cGVHD: T cells, B cells, and profibrotic-inflammatory cytokines.

Donor T cells are necessary for cGVHD [39], and T cell reactions are directly proportional to the grade of human leukocyte antigen mismatch. According to this view, cGVHD can be considered a chronic immune response, driven by persistent stimulation by recipient alloantigens, as may occur in autoimmune disorders, with emergence of autoreactive T cell clone [40]. Loss of tolerance may be sustained by autoreactive $CD4^+$ lymphocytes, which are necessary for maintaining and amplifying the autoimmune reactions [41]. A dysfunction of central tolerance has been theorized, based on the evidence of thymic damage, caused by a combination of preparatory regimens, acute GVHD, and older age [42–44].

Disturbances in the mechanisms of peripheral tolerance have also been invoked. Treg cells have been extensively investigated as potential actors involved in cGVHD, with contradictory findings: a positive correlation between high numbers of circulating $FOXP3^+CD4^+CD25^{hi}$ Treg cells and reduced GVHD incidence has been found in some studies [45, 46], whereas other studies showed inverse correlation [47, 48].

B cells can also contribute to cGVHD through their ability to present alloantigens and produce autoantibodies [49]. Antibody-mediated mechanisms are thought to account for at least some of the clinical manifestations of cGVHD. A wide variety of autoantibodies have been described in cGVHD, many of which are present in rheumatologic conditions [50]. Indeed, clinical responses, observed with B-cell depletion with rituximab (RTX), support the pathogenic role of B cells in cGVHD (see next paragraph). B cells can also work as antigen-presenting cells (APCs), and either donor or host APCs have been implicated in the initiation of skin cGVHD,

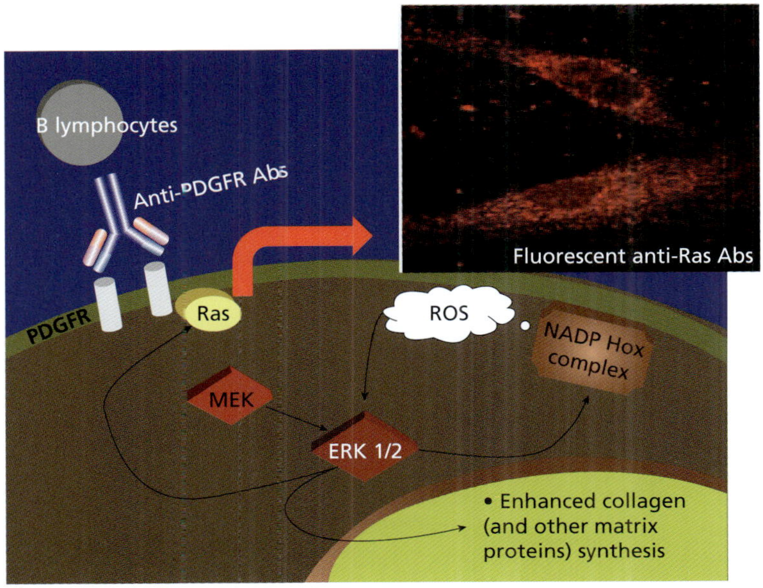

Figure 10.21 PDGF is involved in inflammatory and fibrotic processes in SSc and cGVHD; this cytokine can increase the levels of Ras proteins in human fibroblasts. Stimulating anti-PDGF-R antibodies activates Ras (see upper right: murine fibroblasts, transduced with human PDGF-R and previously incubated with purified immunoglobulins from patients with ScGVHD, show increased expression of Ras) and induces high ROS levels by activating the ERK 1/2 system and the nicotinamide adenine dinucleotide phosphate oxidase (NADPHox) cascade. Moreover, the continuous activation of ERK stabilizes Ha-Ras protein by inhibiting proteasomal degradation. This signaling cascade stimulated collagen synthesis, DNA damage, and accelerated senescence. In scleroderma and cGVHD fibroblasts this loop may be amplified. It is possible to interrupt this loop by blocking RAS farnesylation by PDGF-R inhibition or by using oxidant scavengers as N-acetylcisteine (NAC) or specific inhibitors of this pathway, restoring the normal fibroblast phenotype.

while donor APCs seem to play a dominant role in intestinal cGVHD [51].

Profibrotic cytokines have also been implicated in the pathogenetic mechanisms of fibrotic diseases such as ScGVHD and systemic sclerosis (SSc); SSc is an autoimmune disease characterized by chronic inflammation and fibrosis of the target organs [52]. Many similarities in the clinical picture and pathological description have been noticed between cGVHD and SSc, and several lines of evidence point to a pivotal role of TGF-β in the development of fibrotic changes [38]. Administration of anti-TGF-β antibodies reduced cell infiltrate and reversed skin and lung fibrosis in a mouse model of ScGVHD. Besides TGF-β, PDGF has also been recognized as a pivotal player of fibrotic damage both in SSc and in cGVHD.

Patients with ScGVHD and SSc have stimulatory autoantibodies targeting the PDGF receptor (PDGF-R) and primary fibroblasts from SSc and cGVHD patients, were found to express abnormally high levels of Ha-Ras. Upon engagement of PDGF-R, these antibodies activate a downstream signaling cascade involving Ha-Ras, extracellular-signal-regulated kinases 1 and 2 (ERK 1/2), and reactive oxygen species (ROS). High levels of ROS maintain Ha-Ras upregulated, further perpetuating this loop, leading to increased collagen gene expression and acquisition of the myofibroblast phenotype (Figure 10.21) [53, 54]. Taken together, these data point to a direct involvement of the PDGF pathway in fibrosis and argue for a common pathogenic trait in cGVHD and SSc phenotypes.

Finally, the strongest evidence for the contribution of both cytokines (TGF-β and PDGF) to the development of fibrosis in cGVHD comes from the successful application of a targeted therapy able to inhibit both pathways. Treatment with imatinib, as detailed later in this chapter, has demonstrated substantial efficacy in reducing the

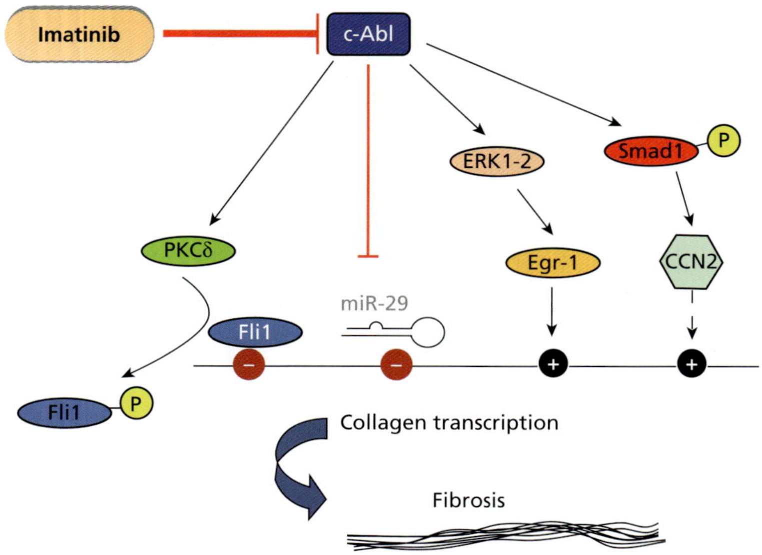

Figure 10.22 Main mechanisms generating the antifibrotic effect of imatinib: c-Abl, the original target of imatinib, is involved in several molecular pathways leading to fibrogenesis. Interference of tyrosine-kinase inhibitor with other molecules involved in fibrotic pathways (PDGFR, Src kinases) are discussed in the text.

fibrotic burden in refractory and resistant ScGVHD. As a broad-spectrum tyrosine-kinase inhibitor, imatinib has several pleiotropic anti-inflammatory and antifibrotic effects (Figure 10.22). However, *in vitro* and *in vivo* studies have clarified that a major antifibrotic role is exerted through the blockade of the PDGF receptor and the intracellular tyrosine kinase c-Abl, which is a key component of the noncanonical TGF-β pathway [55, 56].

Biomarkers

The main risk factors, predictive of poor outcome, in patients with cGVHD are represented by a platelet count <100 000 mm [3], a systemic ScGVHD pattern, and lung involvement, but there are no specific biomarkers for the diagnosis of cGVHD. Recently, several biomarkers have been proposed in cGVHD, not only with the aim of anticipating the diagnosis, but also of monitoring disease activity and response to treatment. The NIH defined a biomarker as "a biological characteristic that can be objectively measured *in vivo*, and evaluated as an indicator of normal or pathogenic processes or responses to a therapeutic intervention" [57].

Among the possible candidates, the imbalance of immune cell populations has been largely investigated and many alterations have been associated with cGVHD: presence of alloreactive helper and cytotoxic T cells, autoreactive T cells [40, 41] or imbalance of helper T cell type 1/cytotoxic T cell type 1 (Th1/Tc1) and helper T cell type 2/cytotoxic T cell type 2 (Th2/Tc2) populations, with an aberrant pattern of interferon (IFN) production, without interleukin-2 production.

cGVHD has also been associated with increased proportions of CD8-cells lacking CD28 [42] and a decreased proportion of natural killer cells in the blood. Some groups have shown that clinical improvement during extracorporeal photopheresis (ECP) occurred more frequently among patients with clonal T-cell receptor rearrangements than among those who had not had such rearrangements [58]. These findings are useful to better understand the immune deregulation and the relationship with the clinical outcome in cGVHD; nevertheless, none of them can be proposed as a diagnostic or prognostic tool in the clinical management of these patients.

Among the cytokines involved in cGVHD symptoms, high concentrations of TGF-β have been associated with ScGVHD, whereas high concentrations tumor necrosis factor (TNF) are associated with fatigue and wasting. An increased expression of IFN-γ-secreting T cells has been reported in skin biopsy specimens from patients with cutaneous cGVHD [59]. The presence of autoantibodies against cytoskeletal proteins (tubulin, actin, myosin) also suggested a role for donor Th2 cells in humans [60]. Stimulating anti-PDGF-R antibodies have been invoked as biomarker of cGVHD, but the functional test reported for the detection is not suitable for clinical use and the preliminary data in cGVHD patients are ambiguous [61, 62].

Although some autoantibodies in cGVHD often lack the specificity seen in classic autoimmune disease, their presence has been proposed to indicate an increased risk of developing extensive ScGVHD. In a study by Patriarca et al. [63] the incidence of ANAs was 70% in patients with limited chronic disease and 94% of patients with extensive chronic disease, compared with 23% of patients who did not develop cGVHD. However, in a large multivariate analysis of 206 patients (including 109 with sclerotic skin disease), ANAs were not associated with risk of skin fibrosis. In this population, composed primarily of patients with severe or treatment-refractory disease, ScGVHD was associated with elevated platelet count ($P < 0.001$) and elevated complement fraction C3 ($P < 0.001$) [4].

Among the nonimmune biomarkers, eosinophilia has often been associated with cGVHD, but it does not carry any prognostic relevance. Other nonimmune biomarkers of cGVHD, such as von Willebrand factor and thrombomodulin, have also been identified as correlating with endothelial damage [64], but the clinical usefulness of these markers, as well the immune biomarkers, has to be proven (Table 10.3).

Table 10.3 Main biomarkers proposed for anticipating the onset of cGVHD and for monitoring the response to treatment

Proposed biomarkers for cGVHD
Soluble markers
Serum BAFF levels [63, 65, 66]
Anti-ds DNA [67]
Anti-PDGF receptor antibodies [54, 61]
Lymphocyte subpopulations
Naive B cells and transitional B cells [63, 68–70]
T regulatory cells [45–48]
Gene-expression profile of lymphocyte subpopulations
In T regulatory cells [71, 72]
In T lymphocytes and in monocytes [73]
In mononuclear cells [74]
Nonimmune biomarkers
Thrombomodulin and von Willebrand factor [64]
Eosinophilia [75]

Histopathology

In the past, cGVHD has traditionally been divided into two major forms: lichen-planus-like and sclerodermiform types. However, it has now become clear that the histopathological picture is far more variable, with possible coexistence of epidermal and dermal alterations and overlap with changes commonly observed in acute GVHD. In addition, histopathological alterations of cutaneous cGVHD evolve over time and are modified by immunosuppressive treatment.

Lichenoid cGVHD

Histopathologically, the interface alterations in lichenoid cGVHD are more prominent than those detected in early acute GVHD. Lichenoid cGVHD shows epidermal hyperplasia, hyperkeratosis, hypergranulosis, and diffuse vacuolar degeneration of the basal cell layer, with numerous apoptotic keratinocytes (usually greater than five apoptotic bodies per section from a 4 mm punch biopsy); nevertheless, the NIH consensus group has suggested that keratinocyte apoptosis without other cGVHD features in day 80 to 100 screening skin biopsy samples does not indicate cGVHD [76]. Such changes are similar to those observed in idiopathic lichen planus. However, focal parakeratosis (associated with clinically evident scaling) can be seen in lichenoid cGVHD, a finding which is hardly ever found in lichen planus. Variable satellitosis may be appreciated and vacuolar changes and dyskeratosis may also be seen in the adnexal epithelia (so-called cytotoxic infundibulitis and/or acrosyringitis). There is a band-like mainly lymphoid infiltrate that obscures that dermo-epidermal junction (Figure 10.23a and b). A sparse to moderate lymphoid infiltrate, with plasma cells, can also be present around eccrine coils. Although the presence of rare eosinophils does not rule out per se a diagnosis of GVHD, their presence, especially in high numbers, is generally more indicative of drug reactions rather than cGVHD.

Sclerodermiform cGVHD

Some histologic features of sclerotic alterations in cGVHD resemble both SSc and, less commonly, morphea, suggesting that c-GVHD and SSc may share common fibrotic mechanisms. It has reported that intimal hyperplasia was present in small and large vessels of both SSc and c-GVHD biopsies and focal capillary proliferation occurs in early c-GVHD. In contrast, loss of canonical

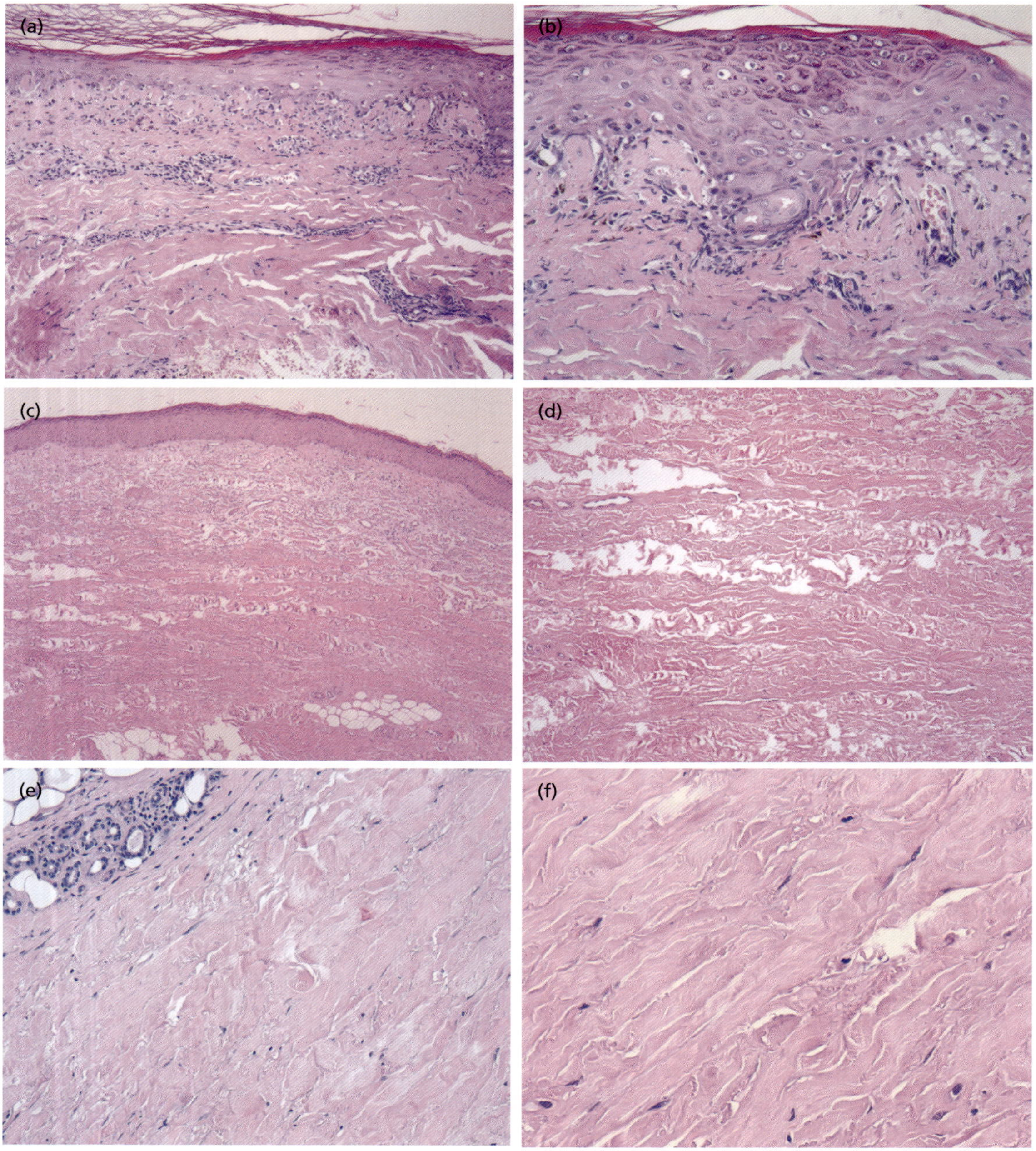

Figure 10.23 (a) Lichenoid cutaneous cGvHD: irregular acantosis and a lichenoid infiltrate obscuring the dermo-epidermal junction; note that there is also dermal fibrosis. (b) Prominent hyperkeratosis, hypergranulosis, and vacuolar basal degeneration with numerous apoptotic keratinocytes. (c) Late sclerodermatous cGVHD: epidermal atrophy; the dermis is diffusely sclerotic.; (d) Absence of adnexal structures; collagen fibers in the reticular dermis appear thickened and homogenized. (e) A deeper biopsy in the subcutaneous septa shows thickening and fibrosis. (f) Collagen bundles appear homogeneously thickened; note the absence of significant inflammation.

endothelial markers and dermal capillaries is seen in SSc but not in c-GVHD [77]. In cGVHD, epidermal alterations often precede the occurrence of dermal sclerotic changes, but some patients develop diffuse dermal sclerosis without an apparent inflammatory lichenoid phase.

Serial biopsies show top-down progression of the fibrosis from the papillary dermis downward, consistent with a pathogenesis related to inflammation and cytokines release.

The suggested minimal criterion for the diagnosis of cutaneous sclerotic cGVHD is represented by sclerosis of papillary dermis or reticular dermis.

The tissue remodeling progresses from loss of the rete ridges to widening of the dermal papillae and discrete superficial fibrosis of the papillary and adventitial dermis. Subsequently, the reticular dermis becomes homogeneneously thickened, and eventually the dermal subcutaneous border becomes straightened with septal fibrosis in the subcutaneous fat. Adnexal structures are frequently atrophic or completely absent (Figure 10.23c and d).

When the sclerotic changes involve deep dermis and subcutaneous structures the picture resembles morphea and systemic sclerosis (Figure 10.23e and f). In the early phases, sclerodermoid changes may be associated with a lymphoplasmacellular infiltrate in the perivascular and interstitial reticular dermis, while in late advanced stages there is no significant dermal inflammation. The epidermis may have minimal apoptosis or vacuolar changes.

Eosinophilic fasciitis

Sclerosis may also extend to the muscular fascia resembling eosinophilic fasciitis. Eosinophilic fasciitis of the skin presents with an acute painful deep groove, or rippling cellulite appearance. A deep incisional biopsy shows edema and fibrosis of the fascia and subcutaneous septae with a mixed infiltrate of lymphocytes, histiocytes, and eosinophils. The infiltration may extend from the fascia into the muscle interstitium.

A lichen sclerosis atrophicus type of cGVHD leads to scarring and stricture when it affects the female genitalia. Histologically, there is epidermal atrophy with vacuolar changes, prominent subepidermal edema with a zone of pale homogenized collagen, a band-like lymphocytic infiltrate. The presence of lichen sclerosus, morphea, septal fibrosis, and fasciitis suggests that the sclerosis can start at and affect any level of the skin.

In cGVHD, full-thickness skin biopsies allow one to accurately assess tissue changes in the eccrine units, subcutaneous fat, and fascia, and to estimate the degree of dermal fibrosis.

NIH pathology consensus

Shulman et al. for the NIH [76] produced a consensus document for pathologists and clinicians about the interpretation of biopsy results in cGVHD. In that document the specific requirements for the diagnosis of skin cGVHD were reported (Table 10.4). The same document recommends, for a final diagnosis, one of the following statements:

1 no GVHD
2 possible GVHD
3 consistent with GVHD (synonymous with probable, favor, or suggestive)
4 GVHD (with no equivocation).

Today, there is a general agreement about the policy of performing a skin biopsy to confirm the initial diagnosis of cGVHD, although a minority of centers do not routinely perform skin biopsy before starting treatment; moreover, the role of histology to assess the response to treatment is still debated. Therefore, the decision to treat cGVHD today, is not based on the histologic criteria, but is established according to the overall clinical assessment.

Clinical management of skin cGVHD

Once diagnosis of GVHD is established, the first step, before starting any treatment, is to distinguish

- classic cGVHD from
- late acute GVHD or
- an overlap syndrome.

The diagnosis of overlap syndrome is based on the simultaneous presence of symptoms of acute GVHD and distinctive or diagnostic features of cGVHD. The diagnosis of classic cGVHD requires the presence of either diagnostic or distinctive symptoms of cGVHD in the absence of features of acute GVHD. As the skin cGVHD is the most common manifestation of cGVHD, and it is often associated with multiorgan involvement, it is crucial to distinguish the different forms of skin cGVHD, not only based on the presence of extensive skin disease (≥50% body surface), but also according to the cGVHD NIH

Table 10.4 Specific histologic criteria for diagnosis of cutaneous cGVHD (modified from Shulman et al. [76])

Organ or system	Minimal criteria for active GVHD	Specific histologic criteria for cGVHD
Skin, any stage	Apoptoses in epidermal basal layer or lower malphigian layer or outer root sheath of hair follicle or acrosyringium ± lichenoid inflammation ± vacuolar change ± lymphocytic satellitosis	
Skin lichen-planus-like		Combination of epidermal orthorkeratosis, hypergranulosis, and acanthosis with lichenoid changes ± syringitis of eccrine units ± panniculitis
Skin sclerotic		Collagenous deposition with thickening throughout the papillary dermis, or pan-dermal collagenosis ± panniculitis
Skin morpheic		Clinically focal or localized lesion predominated by sclerosis in the lower reticular dermis or along the dermal–hypodermal border ± epidermal and appendigeal involvement
Skin fasciitis		Fibrous thickening of fascial septa with adjacent inflammation ± panniculitis

severity score, as reported by the NIH consensus for GVHD [3, 78].

The use of quantifiable and reproducible measurement tools for skin manifestations of cGVHD is crucial for the successful assessment and documentation of therapeutic response.

Several instruments have been proposed for this purpose. Greinix et al. performed a prospective study using a total skin score (TSS) to evaluate cutaneous involvement of cGVHD. TSS combines percentage of involved BSA divided into 10 separate anatomic regions with manifestations of cGVHD coded from 0 (normal skin) to 4 (hidebound skin, unmovable sclerosis) [79]; a modified TSS (Figure 10.24) has also been used in patients with ScGVHD, treated with imatinib [80].

Recently, Jacobsohn reported a prospective multicenter validation of the NIH composite skin score in 458 cGVHD patients. Assessment of the extent and severity of skin involvement using the NIH composite skin score correlated well with severity of symptoms. The same NIH composite skin score also correlated with survival. Worsening in NIH skin score at 6 months was associated with higher mortality, compared with stable NIH skin score, suggesting that this tool could serve as a short-term surrogate end point that predicts for long-term success or failure of experimental drug therapies [17].

Patients with ScGVHD can be eligible for different treatments according to factors such as clinical presentation of cGVHD, other concomitant anatomical localizations, extent of BSA involved, and the severity of cGVHD; schematically, we can make a distinction between topical and systemic therapy, and between primary and secondary therapy of skin cGVHD.

Topical therapy

The topical therapy approach (Table 10.5) plays an important role in alleviating symptoms and treating complications caused by loss of skin integrity and immunosuppression. In the absence of poor prognostic factors, topical agents can serve as the primary treatment for cutaneous cGVHD, but also in moderate and severe cGVHD topical immunosuppression may be added to increase, or accelerate, local response rates. Topical treatment of cutaneous manifestations of cGVHD may be the only treatment given or may be applied in addition to systemic immunosuppression to speed up response or to spare systemic immunosuppression (particularly steroids). Although *topical steroids* are standard of care in numerous skin diseases, they have not been systematically evaluated in cutaneous manifestations of cGVHD. Nonsclerotic skin lesions without erosions or ulcerations (lichen-planus-like or papulosquamous plaques) may

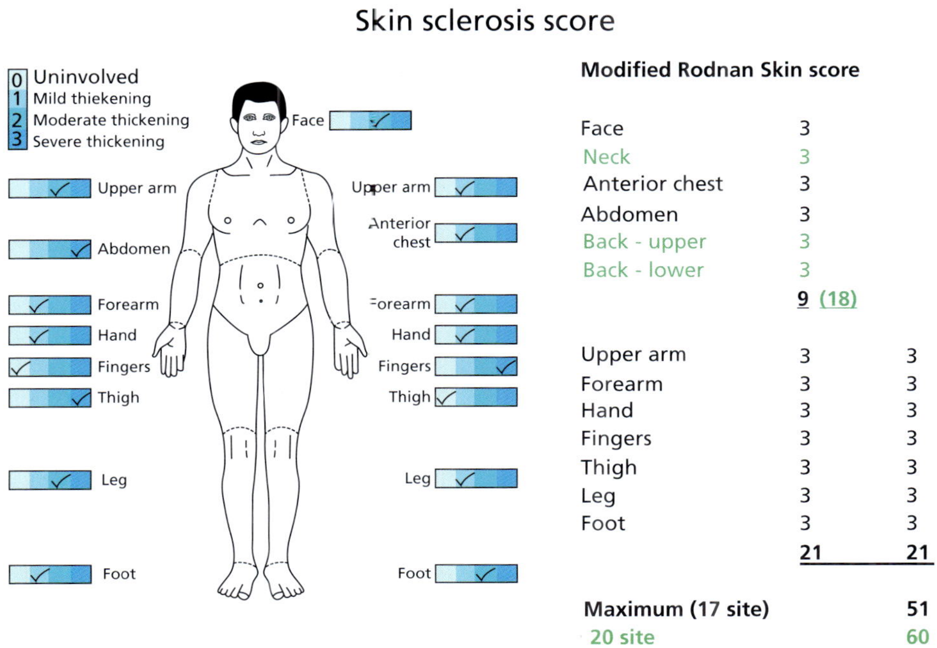

Figure 10.24 Skin sclerosis calculated in the different body area districts in SS. The modified Rodnan skin score utilizes 20 body sites for the measurement of the skin thickness and the maximum score is 60. This score has been utilizied for evaluating skin response in 19 cGVHD patients treated with imatinib [80]. (This research was originally published in *Blood*. Olivieri A, Locatelli F, Zecca M, et al. Imatinib for refractory chronic graft-versus-host disease with fibrotic features. Blood. 2009;114(3):709–718. © the American Society of Hematology.)

Table 10.5 Main topical treatments utilized for skin cGVHD

Topical treatment	Toxicity	Specific indications
Topical steroids [81, 82]	Skin atrophy	Neck down: mid-strength steroids; if no response, higher strength steroids; face: hydrocortisone 1%
Tacrolimus/pimecrolimus [83–85, 104]	Long-term risk for cutaneous malignancies	Should be given twice daily
PUVA [89–94]	Phototoxicity, risk for cutaneous malignancies	Should not be used with phototoxic medication
UVA [95, 105–107]	Phototoxicity, risk for cutaneous malignancies	Requires no UV protection after treatment, should not be used with phototoxic medication
UVB [108]	Phototoxicity, risk for cutaneous malignancies	Only effective in lichenoid cGVHD

respond well to topical steroids and emollients, but long-term use of topical steroids may be complicated by local skin atrophy.

General guidelines regarding topical steroid recommendations for skin GVHD have been extensively reported by Couriel et al. [81] and by Wolff et al. [82]. Alternative *non-steroid topical agents* include tacrolimus [83, 84] and pimecrolimus [85], which achieved encouraging results in small series. Topical calcineurin inhibitors may be useful for sites at high risk of skin atrophy, particularly the lips and intertriginous surfaces, but are poorly tolerated in areas very strongly involved and characterized by loss of integrity of the skin with fissures formations.

Phototherapy of skin lesions may be another example of topical immunosuppression added to systemic treatment. Extensive experience with ultraviolet light phototherapy for the treatment of several inflammatory dermatoses [86, 87] prompted the use of psoralen plus ultraviolet A (PUVA) phototherapy to treat lichen-planus-like cutaneous GVHD [20, 88].

Psoralen is given orally 2 h before UVA exposure at a dose of 0.6–0.8 mg/kg. Alternatively, it may be applied topically. Treatment is given typically on 3–4 days per week with increasing dosage; frequency is then reduced once a stable response is achieved. PUVA has been evaluated in cutaneous manifestations of cGVHD in several retrospective and prospective studies with good clinical response [89–94]. PUVA is generally well tolerated with a high response rate in the skin and mild side effects. UVA1, emitting exclusively in the longwave UVA range (UVA1: 340–400 nm), is a well-established treatment in sclerosing skin diseases and has also been used in skin cGVHD. The advantage of high-dose UVA1 is the avoidance of a photosensitizer without need for UV protection and no systemic side effects associated with the latter [95]. Narrow-band UVB (311 nm) and broad-band UVB (280–320 nm) are increasingly used in the treatment of dermatologic diseases, including cutaneous manifestations of cGVHD. In contrast to UVA1 and PUVA, UVB does not reach the dermal layer involved in ScGVHD. UVB is typically given three to five times per week, and the only short-term risk is phototoxicity, especially when patients are taking photosensitizing drugs.

The potential benefit of phototherapy must be weighed against the elevated risk of cutaneous malignancy in cGVHD patients, particularly those with actinic damage or a history of ionizing radiation. Indeed, the prolonged immunosuppression in these patients increases the risk of secondary malignancies of the skin, including non-melanoma skin cancer [96–99].

Voriconazole, which is commonly used to prevent and treat invasive fungal infections in these patients, is associated with phototoxicity and may predispose susceptible individuals to squamous cell carcinoma [100, 101] and melanoma [102].

Superficial skin erosions at sites of recurrent minor trauma can be treated with protective film coverings. Full-thickness wounds overlying sclerotic skin are often slow to heal, but may respond to topical wound adjuvants, including hyaluronic acid, collagen, fibroblast, keratinocyte, and PDGF products. Hyperbaric oxygen therapy has been used for scleroderma-related ulceration [103].

Other potential causes of skin breakdown, as an alternative to cGVHD involvement, include vasculitis, bullous drug reaction, chronic neuropathy, and cutaneous malignancy; all these causes should be excluded if wounds are not responding to appropriate treatment.

Systemic treatment

In general, systemic immunosuppressive treatment is not needed for patients with mild manifestations of cGVHD involving a single organ, unless adverse risk factors (platelet count <100 000/μL; treatment with prednisone, antecedent acute GVHD, and hyperbilirubinemia) at onset are present.

Mild manifestations of cutaneous cGVHD that need more than a topical treatment, such as fasciitis, may be treated with systemic corticosteroids alone.

Systemic treatment is mandatory for patients with more severe manifestations, especially when multiple sites are involved. Survival at 5 years among patients with "standard-risk" cGVHD is approximately 70%, and is 50% in those with "high-risk" features of thrombocytopenia or antecedent acute GVHD [109, 110]. Conventionally, those patients who have at least three organs involved by cGVHD, or more than 50% of skin involvement (in terms of BSA), or developing cGVHD while taking >0.5 mg/kg of steroids, should be considered for initiation of systemic therapy with prednisone 1 mg/kg per day, for at least 8 weeks. A similar approach is generally recommended for patients with systemic ScGVHD.

Steroids

Systemic glucocorticoids represents the standard *primary treatment for cGVHD*. Combinations of prednisone with a calcineurin inhibitor, such as cyclosporine A or tacrolimus, have been used [82]. Initial doses of 1.0 mg/kg of prednisone per day have been recommended, followed by tapering over a period of several months. Unfortunately, long-term treatment with high-dose prednisone is associated with a high risk of complications and considerable morbidity.

Steroid-sparing treatments would be of enormous benefit for patients with cGVHD, both as a first-line and as a second-line therapy, provided that the net effect between the reduction achieved in glucocorticoid-related toxicity and the adverse effects of the new regimen is advantageous.

Despite several treatment options, very few agents have consistently demonstrated a steroid-sparing effect in patients with cGVHD [111]. Recently ECP, RTX, and imatinib have showed a steroid-sparing effect, but only ECP has been tested in a randomized trial [112, 113].

Steroid refractory cGvHD

While primary treatment of cGVHD is based on controlled trials, evidence for the *secondary management of steroid refractory cGVHD* is limited to phase II trials or retrospective studies. Therefore, it is not surprising that still there is no standard approach for steroid refractory cGVHD [82]. In addition, a standard definition of steroid refractory cGVHD is not available. Generally, accepted criteria for steroid refractory cGVHD include one of the following: cGVHD progression despite treatment with 1 mg/kg per day of prednisone for ≥2 weeks; or no improvement after 4–8 weeks on prednisone 0.5 mg/kg per day; or inability to taper below 0.5 mg/kg per day of prednisone [114].

A number of phase II trials of secondary agents have been published, reporting encouraging response rates. The most promising results have been achieved with RTX [112, 115–123], ECP [113, 124], pentostatin [125], and imatinib [80]. However, most trials are difficult to evaluate as they are based on few patients, with heterogeneous organ involvement and advanced phases of organ manifestations [126–133].

In many studies on second-line treatment of cGVHD, ECP and drugs like mycophenolate and sirolimus were combined with continuous steroid administration. Thus, the contribution of steroids to the reported response rates in these studies remains uncertain. A detailed report of the most significant trials in steroid-refractory cGVHD is reported in Table 10.6, but the most promising results have been reported with ECP, RTX, imatinib, and pentostatin.

Extracorporeal photopheresis

ECP is the process of leukapheresis, followed by *ex vivo* photoactivation with 8-methoxypsoralen and UVA and reinfusion of the buffy coat. Although the mechanism of action of ECP in the treatment of cGVHD is not fully understood, some immune mechanisms of action of ECP are nowadays better characterized. Several clinical and experimental data suggest that ECP basically exerts an immunomodulatory activity, by inducing two main events: PUVA-related massive apoptosis of T lymphocytes and differentiation of monocytes into active dendritic APCs. Moreover, ECP inhibits pro-inflammatory cytokine production and increases anti-inflammatory cytokine production [134–136]. Finally, ECP effectively reduces the stimulation of effector T cells and induces donor-derived Treg cells [137, 138], suggesting that these cells could represent an important immune mediator of cGVHD [139].

Since the initial report by Owisanowski et al. in 1994 of the first case of cGVHD successfully treated with ECP [140], several additional reports and observational studies of ECP treatment in patients with cGVHD have demonstrated that this approach is well tolerated and associated with beneficial treatment effects in multiple organ systems, including ScGVHD [141]. Curiel et al. [124] reported a 59% response rate in 71 patients with skin cGVHD, and 42% of these responses were observed in patients with ScGVHD. More recently, a randomized study in the setting of secondary treatment has formally demonstrated the superiority of ECP, compared with standard therapy alone, in patients with refractory skin cGVHD [113]. The primary efficacy end point was quantitative comparison of percentage change from baseline in TSS of 10 body regions at week 12. Ninety-five patients were randomized to either ECP and standard therapy or standard therapy alone, and ECP was administered three times during week 1 and then twice weekly during weeks 2 through 12.

The median percentage improvement in TSS at week 12 was 14.5% for the ECP arm and 8.5% for the control arm ($P = 0.48$). The proportion of patients who had at least a 50% reduction in steroid dose and at least a 25% decrease from baseline in TSS was 8.3% in the ECP arm at week 12 and 0% in the control arm ($P = 0.04$). The investigator assessment of skin complete or partial responses revealed a significant improvement in favor of ECP ($P < 0.001$), suggesting that ECP is an effective treatment for steroid refractory or steroid-dependent skin cGVHD. However, ECP is a time-consuming procedure that requires a dedicated apheresis center, which is not available in all medical facilities. Treatment is commonly administered on two consecutive days each week for 2–3

Table 10.6 Main clinical options for steroid-refractory cGVHD

Second-line treatment	Response rate (patient number *N*)	Organ-specific (response rate *n*)	Main side effects	References
Mycophenolate mofetil	46–75% (*N* = 21–26)	Skin 53% (*n* = 15) Mouth 67% (*n* = 15) Liver 54 % (*n* = 13)	GI disturbances (diarrhea, nausea, vomiting)	[126, 132, 133]
High-dose cortico-steroids	48% major responses (*N* = 56)	Not reported	Infections, diabetes decompensation, psychological effects (psychosis, insomnia)	[131]
Extracorporeal photopheresis	61% (*N* = 71)	Skin 40% (*n* = 48 + 17) Sclerotic skin 67% (*n* = 21) Mouth 77% (*n* = 7) Eye 64% (*n* = 4) Lung 54% (*n* = 6)	Anemia, requirement for central IV access	[113, 124]
Pentostatin	53% major responses plus 2% minor responses (*N* = 58)	Lichenoid skin 69% (*n* = 39) Sclerotic skin, fascial, mouth 52–57% (*n* = 39)	Nausea, vomiting, infection, renal dysfunction, rash, headache	[125]
Tacrolimus	46% (*N* = 26)	Not reported	Renal dysfunction, thrombotic microangiopathy, neurotoxicity, hypertension	[126]
Rituximab	Metanalysis of seven studies: OR: 66%; CI: 57–74% (*N* = 111)	Skin 60% (*n* = 67) Oral mucosa 36% (*n* = 46) Liver 29% (*n* = 34) Lung 30% (*n* = 14)	Infusion reactions, infections, hepatitis reactivation	[112, 115–123]
Sirolimus	63–94% (*N* = 16–35)	Skin 65% (*n* = 29) Mouth 75% (*n* = 8) Liver 33% (*n* = 6) Eye 64% (*n* = 11) GI 67% (*n* = 6)	Hypertrigliceridemia, renal insufficiency, cytopenias, infections	[128, 129]

CI: confidence interval; IV: intravenous; GI: gastrointestinal; OR: odds ratio.

months, followed by a subsequent taper schedule, with the patient continually reevaluated throughout the therapeutic course [12]. Adverse effects are usually sporadic and mild, including fluid shifts and blood pressure issues. Serious adverse events, such as thrombosis and infection, may occur if a central venous catheter is required for apheresis access.

Rituximab

Evidence that donor B cells play a role in the development of cGVHD in humans led to several trials with RTX, a monoclonal antibody specific for CD20, in steroid-refractory cGVHD [49, 68]. B-cell depletion with RTX has been successful in steroid-refractory cGVHD, showing response rates of 43–80%. In a retrospective GITMO study, RTX was effective in over 50% of 38 patients with refractory cGVHD, with 76% 2-year overall survival. RTX was administered at 375 mg/day every week, for at least four doses [121]. However, the nature of B-cell contribution, as well as to what extent B-cell depletion can restore physiological conditions, has so far not been clarified. Recently, imbalances in B-cell homeostasis have been suggested to identify patients *a priori* with a higher chance of response to RTX treatment [142]. The durability of clinical responses to RTX in patients with cGVHD remains unclear. In patients with autoimmune diseases, initial clinical responses to RTX are inevitably followed by clinical relapse in the majority of patients. Because increased plasma B-cell-activating factor of the tumor necrosis factor family (BAFF) levels are found in patients with autoimmune disease after RTX treatment, concern has been raised that high BAFF in this setting may contribute to clinical relapse [143–146].

Tyrosine kinase inhibitors

Two prospective studies and some retrospective data suggest that imatinib can be useful in cGVHD. We conducted a prospective study in 19, with steroid-refractory cGvHD, with fibrotic features, who received a low-dose imatinib for at least 6 months. All patients had a long history of cGVHD with multiorgan involvement, including skin (17 had scleroderma skin features), lung, and sicca syndrome, and were heavily pretreated.

The overall response rate after 6 months of treatment was 79%, with seven complete responses and eight partial responses. Imatinib allowed the discontinuation or significantly tapered steroid therapy in 10/19 patients. The recently updated outcome of these patients suggests a long-term benefit in terms of overall survival [62] (Figure 10.25).

A similar retrospective study confirmed the activity of imatinib in 14 patients with heavily pretreated refractory fibrotic cGVHD. Imatinib was administered for a median of 6 months. Overall, seven patients responded to imatinib, with four patients improving the Rodnan skin score; also in this series, imatinib therapy allowed for a significant reduction of corticosteroid dosage [147].

Mammalian target of rapamycin inhibitors

Sirolimus and everolimus inhibit T cells via the mammalian target of rapamycin (mTOR) pathway. In addition, mTOR inhibition has been shown to decrease collagen mRNA stability and inhibit platelet-derived and fibroblast growth factors [148]. Animal studies suggest that sirolimus promotes the development and maintenance of Treg cells; therefore, there is considerable interest in this class of agents in cGVHD. A recent retrospective study in patients with ScGVHD found a 76% response rate with either sirolimus or evorolimus given in combination with corticosteroids [149]. These results were comparable to retrospective studies describing a response rate ranging from 63% to 81% [129, 150].

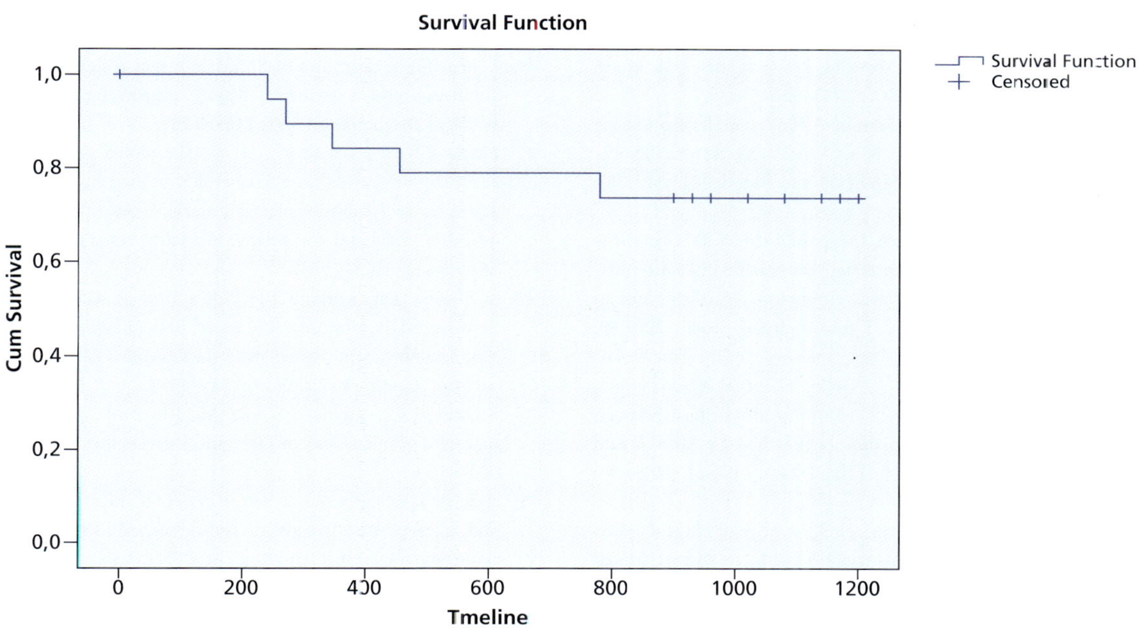

Figure 10.25 Updated overall survival in 19 patients receiving imatinib for steroid-refractory cGVHD [62].

Conclusions

In conclusion, cutaneous cGVHD is a frequent and debilitating complication of allogeneic stem cell transplants. Risk factors such as the combined use of TBI and unmodified peripheral blood cells suggest that ScGVHD is the result of a complex cascade of events, initiating with tissue damage (radiation or high-dose chemotherapy), proceeding with early alloantigen recognition by donor T cells, and culminating in chronic T/B cells activation, production of autoantibodies, and extensive sclerosis of the skin. Once a patient has reached this point, the quality of life is greatly reduced. Early diagnosis, appropriate therapy, and most of all prospective clinical trials are required to better monitor and treat this serious complication.

References

1. Socié G, Veum Stone J, Wingard JR, et al. Long-term survival and late deaths after allogeneic bone marrow transplantation. N Engl J Med. 1999;341:14–21.
2. Vogelsang GB. How I treat chronic graft-versus-host disease. Blood. 2001;97(5):1196–1201.
3. Filipovich AH, Weisdorf D, Pavletic S, et al. National Institutes of Health Consensus Development Project on criteria for clinical trials in chronic graft-versus-host disease: I. Diagnosis and staging working group report. Biol Blood Marrow Transplant. 2005;11:945–956.
4. Martires KJ, Baird K, Steinberg SM, et al. Sclerotic-type chronic GVHD of the skin: clinical risk factors, laboratory markers, and burden of disease. Blood. 2011;118(15): 4250–4257.
5. Ferrara GB, Bacigalupo A, Lamparelli T, et al. Bone marrow transplantation from unrelated donors: the impact of mismatches with substitutions at position 116 of the human leukocyte antigen class I heavy chain. Blood. 2001;98: 3150–3155.
6. Prasad VK, Kernan NA, Heller G, et al. DNA typing for HLA-A and HLA-B identifies disparities between patients and unrelated donors matched by HLA-A and HLA-B serology and HLA-DRB1. Blood. 1999;93: 399–409.
7. Lee SJ, Klein JP, Barrett AJ, et al. Severity of chronic graft-versus-host disease: association with treatment-related mortality and relapse. Blood. 2002;100:406–414.
8. Hymes SR, Alousi AM, Cowen EW. Graft-versus-host disease. Part I. Pathogenesis and clinical manifestations of graft-versus-host disease. J Am Acad Dermatol. 2012;66: 515.e1–515.e18.
9. Hymes SR, Alousi AM, Cowen EW. Graft-versus-host disease. Part II. Management of cutaneous graft-versus-host disease. J Am Acad Dermatol. 2012;66:535.e1–535.e16.
10. Skert C, Patriarca F, Sperotto A, et al. Sclerodermatous chronic graft-versus-host disease after allogeneic hematopoietic stem cell transplantation: incidence, predictors and outcome. Haematologica. 2006;91:258–261.
11. Vassallo C, Brazzelli V, Zecca M, et al. Isomorphic cutaneous graft-versus-host disease reaction after ultraviolet exposure: clinical, histological and direct immunofluorescence studies of four allo-transplanted patients. J Eur Acad Dermatol Venereol. 2009;23:913–918.
12. Pavletic SZ, Martin P, Lee SJ, et al. Measuring therapeutic response in chronic graft-versus-host disease: National Institutes of Health Consensus Development Project on Criteria for Clinical Trials in Chronic Graft-versus-Host Disease: IV. Response Criteria Working Group report. Biol Blood Marrow Transplant. 2006;12:252–266.
13. Hymes SR, Turner ML, Champlin RE, Couriel DR. Cutaneous manifestations of chronic graft versus host disease. Biol Blood Marrow Transplant. 2006;12(11):1101–1113.
14. Ahn HS, Park HJ, Lee JY, Cho BK. A case of chronic cutaneous graft versus host disease with the clinical features of exfoliative dermatitis. Ann Dermatol. 2009;21:319–322.
15. Creamer D, Martyn-Simmons CL, Osborne G, et al. Eczematoid graft-vs-host disease: a novel form of chronic cutaneous graft-vs-host disease and its response to psoralen UV-A therapy. Arch Dermatol. 2007;143:1157–1162.
16. Matsushita T, Hasegawa M, Shirasaki F, et al. A case of acute cutaneous graft-versus-host disease mimicking psoriasis vulgaris. Dermatology. 2008;216:64–67.
17. Pidala J, Kim J, Anasetti C, et al. The global severity of chronic graft-versus-host disease, determined by National Institutes of Health consensus criteria, is associated with overall survival and non-relapse mortality. Haematologica. 2011;96(11):1678–1684.
18. Jacobsohn DA, Kurland BF, Pidala J, et al. Correlation between NIH composite skin score, patient-reported skin score, and outcome: results from the Chronic GVHD Consortium. Blood. 2012;120(13):2545–2552.
19. Schauder CS, Hymes SR, Rapini RP, Zipf TF. Vesicular graft-versus-host disease. Int J Dermatol. 1992;31: 509–510.
20. Aractingi S, Janin A, Devergie A, et al. Histochemical and ultrastructural study of diffuse melanoderma after bone marrow transplantation. Br J Dermatol. 1996;134: 325–331.
21. Kossard S, Ma DD. Acral keratotic graft versus host disease simulating warts. Australas J Dermatol. 1999;40:161–163.

22. Schaffer JV, McNiff JM, Seropian S, et al. Lichen sclerosus and eosinophilic fasciitis as manifestations of chronic graft-versus-host disease: expanding the sclerodermoid spectrum. J Am Acad Dermatol. 2005;53:91–601.
23. Chosidow O, Bagot M, Vernant JP, et al. Sclerodermatous chronic graft-versus-host disease. Analysis of seven cases. J Am Acad Dermatol. 1992;26:49–55.
24. Martires K, Baird K, Citrin D, et al. Localization of sclerotic-type chronic graft-versus-host disease to sites of skin injury: potential insight into the mechanism of isomorphic and isotopic responses. Arch Dermatol. 2011;147:1081–1086.
25. Patel AR, Avila D, Malech HL, et al. Rippled skin, fasciitis, and joint contractures. J Am Acad Dermatol. 2008;59:1070–1074.
26. Man J, Kalisiak M, Birchall IW, Salopek TG. Chronic cutaneous graft-versus-host disease manifesting as calcinosis cutis universalis on a background of widespread sclerodermatoid changes. J Cutan Med Surg. 2010;14:249–253.
27. Carroll CB, Hilton DA, Hamon M, Zajicek JP. Muscle cramps and weakness secondary to graft versus host disease fasciitis. Eur J Neurol. 2005;12:320–322.
28. Janin A, Socié G, Devergie A, et al. Fasciitis in chronic graft-versus-host disease: a clinicopathologic study of 14 cases. Ann Intern Med. 1994;120:993–998.
29. Sullivan KM, Shulman HM, Storb R, et al. Chronic graft-versus-host disease in 52 patients: adverse natural course and successful treatment with combination immunosuppression. Blood. 1981;57:267–276.
30. Spinelli S, Chiodi S, Costantini S, et al. Female genital tract graft-versus-host disease following allogeneic bone marrow transplantation. Haematologica. 2003;88:1163–1168.
31. Spiryda LB, Laufer MR, Soiffer RJ, Antin JA. Graft-versus-host disease of the vulva and/or vagina: diagnosis and treatment. Biol Blood Marrow Transplant. 2003;9:760–765.
32. Sakoda Y, Hashimoto D, Asakura S, et al. Donor-derived thymic-dependent T cells cause chronic graft-versus-host disease. Blood. 2007;109(4):1756–1764. Epub 2006 Oct 10.
33. Martin PJ. Biology of chronic graft-versus-host disease: implications for a future therapeutic approach. Keio J Med. 2008;57(4):177–183.
34. Olivieri J, Coluzzi S, Attolico I, Olivieri A. Tirosin kinase inhibitors in chronic graft versus host disease: from bench to bedside. Sci World J. 2011;11:1908–1931.
35. Chu YW, Gress RE. Murine models of chronic graft-versus-host disease: insights and unresolved issues. Biol Blood Marrow Transplant. 2008;14(4):365–378.
36. Schroeder MA, DiPersio JF. Mouse models of graft-versus-host disease: advances and limitations. Dis Model Mech. 2011;4:318–333.
37. Toubai T, Sun Y, Reddy P. GVHD pathophysiology: is acute different from chronic? Best Pract Res Clin Haematol. 2008;21(2):101–117.
38. McCormick LL, Zhang Y, Tootell E, Gilliam AC. Anti-TGF-beta treatment prevents skin and lung fibrosis in murine sclerodermatous graft-versus-host disease: a model for human scleroderma. J Immunol. 1999;163(10):5693–5699.
39. Korngold R, Sprent J. Lethal graft versus host disease after bone marrow transplantation across minor histocompatibility barriers in mice. Prevention by removing mature T cells from marrow. J Exp Med. 1978;148(6):1687–1698.
40. Tyndall A, Dazzi F. Chronic GVHD as an autoimmune disease. Best Pract Res Clin Haematol. 2008;21(2):281–289.
41. Rozendaal L, Pals ST, Gleichmann E, Melief CJM. Persistence of allospecific helper T cells is required for maintaining autoantibody formation in lupus-like graft-versus-host disease. Clin Exp Immunol. 1990;82(3):527–532.
42. Fukushi N, Arase H, Wang B, et al. Thymus: a direct target tissue in graft-versus-host reaction after allogeneic bone marrow transplantation that results in abrogation of induction of self-tolerance. Proc Natl Acad Sci U S A. 1990;87(16):6301–6305.
43. Ghayur T, Seemayer TA, Xenocostas A, Lapp WS. Complete sequential regeneration of graft-vs.-host-induced severely dysplastic thymuses. Implications for the pathogenesis of chronic graft-vs.-host disease. Am J Pathol. 1988;133(1):39–46.
44. Krenger W, Holländer GA. The immunopathology of thymic GVHD. Semin Immunopathol. 2008;30(4):439–456.
45. Rezvani K, Mielke S, Ahmadzadeh M, et al. High donor FOXP3-positive regulatory T-cell (Treg) content is associated with a low risk of GVHD following HLA-matched allogeneic SCT. Blood. 2006;108(4):1291–1297.
46. Zorn E, Kim HT, Lee SJ, et al. Reduced frequency of FOXP3[+] CD4[+]CD25[+] regulatory T cells in patients with chronic graft-versus-host disease. Blood. 2005;106(8):2903–2911.
47. Miura Y, Thoburn CJ, Bright EC, et al. Association of *Foxp3* regulatory gene expression with graft-versus-host disease. Blood. 2004;104(7):2187–2193.
48. Clark FJ, Gregg R, Piper K, et al. Chronic graft-versus-host disease is associated with increased numbers of peripheral blood CD4[+]CD25high regulatory T cells. Blood. 2004;103(6):2410–2416.
49. Shimabukuro-Vornhagen A, Hallek MJ, Storb RF, von Bergwelt-Baildon MS. The role of B cells in the pathogenesis of graft-versus-host disease. Blood. 2009;114(24):4919–4927.

50. Kapur R, Ebeling S, Hagenbeek A. B-cell involvement in chronic graft-versus-host disease. Haematologica. 2008; 93(11):1702–1711.
51. Anderson BE, McNiff JM, Jain D, Blazar BR, Shlomchik WD, Shlomchik MJ. Distinct roles for donor- and host-derived antigen-presenting cells and costimulatory molecules in murine chronic graft-versus-host disease: requirements depend on target organ. Blood. 2005; 105:2227–2234.
52. Gabrielli A, Avvedimento EV, Krieg T. Scleroderma. N Engl J Med. 2009;360(19):1989–2003.
53. Baroni SS, Santillo M, Bevilacqua F, et al. Stimulatory autoantibodies to the PDGF receptor in systemic sclerosis. N Engl J Med. 2006;354(25):2667–2676.
54. Svegliati S, Olivieri A, Campelli N, et al. Stimulatory autoantibodies to PDGF receptor in patients with extensive chronic graft-versus-host disease. Blood. 2007;110(1): 237–241.
55. Distler JHW, Jungel A, Huber LC, et al. Imatinib mesylate reduces production of extracellular matrix and prevents development of experimental dermal fibrosis. Arthritis Rheum. 2007;56(1):311–322.
56. Zerr P, Distler A, Palumbo-Zerr K, et al. Combined inhibition of c-Abl and PDGF receptors for prevention and treatment of murine sclerodermatous chronic graft-versus-host disease. Am J Pathol. 2012;181(5).
57. Schultz KR, Miklos DB, Fowler D, et al. Toward biomarkers for chronic graft-versus-host disease: National Institutes of Health Consensus Development Project on Criteria for Clinical Trials in Chronic Graft-versus-Host Disease: III. Biomarker Working Group Report. Biol Blood Marrow Transplant. 2006;12:126–137.
58. French LE, Alcindor T, Shapiro M, et al. Identification of amplified clonal T cell populations in the blood of patients with chronic graft-versus-host disease: positive correlation with response to photopheresis. Bone Marrow Transplant. 2002;30:509–515.
59. Tanaka J, Imamura M, Kasai M, et al. The important balance between cytokines derived from type 1 and type 2 helper T cells in the control of graft-vs-host disease. Bone Marrow Transplant. 1997;19:571–576.
60. Tanaka J, Imamura M, Kasai M, et al. Cytokine gene expression by concanavalin A-stimulated peripheral mononuclear cell after bone marrow transplantation, an indicator of immunological abnormality due to chronic graft-vs-host disease. Bone Marrow Transpl. 1994;14:695–701.
61. Chen GL, Arai S, Flowers MED, et al. A phase 1 study of imatinib for corticosteroid-dependent/refractory chronic graft-versus-host disease: response does not correlate with anti-PDGFRA antibodies. Blood. 2011;118(15): 4070–4078.
62. Olivieri A, Cimminiello M, Locatelli F, et al. Imatinib is safe and effective in patients with refractory chronic graft versus host disease: analysis of two consecutive prospective GITMO* studies. *Gruppo Italiano Trapianto Midollo Osseo. Blood. (ASH Annual Meeting Abstracts). 2010; 116:246.
63. Patriarca F, Skert C, Sperotto A, et al. The development of autoantibodies after allogeneic stem cell transplantation is related with chronic graft-vs-host disease and immune recovery. Exp Hematol. 2006;34:389–396.
64. Biedermann BC, Sahner S, Gregor M, et al. Endothelial injury mediated by cytotoxic T lymphocytes and loss of microvessels in chronic graft versus host disease. Lancet. 2002;359:2078–2083.
65. Sarantopoulos S, Stevenson KE, Kim HT, et al. High levels of B-cell activating factor in patients with active chronic graft-versus-host disease. Clin Cancer Res. 2007;13: 6107–6114.
66. Fujii H, Cuvelier G, She K, et al. Biomarkers in newly diagnosed pediatric-extensive chronic graft-versus-host disease: a report from the Children's Oncology Group. Blood. 2008;111:3276–3285.
67. Sarantopoulos S, Stevenson KE, Kim HT, et al. Altered B-cell homeostasis and excess BAFF in human chronic graft-versus-host disease. Blood. 2009;113:3865–3874.
68. Greinix HT, Pohlreich D, Kouba M, et al. Elevated numbers of immature/transitional CD21-B lymphocytes and deficiency of memory $CD27^+$ B cells identify patients with active chronic graft-versus-host disease. Biol Blood Marrow Transplant. 2008;14:208–219.
69. Sarantopoulos S, Stevenson KE, Kim HT, et al. Recovery of B-cell homeostasis after rituximab in chronic graft-versus-host disease. Blood. 2011;117:2275–2283.
70. Fedoriw Y, Samulski TD, Deal AM, et al. Decreased TdT+ bone marrow B cell precursors after allogeneic stem cell transplantation is associated with development of human chronic graft versus host disease (cGVHD). In: Rawlings DJ, Lund FE, Tangye SG, Monroe JG, (eds). B Cells: New Insights into Normal versus Dysregulated Function (D6). Keystone Symposia, Whistler, BC, ,April 12–17, 2011.
71. Ukena SN, Grosse J, Mischak-Weissinger E, et al. Acute but not chronic graft-versus-host disease is associated with a reduction of circulating $CD4^+CD25^{high}CD127^{low/-}$ regulatory T cells. Ann Hematol. 2011;90:213–218.
72. Ukena SN, Geffers R, Buchholz S, et al. Biomarkers for acute and chronic graft-versus-host disease in regulatory T cells. Transpl Immunol. 2012;27:179–183.
73. Poloni A, Sartini D, Emanuelli M, et al. Gene expression profile of cytokines in patients with chronic graft-versus-host disease after allogeneic hematopoietic stem cell

transplantation with reduced conditioning. Cytokine. 2011;53(3):376–383.

74. Lai P, Weng J, Lu Z, et al. Gene expression profiling-based identification of CD28 and PI3K as new biomarkers for chronic graft-versus-host disease. DNA Cell Biol. 2011; 30(12):1019–1025.
75. Ahmad I, Labbé AC, Chagnon M, et al. Incidence and prognostic value of eosinophilia in chronic graft-versus-host disease after nonmyeloablative hematopoietic cell transplantation. Biol Blood Marrow Transplant. 2011;17(11): 1673–1678.
76. Shulman HM, Kleiner D, Lee SJ, et al. Histopathologic diagnosis of chronic graft-versus-host disease: National Institutes of Health Consensus Development Project on Criteria for Clinical Trials in Chronic Graft-versus-Host Disease: II. Pathology Working Group Report. Biol Blood Marrow Transplant. 2006;12(1):31–47.
77. Fleming JN, Shulman HM, Nash RA, et al. Cutaneous chronic graft-versus-host disease does not have the abnormal endothelial phenotype or vascular rarefaction characteristic of systemic sclerosis. PLoS ONE. 2009 4(7):e6203. doi: 10.1371/journal.pone.0006203.
78. Arai S, Jagasia M, Storer B, et al. Global and organ-specific chronic graft-versus-host disease severity according to the 2005 NIH Consensus Criteria. Blood. 2011;118(15): 4242–4249.
79. Greinix HT, Pohlreich D, Maalouf J, et al. A single-center pilot validation study of a new chronic GVHD skin scoring system. Biol Blood Marrow Transplant. 2007;13(6): 715–723.
80. Olivieri A, Locatelli F, Zecca M, et al. Imatinib for refractory chronic graft-versus-host disease with fibrotic features. Blood. 2009;114(3):709–718.
81. Couriel D, Carpenter PA, Cutler C, Bolaños-Meade J, et al. Ancillary therapy and supportive care of chronic graft-versus-host disease: National Institutes of Health Consensus Development Project on Criteria for Clinical Trials in Chronic Graft-versus-Host Disease: V. Ancillary Therapy and Supportive Care Working Group Report. Biol Blood Marrow Transplant. 2006;12:375–396.
82. Wolff D, Gerbitz A, Ayuk F, et al. Consensus conference on clinical practice in chronic graft-versus-host disease (GVHD): first-line and topical treatment of chronic GVHD. Biol Blood Marrow Transplant. 2010;16(12): 1611–1628.
83. Elad S, Or R, Resnick I, Shapira MY. Topical tacrolimus – a novel treatment alternative for cutaneous chronic graft-versus-host disease. Transpl Int. 2003;16:665–670.
84. Choi CJ, Nghiem P. Tacrolimus ointment in the treatment of chronic cutaneous graft-vs-host disease: a case series of 18 patients. Arch Dermatol. 2001;137:1202–1206.
85. Schmook T, Kraft J, Benninghoff B, et al. Treatment of cutaneous chronic graft-versus-host disease with topical pimecrolimus. Bone Marrow Transplant. 2005;36: 87–88.
86. Ozawa M, Ferenczi K, Kikuchi T, et al. 312-nanometer ultraviolet B light (narrow-band UVB) induces apoptosis of T cells within psoriatic lesions. J Exp Med. 1999;189: 711–718.
87. Kripke ML, Morison WL, Parrish JA. Systemic suppression of contact hypersensitivity in mice by psoralen plus UVA radiation (PUVA). J Invest Dermatol. 1983;81:87–92.
88. Hymes SR, Morison WL, Farmer ER, et al. Methoxsalen and ultraviolet A radiation in treatment of chronic cutaneous graft-versus-host reaction. J Am Acad Dermatol. 1985;12:30–37.
89. Vogelsang GB, Wolff D, Altomonte V, et al. Treatment of chronic graft-versus-host disease with ultraviolet irradiation and psoralen (PUVA). Bone Marrow Transplant. 1996;17:1061–1067.
90. Leiter U, Kaskel P, Krahn G, et al. Psoralen plus ultraviolet-A-bath photochemotherapy as an adjunct treatment modality in cutaneous chronic graft versus host disease. Photodermatol Photoimmunol Photomed. 2002;18:183–190.
91. Jampel RM, Farmer ER, Vogelsang GB, et al. PUVA therapy for chronic cutaneous graft-vs-host disease. Arch Dermatol. 1991;127:1673–1678.
92. Ghoreschi K, Thomas P, Penovici M, et al. PUVA-bath photochemotherapy and isotretinoin in sclerodermatous graft-versus-host disease. Eur J Dermatol. 2008;18:667–670.
93. Eppinger T, Ehninger G, Steinert M, et al. 8-Methoxypsoralen and ultraviolet A therapy for cutaneous manifestations of graft-versus-host disease. Transplantation. 1990;50:807–811.
94. Atkinson K, Weller P, Ryman W, Biggs J. PUVA therapy for drug-resistant graft-versus-host disease. Bone Marrow Transplant. 1986;1:227–236.
95. Calzavara PP, Porta F, Izzi T, et al. Prospects for ultraviolet A1 phototherapy as a treatment for chronic cutaneous graft-versus-host disease. Haematologica. 2003;88:1169–1175.
96. Murphy GM. Ultraviolet radiation and immunosuppression. Br J Dermatol. 2009;161(Suppl 3):90–95.
97. Kolb HJ, Socié G, Duell T, et al. Malignant neoplasms in long-term survivors of bone marrow transplantation. Late Effects Working Party of the European Cooperative Group for Blood and Marrow Transplantation and the European Late Effect Project Group. Ann Intern Med. 1999;131: 738–744.
98. Andreani V, Richard MA, Blaise D, et al. Naevi in allogeneic bone marrow transplantation recipients: the effect of

graft-versus-host disease on naevi. Br J Dermatol. 2002;147: 433–441.
99. Curtis RE, Rowlings PA, Deeg HJ, et al. Solid cancers after bone marrow transplantation. N Engl J Med. 1997; 336:897–904.
100. Cowen EW, Nguyen JC, Miller DD, et al. Chronic phototoxicity and aggressive squamous cell carcinoma of the skin in children and adults during treatment with voriconazole. J Am Acad Dermatol. 2010;62:31–37.
101. Vadnerkar A, Nguyen MH, Mitsani D, et al. Voriconazole exposure and geographic location are independent risk factors for squamous cell carcinoma of the skin among lung transplant recipients. J Heart Lung Transplant. 2010;29:1240–1244.
102. Miller DD, Cowen EW, Nguyen JC, et al. Melanoma associated with long-term voriconazole therapy: a new manifestation of chronic photosensitivity. Arch Dermatol. 2010; 146:300–304.
103. Markus YM, Bell MJ, Evans AW. Ischemic scleroderma wounds successfully treated with hyperbaric oxygen therapy. J Rheumatol. 2006;33:1694–1696.
104. Ziemer M, Gruhn B, Thiele JJ, Elsner P. Treatment of extensive chronic cutaneous graft-versus-host disease in an infant with topical pimecrolimus. J Am Acad Dermatol. 2004;50:946–948.
105. Grundmann-Kollmann M, Behrens S, Gruss C, et al. Chronic sclerodermic graft-versus-host disease refractory to immunosuppressive treatment responds to UVA1 phototherapy. J Am Acad Dermatol. 2000;42(1 Pt 1):134–136.
106. Wetzig T, Sticherling M, Simon JC, et al. Medium dose long-wavelength ultraviolet A (UVA1) phototherapy for the treatment of acute and chronic graft-versus-host disease of the skin. Bone Marrow Transplant. 2005;35: 515–519.
107. Ziemer M, Thiele JJ, Gruhn B, Elsner P. Chronic cutaneous graft-versus-host disease in two children responds to UVA1 therapy: improvement of skin lesions, joint mobility, and quality of life. J Am Acad Dermatol. 2004;51:318–319.
108. Enk CD, Elad S, Vexler A, et al. Chronic graft-versus-host disease treated with UVB phototherapy. Bone Marrow Transplant. 1998;22:1179–1183.
109. Akpek G, Zahurak ML, Piantadosi S, et al. Development of a prognostic model for grading chronic graft-versus-host disease. Blood. 2001;97:1219–1226.
110. Pérez-Simón JA, Encinas C, Silva F, et al. Prognostic factors of chronic graft-versus-host disease following allogeneic peripheral blood stem cell transplantation: the National Institutes Health scale plus the type of onset can predict survival rates and the duration of immunosuppressive therapy. Biol Blood Marrow Transplant. 2008;14:1163–1171.
111. Lee SJ, Vogelsang G, Flowers MED. Chronic graft-versus-host disease. Biol Blood Marrow Transplant. 2003;9: 215–223.
112. Cutler C, Miklos D, Kim HT, et al. Rituximab for steroid-refractory chronic graft-versus-host disease. Blood. 2006;108:756–762.
113. Flowers MED, Apperley JF, Van Besien K, et al. A multicenter prospective phase 2 randomized study of extracorporeal photopheresis for treatment of chronic graft-versus-host disease. Blood. 2008;112:2667–2674.
114. Wolff D, Schleuning M, von Harsdorf S, et al. Consensus Conference on Clinical Practice in Chronic GVHD: Second-Line Treatment of Chronic Graft-versus-Host Disease. Biol Blood Marrow Transplant. 2010;17:1–17.
115. Carella AM, Biasco S, Nati S, et al. Rituximab is effective for extensive steroid-refractory chronic graft-vs.-host-disease. Leuk Lymphoma. 2007;48(3):623–624.
116. Mohty M, Marchetti N, El Cheikh J, et al. Rituximab as salvage therapy for refractory chronic GVHD. Bone Marrow Transplant. 2008;41(10):909–911.
117. Canninga-Van Dijk MR, van der Straaten HM, Fijnheer R, et al. Anti-CD20 monoclonal antibody treatment in 6 patients with therapy-refractory chronic graft-versus-host disease. Blood. 2004;104(8):2603–2606.
118. Teshima T, Nagafuji K, Henzan H, et al. Rituximab for the treatment of corticosteroid-refractory chronic graft-versus-host disease. Int J Hematol. 2009;90(2):253–260.
119. Kharfan-Dabaja MA, Mhaskar AR, Djulbegovic B, et al. Efficacy of rituximab in the setting of steroid-refractory chronic graft-versus-host disease: a systematic review and meta-analysis. Biol Blood Marrow Transplant. 2009;15(9): 1005–1013.
120. Von Bonin M, Oelschlagel U, Radke J, et al. Treatment of chronic steroid-refractory graft-versus-host disease with low-dose rituximab. Transplantation. 2008;86(6): 875–879.
121. Zaja F, Bacigalupo A, Patriarca F, et al. Treatment of refractory chronic GVHD with rituximab: a GITMO study. Bone Marrow Transplant. 2007;40(3):273–277.
122. Ratanatharathorn V, Ayash L, Reynolds C, et al. Treatment of chronic graft-versus-host disease with anti-CD20 chimeric monoclonal antibody. Biol Blood Marrow Transplant. 2003;9(8):505–511.
123. Okamoto M, Okano A, Akamatsu S, et al. Rituximab is effective for steroid-refractory sclerodermatous chronic graft-versus-host disease. Leukemia. 2006;20(1):172–173.
124. Couriel DR, Hosing C, Saliba R, et al. Extracorporeal photochemotherapy for the treatment of steroid-resistant chronic GVHD. Blood. 2006;107(8):3074–3080.
125. Jacobsohn DA, Chen AR, Zahurak M, et al. Phase II study of pentostatin in patients with corticosteroid-refractory

chronic graft-versus-host disease. J Clin Oncol. 2007; 25(27):4255–4261.

126. Mookerjee B, Altomonte V, Vogelsang G. Salvage therapy for refractory chronic graft-versus-host disease with mycophenolate mofetil and tacrolimus. Bone Marrow Transplant. 1999;24(5):517–520.
127. Greinix HT, Volc-Platzer B, Kalhs P, et al. Extracorporeal photochemotherapy in the treatment of severe steroid-refractory acute graft-versus-host disease: a pilot study. Blood. 2000;96(7):2426–2431.
128. Johnston LJ, Brown J, Shizuru JA, et al. Rapamycin (sirolimus) for treatment of chronic graft-versus-host disease. Biol Blood Marrow Transplant. 2005;11(1): 47–55.
129. Couriel DR, Saliba R, Escalan MP, et al. Sirolimus in combination with tacrolimus and corticosteroids for the treatment of resistant chronic graft-versus-host disease. Br J Haematol. 2005;130(3):409–417.
130. Kanamaru A, Takemoto Y, Kakishita E, et al. FK506 treatment of graft-versus-host disease developing or exacerbating during prophylaxis and therapy with cyclosporin and/or other immunosuppressants. Japanese FK506 BMT Study Group. Bone Marrow Transplant. 1995;15(6): 885–889.
131. Akpek G, Lee SM, Anders V, Vogelsang GB. A high-dose pulse steroid regimen for controlling active chronic graft-versus-host disease. Biol Blood Marrow Transplant. 2001; 7(9):495–502.
132. Busca A, Locatelli F, Marmont F, et al. Response to mycophenolate mofetil therapy for refractory chronic graft-versus-host disease. Haematologica. 2003;88(7):837–839.
133. Lopez F, Parker P, Nademanee A, et al. Efficacy of mycophenolate mofetil in the treatment of chronic graft-versus-host disease. Biol Blood Marrow Transplant. 2005;11(4): 307–313.
134. Girardi M, Schechner J, Glusac E, et al. Transimmunization and the evolution of extracorporeal photochemotherapy. Transfus Apher Sci. 2002;26:181–190.
135. Berger CL, Xu AL, Hanlon D, et al. Induction of human tumor-loaded dendritic cells. Int J Cancer. 2001;91: 438–447.
136. Fimiani M, Di Renzo M, Rubegni P. Mechanism of action of extracorporeal photochemotherapy in chronic graft-versus-host disease. Br J Dermatol. 2004;150:1055–1060.
137. Peritt D. Potential mechanisms of photopheresis in hematopoietic stem cell transplantation. Biol Blood Marrow Transplant. 2006;12:7–12.
138. Gatza E, Rogers CE, Clouthier SG, et al. Extracorporeal photopheresis reverses experimental graft-versus-host disease through regulatory T cells. Blood. 2008;112:1515–1521.
139. Di Biaso I, Di Maio L, Bugarin C, et al. Regulatory T cells and extracorporeal photochemotherapy: correlation with clinical response and decreased frequency of proinflammatory T cells. Transplantation. 2009;87(9):1422–1425.
140. Owisanowski M, GololLnick H, Siegert W, et al. Successful treatment of chronic graft-versus-host disease with extracorporeal photopheresis. Bone Marrow Transplant. 1994; 14:845–848.
141. Apisarnthanarax N, Donato M, Korbling M, et al. Extracorporeal photopheresis therapy in the management of steroid-refractory or steroid-dependent cutaneous chronic graft-versus-host disease after allogeneic stem cell transplantation: feasibility and results. Bone Marrow Transplant. 2003;31:459–465.
142. Van Dorp S, Resemann H, Te Boome L, et al. The immunological phenotype of rituximab-sensitive chronic graft-versus-host disease: a phase II study. Haematologica. 2011;96(9):1380–1384.
143. Kuzima Z, Greinix HT, Weigl R, et al. Significant differences in B-cell subpopulations characterize patients with chronic graft-versus-host disease associated dysgammaglobulinemia. Blood. 2011;117(7):2265–2274.
144. Batten M, Groom J, Cachero TG, et al. BAFF mediates survival of peripheral immature B lymphocytes. J Exp Med. 2000;192:1453–1466.
145. Mariette X, Roux S, Zhang J, et al. The level of BLyS (BAFF) correlates with the titre of autoantibodies in human Sjögren's syndrome. Ann Rheum Dis. 2003;62:168–171.
146. Mackay F, Woodcock SA, Lawton P, et al. Mice transgenic for BAFF develop lymphocytic disorders along with autoimmune manifestations. J Exp Med 1999;190 1697–1710.
147. Magro L, Mohty M, Catteau B, et al. Imatinib mesylate as salvage therapy for refractory sclerotic chronic graft-versus-host disease. Blood. 2009;114(3):719–722.
148. Park J, Ha H, Ahn HJ, et al. Sirolimus inhibits platelet-derived growth factor-induced collagen synthesis in rat vascular smooth muscle cells. Transplant Proc. 2005;37: 3459–3462.
149. Jedlickova Z, Burlakova I, Bug G, et al. Therapy of sclerodermatous chronic graft-versus-host disease with mammalian target of rapamycin inhibitors. Biol Blood Marrow Transplant. 2011;17:657–663.
150. Jurado M, Vallejo C, Perez-Simon JA, et al. Sirolimus as part of immunosuppressive therapy for refractory chronic graft-versus-host disease. Biol Blood Marrow Transplant. 2007;13:701–706.

CHAPTER 11

Anti-infective prophylaxis, immunization and prevention of recurrent infectious complications in long-term survivors

John P Galvin[1] *and Jayesh Mehta*[2]

[1]Division of Hematology/Oncology, Department of Medicine, Feinberg School of Medicine, Northwestern University, Chicago, IL, USA

[2]Northwestern Memorial Hospital, Chicago, IL, USA

Introduction

The risks for infection after hematopoietic stem cell transplantation (HSCT) are associated with the specific post-HSCT phases of engraftment (Figure 11.1). The major compromise of the pre-engraftment phase is neutropenia and mucosal injury from cytotoxic chemotherapy. During the early and late postengraftment phases the main vulnerabilities are a naive immune system and the presence of graft-versus-host disease (GVHD). The late postengraftment phase begins at about 3 months after HSCT. During this period, there is a restoration of cellular and humoral immunity. The presence of chronic GVHD during the late postengraftment phase is common and often requires the continuation of immunosuppressive treatment. The combination of mucosal damage from GVHD and T- and B-cell dysfunction from immunosuppression therapy increases the risk for infections. During this late period, bacteria are responsible for about 33% of infections, viral infections account for more than 40%, and another 20% have been attributed to fungi [1].

Late bacterial infections

The presence of chronic GVHD often leads to a functional asplenia, which contributes to a higher susceptibility to encapsulated bacteria such as *Streptococcus pneumoniae*, *Haemophilus influenzae*, or *Neisseria meningitidis* [2, 3]. Pneumococcus prophylaxis is recommended for patients with chronic GVHD [4, 5]. *Nocardia* is an occasional pathogen seen in the late post-HSCT phase and can be difficult to distinguish from the clinical and radiographic features of pulmonary aspergillosis [6]. Therefore, in the late post-HSCT phase the work-up for pulmonary infiltrates should include cultures from a bronchial lavage and/or biopsy.

Enteritis caused by *Clostridium difficile* is one of most common nosocomial infections and may occur any time after HSCT. Some *C. difficile* strains can produce highly potent toxins and lead to perforation, shock, and death [7, 8]. In addition to the frequent exposures to healthcare environments (hospitals, clinics, blood centers), the exposure to fluoroquinolones (commonly used prophylactically or empirically post-HSCT) is a known risk

Blood and Marrow Transplantation Long-Term Management: Prevention and Complications, First Edition. Edited by Bipin N Savani.

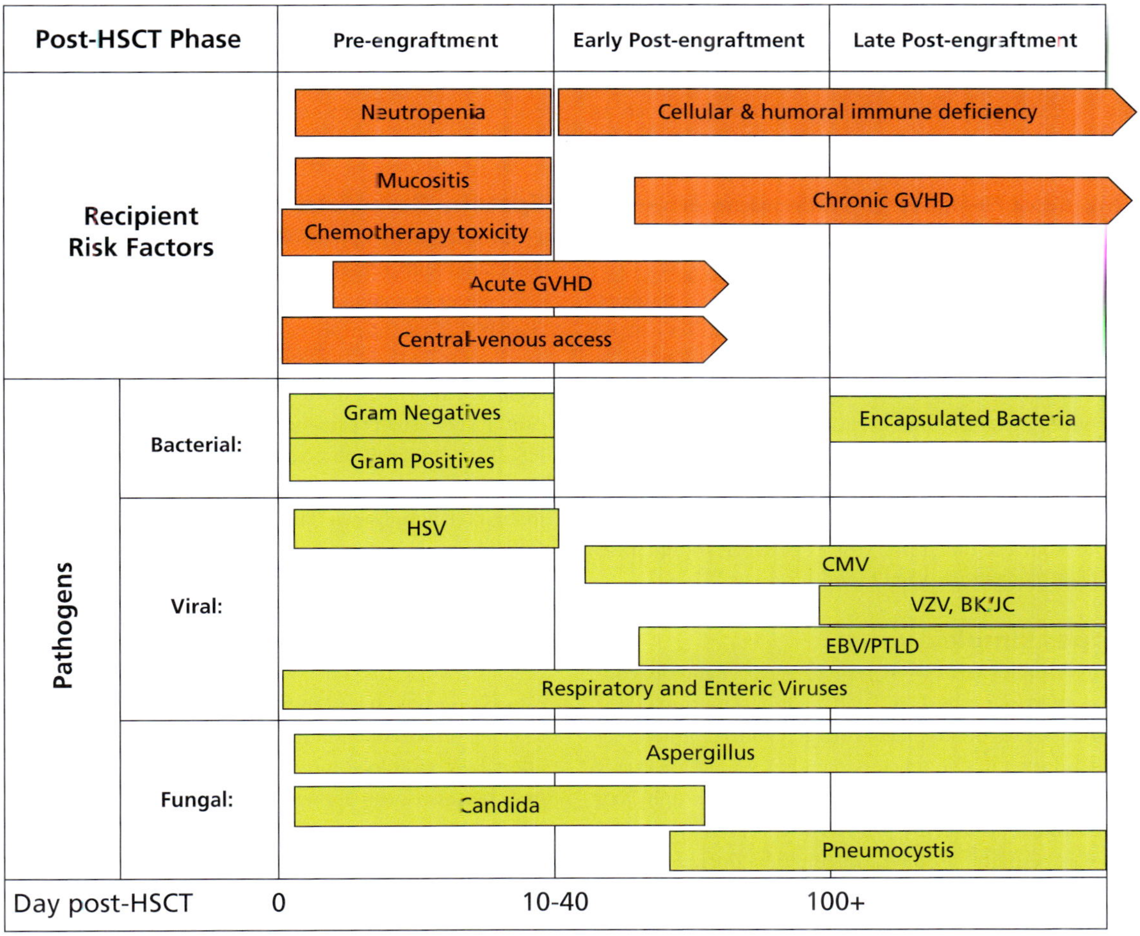

Figure 11.1 Risk factors and common pathogens post-HSCT.

factor for *C. difficile* infection [7, 8]. Therefore, the differential for chronic diarrhea post-HSCT should always include *C. difficile* colitis.

Late viral infections

Cytomegalovirus

Late-occurring cytomegalovirus (CMV) infection is associated with delayed and incomplete reconstitution of specific immunity [9, 10]. Several factors, including chronic GVHD, early CMV reactivation, and persistent lymphopenia, have been shown to predict the development of late CMV infection [11–15]. The control and treatment of CMV post-HSCT is essential, owing to its strong association with nonrelapse mortality [15].

There are two approaches to preventing CMV disease that have proved effective: close monitoring and preemptive treatment with or without prophylactic antiviral treatment [11, 16, 17]. Prophylactic therapy with acyclovir or valacyclovir has been shown to reduce the risk for CMV infection [18–21]. Prophylactic use of valacyclovir has been shown to reduce the need for preemptive therapy to approximately 50% [18]. Ganciclovir and valganciclovir are also effective for the prevention of CMV disease [22, 23]; however, they are less tolerated owing to myelotoxicity.

Preemptive therapy based on early detection of CMV has become an effective strategy for the prevention of CMV infection post-HSCT [24, 25]. The close monitoring of CMV status through sensitive methods such as CMV antigen assays or CMV quantitative polymerase chain reaction accurately identifies patients at risk for CMV disease [26–30]. Patients with evidence of reactivation are preemptively treated with ganciclovir or valganciclovir, which have similar efficacy in treating CMV [31]. Antiviral resistance is possible but rare in HSCT patients, and a slow response to treatment often indicates a rapid replication of CMV in an immunocompromised patient [30, 32]. A CMV reactivation should be treated until the monitoring tests become negative [33, 34].

In addition to active surveillance and treatment of CMV, reducing the risk of CMV transmission from blood products is also important. CMV is mainly harbored in the leukocytes; therefore, HSCT patients should only receive leukocyte-depleted blood products [35–37].

Herpes simplex virus

Herpes simplex virus (HSV) can cause local and disseminated infections after HSCT. The manifestation in HSCT recipients can be atypical with generalized inflammation and pain of the mucous membranes and/or classic vesicular or ulcerative lesions. Antiviral prophylaxis is indicated in all HSV seropositive HSCT recipients [38–41]. Antiviral prophylaxis should be during the pre-engraftment phase and continue postengraftment in patients with GVHD or a history of frequent reactivation before HSCT [42].

Varicella zoster virus

Varicella zoster virus (VZV) is a serious pathogen in immunocompromised patients. In the absence of prophylaxis, reactivated VZV infection develops in approximately a third of HSCT recipients [43, 44]. The risk for VZV infection is greatest between 3 and 6 months post-HSCT and decreases over the first 2 years post-HSCT [45]. Antiviral prophylaxis for at least a year post-HSCT is often used to prevent VZV reactivation. A 12-month regimen of acyclovir has been shown to be highly effective in reducing the risk of VZV disease [45–47]. Antiviral prophylaxis may exceed 12 months in the setting of chronic GVHD [45, 48]. Clinical manifestations can vary from dermatomal herpes zoster to visceral disseminated disease, which is associated with a high mortality rate [43, 49, 50]. Visceral disease can also occur without cutaneous manifestations and, therefore, may be difficult to diagnose. Early initiation of antiviral therapy is essential when disseminated, or visceral VZV disease is suspected.

Epstein–Barr virus

Posttransplant lymphoproliferative disorder (PTLD) is associated with Epstein–Barr virus (EBV) infection of B cells, either as a consequence of reactivation of the virus post-HSCT or from primary post-HSCT EBV infection acquired from the donor. Prior to the availability of rituximab, the mortality from PTLD after HSCT was significant. PTLD usually presents during the first months after HSCT as a polymorphic polyclonal B-lymphocyte proliferation with the potential to develop into a monoclonal malignant lymphoma. The incidence of PTLD is unaffected by antiviral prophylaxis [51]. Therefore, the use of antivirals for EBV is currently not recommended [47, 52–54]. However, EBV viral load monitoring in high-risk patients with the preemptive reduction of immunosuppression when the EBV viral load reaches a predetermined threshold has been reported to reduce PTLD rates [55, 56]. If the reduction in immunosuppression does not affect EBV viral load, preemptive treatment with rituximab has also been shown to decrease the incidence of PTLD [57].

Respiratory viruses

Respiratory viruses, especially influenza, can be seen late post-HSCT. The primary mode for prevention of influenza is vaccination and should be given to all transplant patients starting at about 4 months post-HSCT and then annually while the patients are immunosuppressed [47, 58]. Vaccinations of family and close household contacts as well as health-care staff are important in reducing risk for transmitting influenza [59, 60]. There is no evidence supporting the use of antiviral prophylaxis or preemptive treatment for parainfluenza or respiratory syncytial virus [61, 62]. The use of intravenous immunoglobulins is indicated for those with evidence of hypogammaglobulinemia (IgG levels <400 mg/dL) [63, 64].

Adenovirus

There is neither established prophylaxis nor treatment for adenovirus infections in HSCT recipients. Few antiviral agents have *in vivo* activity against adenoviruses, and there are no studies supporting the use of antiviral therapy for adenoviral infections. Ribavirin has been used in case reports with varying results [65–72].

Hepatitis B and C viruses

Hepatitis B virus (HBV) infection can reactivate in previously HBV-infected patients, especially during prolonged treatment for GVHD. Reactivation can result in a potentially severe acute hepatitis, and patients should be carefully monitored. If signs of HBV reactivation develop, HSCT recipients should be given antiviral therapy [73–75]. An effort should be made prior to HSCT to provide hepatitis B immunization to HBV-seronegative HSCT candidates, preferably prior to chemotherapy. HSCT recipients who fail to respond to pretransplant vaccination should be revaccinated post-HSCT after immune recovery [42]. If the HSCT recipient is HBV-seropositive, the risk of HBV reactivation can increase following a prolonged treatment with steroids; therefore, these patients should be closely monitored for liver abnormalities. The incidence of HBV-associated cirrhosis and hepatocellular carcinoma, however, does not appear to be higher in HBV-seropositive HSCT patients in comparison with non-HSCT patients [76].

There is no evidence of short-term adverse effects of hepatitis C virus (HCV) infection in HSCT recipients, and HCV-infected HSCT recipients have similar morbidity up to 10 years after transplant [77]. Subsequently, however, these patients appear to be at risk for progression to cirrhosis, which may occur more rapidly than in non-HSCT patients [78]. Treatment for chronic HCV should be considered in all HCV-infected HCT recipients because studies suggest improved outcome in those who respond to combination therapy with interferon and ribavirin [79].

Polyomaviruses: BK and JC

Polyomavirus-associated hemorrhagic cystitis (PVHC), which affects up to 15% of HSCT recipients during pre-engraftment to early postengraftment periods, is associated with the polyomavirus BK [80, 81]. BK virus (BKV) and JC virus (JCV) infect a majority of people worldwide in early childhood [82, 83]. Urinary shedding of BKV and JCV occurs in up to 20% of healthy immunocompetent people [84]. Urinary shedding of BKV occurs in up to 80% of HSCT recipients [80, 85]. Owing to its prevalence in the population, there is no evidence to support routine testing of HSCT recipients or donors for the presence of BKV-specific or JCV-specific antibodies. Fluoroquinolones have been shown to inhibit BKV replication in tissue culture and reduce BK viral loads in HSCT patients. However, the prophylactic use of fluoroquinolones has not proven to reduce the incidence of PVHC and is not recommended [86]. The use of an antiviral agent such as cidofovir as prophylaxis for PVHC is also not recommended [42].

Late fungal infections

Invasive fungal infections (IFIs) in HSCT recipients are associated with significant morbidity and mortality. HSCT patients with IFIs have a high mortality rate and a low 1-year survival [87–90]. *Candida*, *Aspergillus*, and *Pneumocystis* are the primary fungal pathogens and have accounted for the majority of IFIs in late-phase HSCT recipients. Many factors affect the risk for late onset fungal disease, including neutropenia, GVHD, and CMV disease [91].

Candida

Candida colonizes the skin and mucosal surfaces in most immunocompetent people. The mucosal injury that results from chemotherapy and/or GVHD allows for entry of candida organisms into the tissues and bloodstream. This vulnerability is magnified in a neutropenic setting, which sets the stage for an invasive *Candida* infection. Antifungal prophylaxis for HSCT recipients has been extensively studied [92]. Clinical trials have shown that the triazoles, specifically fluconazole, are well tolerated and are highly effective as prophylaxis against most *Candida* species. Therefore, fluconazole is recommended as routine prophylaxis after HSCT until the discontinuation of immunosuppression therapy and resolution of GVHD [42].

Aspergillus

Aspergillosis most commonly occurs during the early and late postengraftment phases. These periods are associated with profound T-cell immunodeficiency, due to acute and/or chronic GVHD and high-dose steroid use.

Itraconazole, voriconazole, and posaconazole have been evaluated as prophylaxis for aspergillosis. Posaconazole and voriconazole have been found to be well tolerated and effective in patients with GVHD and offer better mold coverage for high risk patients [93–96]. Lipid amphotericin B formulations and echinocandins also have anti-aspergillosis activity and have been studied in limited trials, but are less attractive due to the requirement for intravenous administration. The detection of galactomannan, a substance released by active *Aspergillus*, provides a marker for *Aspergillus* infection. The presence of galactomannan post-HSCT has been shown to be useful in detecting active *Aspergillus* infection [97–99]. The clinical suspicion of a fungal pneumonia in HSCT patients should prompt CT imaging and empiric therapy with voriconazole, which is the treatment of choice for aspergillosis [100, 101].

Pneumocystis jiroveci

Pneumocystis jiroveci (formerly *Pneumocystis carinii*) is a common pathogen of interstitial pneumonia in the late postengraftment phase. Without specific prophylaxis, about 30% of patients with chronic GVHD develop *Pneumocystis* pneumonia [102]. Prophylaxis with trimethoprim–sulfamethoxazole (TMP–SMZ) is recommended for as long as HSCT patients are on immunosuppression. If TMP–SMZ is not well tolerated, atovaquone, dapsone, or inhaled pentamidine can also be used for prophylaxis [42].

Table 11.1 Vaccination recommendations after HSCT[a]

Vaccine	Recommendation	Administration time post-HSCT (months)
Pneumoccocal (PCV)	Yes	3–6
Tetanus, diphtheria, pertussis (DTaP)[b]	Yes	6–12
H. influenzae	Yes	6–12
Meningococcal	Depends on country	6–12
Inactivated polio	Yes	6–12
Hepatitis B	Depends on country	6–12
Influenza	Yes	4–6, then lifelong
Measles–mumps–rubella	For children and seronegative adults	24
Varicella (Varivax)[c]	Optional	24
Hepatitis A	Optional, depends on country	Limited data
Human papillomavirus	Optional	Limited data

[a] Based on the most recent guidelines [42].
[b] Full dose diphtheria, tetanus, and pertussis vaccines preferred if available (DTaP).
[c] The Varivax vaccine is preferred; there are limited data to support the Zostavax "shingles" vaccine.

Vaccines

Re-immunization is required for HSCT recipients because they lose immunity to common childhood illnesses (Table 11.1). Specific diseases that can be prevented with immunizations, like pneumococcal, *Haemophilus influenzae*, measles, varicella, and influenza infections have been shown to pose an increased risk for HSCT recipients [49, 103–107]. This increased risk is due to the decreased quantity and functionality of T and B cells after an HSCT. Newly generated B cells have a limited capability to undergo somatic mutation and isotype switching during the first year after transplant. Naive T cells capable of responding to new antigens start to be generated only at 6–12 months posttransplant. The recovery of T cells is also influenced by patient age, T cell depletion of the graft, and the presence of chronic GVHD. In the absence of chronic GVHD, re-immunization of childhood illnesses should start at about 1 year post-HSCT [108]. Pneumococcal and seasonal influenza vaccinations can be given as early as 4 months after HSCT. Household contacts and care providers should also receive lifelong seasonal influenza vaccinations [42]. Live virus vaccines should be given at about 2 years following HSCT and in the absence of active GVHD and immunosuppressive therapy [42].

References

1. Sable CA, Donowitz GR. Infections in bone marrow transplant recipients. Clin Infect Dis. 1994;18(3):273–281; quiz 282–284.
2. Atkinson K, Storb R, Prentice RL, et al. Analysis of late infections in 89 long-term survivors of bone marrow transplantation. Blood. 1979;53(4):720–731.

3. Ochs L, Shu XO, Miller J, et al. Late infections after allogeneic bone marrow transplantations: comparison of incidence in related and unrelated donor transplant recipients. Blood. 1995;86(10):3979–3986.
4. Kulkarni S, Powles R, Treleaven J, et al. Chronic graft versus host disease is associated with long-term risk for pneumococcal infections in recipients of bone marrow transplants. Blood. 2000;95(12):3683–3686.
5. Mehta J, Powles R, Singhal S, et al. Antimicrobial prophylaxis to prevent opportunistic infections in patients with chronic lymphocytic leukemia after allogeneic blood or marrow transplantation. Leuk Lymphoma. 1997;26(1–2): 83–88.
6. Daly AS, McGeer A, Lipton JH. Systemic nocardiosis following allogeneic bone marrow transplantation. Transpl Infect Dis. 2003;5(1):16–20.
7. Loo VG, Poirier L, Miller MA, et al. A predominantly clonal multi-institutional outbreak of *Clostridium difficile*-associated diarrhea with high morbidity and mortality. N Engl J Med. 2005;353(23):2442–2449.
8. McDonald LC, Killgore GE, Thompson A, et al. An epidemic, toxin gene-variant strain of *Clostridium difficile*. N Engl J Med. 2005;353(23):2433–2441.
9. Maris M, Boeckh M, Storer B, et al. Immunologic recovery after hematopoietic cell transplantation with nonmyeloablative conditioning. Exp Hematol. 2003;31(10):941–952.
10. van Burik JA, Brunstein CG. Infectious complications following unrelated cord blood transplantation. Vox Sang. 2007;92(4):289–296.
11. Boeckh M, Leisenring W, Riddell SR, et al. Late cytomegalovirus disease and mortality in recipients of allogeneic hematopoietic stem cell transplants: importance of viral load and T-cell immunity. Blood. 2003;101(2):407–414.
12. Krause H, Hebart H, Jahn G, et al. Screening for CMV-specific T cell proliferation to identify patients at risk of developing late onset CMV disease. Bone Marrow Transplant. 1997;19(11):1111–1116.
13. Li CR, Greenberg PD, Gilbert MJ, et al. Recovery of HLA-restricted cytomegalovirus (CMV)-specific T-cell responses after allogeneic bone marrow transplant: correlation with CMV disease and effect of ganciclovir prophylaxis. Blood. 1994;83(7):1971–1979.
14. Ljungman P, Aschan J, Lewensohn-Fuchs I, et al. Results of different strategies for reducing cytomegalovirus-associated mortality in allogeneic stem cell transplant recipients. Transplantation. 1998;66(10):1330–1334.
15. Ozdemir E, Saliba RM, Champlin RE, et al. Risk factors associated with late cytomegalovirus reactivation after allogeneic stem cell transplantation for hematological malignancies. Bone Marrow Transplant. 2007;40(2):125–136.
16. Junghanss C, Boeckh M, Carter RA, et al. Incidence and outcome of cytomegalovirus infections following nonmyeloablative compared with myeloablative allogeneic stem cell transplantation, a matched control study. Blood. 2002;99(6):1978–1985.
17. Peggs KS, Preiser W, Kottaridis PD, et al. Extended routine polymerase chain reaction surveillance and pre-emptive antiviral therapy for cytomegalovirus after allogeneic transplantation. Br J Haematol. 2000;111(3):782–790.
18. Ljungman P, de La Camara R, Milpied N, et al. Randomized study of valacyclovir as prophylaxis against cytomegalovirus reactivation in recipients of allogeneic bone marrow transplants. Blood. 2002;99(8):3050–3056.
19. Meyers JD, Reed EC, Shepp DH, et al. Acyclovir for prevention of cytomegalovirus infection and disease after allogeneic marrow transplantation. N Engl J Med. 1988; 318(2):70–75.
20. Prentice HG, Gluckman E, Powles RL, et al. Impact of long-term acyclovir on cytomegalovirus infection and survival after allogeneic bone marrow transplantation. European Acyclovir for CMV Prophylaxis Study Group. Lancet. 1994;343(8900):749–753.
21. Prentice HG, Gluckman E, Powles RL, et al. Long-term survival in allogeneic bone marrow transplant recipients following acyclovir prophylaxis for CMV infection. The European Acyclovir for CMV Prophylaxis Study Group. Bone Marrow Transplant. 1997;19(2):129–133.
22. Goodrich JM, Bowden RA, Fisher L, et al. Ganciclovir prophylaxis to prevent cytomegalovirus disease after allogeneic marrow transplant. Ann Intern Med. 1993; 118(3):173–178.
23. Winston DJ, Ho WG, Bartoni K, et al. Ganciclovir prophylaxis of cytomegalovirus infection and disease in allogeneic bone marrow transplant recipients. Results of a placebo-controlled, double-blind trial. Ann Intern Med. 1993; 118(3):179–184.
24. Avery RK, Adal KA, Longworth DL, Bolwell BJ. A survey of allogeneic bone marrow transplant programs in the United States regarding cytomegalovirus prophylaxis and pre-emptive therapy. Bone Marrow Transplant. 2000;26(7): 763–767.
25. Ljungman P, De Bock R, Cordonnier C, et al. Practices for cytomegalovirus diagnosis, prophylaxis and treatment in allogeneic bone marrow transplant recipients: a report from the Working Party for Infectious Diseases of the EBMT. Bone Marrow Transplant. 1993;12(4):399–403.
26. Emery VC, Sabin CA, Cope AV, et al. Application of viral-load kinetics to identify patients who develop cytomegalovirus disease after transplantation. Lancet. 2000;355(9220):2032–2036.

27. Gor D, Sabin C, Prentice HG, et al. Longitudinal fluctuations in cytomegalovirus load in bone marrow transplant patients: relationship between peak virus load, donor/recipient serostatus, acute GVHD and CMV disease. Bone Marrow Transplant. 1998;21(6):597–605.
28. Lilleri D, Gerna G, Furione M, et al. Use of a DNAemia cut-off for monitoring human cytomegalovirus infection reduces the number of preemptively treated children and young adults receiving hematopoietic stem-cell transplantation compared with qualitative pp65 antigenemia. Blood. 2007;110(7):2757–2760.
29. Ljungman P, Perez-Bercoff L, Jonsson J, et al. Risk factors for the development of cytomegalovirus disease after allogeneic stem cell transplantation. Haematologica. 2006;91(1):78–83.
30. Nichols WG, Corey L, Gooley T, et al. Rising pp65 antigenemia during preemptive anticytomegalovirus therapy after allogeneic hematopoietic stem cell transplantation: risk factors, correlation with DNA load, and outcomes. Blood. 2001;97(4):867–874.
31. Einsele H, Reusser P, Bornhauser M, et al. Oral valganciclovir leads to higher exposure to ganciclovir than intravenous ganciclovir in patients following allogeneic stem cell transplantation. Blood. 2006;107(7):3002–3008.
32. Gerna G, Lilleri D, Zecca M, et al. Rising antigenemia levels may be misleading in pre-emptive therapy of human cytomegalovirus infection in allogeneic hematopoietic stem cell transplant recipients. Haematologica. 2005;90(4):526–533.
33. Einsele H, Ehninger G, Hebart H, et al. Polymerase chain reaction monitoring reduces the incidence of cytomegalovirus disease and the duration and side effects of antiviral therapy after bone marrow transplantation. Blood. 1995;86(7):2815–2820.
34. Reusser P, Einsele H, Lee J, et al. Randomized multicenter trial of foscarnet versus ganciclovir for preemptive therapy of cytomegalovirus infection after allogeneic stem cell transplantation. Blood. 2002;99(4):1159–1164.
35. Bowden RA, Slichter SJ, Sayers M, et al. A comparison of filtered leukocyte-reduced and cytomegalovirus (CMV) seronegative blood products for the prevention of transfusion-associated CMV infection after marrow transplant. Blood. 1995;86(9):3598–3603.
36. Ljungman P, Larsson K, Kumlien G, et al. Leukocyte depleted, unscreened blood products give a low risk for CMV infection and disease in CMV seronegative allogeneic stem cell transplant recipients with seronegative stem cell donors. Scand J Infect Dis. 2002;34(5):347–350.
37. Nichols WG, Price TH, Gooley T, et al. Transfusion-transmitted cytomegalovirus infection after receipt of leukoreduced blood products. Blood. 2003;101(10):4195–4200.
38. Gluckman E, Lotsberg J, Devergie A, et al. Prophylaxis of herpes infections after bone-marrow transplantation by oral acyclovir. Lancet. 1983;2(8352):706–708.
39. Saral R, Burns WH, Laskin OL, et al. Acyclovir prophylaxis of herpes-simplex-virus infections. N Engl J Med. 1981;305(2):63–67.
40. Wade JC, Newton B, Flournoy N, Meyers JD. Oral acyclovir for prevention of herpes simplex virus reactivation after marrow transplantation. Ann Intern Med. 1984;100(6):823–828.
41. Wade JC, Newton B, McLaren C, et al. Intravenous acyclovir to treat mucocutaneous herpes simplex virus infection after marrow transplantation: a double-blind trial. Ann Intern Med. 1982;96(3):265–269.
42. Tomblyn M, Chiller T, Einsele H et al. Guidelines for preventing infectious complications among hematopoietic cell transplant recipients: a global perspective. Bone Marrow Transplant. 2009;44(8):453–558.
43. Steer CB, Szer J, Sasadeusz J, et al. Varicella–zoster infection after allogeneic bone marrow transplantation: incidence, risk factors and prevention with low-dose aciclovir and ganciclovir. Bone Marrow Transplant. 2000;25(6):657–664.
44. Wacker P, Hartmann O, Benhamou E, et al. Varicella–zoster virus infections after autologous bone marrow transplantation in children. Bone Marrow Transplant. 1989;4(2):191–194.
45. Erard V, Guthrie KA, Varley C, et al. One-year acyclovir prophylaxis for preventing varicella–zoster virus disease after hematopoietic cell transplantation: no evidence of rebound varicella–zoster virus disease after drug discontinuation. Blood. 2007;110(8):3071–3077.
46. Boeckh M, Kim HW, Flowers ME, et al. Long-term acyclovir for prevention of varicella zoster virus disease after allogeneic hematopoietic cell transplantation – a randomized double-blind placebo-controlled study. Blood. 2006;107(5):1800–1805.
47. Centers for Disease Control and Prevention, Infectious Disease Society of America, American Society of Blood and Marrow Transplantation. Guidelines for preventing opportunistic infections among hematopoietic stem cell transplant recipients. MMWR Recomm Rep. 2000;49(RR–10):1–125, CE1–CE7.
48. Thomson KJ, Hart DP, Banerjee L, et al. The effect of low-dose aciclovir on reactivation of varicella zoster virus after allogeneic haemopoietic stem cell transplantation. Bone Marrow Transplant. 2005;35(11):1065–1069.
49. Locksley RM, Flournoy N, Sullivan KM, Meyers JD. Infection with varicella–zoster virus after marrow transplantation. J Infect Dis 1985;152(6):1172–1181.

50. Martino R, Rovira M, Carreras E et al. Severe infections after allogeneic peripheral blood stem cell transplantation: a matched-pair comparison of unmanipulated and CD34+ cell-selected transplantation. Haematologica. 2001;86(10):1075–1086.
51. Green M, Kaufmann M, Wilson J, Reyes J. Comparison of intravenous ganciclovir followed by oral acyclovir with intravenous ganciclovir alone for prevention of cytomegalovirus and Epstein–Barr virus disease after liver transplantation in children. Clin Infect Dis. 1997;25(6):1344–1349.
52. Gerritsen EJ, Stam ED, Hermans J, et al. Risk factors for developing EBV-related B cell lymphoproliferative disorders (BLPD) after non-HLA-identical BMT in children. Bone Marrow Transplant. 1996;18(2):377–382.
53. Shapiro RS, McClain K, Frizzera G, et al. Epstein–Barr virus associated B cell lymphoproliferative disorders following bone marrow transplantation. Blood. 1988; 71(5):1234–1243.
54. Zutter MM, Martin PJ, Sale GE et al. Epstein–Barr virus lymphoproliferation after bone marrow transplantation. Blood. 1988;72(2):520–529.
55. Bakker NA, Verschuuren EA, Erasmus ME, et al. Epstein–Barr virus-DNA load monitoring late after lung transplantation: a surrogate marker of the degree of immunosuppression and a safe guide to reduce immunosuppression. Transplantation. 2007;83(4):433–438.
56. Tsai DE, Douglas L, Andreadis C, et al. EBV PCR in the diagnosis and monitoring of posttransplant lymphoproliferative disorder: results of a two-arm prospective trial. Am J Transplant. 2008;8(5):1016–1024.
57. Meerbach A, Wutzler P, Hafer R, et al. Monitoring of Epstein–Barr virus load after hematopoietic stem cell transplantation for early intervention in post-transplant lymphoproliferative disease. J Med Virol. 2008;80(3):441–454.
58. Ljungman P, Cordonnier C, Einsele H, et al. Vaccination of hematopoietic cell transplant recipients. Bone Marrow Transplant. 2009;44(8):521–526.
59. Centers for Disease Control and Prevention. Immunization of health-care workers: recommendations of the Advisory Committee on Immunization Practices (ACIP) and the Hospital Infection Control Practices Advisory Committee (HICPAC). MMWR Recomm Rep. 1997; 46(RR-18):1–42.
60. Fiore AE, Uyeki TM, Broder K, et al. Prevention and control of influenza with vaccines: recommendations of the Advisory Committee on Immunization Practices (ACIP), 2010. MMWR Recomm Rep. 2010;59(RR-8):1–62.
61. Englund JA, Piedra PA, Whimbey E. Prevention and treatment of respiratory syncytial virus and parainfluenza viruses in immunocompromised patients. Am J Med. 1997;102(3A):61–70; discussion 75–76.
62. Ljungman P, Ward KN, Crooks BN, et al. Respiratory virus infections after stem cell transplantation: a prospective study from the Infectious Diseases Working Party of the European Group for Blood and Marrow Transplantation. Bone Marrow Transplant. 2001;28(5):479–484.
63. Orange JS, Hossny EM, Weiler CR, et al. Use of intravenous immunoglobulin in human disease: a review of evidence by members of the Primary Immunodeficiency Committee of the American Academy of Allergy, Asthma and Immunology. J Allergy Clin Immunol. 2006;117(4 Suppl): S525–S553.
64. Buckley RH, Schiff RI. The use of intravenous immune globulin in immunodeficiency diseases. N Engl J Med. 1991;325(2):110–117.
65. Baldwin A, Kingman H, Darville M, et al. Outcome and clinical course of 100 patients with adenovirus infection following bone marrow transplantation. Bone Marrow Transplant. 2000;26(12):1333–1338.
66. Cassano WF. Intravenous ribavirin therapy for adenovirus cystitis after allogeneic bone marrow transplantation. Bone Marrow Transplant. 1991;7(3):247–248.
67. Chakrabarti S, Collingham KE, Fegan CD, Milligan DW. Fulminant adenovirus hepatitis following unrelated bone marrow transplantation: failure of intravenous ribavirin therapy. Bone Marrow Transplant. 1999;23(11): 1209–1211.
68. Hromas R, Clark C, Blanke C, et al. Failure of ribavirin to clear adenovirus infections in T cell-depleted allogeneic bone marrow transplantation. Bone Marrow Transplant. 1994;14(4):663–664.
69. Kapelushnik J, Or R, Delukina M, et al. Intravenous ribavirin therapy for adenovirus gastroenteritis after bone marrow transplantation. J Pediatr Gastroenterol Nutr. 1995;21(1):110–112.
70. Liles WC, Cushing H, Holt S, et al. Severe adenoviral nephritis following bone marrow transplantation: successful treatment with intravenous ribavirin. Bone Marrow Transplant. 1993;12(4):409–412.
71. Mann D, Moreb J, Smith S, Gian V. Failure of intravenous ribavirin in the treatment of invasive adenovirus infection following allogeneic bone marrow transplantation: a case report. J Infect. 1998;36(2):227–228.
72. Miyamura K, Hamaguchi M, Taji H, et al. Successful ribavirin therapy for severe adenovirus hemorrhagic cystitis after allogeneic marrow transplant from close HLA donors rather than distant donors. Bone Marrow Transplant. 2000;25(5):545–548.
73. Hsiao LT, Chiou TJ, Liu JH, et al. Extended lamivudine therapy against hepatitis B virus infection in hematopoietic

stem cell transplant recipients. Biol Blood Marrow Transplant. 2006;12(1):84–94.
74. Kitano K, Kobayashi H, Hanamura M, et al. Fulminant hepatitis after allogenic bone marrow transplantation caused by reactivation of hepatitis B virus with gene mutations in the core promotor region. Eur J Haematol. 2006;77(3):255–258.
75. Locasciulli A, Bruno B, Alessandrino EP, et al. Hepatitis reactivation and liver failure in haemopoietic stem cell transplants for hepatitis B virus (HBV)/hepatitis C virus (HCV) positive recipients: a retrospective study by the Italian Group for Blood and Marrow Transplantation. Bone Marrow Transplant. 2003;31(4):295–300.
76. Hui CK, Lie A, Au WY, et al. A long-term follow-up study on hepatitis B surface antigen-positive patients undergoing allogeneic hematopoietic stem cell transplantation. Blood. 2005;106(2):464–469.
77. Strasser SI, Myerson D, Spurgeon CL, et al. Hepatitis C virus infection and bone marrow transplantation: a cohort study with 10-year follow-up. Hepatology. 1999;29(6):1893–1899.
78. Peffault de Latour R, Levy V, Asselah T, et al. Long-term outcome of hepatitis C infection after bone marrow transplantation. Blood. 2004;103(5):1618–1624.
79. Peffault de Latour R, Asselah T, Levy V, et al. Treatment of chronic hepatitis C virus in allogeneic bone marrow transplant recipients. Bone Marrow Transplant. 2005;36(8):709–713.
80. Arthur RR, Shah KV, Baust SJ, et al. Association of BK viruria with hemorrhagic cystitis in recipients of bone marrow transplants. N Engl J Med. 1986;315(4):230–234.
81. Bedi A, Miller CB, Hanson JL, et al. Association of BK virus with failure of prophylaxis against hemorrhagic cystitis following bone marrow transplantation. J Clin Oncol. 1995;13(5):1103–1109.
82. Hirsch HH, Steiger J. Polyomavirus BK. Lancet Infect Dis. 2003;3(10):611–623.
83. Knowles WA. Discovery and epidemiology of the human polyomaviruses BK virus (BKV) and JC virus (JCV). Adv Exp Med Biol. 2006;577:19–45.
84. Egli A, Infanti L, Dumoulin A, et al. Prevalence of polyomavirus BK and JC infection and replication in 400 healthy blood donors. J Infect Dis. 2009;199(6):837–846.
85. Arthur RR, Shah KV, Charache P, Saral R. BK and JC virus infections in recipients of bone marrow transplants. J Infect Dis. 1988;158(3):563–569.
86. Rinaldo CH, Hirsch HH. Antivirals for the treatment of polyomavirus BK replication. Expert Rev Anti Infect Ther. 2007;5(1):105–115.
87. Gudlaugsson O, Gillespie S, Lee K, et al. Attributable mortality of nosocomial candidemia, revisited. Clin Infect Dis. 2003;37(9):1172–1177.
88. Husain S, Munoz P, Forrest G, et al. Infections due to *Scedosporium apiospermum* and *Scedosporium prolificans* in transplant recipients: clinical characteristics and impact of antifungal agent therapy on outcome. Clin Infect Dis. 2005;40(1):89–99.
89. Marr KA, Carter RA, Crippa F, et al. Epidemiology and outcome of mould infections in hematopoietic stem cell transplant recipients. Clin Infect Dis. 2002;34(7):909–917.
90. Nucci M, Marr KA, Queiroz-Telles F, et al. *Fusarium* infection in hematopoietic stem cell transplant recipients. Clin Infect Dis. 2004;38(9):1237–1242.
91. Marr KA, Carter RA, Boeckh M, et al. Invasive aspergillosis in allogeneic stem cell transplant recipients: changes in epidemiology and risk factors. Blood. 2002;100(13):4358–4366.
92. Wingard JR. Antifungal chemoprophylaxis after blood and marrow transplantation. Clin Infect Dis. 2002;34(10):1386–1390.
93. Marr KA, Crippa F, Leisenring W, et al. Itraconazole versus fluconazole for prevention of fungal infections in patients receiving allogeneic stem cell transplants. Blood. 2004;103(4):1527–1533.
94. Torres A, Serrano J, Rojas R, et al. Voriconazole as primary antifungal prophylaxis in patients with neutropenia after hematopoietic stem cell transplantation or chemotherapy for acute myeloid leukemia. Eur J Haematol. 2010;84(3):271–273.
95. Ullmann AJ, Lipton JH, Vesole DH, et al. Posaconazole or fluconazole for prophylaxis in severe graft-versus-host disease. N Engl J Med. 2007;356(4):335–347.
96. Winston DJ, Maziarz RT, Chandrasekar PH, et al. Intravenous and oral itraconazole versus intravenous and oral fluconazole for long-term antifungal prophylaxis in allogeneic hematopoietic stem-cell transplant recipients. A multicenter, randomized trial. Ann Intern Med. 2003;138(9):705–713.
97. Maertens J, Theunissen K, Verhoef G, et al. Galactomannan and computed tomography-based preemptive antifungal therapy in neutropenic patients at high risk for invasive fungal infection: a prospective feasibility study. Clin Infect Dis. 2005;41(9):1242–1250.
98. Maertens J, Van Eldere J, Verhaegen J, et al. Use of circulating galactomannan screening for early diagnosis of invasive aspergillosis in allogeneic stem cell transplant recipients. J Infect Dis. 2002;186(9):1297–1306.
99. Pfeiffer CD, Fine JP, Safdar N. Diagnosis of invasive aspergillosis using a galactomannan assay: a meta-analysis. Clin Infect Dis. 2006;42(10):1417–1427.

100. Herbrecht R, Denning DW, Patterson TF, et al. Voriconazole versus amphotericin B for primary therapy of invasive aspergillosis. N Engl J Med. 2002;347(6):408–415.
101. Walsh TJ, Anaissie EJ, Denning DW, et al. Treatment of aspergillosis: clinical practice guidelines of the Infectious Diseases Society of America. Clin Infect Dis. 2008; 46(3):327–360.
102. De Castro N, Neuville S, Sarfati C, et al. Occurrence of *Pneumocystis jiroveci* pneumonia after allogeneic stem cell transplantation: a 6-year retrospective study. Bone Marrow Transplant. 2005;36(10):879–883.
103. Engelhard D, Cordonnier C, Shaw PJ, et al. Early and late invasive pneumococcal infection following stem cell transplantation: a European Bone Marrow Transplantation survey. Br J Haematol. 2002;117(2):444–450.
104. Kumar D, Chen MH, Welsh B, et al. A randomized, double-blind trial of pneumococcal vaccination in adult allogeneic stem cell transplant donors and recipients. Clin Infect Dis. 2007;45(12):1576–1582.
105. Nakano T, Shimono Y, Sugiyama K, et al. Clinical features of measles in immunocompromised children. Acta Paediatr Jpn. 1996;38(3):212–217.
106. Nichols WG, Guthrie KA, Corey L, Boeckh M. Influenza infections after hematopoietic stem cell transplantation: risk factors, mortality, and the effect of antiviral therapy. Clin Infect Dis. 2004;39(9):1300–1306.
107. Youssef S, Rodriguez G, Rolston KV, et al. *Streptococcus pneumoniae* infections in 47 hematopoietic stem cell transplantation recipients: clinical characteristics of infections and vaccine-breakthrough infections, 1989–2005. Medicine (Baltimore). 2007;86(2):69–77.
108. van Burik JA, Weisdorf DJ. Infections in recipients of blood and marrow transplantation. Hematol Oncol Clin North Am. 1999;13(5):1065–1089, viii.

12

CHAPTER 12
Seasonal virus infections: prevention and management guidelines

Gaurav Trikha[1] *and John R Wingard*[2]

[1]Division of Cardiovascular Medicine, Shands Hospital at University of Florida, Gainesville, FL, USA
[2]Division of Hematology/Oncology, University of Florida College of Medicine, Gainesville, FL, USA

Introduction

Preventing and treating infectious diseases in hematopoietic stem cell transplant (HCT) recipients presents special challenges, as current treatments and vaccines may have limited efficacy in this population. Immune suppression is an inevitable component of HCT. The recipients undergo ablation of the immune system prior to transplantation, and immune reconstitution occurs only after successful engraftment of the transplant. Recipients routinely receive immune suppressants during the first 6 months post-transplant period (e.g., tacrolimus, cyclosporine, prednisone) in order to prevent and treat graft-versus-host disease (GVHD). The occurrence of acute or chronic GVHD intensifies the immunodeficiency and prolongs the time to immune reconstitution. Therefore, HCT patients are severely immunosuppressed for a significant period and are at high risk for various opportunistic infections that can cause significant morbidity and mortality.

Community respiratory viral (CRV) infections occur in both immunocompetent and immunosuppressed populations. The emergence of the novel 2009 H1N1 (2009H1N1v) influenza virus (IFV) has illustrated many challenges in preventing and treating respiratory viral infections and underscores the need for appropriate unique strategies for this at-risk population. Some of these challenges include the lack of population immunity to a novel influenza strain that led to pandemic outbreaks as well as the potential for the development of drug resistance that has rendered existing therapeutic modalities less effective [1, 2]. Differences in the magnitude of risk of lower tract disease, duration of viral shedding, and the types of risk factors for lower tract disease with the 2009 H1N1v strain became apparent in HCT recipients, but only in hindsight [3, 4].

Preventing exposure

CRV pathogens predominate in different seasons. Community outbreaks of respiratory syncytial virus (RSV) infections typically occur during the late fall, winter, and early spring, frequently followed by outbreaks of human metapneumovirus (HMPV). Influenza outbreaks typically occur during the winter in temperate climates, but may occur throughout the year in more tropical areas. Human parainfluenza virus (HPIV) infections occur throughout the year, with infections occurring primarily in the spring, summer, and fall. Other viruses, such as rhinoviruses and coronaviruses, tend to take place throughout the year, although sporadic outbreaks of all these respiratory viruses may occur. Nosocomial transmission of CRVs is common, and widespread hospital outbreaks of CRVs have occurred with sometimes devastating sequelae [5, 6].

HCT centers should maintain appropriate precautions and infection control measures for preventing the

Blood and Marrow Transplantation Long-Term Management: Prevention and Complications, First Edition. Edited by Bipin N Savani.

transmission of CRV among hospitalized HCT recipients and candidates undergoing conditioning therapy [7–11]. HCT recipients or candidates with upper respiratory tract infection (URI) or lower respiratory tract infection (LRI) symptoms due to CRV infection should be placed on contact plus droplet precautions until a specific pathogen has been identified. Pathogen-specific CRV isolation precautions can be instituted after the organism has been identified, and with guidelines should address:

- contact precautions for RSV and HPIV;
- droplet precautions for influenza.

Personal protective equipment (for example, gown, gloves, surgical mask, and eye protection) should be donned before entering and discarded on exiting a patient's room to ensure that personal protective equipment is always changed between patients . When caring for an HCT recipient with documented or suspected CRV infection, health-care workers and visitors should disinfect hands with an alcohol-based gel or, if hands are visibly soiled, with soap and water [8, 12].

Respiratory secretions of any hospitalized HCT candidate or recipient with signs or symptoms of CRV infection should be tested promptly for CRV. This practice permits the timely initiation of isolation precautions to prevent transmission to other patients and health-care workers, as well as preemptive treatment of certain CRVs (for example, influenza) that might prevent severe disease and death among HCT recipients [8].

To prevent nosocomial transmission of CRV, HCT centers should recognize that prolonged CRV shedding may occur [5]. Viral shedding has been reported to last >4 months for influenza [13], >2 years for adenovirus [14, 15], and >22 days for RSV [5].

Immunization of household contacts, notably for influenza, can produce herd immunity and reduce the risk that the HCT recipient can be exposed from this important source. This is discussed later in the section entitled "Prevention."

Preventing disease

Where possible, an etiology of URIs should be ascertained to optimize management. In particular, patients exhibiting URI symptoms at the time conditioning therapy is scheduled to start should postpone their conditioning regimen until the URIs resolve, if possible, because certain URIs might progress to LRI during immunosuppression [5, 16–18].

Influenza virus (IFV)

IFV is genetically a distinct, single-stranded RNA virus of the *Orthomyxoviridae* family. It is tropic for the human respiratory tract and utilizes sialic acid as its receptor [19, 20]. IFV is typically caused by infection with either influenza A virus (IFV A) or influenza B virus (IFV B), each composed of 11 genes encoded by 8 negative-stranded RNA segments enclosed in a lipid envelope derived from the host cell. The envelope displays three key viral proteins: hemagglutinin (HA) attaches the virus to host cell receptors and mediates fusion of viral and cellular membranes; neuraminidase (NA) facilitates release of new viruses from the host cell; and M2 proteins serve as ion channels. Only IFV A is further classified by subtype on the basis of the two main surface glycoproteins HA and NA. There are 16 known HA subtypes and 9 known NA subtypes of IFV A. Subtypes of IFV A that are circulating worldwide include 2009H1N1v, seasonal H1N1, and H3N2v. Approved antiviral drugs target two of the three aforementioned viral proteins, M2 and NA. They include the M2 inhibitors adamantanes (amantadine and rimantadine), and the NA inhibitors (NAIs) oseltamivir (Tamiflu), peramivir, and zanamivir (Relenza).

There are multiple causes for the increased susceptibility to influenza infection in immunosuppressed patients. In HCT, the intensity of myeloablation and consequent lymphopenia increases susceptibility to respiratory infections, including influenza [21]. IFV in the immunocompetent individual usually results in viral shedding that is self-limited, lasting 5–6 days. In contrast, viral shedding prolonged for over 2 weeks is common in immunosuppressed hosts and has reportedly lasted as long as 6 months [22, 23]. Prolonged viral replication and shedding of IFV has been associated with selection of resistant virus. For example, in a small series of HCT subjects, the incidence of NAI resistance was 67% [24]. Additional studies suggest that the incidence of resistance may be higher in immunosuppressed patients than in immunocompetent adults or children [22, 25].

Transmission among humans occurs primarily through respiratory droplets containing infectious virions. After a susceptible person inhales infectious virus, an incubation period of 1–2 days occurs before onset of symptoms. Influenza manifests clinically primarily as a URI. Initially, systemic symptoms such as high fever, myalgias, headache, and lassitude predominate, followed 2–3 days later by dry cough, oropharyngeal pain, and nasal discharge in non-HCT patients. Two major complications that can occur are viral pneumonia and secondary bacterial pneumonia. The influenza syndrome is similar in patients with cancer and HCT recipients, but high fever and myalgias may be less prominent. The degrees of risk of influenza complications are influenced by the depth of immunosuppression. Children with cancer, adults with acute leukemia, and HCT recipients are most susceptible to severe complications and death [25].

The impact of seasonal influenza on immunosuppressed individuals has been clinically characterized primarily through case studies. Complications from influenza in this population include high rates of mortality, a need for mechanical ventilation, progression to lower airway disease, high rates of secondary bacterial infection, and persistent viral shedding [26, 27]. Factors associated with greater risk for progression to pneumonia include older age (>65 years) and the presence of severe neutropenia or lymphopenia. Among HCT patients who develop pneumonia, severe lymphopenia (absolute lymphocyte count <200 cells/ml) is associated with a higher risk for death. Death has been noted in 15–30% of patients with pneumonia. Even in survivors of influenza, residual sequelae may include long-lasting pulmonary impairment [26].

2009H1N1v infection

Emergence of the pandemic 2009H1N1v unveiled many of the challenges in preventing and treating respiratory viral infections. The 2009H1N1v originated from genetic reassortment between IFVs from humans, birds, and pigs. Both of the US Food and Drug Administration (FDA)-approved adamantanes lacked inhibitory activity towards the M2 channel of 2009H1N1v, owing to mutation in amino acid Ser31 [28, 29]. The M gene encoded by this new pandemic IFV is reportedly similar to the M gene in the Eurasian swine virus, which confers resistance to both amantadine and rimantidine. Fortunately, the majority of 2009H1N1v isolates tested to date do remain sensitive to the NAIs. However, drug resistance in 2009H1N1v has been described in the immunocompetent host. As of August 2010, the World Health Organization had documented 304 cases associated with the H274Y mutations (histidine to tyrosine at codon 274 in N2 nomenclature or H275Y in N1 nomenclature) in H1N1v with reduced sensitivity to oseltamivir [30, 31]. The concern for the potential for increased resistance is also exemplified by a report of several genetic changes in 2009H1N1v isolates from the Southern Hemisphere that have been associated with vaccine breakthroughs and a number of fatalities in both Singapore and Australia [32]. Thus, there is concern that drug resistance could become prevalent, as occurred with seasonal IFV strains in 2009, when mutations associated with resistance to oseltamivir were found in almost all isolates [33].

A number of cases of severe 2009H1N1v infection resulting in significant morbidity and mortality have been described in HCT patients, and in some they were associated with drug resistance. A study examined the outcome of 27 H1N1v patients post-HCT [34]. Influenza-related 30-day overall mortality was 22%, while patients with LRI had a 43% mortality rate. Chronic steroid use (≥20 mg/day of prednisone equivalent) at the time of presentation was a risk factor for LRI and death.

Possible risk factors and poorer outcomes were examined in 13 patients with 2009H1N1v infection post-HCT [35]. Five of 13 patients had 2009H1N1 influenza-induced LRI and only one survived. The authors noted that lower respiratory tract disease and poorer outcomes occurred in patients receiving intense immunosuppressive therapy who were neutropenic and had GVHD.

In a series of 2009H1N1v cases compared with seasonal influenza A, the 2009H1N1v cases were associated with greater likelihood of LRI, hypoxemia, and prolonged viral shedding compared with seasonal influenza when controlled for confounding factors. Lymphopenia, delay in institution of antiviral therapy, and viremia were associated with severe complications and death [3, 4].

Although most strains of H1N1 virus exhibit sensitivity to the NAIs, resistance has been noted and this phenomenon has influenced treatment choices. Antón et al. described the development of drug resistance and the associated viral kinetics after infection with 2009H1N1v in an immunosuppressed patient [36]. Resistance to oseltamivir was observed after 10 days of treatment. During subsequent treatment with zanamivir, viral loads remained elevated for 5 days but then declined over an additional 7 days.

The United States Centers for Disease Control and Prevention (US CDC) described infections in two immunosuppressed individuals early in the 2009H1N1v pandemic [37]. The first patient developed influenza-like symptoms approximately 30 days after HCT and was treated with oseltamivir for >6 weeks, with evidence of persistence infection by polymerase chain reaction (PCR) assay. Sequence analysis revealed variants containing H274Y mutation within 2 weeks after beginning oseltamivir treatment began. A second patient developed respiratory symptoms after two cycles of chemotherapy and was initially treated with oseltamivir and rimantadine. H274Y was detected and oseltamivir discontinued. Treatment with inhaled zanamivir was attempted but poorly tolerated. The patient was subsequently treated with intravenous (IV) zanamivir and ribavirin in combination. She remained symptomatic at the time of the report with no additional follow up on the patient's clinical status.

Memol et al. described two HCT patients who rapidly developed resistance to oseltamivir and peramivir after infection with 2009H1N1v [38]. One developed respiratory symptoms and was treated for 30 days with oseltamivir. The H274Y mutation was detected by day 9 posttreatment. The other developed mild upper respiratory symptoms and was treated with oseltamavir. After 24 days of continuous oseltamivir therapy the patient developed respiratory distress, and bronchoscopy revealed the presence of IFV. The patient then received 10 days of inhaled zanamivir with symptomatic improvement.

Selection of multidrug resistance to all available NAIs (oseltamivir, zanamivir, and peramivir) was described in a pediatric patient who developed influenza-like symptoms just prior to HCT [39]. Influenza was confirmed by PCR and the patient was treated with oseltamivir. Twelve days later the H274Y mutation was detected and the patient received zanamivir intravenously. The viral load decreased and the patient was discharged but returned approximately 3 weeks later with upper respiratory symptoms. IV zanamivir was reinitiated; however, the virus persisted and a new mutation, I223R, was detected on day 55, exhibiting decreased sensitivity to oseltamivir, zanamivir, and peramivir. Respiratory status of this patient worsened, eventually leading to death.

Renaud et al. described a patient who developed respiratory symptoms and fever approximately 2 years after allogeneic HCT [40]. The patient received oseltamivir, but his respiratory status declined and bronchoalveolar lavage fluid revealed a high viral load for 2009H1N1v. PCR revealed that >90% of viral RNA was wild type, encoding histidine at position 274. On day 7 the patient began IV peramivir. However, on day 17, because of continued viral shedding, peramivir was discontinued and H274Y confirmed as present by PCR, illustrating the emergence of resistance to NAIs during therapy.

Redelman-Sidi et al. characterized 45 cancer and HCT patients with 2009H1N1v [41]. They responded well to oseltamivir and had mild respiratory symptoms. However, no patient in this cohort was less than 5 months posttransplantation. The mild clinical presentation was likely due to immune reconstitution expected beyond the first 100 days posttransplant. In another study, 2/6 (33%) patients who acquired the 2009 H1N1 influenza at <100 days post-HSCT developed respiratory failure requiring mechanical ventilation versus 1/33 (3%) patients who developed the infection at >100 days posttransplantation [42].

A concerning report described the first documented person-to-person transmission of oseltamivir-resistant 2009H1N1v in an inpatient stem-cell transplant unit [43]. Eleven patients were infected with 2009H1N1v, 10 strains of which were genetically related. Eight of the 10 displayed the identical H274Y mutation.

Overall, the incidence of 2009H1N1v resistance to NAIs remains low even in the HCT patient population. Given that prolonged shedding in the respiratory secretions is well documented, the risk is higher than for the immunocompetent population. As a result, we suggest that HCT recipients diagnosed with 2009H1N1v LRI and on a prolonged treatment course of oseltamivir (>7 days) showing worsening clinical signs or symptoms be checked for resistance. The impact of the resistance on treatment is discussed below.

Diagnostics

HCT patients of any age with IFV infection may shed influenza viruses for weeks to months, even without fever or respiratory symptoms. Therefore, collection of upper and lower respiratory tract specimens (e.g., with bronchoalveolar lavage) within 5 days after illness onset may still be useful for influenza testing in these persons. In order of priority, the following influenza tests are recommended, if available:

1. RT-PCR (real time-PCR). This is currently the most sensitive and specific of testing modalities for influenza, with results available within 4–6 h after specimen submission. RT-PCR shows greater sensitivity than viral culture, may be used as a confirmatory test, and is useful for quickly differentiating between influenza types and subtypes. RT-PCR is also the preferred test for specimens obtained from persons with a history of exposure to animals with possible influenza illness (e.g., influenza A [H5N1] in poultry in Eurasia or Africa or swine influenza in any part of the world, including North America).

2. Immunofluorescence. Direct fluorescent antibody and indirect fluorescent antibody staining for influenza antigen detection are used as screening tests. Immunofluorescence exhibits slightly lower sensitivity and specificity than viral isolation in cell culture, but results are available within hours after specimen submission. Performance of these assays depends heavily on laboratory expertise and the quality of the specimen collected (i.e., specimens must include respiratory epithelium cells).

3. Commercial rapid influenza diagnostic tests. The currently available antigen detection tests provide results in 10–30 min but exhibit decreased sensitivity (70–90% in children and <40% to 60% in adults), compared with RT-PCR and with viral culture. Performance of these assays depends heavily on patient age, duration of illness, sample type, and perhaps viral type. Given the lower sensitivity of immunofluorescence and commercial rapid tests, follow-up testing with RT-PCR is required.

4. Viral isolation (in standard cell culture and shell vial culture) is not a screening test, but during periods of low influenza activity (late spring, summer, and early fall) it should be performed on respiratory specimens collected from persons with suspected influenza that present for medical care within 5 days after illness onset, especially if such persons are known to be epidemiologically linked to an influenza outbreak. During the influenza season, viral culture should be performed with respiratory specimens obtained from a subset of persons for routine virologic surveillance purposes and to confirm some negative test results from rapid antigen and immunofluorescence testing, particularly in the setting of institutional outbreaks.

5. Serologic testing is usually not recommended to detect evidence of human influenza virus infection for management of acute illness. Influenza serologic test data for a single serum specimen cannot be reliably interpreted. Paired acute and convalescent-phase serum samples are needed for determination of antibody titers (by hemagglutinin inhibition, enzyme-linked immunosorbent assay, or complement fixation, available only through reference laboratories), but results cannot be obtained in a timely fashion and will not influence clinical management. Paired serum specimens are useful only for retrospective diagnosis and for research purposes.

In a study of patients with severe influenza, specimens from the nasopharyngeal area were felt to be the highest yield, followed by nasal swab and then throat swab [44]. Also, a recent US CDC evaluation of 11 commercially available rapid influenza diagnostic tests showed collecting specimens in the first 24–72 h after illness onset can maximize the concentration of virus antigen in the sample.

In our institution, patients presenting with symptoms or signs consistent with IFV are screened by influenza antigen (quick turn around time) and followed by RT-PCR (greater sensitivity). If the presentation is in the middle of a community outbreak of seasonal IFV and clinical impression is felt consistent with influenza, presumptive treatment should be strongly considered at time of presentation, rather than awaiting the results of the diagnostic testing.

Treatment options

Limited data exist from randomized controlled trials on the utility and optimal duration of use of licensed antivirals in immunosuppressed individuals.

Neuraminidase inhibitors

At present, the predominant class of antivirals used for the treatment and prophylaxis of influenza are the NAIs, which interfere with the release of IFV particles from infected cells, preventing the spread of infection to other cells. The licensed NAIs include oseltamivir, inhaled zanamivir, and recently, under emergency use authorization, IV peramivir. IV zanamivir had been available through an Investigational New Drug (IND) application with the US FDA [45].

The antiviral treatment options for HCT patients are empiric and tailored to the particular strain and its known sensitivity. As discussed above, HCT recipients infected with IFV can have prolonged infections lasting for more than 5 days, and longer duration NAI treatment might be warranted. The specific duration of treatment is often empiric. While NAIs are well tolerated, postlicensing reports have indicated that zanamivir may cause cough, bronchospasm, or even death in patients with preexisting pulmonary disease. Hence, this antiviral should be used with caution in patients with serious underlying respiratory diseases.

Oseltamivir is recommended for infection caused by 2009H1N1v in the immunocompetent host, as this virus is typically resistant to the adamantanes [46], in contrast to the previous 2008–2009 seasonal H1N1 strain, which was characterized by oseltamivir resistance but susceptible to amantadine [47]. As the development of resistance is more complex in immunosuppressed individuals, the US CDC has recommended that patients with suspected or confirmed oseltamivir-resistant 2009H1N1v be treated with zanamivir [48]. If inhaled zanamivir is contraindicated or not well tolerated, then IV zanamivir is available for compassionate use from its manufacturer via an emergency IND application to the US FDA. The US CDC also recommends that patients infected with IFV suspected or documented to have H274Y mutation should not be treated with peramivir, as clinical isolates expressing the oseltamivir resistance-associated substitution H274Y demonstrate reduced peramivir susceptibility in vitro. The US CDC had tested seasonal influenza A(H1N1) viruses collected in 2008–2010 from the USA and globally for resistance to antivirals approved by the FDA. They reported 28 viruses with both adamantane and oseltamivir (dual) resistance from five countries belonging to four distinct genotypes [49].

The optimal therapy for severely immunosuppressed patients with oseltamivir-resistant 2009H1N1v has not been clearly defined. Some severely immunosuppressed patients with 2009H1N1v have been treated with a combination of IV zanamivir and aerosolized ribavirin [50] or IV zanamivir monotherapy. No controlled studies, however, have confirmed the efficacy of this combination approach [51]. A study of 541 patients with confirmed IFV investigated the use of combination therapy (zanamivir and oseltamivir) versus either oseltamivir or zanamivir monotherapy [52]. For the primary endpoints of declining viral load and time to alleviation of symptoms, combination therapy was less effective than oseltamivir monotherapy and not significantly more effective than zanamivir monotherapy.

Clinical investigational treatments other than NAIs

Favipiravir (T705, Toyama Chemical) is an investigational antiviral drug that functions as a nucleotide analog and inhibitor of viral RNA polymerase (PB1, PB2, and PA) [53, 54]. Preclinical studies by Itoh and colleagues suggest that favipiravir is active against pandemic H1N1 strains both in vitro and in vivo [55].

A recent study demonstrated that favipiravir was effective against oseltamivir-resistant seasonal and pandemic-viruses in vitro [56]. In addition, the drug has potent activity against H5N1 IFV in vivo [57]. Favipiravir, alone or in combination with licensed NAIs, is being investigated in phase II clinical studies for the treatment of influenza. There are currently no reports of the use of favipiravir in immunosuppressed patients.

DAS181 (Fludase, NexBio Inc.) is a recombinant fusion protein with sialidase activity and carrying a cationic sequence tag on the C-terminus [58]. This drug selectively cleaves sialic acids from host cells, rendering them inaccessible to IFV, which seeks sialic acid as its receptor.

DAS181 has activity against numerous seasonal IFV strains *in vitro* and *in vivo* as well as highly pathogenic avian influenza strains (H5N1) [59] and against the 2009H1N1v pandemic strains *in vitro*, *in vivo*, and *ex vivo* [60]. It also has antiviral activity against clinical IFV isolates with the H274Y mutation. DAS181 is currently in phase II trials for the treatment of influenza in immunocompetent subjects.

Prevention

Influenza vaccination is the most widely studied amongst CRV. Lifelong seasonal influenza vaccine is recommended for all HCT candidates and recipients. Inactivated influenza vaccine should be administered beginning at least 6 months after HCT and annually thereafter for the life of the patient [10]. A dose of inactivated influenza vaccine can be given as early as 4 months after HCT, but a second dose should be considered in this situation. Two doses are recommended routinely for the initial vaccination for all children receiving influenza vaccine for the first time.

Data demonstrating efficacy of inactivated (killed) IFV vaccine for HCT recipients are limited. The protective effect is lower in the patients in general, and one study reported 29% protective antibody levels to influenza A H1/N1 serotype in the recipients. It is widely accepted that transplant-to-vaccination interval has an important impact on vaccine immunogenicity [61]. A study in pediatric allogeneic HCT recipients showed higher response rates in patients >1 year post-HCT, but the enrolled patients were found to have increasing antibody response even at 6 months post-HCT [62]. The correlation of CD4 counts and response to vaccination has been inconsistent. A few studies have reported correlation of naive-CD4 cells and antibody response [63, 64], but these are limited by low patient numbers and are nonrandomized.

Vaccination of close contacts of immunosuppressed persons, including healthcare practitioners (HCPs), might reduce the risk for influenza transmission. In 2006 and then again in 2010, a joint recommendation from the Advisory Committee on Immunization Practices and the Hospital Infection Control Practices Advisory Committee (HICPAC) recommended that trivalent inactivated vaccine (TIV) be used for vaccinating household members, HCPs, and others who have close contact with HCT recipients during those periods in which the immunosuppressed person requires care in a protective environment (typically defined as a specialized patient-care area with a positive airflow relative to the corridor, high-efficiency particulate air filtration, and frequent air changes).

Since responses to vaccines are impaired early after HCT, immunization of family members and care providers in close contact with the patient can offer some protection that such individuals will not infect the patient. Since vaccination cannot be assured of providing the HCT recipient with early protection after transplant if exposed or in the midst of a community or nosocomial outbreak, chemoprophylaxis with an NAI should be strongly considered.

Respiratory syncytial virus infections

In the USA, RSV infections occur in the fall, winter, and spring, with an attack rate up to 10% during winter time [65, 66]. Allogeneic HCT recipients are more likely to experience RSV pneumonia if they received a myeloablative, mismatched, or unrelated transplant and have advanced age [67, 68]. Patients who remain lymphopenic and acquire RSV infection are at high risk of progressing to pneumonia during the first 3 months after HCT [7, 69]. HCT recipients with influenza-like symptoms (i.e., runny nose, fever, nasal congestion, sore throat, and cough) during the cold season should be tested for RSV and other respiratory viruses. Viral isolation by conventional culture is the "gold standard" for diagnosis of RSV infection; however, it may take up to 1 week to finalize the culture and it has a low sensitivity [70, 71]. Rapid diagnosis of RSV infection can be made by direct antigen testing on clinical specimens (i.e., direct immunofluorescence staining), using the shell vial culture technique, which provides results within 48 h, with a sensitivity of 93% and a specificity of 97% [72], and by RT-PCR assays for detection of RSV RNA with a higher sensitivity and specificity [70, 71]. In our institution, any patient presenting with URI symptoms should be screened by direct antigen testing and followed by viral respiratory polymerase chain reaction.

Prevention of RSV transmission in a hospital setting, especially where immunosuppressed patients are housed, is considered a basic standard of care in many hospitals. Strict infection control precautions considered critical to preventing spread within a hospital ward include respiratory isolation of infected patients, hand washing before and after contact with patients, and educational efforts targeting healthcare workers and family members.

RSV-associated mortality in HCT patients has been reported to range from 7% to 83% in patients whose infection progresses to LRI [5, 73–75]. Chemoprophylaxis in susceptible HCT patients may be considered, especially in outbreak situations when horizontal transmission is occurring [76]. Palivizumab (PVZ) is the only commercially available drug that has been licensed (June 1998) for prevention of RSV infection in high-risk children [77, 78]. To date, there are no randomized trials of chemoprophylaxis in HCT patients, and it remains uncertain as to how effective this approach is. A newer drug, motavizumab, has been studied for prophylaxis in high-risk children and appears to be non-inferior to PVZ [79]. However, this drug is not yet approved by the FDA for prophylaxis in high-risk children. Currently, there is no commercially available vaccine that can prevent RSV infection.

Management of RSV infection should target (1) viral replication, (2) virus-induced lung inflammation (3) co-infections or superimposed infections, and (4) respiratory dysfunction [80]. Available therapies that have been used for treatment of RSV infections are limited to ribavirin, intravenous immunoglobulin (IVIG), and PVZ. The lack of well-designed randomized controlled trials leaves clinicians with a few studies, mostly retrospective and from single centers, as the only available clinical data.

The aerosolized form of ribavirin was approved by the FDA in 1986 for treatment of RSV LRI in hospitalized high-risk infants and young children, and it is still the only drug approved for this indication [81]. Data on the use of oral ribavirin are very limited, but Khanna et al. [82], in the largest published study to date on the use of oral ribavirin in HSCT recipients for RSV infection, reported a rather similar outcome from a single center.

Since RSV URI often progresses to LRI, there has been considerable interest in preemptive treatment of patients with RSV URI to prevent LRI. Regardless of the form or duration of therapy or the addition of an immunomodulator, in uncontrolled studies, the rate of progression to LRI and mortality rate appeared to be lower in patients who received ribavirin than in patients who did not receive any form of RSV therapy [5, 67–69, 83–89]. In those studies, a higher proportion (47%; range: 27–100%) of cases that were not treated at URI stage progressed to LRI , and 46% of these died of RSV infection. Patients whose infection progressed to LRI and were not treated had a higher mortality rate than those whose infection was treated (deaths among treated: 50%, range: 33–88%; deaths among untreated: 89%, range: 50–100%). There was also a difference in mortality rate, which was lower in patients who were treated at the URI stage. In conclusion, the data in support of preemptive RSV are as yet inconclusive since adequate prospective randomized trials are lacking. However, some experts advocate preemptive approaches in high-risk patients, particularly in those with lymphopenia. In a meta-analysis [90] comparing various combination regimens, a better outcome was noted in regard to progression to LRI and death among patients treated with aerosolized ribavirin (AR) and an immunomodulator than in those treated with aerosolized ribavirin alone, although there has been only one randomized control study ever done [85]. Among patients whose infection progressed to LRI, those treated with aerosolized ribavirin and an immunomodulator had a lower mortality rate of 24% than those treated with aerosolized ribavirin alone (50%) or with IV or oral ribavirin with or without an immunomodulator (54%) [90].

Human parainfluenza virus (HPIV)

HPIV infections encompass four serotypes that cause mostly mild URI throughout the year with seasonal increases in fall and spring in children [91]. Several studies have documented a high occurrence of HPIV type III infection in HCT recipients [7, 92, 93]. In adult and pediatric leukemia and HCT patients, symptomatic HPIV infections have been reported to range from 2% to 7%, of which at least one-third are manifest as LRI [94–101]. Most of the outbreaks of HPIV type III infection occurred in spring and summer, as has been described by other studies [93, 102, 103]. URIs cause significant persistent air flow decline in 40%, and a single-center study shows that almost half of the patients progressed to HPIV pneumonia, with a subsequent mortality rate of 17% [104, 105]. Risk factors for LRI include higher dose steroids and lymphopenia <200 cells/ml [7].

The role of treatment is limited by the lack of effective agents and randomized control trials (RCT), although some centers consider treating HPIV LRI. Treatment with aerosolized ribavirin and or IVIG did not prevent progression to pneumonia and did not affect duration of illness or survival in either group [16, 95, 106]. DAS181 is a recombinant fusion protein containing the catalytic domain of actinomyces viscosus sialidase, which effectively removes sialic acids from the surface of respiratory epithelial cells, thereby inhibiting infection by different parainfluenza virus strains. In cultured human airway epithelial cells and in a cotton rat parainfluenza virus infection model, DAS181 has been shown to remove sialic acid receptors, inhibit parainfluenza virus genome replication and progeny virion formation, and significantly reduce viral titers in the infected lungs [107]. Experience with DAS181 for the treatment of parainfluenza virus infections in humans is limited. There have been three case reports in immunosuppressed patients two patients post-HCT and one after lung transplant. The patients were diagnosed by quantitative HPIV PCR of nasal and oral washings and subsequently treated with

DAS181 for 3–5 days. All three patients had interval clinical improvement, but only one of them had a concurrent decline in the (0.5 log) in the viral titer in oropharyngeal swabs. Given that DAS181 has substantial anti-inflammatory effects, further formal clinical studies should be performed in immunosuppressed patients with moderate-to-severe parainfluenza virus type 3 infections to evaluate the true antiviral therapeutic efficacy and safety of this agent [108].

Human metapneumovirus (HMPV)

HMPV infection rates in HCT patients range from 5% to 9% during the first 2 years posttransplant [99]. The winter and spring prominence of HMPV infections reflects the seasonal incidence of HMPV infections and has been well described in studies [100, 101, 109–111]. Progression to HPMV LRI is rare, and rates and risk factors are not well described. In HCT patients with pneumonia, HMPV is frequently co-detected with other pathogens, including bacteria, fungi, and other community-acquired respiratory viruses (CARVs), as well as cytomegalovirus, all which obscure the attributable morbidity [67, 112]. Recipient cytomegalovirus seropositivity was a risk factor in one study of HCT patients [67].

Ribavirin has *in vitro* and animal model activity against human metapneumovirus [113, 114]. However, there have been no trials to assess its clinical efficacy.

Human coronavirus (HCoV)

Human coronaviruses (HCoVs) circulate throughout the year with a predominance in winter, which may reflect in part the increasing testing for respiratory viral infections [115–117]. In HCT patients, HCoV has been detected in 6.7–15.4%, in a recent prospective study of patients post-allogeneic transplant HCoV incidence was second highest at 100 days post-transplant [63]. In spite of a high incidence, the rate of pneumonia and death attributable to these viruses was low compared with other common respiratory viruses. Few cases of fatal pneumonia attributed to HCoV infection in immunosuppressed patients have been reported [18, 118, 119]. The role of treatment is limited in view of the largely benign course, the lack of effective agents and RCTs, and only few centers consider treating HCoV LRI [120].

Human rhinovirus (HRhV)

Human rhinoviruses (HRhVs) belong to the *Picornaviridae* family and are divided into three species called A, B, and C encompassing more than 100 serotypes. HRhVs circulate throughout the year and are the most common cause of URI disease (rhinorrhea, postnasal drip, cough) and occasionally tracheobronchitis [121]. In allogeneic HCT recipients, HRhV is the most frequent CARV, reaching a cumulative incidence of 22.3% by day 100 [117]. HRhV infection may be asymptomatic in 13% of HCT patients, and prolonged shedding over 4 weeks is frequent, with co-infections with other CARVs occurring in 19% of patients [117, 122]. The nucleic acid amplification test has been seen as the best test for detecting virus compared with viral culture. One study reports that higher HRhV loads correlate with symptomatic presentations [123].

LRI with frank pneumonia is rare and may occur in <10% of allogeneic HCT infected with HRhV, usually after myeloablative conditioning, with an estimated mortality of less than 10% [67, 68, 122, 124]. The role of HRhV treatment is limited by the lack of agents and clinical trials, and only a few centers consider treating HRhV LRI [86].

Other community respiratory viral infections

Human bocavirus (HBoV), human enterovirus, and human polyomavirus have been detected in patients with hematologic malignancies or HCT, but risk factors for disease and the need for therapy have been difficult to assess owing to the lack of studies and co-detection of other pathogens [122, 125, 126]. In bronchoalveolar lavage from adult patients, HBoV was detected in 0–3% of cases. Recent studies suggest that HBoV loads above 5 log10 copies/mL in respiratory fluids are more likely to indicate clinically significant replication [125].

References

1. Leung TWC, Tai ALS, Cheng PKC, et al. Detection of an oseltamivir-resistant pandemic influenza A/H1N1 virus in Hong Kong. J Clin Virol. 2009;46(3):298–299.

2. Centers for Disease Control and Prevention. Oseltamivir-resistant 2009 pandemic influenza A(H1N1) virus infection in two summer campers receiving prophylaxis – North Carolina, 2009. MMWR Morb Mortal Wkly Rep. 2009; 58(35):969–972.
3. Choi SM, Xie H, Campbell AP, et al. Influenza viral RNA detection in blood as a marker to predict disease severity in hematopoietic cell transplant recipients. J Infect Dis. 2012;206(12):1872–1877.
4. Choi SM, Boudreault AA, Xie H, et al. Differences in clinical outcomes after 2009 influenza A/H1N1 and seasonal influenza among hematopoietic cell transplant recipients. Blood. 2011;117(19):5050–5056.
5. Harrington RD, Hooton TM, Hackman RC, et al. An outbreak of respiratory syncytial virus in a bone marrow transplant center. J Infect Dis. 1992;165(6):987–993.
6. Raad I, Abbas J, Whimbey E. Infection control of nosocomial respiratory viral disease in the immunosuppressed host. Am J Med. 1997;102(3A):48–52.
7. Chemaly RF, Ghosh S, Bodey GP, et al. Respiratory viral infections in adults with hematologic malignancies and human stem cell transplantation recipients: a retrospective study at a major cancer center. Medicine (Baltimore). 2006;85:278–287.
8. Tablan OC, Anderson LJ, Besser R, et al. Guidelines for preventing health-care-associated pneumonia, 2003: recommendations of CDC and the Healthcare Infection Control Practices Advisory Committee. MMWR Recomm Rep. 2004;53:1–36.
9. Lee I, Barton TD. Viral respiratory tract infections in transplant patients: epidemiology, recognition and management. Drugs. 2007;67:1411–1427.
10. Tomblyn M, Chiller T, Einsele H, et al. Guidelines for preventing infectious complications among hematopoietic cell transplant recipients: a global perspective. Biol Blood Marrow Transplant. 2009;15(10):1143–1238.
11. Wingard JR. Influenza: preparedness for an inevitable "Emergency" for oncology and BMT units. J Natl Compr Canc Netw. 2008;6(2):215–222.
12. Boyce JM, Pittet D. Guideline for hand hygiene in health-care settings. Recommendations of the Healthcare Infection Control Practices Advisory Committee and the HICPAC/SHEA/ APIC/IDSA Hand Hygiene Task Force. Society for Healthcare Epidemiology of America/ Association for Professionals in Infection Control/ Infectious Diseases Society of America. MMWR Recomm Rep. 2002;51:1–45.
13. Hayden FG. Prevention and treatment of influenza in immunosuppressed patients. Am J Med. 1997;102:55–60.
14. Fox JP, Brandt CD, Wassermann FE, et al. The virus watch program: a continuing surveillance of viral infections in metropolitan New York families. VI. Observations of adenovirus infections: virus excretion patterns, antibody response, efficiency of surveillance, patterns of infections, and relation to illness. Am J Epidemiol. 1969;89:25–50.
15. Hillis WO, Cooper MR, Bang FB. Adenovirus infection in West Bengal. I: persistence of viruses in infants and young children. Indian J Med Res. 1973;61:980–988.
16. Whimbey E, Champlin RE, Couch RB, et al. Community respiratory virus infections among hospitalized adult bone marrow transplant recipients. Clin Infect Dis. 1996; 22:778–782.
17. Whimbey E, Champlin RE, Englund JA, et al. Combination therapy with aerosolized ribavirin and intravenous immunoglobulin for respiratory syncytial virus disease in adult bone marrow transplant recipients. Bone Marrow Transplant. 1995;16:393–399.
18. Folz RJ, Elkordy MA. Coronavirus pneumonia following autologous bone marrow transplantation for breast cancer. Chest. 1999;115:901–905.
19. Suzuki T, Portner A, Scroggs RA, et al. Receptor specificities of human respiroviruses. J Virol. 2001;75:4604–4613.
20. Ito T. Interspecies transmission and receptor recognition of influenza A viruses. Microbiol Immunol. 2000;44(6): 423–430.
21. Martino R, Porras RP, Rabella N, et al. Prospective study of the incidence, clinical features, and outcome of symptomatic upper and lower respiratory tract infections by respiratory viruses is adult recipients of hematopoietic stem cell transplants for hematologic malignancies. Biol Blood Marrow Transplant. 2005;11(10):781–796.
22. Boivin G, Goyette N, Bernatchez H. Prolonged excretion of amantadine-resistant influenza A virus quasi species after cessation of antiviral therapy in an immunosuppressed patient. Clin Infect Dis. 2002;34(5):E23–E25.
23. Klimov AI, Rocha E, Hayden FG, et al. Prolonged shedding of amantadine-resistant influenza A viruses by immunodeficient patients: detection by polymerase chain reaction-restriction analysis. J Infect Dis. 1995;172(5): 1352–1355.
24. Gooskens J, Jonges M, Claas ECJ, et al. Prolonged influenza virus infection during lymphocytopenia and frequent detection of drug-resistant viruses. J Infect Dis. 2009; 199(10):1435–1441.
25. Gooskens J, Jonges M, Claas ECJ, et al. Morbidity and mortality associated with nosocomial transmission of oseltamivir-resistant influenza A(H1N1) virus. J Am Med Assoc. 2009;301(10):1042–1046.
26. Nichols WG, Guthrie KA, Corey L, et al. Influenza infections after hematopoietic stem cell transplantation: risk factors, mortality, and the effect of antiviral therapy. Clin Infect Dis. 2004;39(9):1300–1306.

27. Kumar D, Humar A. Respiratory viral infections in transplant and oncology patients. Infect Dis Clin North Am. 2010;24(2):395–412.
28. Shinde V, Bridges CB, Uyeki TM, et al. Triple-reassortant swine influenza A (H1) in humans in the United States, 2005–2009. N Engl J Med. 2009;360(25):2616–2625.
29. Dawood FS, Jain S, Finelli L, et al. Emergence of a novel swine-origin influenza A (H1N1) virus in humans. N Engl J Med. 2009;360(25):2605–2615.
30. Rungrotmongkol T, Intharathep P, Malaisree M, et al. Susceptibility of antiviral drugs against 2009 influenza A (H1N1) virus. Biochem Biophys Res Commun. 2009; 385(3):390–394.
31. Weekly update on oseltamivir resistance to influenza A (H1N1) 2009 viruses. 2010. Available from: http://www.who.int/csr/disease/swineflu/oseltamivirresistant20100820.pdf (accessed 3 May 2013).
32. Barr IG, Cui L, Komadina N, et al. A new pandemic influenza A(H1N1) genetic variant predominated in the winter 2010 influenza season in Australia, New Zealand and Singapore. Euro Surveill. 2010;15(42):1–6.
33. Moss RB, Davey RT, Steigbigel RT, et al. Targeting pandemic influenza: a primer on influenza antivirals and drug resistance. J Antimicrob Chemother. 2010;65(6): 1086–1093.
34. Espinosa-Aguilar L, Green JS, Forrest GN, et al. Novel H1N1 influenza in hematopoietic stem cell transplantation recipients: two centers' experiences. Biol Blood Marrow Transplant. 2011;17(4):566–573.
35. George B, Ferguson P, Kerridge I, et al. The clinical impact of infection with swine flu (H1N109) strain of influenza virus in hematopoietic stem cell transplant recipients. Biol Blood Marrow Transplant. 2011;17(1):147–153.
36. Antón A, López-Iglesias AA, Tórtola T, et al. Selection and viral load kinetics of an oseltamivir-resistant pandemic influenza A (H1N1) virus in an immunosuppressed patient during treatment with neuraminidase inhibitors. Diagn Microbiol Infect Dis. 2010;68(3):214–219.
37. Centers for Disease Control and Prevention. Oseltamivir-resistant novel influenza A (H1N1) virus infection in two immunosuppressed patients – Seattle, Washington, 2009. MMWR Morb Mortal Wkly Rep. 2009;58:893–896.
38. Memoli MJ, Hrabal RJ, Hassantoufighi A, et al. Rapid selection of oseltamivir- and peramivir-resistant pandemic H1N1 virus during therapy in 2 immunosuppressed hosts. Clin Infect Dis. 2010;50(9):1252–1255.
39. Van der Vries E, Stelma FF, Boucher CAB. Emergence of a multidrug-resistant pandemic influenza A (H1N1) virus. N Engl J Med. 2010;363(14):1381–1382.
40. Renaud C, Pergam SA, Polyak C, et al. Early emergence of an H275Y mutation in a hematopoietic cell transplant recipient treated with intravenous peramivir. Transpl Infect Dis. 2010;12(6):513–517.
41. Redelman-Sidi G, Sepkowitz KA, Huang CK, et al. H1N1 influenza infection in cancer patients and hematopoietic stem cell transplant recipients. J Infect. 2009;60(4): 257–263.
42. Rihani R, Hayajneh W, Sultan I, et al. Infections with the 2009 H1N1 influenza virus among hematopoietic SCT recipients: a single center experience. Bone Marrow Transplant. 2011;46:1430–1436.
43. Moore C, Galiano M, Lackenby A, et al. Evidence of person-to-person transmission of oseltamivir-resistant pandemic influenza A(H1N1) 2009 virus in a hematology unit. J Infect Dis. 2011;203(1):18–24.
44. Ngaosuwankul J, Noisumdaeng P, Komolsiri P, et al. Influenza A viral loads in respiratory samples collected from patients infected with pandemic H1N1, seasonal H1N1 and H3N2 viruses. Virol J. 2010;7:75.
45. Kidd IM, Down J, Nastouli E, et al. H1N1 pneumonitis treated with intravenous zanamivir. Lancet. 2009; 374(9694):1036.
46. Centers for Disease Control and Prevention. 2009. Updated interim recommendations for the use of antiviral medications in the treatment and prevention of influenza for the 2009–2010 season. Available from: http://www.cdc.gov/H1N1flu/recommendations.htm (accessed 3 May 2013).
47. Moscona A. Global transmission of oseltamivir-resistant influenza. N Engl J Med. 2009;360(10):953–956.
48. Centers for Disease Control and Prevention. 2009. Updated Interim recommendations: special considerations for clinicians regarding 2009 H1N1 influenza in severely immunosuppressed patients. Available from: http://www.cdc.gov/h1n1flu/immunosuppression/index.htm (accessed 3 May 2013).
49. Sheu TG, Fry AM, Garten RJ, et al. Dual resistance to adamantanes and oseltamivir among seasonal influenza A(H1N1) viruses: 2008–2010. J Infect Dis. 2011;203(1): 13–17.
50. Chan-Tack KM, Murray JS, Birnkrant DB. Use of ribavirin to treat influenza. N Engl J Med. 2009;361(17): 1713–1714.
51. Gaur AH, Bagga B, Barman S, et al. Intravenous zanamivir for oseltamivir-resistant 2009 H1N1 influenza. N Engl J Med. 2010;362(1):88–89.
52. Duval X, Van der Werf S, Blanchon T, et al. Efficacy of oseltamivir–zanamivir combination compared to each monotherapy for seasonal influenza: a randomized placebo-controlled trial. PLoS Med. 2010;7(11):Article ID e1000362.
53. Smee DF, Hurst BL, Egawa H, et al. Intracellular metabolism of favipiravir (T-705) in uninfected and influenza A

(H5N1) virus-infected cells. J Antimicrob Chemother. 2009;64(4):741–746.
54. Furuta Y, Takahashi K, Shiraki K, et al. T-705 (favipiravir) and related compounds: novel broad-spectrum inhibitors of RNA viral infections. Antiviral Res. 2009;82(3):95–102.
55. Itoh Y, Shinya K, Kiso M, et al. *In vitro* and *in vivo* characterization of new swine-origin H1N1 influenza viruses. Nature. 2009;460(7258):1021–1025.
56. Sleeman K, Mishin VP, Deyde VM, et al. *In vitro* antiviral activity of favipiravir (T-705) against drug-resistant influenza and 2009 A(H1N1) viruses. Antimicrob Agents Chemother. 2010;54(6):2517–2524.
57. Kiso M, Takahashi K, Sakai-Tagawa Y, et al. T-705 (favipiravir) activity against lethal H5N1 influenza A viruses. Proc Natl Acad Sci U S A. 2010;107(2):882–887.
58. Malakhov MP, Aschenbrenner LM, Smee DF, et al. Sialidase fusion protein as a novel broad-spectrum inhibitor of influenza virus infection. Antimicrob Agents Chemother. 2006;50(4):1470–1479.
59. Belser JA, Lu X, Szretter KJ, et al. DAS181, a novel sialidase fusion protein, protects mice from lethal avian influenza H5N1 virus infection. J Infect Dis. 2007;196(10):1493–1499.
60. Triana-Baltzer GB, Gubareva LV, Klimov AI, et al. Inhibition of neuraminidase inhibitor-resistant influenza virus by DAS181, a novel sialidase fusion protein. PLoS ONE. 2009;4(11):Article ID e7838.
61. Avetisyan G, Aschan J, Hassan M, et al. Evaluation of immune responses to seasonal influenza vaccination in healthy volunteers and in patients after stem cell transplantation. Transplantation. 2008;2:257–263.
62. Karras NA, Weeres M, Sessions W, et al. A randomized trial of one versus two doses of influenza vaccine after allogeneic transplantation. Biol Blood Marrow Transplant. 2013;19:109–116.
63. Roux E, Dumont-Girard F, Starobinski M, et al Recovery of immune reactivity after T-cell-depleted bone marrow transplantation depends on thymic activity. Blood. 2000;6:2299–2303.
64. Mohty B, Bel M, Vukicevic M, et al. Graft-versus-host disease is the major determinant of humoral responses to the AS03-adjuvanted influenza A/09/H1N1 vaccine in allogeneic hematopoietic stem cell transplant recipients. Haematologica. 2011;96:896–904.
65. Nichols WG, Gooley T, Boeckh M. Community-acquired respiratory syncytial virus and parainfluenza virus infections after hematopoietic stem cell transplantation: the Fred Hutchinson Cancer Research Center experience. Biol Blood Marrow Transplant. 2001;7(Suppl):11S–15S.
66. Welliver RC. Pharmacotherapy of respiratory syncytial virus infection. Curr Opin Pharmacol. 2010;10:289–293.
67. Martino R, Porras RP, Rabella N, et al. Prospective study of the incidence, clinical features, and outcome of symptomatic upper and lower respiratory tract infections by respiratory viruses in adult recipients of hematopoietic stem cell transplants for hematologic malignancies. Biol Blood Marrow Transplant. 2005;11(10):781–796.
68. Schiffer JT, Kirby K, Sandmaier B, et al. Timing and severity of community acquired respiratory virus infections after myeloablative versus non-myeloablative hematopoietic stem cell transplantation. Haematologica. 2009;94(8):1101–1108.
69. Ljungman P, Ward KN, Crooks BN, et al. Respiratory virus infections after stem cell transplantation: a prospective study from the Infectious Diseases Working Party of the European Group for Blood and Marrow Transplantation. Bone Marrow Transplant. 2001;28(5):479–484.
70. Kuypers J, Campbell AP, Cent A, et al. Comparison of conventional and molecular detection of respiratory viruses in hematopoietic cell transplant recipients. Transpl Infect Dis. 2009;11(4):298–303.
71. Kuypers J, Wright N, Ferrenberg J, et al. Comparison of real-time PCR assays with fluorescent-antibody assays for diagnosis of respiratory virus infections in children. J Clin Microbiol. 2006;44(7):2382–2388.
72. Ohm-Smith MJ, Nassos PS, Haller BL. Evaluation of the Binax NOW, BD Directigen, and BD Directigen EZ assays for detection of respiratory syncytial virus. J Clin Microbiol. 2004;42(7):2996–2999.
73. McCarthy AJ, Kingman HM, Kelly C, et al. The outcome of 26 patients with respiratory syncytial virus infection following allogeneic stem cell transplantation. Bone Marrow Transplant. 1999;24(12):1315–1322.
74. Lewinsohn DM, Bowden RA, Mattson D, et al. Phase I study of intravenous ribavirin treatment of respiratory syncytial virus pneumonia after marrow transplantation. Antimicrob Agents Chemother. 1996;40(11):2555–2556.
75. Machado CM, Boas LS, Mendes AV, et al. Low mortality rates related to respiratory virus infections after bone marrow transplantation. Bone Marrow Transplant. 2003;31(8):695–700.
76. Kassis C, Champlin RE, Hachem RY, et al. Detection and control of a nosocomial respiratory syncytial virus outbreak in a stem cell transplantation unit: the role of palivizumab. Biol Blood Marrow Transplant. 2010;16(9):1265–1271.
77. American Academy of Pediatrics Committee on Infectious Diseases, Committee on Fetus and Newborn. Prevention of respiratory syncytial virus infections: indications for the use of palivizumab and update on the use of RSV-IGIV. Pediatrics. 1998;102:1211–1216.

78. Impact-RSV Study Group. Palivizumab, a humanized respiratory syncytial virus monoclonal antibody, reduces hospitalization from respiratory syncytial virus infection in high-risk infants. Pediatrics. 1998;102:531–537.
79. Carbonell-Estrany X, Simões EAF, Dagan R, et al. Motavizumab Study Group: motavizumab versus palivizumab for the prophylaxis of serious respiratory syncytial virus disease in high-risk children: a randomized controlled noninferiority trial. Pediatrics. 2010;125(1):e35–e51.
80. Crooks BN, Taylor CE, Turner AJ, et al. Respiratory viral infections in primary immune deficiencies: significance and relevance to clinical outcome in a single BMT unit. Bone Marrow Transplant. 2000;26(10):1097–1102.
81. Food and Drug Administration. Ribavirin aerosol approved for severe cases of RSV in infants and young children. FDA Drug Bull. 1986;16:7.
82. Khanna N, Widmer AF, Decker M, et al. Respiratory syncytial virus infection in patients with hematological diseases: single-center study and review of the literature. Clin Infect Dis. 2008;46(3):402–412.
83. Ebbert JO, Limper AH. Respiratory syncytial virus pneumonitis in immunosuppressed adults: clinical features and outcome. Respiration. 2005;72:263–269.
84. Hertz MI, Englund JA, Snover D, et al. Respiratory syncytial virus-induced acute lung injury in adult patients with bone marrow transplants: a clinical approach and review of the literature. Medicine (Baltimore). 1989;68(5):269–281.
85. Boeckh M, Englund J, Li Y, et al. Randomized controlled multicenter trial of aerosolized ribavirin for respiratory syncytial virus upper respiratory tract infection in hematopoietic cell transplant recipients: NIAID Collaborative Antiviral Study Group. Clin Infect Dis. 2007;44(2):245–249.
86. Hassan IA, Chopra R, Swindell R, et al. Respiratory viral infections after bone marrow/peripheral stem-cell transplantation: the Christie Hospital experience. Bone Marrow Transplant. 2003;32(1):73–77.
87. McColl MD, Corser RB, Bremner J, et al. Respiratory syncytial virus infection in adult BMT recipients: effective therapy with short duration nebulised ribavirin. Bone Marrow Transplant. 1998;21(4):423–425.
88. Bowden RA. Respiratory virus infections after marrow transplant: the Fred Hutchinson Cancer Research Center experience. Am J Med. 1997;102(3A):27–30; discussion 42–43.
89. Englund JA, Sullivan CJ, Jordan MC, et al. Respiratory syncytial virus infection in immunosuppressed adults. Ann Intern Med. 1988;109(3):203–208.
90. Shah JN, Chemaly RF. Management of RSV infections in adult recipients of hematopoietic stem cell transplantation. Blood. 2011;117(10):2755–2763. Epub 2010 Dec 7.
91. Hall CB. Respiratory syncytial virus and parainfluenza virus. N Engl J Med. 2001;344:1917–1928.
92. Vartivarian SE, Champlin RE, Elting LS, et al. Parainfluenza virus infection in adult bone marrow transplant recipients. Eur J Clin Microbiol Infect Dis. 1993;12(9):699–701.
93. Marcolini JA, Malik S, Suki D, et al. Respiratory disease due to parainfluenza virus in adult leukemia patients. Eur J Clin Microbiol Infect Dis. 2003;22(2):79–84.
94. Chen YB, Driscoll J, McAfee SL, et al. Treatment of parainfluenza 3 infection with DAS181 in a patient after allogeneic stem cell transplantation. Clin Infect Dis. 2011;53(7):e77–e80.
95. Guzmán-Suarez BB, Buckley MW, Gilmore ET, et al. Clinical potential of DAS181 for treatment of parainfluenza-3 infections in transplant recipients. Transpl Infect Dis. 2012;14(4):427–433.
96. Srinivasan A, Wang C, Yang J, et al. Parainfluenza virus infections in children with hematologic malignancies. Pediatr Infect Dis J. 2011;30:855–859.
97. Srinivasan A, Wang C, Yang J, et al. Symptomatic parainfluenza virus infections in children undergoing hematopoietic stem cell transplantation. Biol Blood Marrow Transplant. 2011;17:1520–1527.
98. Ustun C, Slaby J, Shanley RM, et al. Human parainfluenza virus infection after hematopoietic stem cell transplantation: risk factors, management, mortality, and changes over time. Biol Blood Marrow Transplant. 2012;18:1580–1588.
99. Williams JV, Martino R, Rabella N, et al. A prospective study comparing human metapneumovirus with other respiratory viruses in adults with hematologic malignancies and respiratory tract infections. J Infect Dis. 2005;192(6):1061–1065. Epub 2005 Aug 12.
100. Van den Hoogen BG, van Doornum GJ, Fockens JC, et al. Prevalence and clinical symptoms of human metapneumovirus infection in hospitalized patients. J Infect Dis. 2003;188:1571–1577.
101. Boivin G, Abed Y, Pelletier G, et al. Virological features and clinical manifestations associated with human metapneumovirus: a new paramyxovirus responsible for acute respiratory-tract infections in all age groups. J Infect Dis. 2002;186:1330–1334.
102. Nichols WG, Corey L, Gooley T, et al. Parainfluenza virus infections after hematopoietic stem cell transplantation: risk factors, response to antiviral therapy, and effect on transplant outcome. Blood. 2001;98(3):573–578.
103. Lewis VA, Champlin R, Englund J, et al. Respiratory disease due to parainfluenza virus in adult bone marrow transplant recipients. Clin Infect Dis. 1996;23(5):1033–1037.

104. Erard V, Chien JW, Kim HW, et al. Airflow decline after myeloablative allogeneic hematopoietic cell transplantation: the role of community respiratory viruses. J Infect Dis. 2006;193:1619–1625.
105. Chemaly RF, Hanmod SS, Rathod DB, et al. The characteristics and outcomes of parainfluenza virus infections in 200 patients with leukemia or recipients of hematopoietic stem cell transplantation. Blood. 2012;119(12):2738–2745; quiz 2969. Epub 2012 Jan 12.
106. Wendt CH, Weisdorf DJ, Jordan MC, et al. Parainfluenza virus respiratory infection after bone marrow transplantation. N Engl J Med. 1992;326(14):921–926.
107. Elizaga J, Olavarria E, Apperley J, et al. Parainfluenza virus 3 infection after stem cell transplant: relevance to outcome of rapid diagnosis and ribavirin treatment. Clin Infect Dis. 2001;32(3):413–418.
108. Moscona A, Porotto M, Palmer S, et al. A recombinant sialidase fusion protein effectively inhibits human parainfluenza viral infection *in vitro* and *in vivo*. J Infect Dis. 2010;202(2):234–241.
109. Esper F, Boucher D, Weibel C, et al. Human metapneumovirus infection in the United States: clinical manifestations associated with a newly emerging respiratory infection in children. Pediatrics. 2003;111:1407–1410.
110. Peiris JS, Tang WH, Chan KH, et al. Children with respiratory disease associated with metapneumovirus in Hong Kong. Emerg Infect Dis. 2003;9:628–633.
111. Williams JV, Harris PA, Tollefson SJ, et al. Human metapneumovirus and lower respiratory tract disease in otherwise healthy infants and children. N Engl J Med. 2004;350:443–450.
112. Debur MC, Vidal LR, Stroparo E, et al. Human metapneumovirus infection in hematopoietic stem cell transplant recipients. Transpl Infect Dis. 2010;12:173–179.
113. Wyde PR, Chetty SN, Jewell AM, et al. Comparison of the inhibition of human metapneumovirus and respiratory syncytial virus by ribavirin and immune serum globulin in vitro. Antiviral Res. 2003;60:51–59.
114. Hamelin ME, Prince GA, Boivin G. Effect of ribavirin and glucocorticoid treatment in a mouse model of human metapneumovirus infection. Antimicrob Agents Chemother. 2006;50:774–777.
115. Kuypers J, Martin ET, Heugel J, et al. Clinical disease in children associated with newly described coronavirus subtypes. Pediatrics. 2007;119(1):e70–e76.
116. Leung TF, Li CY, Lam WY, et al. Epidemiology and clinical presentations of human coronavirus NL63 infections in Hong Kong children. J Clin Microbiol. 2009;47(11): 3486–3492.
117. Milano F, Campbell AP, Guthrie KA, et al. Human rhinovirus and coronavirus detection among allogeneic hematopoietic stem cell transplantation recipients. Blood. 2010; 115:2088–294.
118. Oosterhof L, Christensen CB, Sengeløv H. Fatal lower respiratory tract disease with human corona virus NL63 in an adult haematopoietic cell transplant recipient. Bone Marrow Transplant. 2010;45:1115–1116.
119. Van Kraaij MG, van Elden LJ, van Loon AM, et al. Frequent detection of respiratory viruses in adult recipients of stem cell transplants with the use of real-time polymerase chain reaction, compared with viral culture. Clin Infect Dis. 2005;40(5):662–669.
120. Pene F, Merlat A, Vabret A, et al. Coronavirus 229E-related pneumonia in immunocompromised patients. Clin Infect Dis. 2003;37:929–932.
121. Turner RB. Upper respiratory tract infections section B. In: Mandell GL, Bennett JE, Dolin R (eds). Principles and practice of infectious diseases. 7th edn. Philadelphia: Elsevier; 2010, pp. 809–813.
122. Parody R, Rabella N, Martino R, et al. Upper and lower respiratory tract infections by human enterovirus and rhinovirus in adult patients with hematological malignancies. Am J Hematol. 2007;82:807–811.
123. Gerna G, Piralla A, Rovida F, et al. Correlation of rhinovirus load in the respiratory tract and clinical symptoms in hospitalized immunocompetent and immunosuppressed patients. J Med Virol. 2009;81(8):1498–1507.
124. Gutman JA, Peck AJ, Kuypers J, et al. Rhinovirus as a cause of fatal lower respiratory tract infection in adult stem cell transplantation patients: a report of two cases. Bone Marrow Transplant. 2007;40(8):809–811.
125. Gerna G, Piralla A, Campanini G, et al. The human bocavirus role in acute respiratory tract infections of pediatric patients as defined by viral load quantification. New Microbiol. 2007;30:383–392.
126. Mourez T, Bergeron A, Ribaud P, et al. Polyomaviruses KI and WU in immunosuppressed patients with respiratory disease. Emerg Infect Dis. 2009;15:107–109.

13

CHAPTER 13

Exposure to family members: infections and recent live vaccinations

Brian G Engelhardt[1] *and James E Crowe, Jr*[2,3]

[1]Division of Hematology and Oncology, Department of Medicine, Vanderbilt University Medical Center, Nashville, TN, USA

[2]Department of Pediatrics, Vanderbilt University Medical Center, Nashville, TN, USA

[3]Department of Pathology, Microbiology, and Immunology, Vanderbilt University Medical Center, Nashville, TN, USA

An ounce of prevention is worth a pound of cure.

Benjamin Franklin

Introduction

Long-term survivors of allogeneic hematopoietic stem cell transplantation (HCT) are exposed frequently to infectious pathogens through interactions with family members, health-care providers, and other close contacts. Delayed immune reconstitution, chronic graft-versus-host disease (GVHD), prolonged immunosuppression, and variable responses to vaccination all contribute to the susceptibility of long-term transplant survivors to infectious diseases [1–9]. Of these problems, chronic GVHD is probably the most important risk factor for late immune dysregulation [10, 11].

Chronic GVHD is common after HCT and is characterized by well-described defects in both cellular and humoral immunity [4, 12, 13]. Classically, patients with chronic GVHD have been noted to have an impaired ability to respond to capsular polysaccharide antigens and, therefore, are predisposed to infections with encapsulated bacteria (e.g., *Streptococcus pneumoniae*) [10, 14]. In actuality, long-term HCT survivors are susceptible not only to encapsulated bacteria but also to a broad range of opportunistic and community-acquired pathogens [5, 10, 15]. Of particular concern are respiratory viruses, owing to their prevalence in the community, high transmission rates, and virulence within this susceptible group of patients [16–23]. Infection control represents an efficient and cost-effective mechanism to limit the excessive morbidity and mortality associated with these infectious complications. Immunization of not only the HCT recipient but also their close contacts is another method for preventing disease transmission. Health-care personnel are often asked to comment on the safety considerations for the transplant recipient or the implementation of isolation precautions when family members are sick or when a live vaccine is given. This chapter will review current guidelines on disease prevention strategies when HCT recipients are exposed to sick contacts within the household or when family members receive live virus vaccines. Immunization schedules and the management of viral respiratory tract infections in HCT recipients are considered separately in Chapters 11 and 12, respectively.

Blood and Marrow Transplantation Long-Term Management: Prevention and Complications, First Edition. Edited by Bipin N Savani.

Exposure to family members: infections

Community-acquired respiratory viruses

The most commonly acquired viral respiratory tract infections following HCT include those caused by rhinoviruses, parainfluenza viruses (primarily serotype 3), respiratory syncytial virus (RSV), and influenza A or B viruses [16, 19, 20, 24–27]. Human metapneumovirus (hMPV) is a recently discovered virus that is genetically similar to RSV and causes symptomatic upper and lower respiratory tract infections primarily in young children and older adults [28–31]. hMPV has also been identified as an emerging pathogen within HCT recipients [32, 33]. With the exception of some parainfluenza viruses, which cause infection in the population throughout the year, most respiratory viruses exhibit a seasonal distribution. The majority of documented respiratory virus cases occur in the winter months and early spring in the USA [20, 29]. RSV, parainfluenza, influenza, and hMPV can cause pneumonia frequently in HCT recipients with an associated high frequency of mortality [16, 19, 20, 27, 33]. Even with appropriate treatment and supportive care, the case-fatality rate can approach 25–45% for these viral pneumonias [19–21, 26, 27, 33, 34]. Owing to the morbidity and mortality associated with severe infections, prevention of viral spread to susceptible hosts is critical.

These ubiquitous community-acquired viruses are spread mostly by direct contact with infected secretions, and possibly also by large-particle aerosols. Typically, they are not spread by small-particle aerosols. Transmission rates can be high, and brisk outbreaks of influenza, parainfluenza, and RSV have been reported within the community and in the hospital setting [17, 20, 34–37]. The key fundamentals for prevention of pathogen spread include education of the HCT recipient and their family members, avoidance of individuals with respiratory symptoms, and cleanliness with frequent hand washing [17, 18, 37–40].

Infection containment

Education is a critical component of prevention. HCT recipients, family members, and other close contacts should be taught standard infection control measures, symptoms of contagion (i.e., fever, rhinorrhea, sore throat, cough, etc.), and the significant risk that respiratory viruses pose to transplant patients [17, 41, 42]. In general, the transplant patient should limit frequent touching of mucocutaneous tissues, including the eyes, nares, and mouth when in public. HCT recipients should avoid direct contact with visitors and friends with signs or symptoms of a communicable infection. Household contacts with infectious symptoms are most likely to transmit viruses to patients; minimizing contact in this setting is desirable but may be difficult to achieve [37, 40]. When possible, contacts with documented RSV, parainfluenza, influenza, or hMPV infection should be isolated from HCT recipients [17, 20, 43]. If interaction is inevitable, those persons with respiratory symptoms or disease should maintain scrupulously clean hand hygiene and wear surgical masks when near transplant patients, especially if the HCT survivor is immunocompromised due to chronic GVHD [17, 44]. Alternatively, the HCT recipient can wear a mask. Since most of these viruses are spread principally by contact, a paper (surgical) mask is probably sufficient in most cases. N95-level particulate respirators restrict contact with small-particle aerosols, but this type of protection usually is not necessary and these masks are difficult to wear properly for prolonged periods.

Even with strict adherence to infection control, these methods are limited by prolonged viral shedding from asymptomatic persons without illness or from contacts recently recovered from a viral infection [37]. Viral shedding has been reported for over 4 months in transplant patients with influenza, over 20 days for RSV and over 40 days for parainfluenza [36, 37, 45, 46]. Therefore, exposure to a pathogen can occur before symptoms of contagion develop and thus before necessary precautions can be taken.

Although wearing a surgical mask seems logical and is generally recommended when HCT patients are interacting with a contagious individual, the actual data on mask usage is conflicted. With regard to HCT patients, a recent observational study examined the impact of surgical mask usage by all individuals with direct patient contact (caregivers, visitors, and medical staff) when within 3 feet of the patient regardless of symptomatology. The study revealed a significant reduction in respiratory viral infections when compared with the historical control period during which standard infection control measures were used (10.3% in pre-mask era versus 3.3% in the mask era; $p < 0.001$). The mask was most effective in limiting the transmission of parainfluenza virus 3 [44]. In a prospective clinical trial, health-care workers in a tertiary care hospital were randomized to either wear face masks or not. The incidence of symptomatic viral infections did not differ between the groups [47]. The overall risk of viral transmission likely depends on multiple factors, including the immunocompetence of the individual at risk, the virulence of the pathogen circulating within the community, and the length of exposure. Since many viral illnesses are spread by both aerosolized droplets and by contact from hand to nose or eye, a surgical mask without proper hand hygiene likely limits the efficacy of this procedure.

Hand hygiene

Hand washing is probably the most important method to prevent the spread of infectious diseases, especially for respiratory viruses that are transmitted primarily by contact [48–52]. Hand washing is effective for limiting both nosocomial and community-acquired infections and it works regardless of whether the close contact is known to be infectious or not [53–59]. In general, all HCT recipients should be encouraged to wash their hands frequently and diligently. Proper hand hygiene includes the use of alcohol-based hand gel/foam and routine washing with either plain or antimicrobial soap and water. Current guidelines recommend that HCT patients should wash their hands before eating/preparing food, after using the toilet or changing diapers, before/after touching a wound, before mucocutaneous self-contact, after gardening, after touching pets/humans/animals, after contact with bodily fluids, after going outdoors, and especially after contact with contagious individuals [40]. Pediatric HCT patients should be taught proper hand washing techniques and should be observed by adults to ensure appropriate sanitation. Recent data from the literature indicate that when hands are not visibly dirty, an alcohol-based hand rub could be the optimal method to prevent the transmission of pathogens in both community and hospital settings [53–59]. In a prospective, observational cohort study of families with young children, the use of alcohol-based hand gels was independently associated with the prevention of secondary transmission of respiratory illness in the home (incidence rate ratio, IRR: 0.6; 95% CI: 0.4–0.9; $P = 0.01$) [58]. In a randomized trial, the use of alcohol-based hand sanitizers by families was associated with a significant decrease in the rate of secondary gastrointestinal illness when compared to control families (IRR: 0.41; 95% CI: 0.19–0.90; $P = 0.03$) [59]. Overall, alcohol-based hand sanitizers are convenient, portable, and offer significant microbiocidal activity. For the long-term HCT survivor, the importance of hand hygiene by any method cannot be stressed enough. Frequent and thorough hand washing with soap and water or cleaning with an alcohol-based rub are all effective means to prevent the transmission of infectious disease.

Postexposure prophylaxis and other strategies

Immunosuppression is a major risk factor for viral infections. Previous data indicate that lymphopenia and higher doses of systemic steroids are associated with increased risk for pneumonia following RSV or parainfluenza infection in patients early after transplant [20, 34, 60]. Cytopenias and immunosuppressive medications also are common in long-term survivors with chronic GVHD. Therefore, immunosuppression withdrawal has been proposed as a means to prevent severe viral infection [61]. However, a systematic analysis of accelerated immunosuppression taper in exposed individuals has not been undertaken and, therefore, cannot be recommended uniformly.

To decrease the risk of recurrent infections, prophylactic intravenous immunoglobulin (IVIG) is commonly given to HCT patients with chronic GVHD and hypogamaglobulinemia (serum IgG <400 mg/dL) [39]. To prevent RSV disease during its typical season in the Northern Hemisphere from November through April, some transplant centers previously used RSV-specific immunoglobulin (RSVIG) in lieu of standard IVIG preparations or added RSV-specific monoclonal antibody treatment (palivizumab) to IVIG for pediatric HCT patients receiving passive immune therapy [37, 40, 62]. The ability of prophylactic IVIG to prevent infections when given universally to all HCT recipients beyond 3 months of transplant is unclear [63]. In addition, the efficacy of preemptive IVIG therapy to abort infection in an exposed long-term survivor also is unknown.

Treatment of RSV pneumonia in immunocompromised patients is challenging. Most centers treat such patients with aerosolized ribavirin with or without antibody immunotherapy [20, 23, 64–66]. Ribavirin also has activity against hMPV *in vitro* and has been shown to reduce viral replication in animal models [67, 68]. Some data are available on the preemptive use of inhaled ribavirin on HCT patients with RSV upper respiratory tract infections [69–71]; however, there is no information on the use of ribavirin prophylactically in asymptomatic long-term HCT survivors exposed to RSV or hMPV by family members or close contacts.

Treatment with inhaled ribavirin is technically complex, which limits the feasibility of this procedure for routine postexposure chemoprophylaxis. Long-term HCT survivors should monitor themselves for new symptoms after exposure to an individual with known RSV, hMPV, or parainfluenza infection. If new symptoms develop, they should see seek prompt medical attention and undergo evaluation for routine respiratory viruses using standard methods (i.e., nasal washes or swabs can be submitted for viral culture, enzyme-linked immunosorbent assays, direct immunofluorescence testing, or molecular diagnostic testing by reverse transcription-polymerase chain reaction). Appropriate treatment is dictated by the test results (i.e., the identity of the virus), length of time from transplant, severity of the infection (i.e., upper versus lower respiratory tract infection), and the degree of immunosuppression. A notable exception to this rule is influenza, which requires special precautions following known exposures.

Influenza prevention and chemoprophylaxis

Of the respiratory viruses discussed, only influenza has an US Food and Drug Administration (FDA)-approved vaccine and a chemoprophylaxis strategy with demonstrated efficacy. Starting prior to transplant, the trivalent inactivated influenza vaccine should be administered annually to all HCT recipients, their family members, and close contacts. Seasonal vaccination should be indefinite for the transplant patient and should continue for at least 2 years after HCT for their close contacts, unless there is ongoing immunosuppression, in which case immunization should continue [37, 40, 72]. A strong argument can be made for lifelong influenza vaccination for not only the HCT recipient but also for their family members and close contacts to prevent inadvertent transmission of virus.

Response to influenza vaccination can be variable in HCT recipients [8, 9, 45, 73–75]. Therefore, chemoprophylaxis with M2 channel inhibitors (amantadine or rimantadine) or neuramidase inhibitors (zanamivir and oseltamivir) is indicated for all HCT recipients exposed to influenza within 2 years of their transplant or if they are over 2 years posttransplant and remain immunosuppressed from medications or chronic GVHD [8, 37, 40, 45, 60]. Owing to the antigenic drift of influenza strains and the occasional major antigenic shifts characteristic of pandemics, yearly vaccination does not necessarily convey protection from all infectious strains of influenza in a season. Family members, household contacts, and long-term HCT survivors also should receive appropriate chemoprophylaxis during outbreaks by influenza strains not included in the seasonal influenza vaccine [37, 40, 72]. It is important to remember that amantadine or rimantadine have activity against influenza A, but not B, while zanamivir and oseltamivir are effective against both influenza A and B. Some strains of influenza are completely resistant to amantadine and rimantadine; updated information on the resistance patterns and treatment recommendations are available from the website of the US Centers for Disease Control and Prevention. Chemoprophylaxis in the HCT recipient should begin as soon as possible after contact with the index case (preferably within 36–48 h) and continue for 7–10 days after known exposure. Starting the medication more than 48 h after inoculation may decrease the clinical benefit because of the rapid replication kinetics of influenza virus. In the setting of an influenza outbreak, chemoprophylaxis should continue for 14–28 days or until the end of the community outbreak [40, 72, 76].

Exposure to family members: recent live vaccinations

HCT recipients are susceptible to vaccine-preventable diseases [14, 19, 77]. To prevent the transmission of pathogens, HCT survivors and their family members or close contacts should be immunized as per the usual schedules developed for the immunocompromised and immunocompetent hosts, respectively [40]. Some special precautions are necessary when live vaccines are administered. After transplant, antibody titers induced by prior vaccines decline, leaving patients susceptible not only to wild-type infections but also in some cases to infection by vaccine virus shed by immunized contacts [78–80]. Therefore, inactivated vaccines should be administered to family members and close contacts of HCT patients when available. If no alternative to the live vaccine exists, the following recommendations have been developed to limit the potential transmission of vaccine virus from the close contact to the long-term HCT survivor [40].

Measles, mumps, rubella vaccine

Measles, mumps, rubella (MMR) vaccine can be administered to family members and close contacts as per usual schedules. There are no significant data indicating that the viruses contained in the MMR vaccine are transmissible with the exception of the rubella virus component. There is a report of rubella virus vaccine being transmitted from a vaccinated mother to her breast-feeding child [81]. If fever, myalgias, or rash develop in a vaccine recipient, these subjects should limit their interaction with the long-term HCT survivor until resolution of all symptoms [40].

Oral polio vaccine

Family members and close contacts of the HCT patient should be immunized with the inactivated polio vaccine. Oral polio vaccine (OPV) contains three live attenuated viruses with a limited number of attenuating mutations that have propensity to revert to wild-type residues when shed by a vaccinee. Virus shed from the gastrointestinal tract following oral vaccination rarely can cause paralytic poliomyelitis in the vaccinee or their close contacts [82, 83]. Recipients of the OPV should avoid interaction with the HCT survivor for at least 4–6 weeks after immunization, during which time viral shedding is possible. Some children and also adults with HIV infection have been documented to shed OPV in stools for months. If interaction with immunized subjects is inevitable, then the HCT patient should maintain strict hand hygiene, since the virus is spread by the fecal–oral route. HCT patients should minimize contact with feces or saliva from the vaccine recipient (i.e., changing diapers, toileting of toddlers, sharing food, etc.) [82, 83]. OPV is no longer licensed for use in the USA; however, the oral formulation remains the vaccine of choice in developing countries by the World Health Organization Expanded Program on Immunization.

Rotavirus vaccine

There are two commercially available rotavirus vaccines, and both can be administered to HCT family members or close household contacts as per age-appropriate vaccination schedules [40, 84–86]. RotaTeq (Merck) is a live, attenuated oral pentavalent vaccine that contains five rotaviruses produced by reassortment; Rotarix (GlaxoSmithKline) is a live, attenuated oral monovalent vaccine containing a rotavirus strain of G1P[8] specificity. Although both vaccines contain live attenuated viruses, there have been no reported cases of vaccine virus transmission [84, 87]. Viral shedding can occur for 2–4 weeks after vaccination, and the HCT survivor should try to avoid or at least minimize contact with feces from the vaccinated infant while maintaining stringent hand hygiene during this time.

Varicella virus vaccines

Live virus vaccines are available for the prevention of chickenpox in children (Varivax) or shingles in adults over the age of 60 (Zostavax) [88, 89]. Family members and close household contacts are encouraged to receive the chickenpox vaccine as indicated, which can serve to prevent exposure of the HCT recipient to wild-type virus. Although exceedingly rare, transmission of vaccine virus has been reported; however, this risk is low even among immunocompromised individuals [88, 90]. If the vaccine recipient develops a rash within 1 month of immunization, they should keep the affected area containing vesicles covered and avoid contact with the long-term HCT survivor until all lesions are crusted over.

The quantity of attenuated virus in the shingles vaccine is greater than the chickenpox vaccine and, therefore, may represent an increased risk to the HCT patient. Some experts recommend delaying administration of the shingles vaccine to household members for 2 years after transplant and longer if the HCT survivor remains immunosuppressed. Despite this risk, there have not been any documented cases of secondary transmission of varicella zoster vaccine viruses. As with the chickenpox vaccine, the same precautions should be instituted when a household contact develops a vaccine-associated rash following herpes zoster vaccination.

Varicella-seronegative patients transplanted less than 2 years prior and those with chronic GVHD or who are on immunosuppression require treatment with human varicella-zoster immune globulin (VariZIG; Cangene) after exposure to a household member with chickenpox or shingles. Alternatively, prophylaxis with acyclovir or valacyclovir can be prescribed if VariZIG is unavailable in this situation [40]. Additionally, varicella-seropositive HCT patients who are significantly immunosuppressed due to high-dose steroids also should be considered for passive immunization or anti-viral prophylaxis after exposure to wild-type varicella virus disease or even a vaccine-associated varicella-like rash [40]. Uniform and definite chemoprophylaxis guidelines for all long-term HCT survivors exposed to a varicella vaccinee rash have not been developed, but prophylactic measures should be considered strongly, including the above recommendations.

Live attenuated influenza vaccine (LAIV)

The FDA has approved an intranasally delivered live attenuated influenza vaccine (LAIV – FluMist; MedImmune) for healthy individuals from 2 to 49 years of age; however, it is not recommended for close contacts of immunocompromised people [40, 91]. Similar to polio vaccination, family members and close contacts of the HCT patient should be immunized only with the inactivated influenza vaccine. Vaccine virus is typically shed for about 3–7 days in adults and children, with longer shedding in pediatric individuals [92, 93]. Reversion of the attenuated virus to a wild-type virulent strain has not been reported, but transmission of vaccine virus has been detected [92, 94, 95]. On account of viral shedding, it is reasonable for the HCT patient to avoid close contact with the recipient of the LAIV for about 1 week, especially if severely immunocompromised due to chronic GVHD or immunosuppression [40, 91]. In adults, the trivalent inactivated influenza vaccine and the LAIV likely have equivalent efficacy [96–99]. There is no risk for transmission of the inactivated influenza vaccine virus. Therefore, inactivated vaccine is the preferred influenza vaccine for household contacts of HCT survivors [40].

Additional live vaccines

Other live vaccines that are encountered occasionally include: bacillus Calmette–Guerin vaccine for tuberculosis, cholera vaccine, oral typhoid vaccine, and smallpox (vaccinia) vaccine. These vaccines are administered less frequently in the USA and are usually given for special indications or for travel. These vaccines generally are contraindicated for the HCT recipient, especially within the first 24 months of transplant or in the setting of active immunosuppression. Therefore, there is also some risk when close contacts are immunized with these vaccines. Formal recommendations to prevent or limit transmission of these vaccine viruses to HCT survivors have not been developed.

Conclusion

Infections are one of the leading causes for non-relapse mortality among long-term survivors of HCT [100]. Minimizing infectious complications and thereby preventing unnecessary deaths is a major goal for health-care providers treating transplant patients. The mainstays of pathogen containment have changed little from the time of Semmelweis and Lister and include minimizing exposure to contagious individuals, maintaining a hygienic environment, and diligent hand-washing practices. Immunization of family members and close household contacts of HCT recipients as per standard guidelines is another method to minimize infectious complications. Owing to concerns about transmission of attenuated vaccine viruses to transplant patients, inactivated vaccines are preferred when available. However, under most circumstances the routine immunization of close contacts and family members with a live virus vaccine presents only modest risk to the HCT recipient and may offer substantial protection in the form of herd immunity. In general, HCT patients and their close contacts should be immunized as per the usual schedules developed for the immunocompromised and immunocompetent hosts, respectively [40]. Notable exceptions include OPV and LAIV, which are contraindicated for the close contacts of HCT patients. The use of rational strategies to minimize the spread of infectious pathogens from close contacts and family members to the transplant patient should improve the quality of life and survival of long-term HCT survivors if compliance levels are high.

References

1. Small TN, Papadopoulos EB, Boulad F, et al. Comparison of immune reconstitution after unrelated and related T-cell-depleted bone marrow transplantation: effect of patient age and donor leukocyte infusions. Blood. 1999;93(2):467–480.

2. Le RQ, Melenhorst JJ, Battiwalla M, et al. Evolution of the donor T-cell repertoire in recipients in the second decade after allogeneic stem cell transplantation. Blood. 2011; 117(19):5250–5256.
3. Noel DR, Witherspoon RP, Storb R, et al. Does graft-versus-host disease influence the tempo of immunologic recovery after allogeneic human marrow transplantation? An observation on 56 long-term survivors. Blood. 1978; 51(6):1087–1105.
4. Witherspoon RP, Storb R, Ochs HD, et al. Recovery of antibody production in human allogeneic marrow graft recipients: influence of time posttransplantation, the presence or absence of chronic graft-versus-host disease, and antithymocyte globulin treatment. Blood. 1981;58(2): 360–368.
5. Ochs L, Shu XO, Miller J, et al. Late infections after allogeneic bone marrow transplantations: comparison of incidence in related and unrelated donor transplant recipients. Blood. 1995;86(10):3979–3986.
6. Patel SR, Ortin M, Cohen BJ, et al. Revaccination with measles, tetanus, poliovirus, *Haemophilus influenzae* type B, meningococcus C, and pneumococcus vaccines in children after hematopoietic stem cell transplantation. Clin Infect Dis. 2007;44(5):625–634.
7. Cordonnier C, Labopin M, Chesnel V, et al. Influence of immunisation timing on the response to conjugate-pneumococcal vaccine after allogeneic stem cell transplant: final results of the EBMT IDWP01 Trial. Bone Marrow Transplant. 2008;45(Suppl 1):S2.
8. Engelhard D, Nagler A, Hardan I, et al. Antibody response to a two-dose regimen of influenza vaccine in allogeneic T cell-depleted and autologous BMT recipients. Bone Marrow Transplant. 1993;11(1):1–5.
9. Mohty B, Bel M, Vukicevic M, et al. Graft-versus-host disease is the major determinant of humoral responses to the AS03-adjuvanted influenza A/09/H1N1 vaccine in allogeneic hematopoietic stem cell transplant recipients. Haematologica. 2011;96(6):896–904.
10. Atkinson K, Storb R, Prentice RL, et al. Analysis of late infections in 89 long-term survivors of bone marrow transplantation. Blood. 1979;53(4):720–731.
11. Bjorklund A, Aschan J, Labopin M, et al. Risk factors for fatal infectious complications developing late after allogeneic stem cell transplantation. Bone Marrow Transplant. 2007;40(11):1055–1062.
12. Lum LG, Seigneuret MC, Storb RF, et al. *In vitro* regulation of immunoglobulin synthesis after marrow transplantation. I. T-cell and B-cell deficiencies in patients with and without chronic graft-versus-host disease. Blood. 1981; 58(3):431–439.
13. Graze PR, Gale RP. Chronic graft versus host disease: a syndrome of disordered immunity. Am J Med. 1979; 66(4):611–620.
14. Engelhard D, Cordonnier C, Shaw PJ, et al. Early and late invasive pneumococcal infection following stem cell transplantation: a European Bone Marrow Transplantation survey. Br J Haematol. 2002;117(2):444–450.
15. Khushalani NI, Bakri FG, Wentling D, et al. Respiratory syncytial virus infection in the late bone marrow transplant period: report of three cases and review. Bone Marrow Transplant. 2001;27(10):1071–1073.
16. Kim YJ, Boeckh M, Englund JA. Community respiratory virus infections in immunocompromised patients: hematopoietic stem cell and solid organ transplant recipients, and individuals with human immunodeficiency virus infection. Semin Respir Crit Care Med. 2007;28(2): 222–242.
17. Raad I, Abbas J, Whimbey E. Infection control of nosocomial respiratory viral disease in the immunocompromised host. Am J Med. 1997;102(3A):48–52; discussion 53–54.
18. Lee I, Barton TD. Viral respiratory tract infections in transplant patients: epidemiology, recognition and management. Drugs. 2007;67(10):1411–1427.
19. Nichols WG, Guthrie KA, Corey L, Boeckh M. Influenza infections after hematopoietic stem cell transplantation: risk factors, mortality, and the effect of antiviral therapy. Clin Infect Dis. 2004;39(9):1300–1306.
20. Nichols WG, Gooley T, Boeckh M. Community-acquired respiratory syncytial virus and parainfluenza virus infections after hematopoietic stem cell transplantation: the Fred Hutchinson Cancer Research Center experience. Biol Blood Marrow Transplant. 2001;7(Suppl):11S–15S.
21. Whimbey E, Vartivarian SE, Champlin RE, et al. Parainfluenza virus infection in adult bone marrow transplant recipients. Eur J Clin Microbiol Infect Dis. 1993;12(9): 699–701.
22. Whimbey E, Champlin RE, Couch RB, et al. Community respiratory virus infections among hospitalized adult bone marrow transplant recipients. Clin Infect Dis. 1996; 22(5):778–782.
23. Ljungman P. Respiratory virus infections in stem cell transplant patients: the European experience. Biol Blood Marrow Transplant. 2001;7(Suppl):5S–7S.
24. Ghosh S, Champlin R, Couch R, et al. Rhinovirus infections in myelosuppressed adult blood and marrow transplant recipients. Clin Infect Dis. 1999;29(3):528–532.
25. Bowden RA. Respiratory virus infections after marrow transplant: the Fred Hutchinson Cancer Research Center experience. Am J Med. 1997;102(3A):27–30; discussion 42–43.

26. Martin MA, Bock MJ, Pfaller MA, Wenzel RP. Respiratory syncytial virus infections in adult bone marrow transplant recipients. Lancet. 1988;1(8599):1396–1397.
27. Hertz MI, Englund JA, Snover D, et al. Respiratory syncytial virus-induced acute lung injury in adult patients with bone marrow transplants: a clinical approach and review of the literature. Medicine (Baltimore). 1989; 68(5):269–281.
28. van den Hoogen BG, de Jong JC, Groen J, et al. A newly discovered human pneumovirus isolated from young children with respiratory tract disease. Nat Med. 2001; 7(6):719–724.
29. Boivin G, Abed Y, Pelletier G, et al. Virological features and clinical manifestations associated with human metapneumovirus: a new paramyxovirus responsible for acute respiratory-tract infections in all age groups. J Infect Dis. 2002;186(9):1330–1334.
30. Williams JV, Harris PA, Tollefson SJ, et al. Human metapneumovirus and lower respiratory tract disease in otherwise healthy infants and children. N Engl J Med. 2004; 350(5):443–450.
31. Esper F, Martinello RA, Boucher D, et al. A 1-year experience with human metapneumovirus in children aged <5 years. J Infect Dis. 2004;189(8):1388–1396.
32. Englund JA, Boeckh M, Kuypers J, et al. Brief communication: fatal human metapneumovirus infection in stem-cell transplant recipients. Ann Intern Med. 2006;144(5): 344–349.
33. Williams JV, Martino R, Rabella N, et al. A prospective study comparing human metapneumovirus with other respiratory viruses in adults with hematologic malignancies and respiratory tract infections. J Infect Dis. 2005; 192(6):1061–1065.
34. Nichols WG, Corey L, Gooley T, et al. Parainfluenza virus infections after hematopoietic stem cell transplantation: risk factors, response to antiviral therapy, and effect on transplant outcome. Blood. 2001;98(3):573–578.
35. Novel Swine-Origin Influenza A (H1N1) Virus Investigation Team, Dawood FS, Jain S, et al. Emergence of a novel swine-origin influenza A (H1N1) virus in humans. N Engl J Med. 2009;360(25):2605–2615.
36. Harrington RD, Hooton TM, Hackman RC, et al. An outbreak of respiratory syncytial virus in a bone marrow transplant center. J Infect Dis. 1992;165(6):987–993.
37. Dykewicz CA, National Center for Infectious Diseases, Centers for Disease Control and Prevention, et al. Guidelines for preventing opportunistic infections among hematopoietic stem cell transplant recipients: focus on community respiratory virus infections. Biol Blood Marrow Transplant. 2001;7(Suppl):19S–22S.
38. Sehulster L, Chinn RY. Guidelines for environmental infection control in health-care facilities. Recommendations of CDC and the Healthcare Infection Control Practices Advisory Committee (HICPAC). MMWR Recomm Rep. 2003;52(RR-10):1–42.
39. Couriel D, Carpenter PA, Cutler C, et al. Ancillary therapy and supportive care of chronic graft-versus-host disease: National Institutes of Health consensus development project on criteria for clinical trials in chronic graft-versus-host disease: V. Ancillary Therapy and Supportive Care Working Group Report. Biol Blood Marrow Transplant. 2006;12(4):375–396.
40. Tomblyn M, Chiller T, Einsele H, et al. Guidelines for preventing infectious complications among hematopoietic cell transplantation recipients: a global perspective. Biol Blood Marrow Transplant. 2009;15(10): 1143–1238.
41. Garcia R, Raad I, Abi-Said D, et al. Nosocomial respiratory syncytial virus infections: prevention and control in bone marrow transplant patients. Infect Control Hosp Epidemiol. 1997;18(6):412–416.
42. Sable CA, Hayden FG. Orthomyxoviral and paramyxoviral infections in transplant patients. Infect Dis Clin North Am. 1995;9(4):987–1003.
43. CDC. Infection Control Guidance for the Prevention and Control of Influenza in Acute-Care Facilities. Atlanta, GA: Centers for Disease Control and Prevention (CDC), 2007.
44. Sung AD, Sung JA, Corbet K, et al. Surgical mask usage reduces the incidence of parainfluenza virus 3 in recipients of stem cell transplantation. Blood (ASH Annual Meeting Abstracts). 2012;120:462a.
45. Hayden FG. Prevention and treatment of influenza in immunocompromised patients. Am J Med. 1997;102(3A): 55–60; discussion 75–76.
46. Peck AJ, Englund JA, Kuypers J, et al. Respiratory virus infection among hematopoietic cell transplant recipients: evidence for asymptomatic parainfluenza virus infection. Blood. 2007;110(5):1681–1688.
47. Jacobs JL, Ohde S, Takahashi O, et al. Use of surgical face masks to reduce the incidence of the common cold among health care workers in Japan: a randomized controlled trial. Am J Infect Control. 2009;37(5):417–419.
48. Siegel JD, Rhinehart E, Jackson M, et al. 2007 guideline for isolation precautions: preventing transmission of infectious agents in healthcare settings. Am J Infect Control 2007;35(10 Suppl 2):S65–S164.
49. Luby SP, Agboatwalla M, Feikin DR, et al. Effect of handwashing on child health: a randomised controlled trial. Lancet. 2005;366(9481):225–233.

50. Roberts L, Smith W, Jorm L, et al. Effect of infection control measures on the frequency of upper respiratory infection in child care: a randomized, controlled trial. Pediatrics. 2000;105(4 Pt 1):738–742.
51. Ryan MA, Christian RS, Wohlrabe J. Handwashing and respiratory illness among young adults in military training. Am J Prev Med. 2001;21(2):79–83.
52. White C, Kolble R, Carlson R, et al. The effect of hand hygiene on illness rate among students in university residence halls. Am J Infect Control. 2003;31(6):364–370.
53. Pittet D, Hugonnet S, Harbarth S, et al. Effectiveness of a hospital-wide programme to improve compliance with hand hygiene. Infection Control Programme. Lancet. 2000;356(9238):1307–1312.
54. Widmer AF. Replace hand washing with use of a waterless alcohol hand rub? Clin Infect Dis. 2000;31(1): 136–143.
55. Boyce JM, Pittet D, Healthcare Infection Control Practices Advisory Committee, HICPAC/SHEA/APIC/IDSA Hand Hygiene Task Force Guideline for hand hygiene in healthcare settings. Recommendations of the Healthcare Infection Control Practices Advisory Committee and the HICPAC/SHEA/APIC/IDSA Hand Hygiene Task Force. Society for Healthcare Epidemiology of America/ Association for Professionals in Infection Control/ Infectious Diseases Society of America. MMWR Recomm Rep. 2002;51(RR-16):1–45; quiz CE1–CE4.
56. Bischoff WE, Reynolds TM, Sessler CN, et al. Handwashing compliance by health care workers: the impact of introducing an accessible, alcohol-based hand antiseptic. Arch Intern Med. 2000;160(7):1017–1021.
57. Hugonnet S, Perneger TV, Pittet D. Alcohol-based handrub improves compliance with hand hygiene in intensive care units. Arch Intern Med. 2002;162(9):1037–1043.
58. Lee GM, Salomon JA, Friedman JF, et al. Illness transmission in the home: a possible role for alcohol-based hand gels. Pediatrics. 2005;115(4):852–860.
59. Sandora TJ, Taveras EM, Shih MC, et al. A randomized, controlled trial of a multifaceted intervention including alcohol-based hand sanitizer and hand-hygiene education to reduce illness transmission in the home. Pediatrics. 2005;116(3):587–594.
60. Chakrabarti S, Avivi I, Mackinnon S, et al. Respiratory virus infections in transplant recipients after reduced-intensity conditioning with Campath-1H: high incidence but low mortality. Br J Haematol. 2002;119(4):1125–1132.
61. Englund JA, Piedra PA, Whimbey E. Prevention and treatment of respiratory syncytial virus and parainfluenza viruses in immunocompromised patients. Am J Med. 1997;102(3A):61–70; discussion 75–76.
62. American Academy of Pediatrics. Respiratory syncytial virus. In: Pickering LK, Baker CJ, Long SS, McMillan JA (eds). Red Book: 2006 Report of the Committee on Infectious Diseases. Elk Grove Village, IL: American Academy of Pediatrics, 2006; pp. 560–566.
63. Sullivan KM, Storek J, Kopecky KJ, et al. A controlled trial of long-term administration of intravenous immunoglobulin to prevent late infection and chronic graft-vs.-host disease after marrow transplantation: clinical outcome and effect on subsequent immune recovery. Biol Blood Marrow Transplant. 1996;2(1):44–53.
64. Whimbey E, Champlin RE, Englund JA, et al. Combination therapy with aerosolized ribavirin and intravenous immunoglobulin for respiratory syncytial virus disease in adult bone marrow transplant recipients. Bone Marrow Transplant. 1995;16(3):393–399.
65. De Vincenzo JP, Leombruno D, Soiffer RJ, Siber GR. Immunotherapy of respiratory syncytial virus pneumonia following bone marrow transplantation. Bone Marrow Transplant. 1996;17(6):1051–1056.
66. de Fontbrune FS, Robin M, Porcher R, et al. Palivizumab treatment of respiratory syncytial virus infection after allogeneic hematopoietic stem cell transplantation. Clin Infect Dis. 2007;45(8):1019–1024.
67. Wyde PR, Chetty SN, Jewell AM, et al. Comparison of the inhibition of human metapneumovirus and respiratory syncytial virus by ribavirin and immune serum globulin in vitro. Antiviral Res. 2003;60(1):51–59.
68. Hamelin ME, Prince GA, Boivin G. Effect of ribavirin and glucocorticoid treatment in a mouse model of human metapneumovirus infection. Antimicrob Agents Chemother. 2006;50(2):774–777.
69. Adams R, Christenson J, Petersen F, Beatty P. Preemptive use of aerosolized ribavirin in the treatment of asymptomatic pediatric marrow transplant patients testing positive for RSV. Bone Marrow Transplant. 1999;24(6): 661–664.
70. Chemaly RF, Ghosh S, Bodey GP, et al. Respiratory viral infections in adults with hematologic malignancies and human stem cell transplantation recipients: a retrospective study at a major cancer center. Medicine (Baltimore). 2006;85(5):278–287.
71. Boeckh M, Englund J, Li Y, et al. Randomized controlled multicenter trial of aerosolized ribavirin for respiratory syncytial virus upper respiratory tract infection in hematopoietic cell transplant recipients. Clin Infect Dis. 2007; 44(2):245–249.
72. Fiore AE, Shay DK, Haber P, et al. Prevention and control of influenza. Recommendations of the Advisory Committee on Immunization Practices (ACIP), 2007. MMWR Recomm Rep. 2007;56(RR-6):1–54.

73. de Lavallade H, Garland P, Sekine T, et al. Repeated vaccination is required to optimize seroprotection against H1N1 in the immunocompromised host. Haematologica. 2011;96(2):307–314.
74. Avetisyan G, Aschan J, Hassan M, Ljungman P. Evaluation of immune responses to seasonal influenza vaccination in healthy volunteers and in patients after stem cell transplantation. Transplantation. 2008;86(2):257–263.
75. Issa NC, Marty FM, Gagne LS, et al. Seroprotective titers against 2009 H1N1 influenza A virus after vaccination in allogeneic hematopoietic stem cell transplantation recipients. Biol Blood Marrow Transplant. 2011;17(3): 434–438.
76. Glezen WP. Clinical practice. Prevention and treatment of seasonal influenza. N Engl J Med. 2008;359(24): 2579–2585.
77. Machado CM, Goncalves FB, Pannuti CS, et al. Measles in bone marrow transplant recipients during an outbreak in Sao Paulo, Brazil. Blood. 2002;99(1):83–87.
78. Ljungman P, Fridell E, Lonnqvist B et al. Efficacy and safety of vaccination of marrow transplant recipients with a live attenuated measles, mumps, and rubella vaccine. J Infect Dis. 1989;159(4):610–615.
79. Pauksen K, Duraj V, Ljungman P, et al. Immunity to and immunization against measles, rubella and mumps in patients after autologous bone marrow transplantation. Bone Marrow Transplant. 1992;9(6):427–432.
80. Pauksen K, Hammarstrom V, Ljungman P, et al. Immunity to poliovirus and immunization with inactivated poliovirus vaccine after autologous bone marrow transplantation. Clin Infect Dis. 1994;18(4):547–552.
81. Centers for Disease Control and Prevention Measles, mumps, and rubella-vaccine use and stategies for elimination of measles, rubella, and congenital rubella syndrome and control of mumps: recommendations of the Advisory Committee on Immunization Practices (ACIP). MMWR Recomm Rep. 1998;47(RR-8):1–48.
82. Prevots DR, Burr RK, Sutter RW, et al. Poliomyelitis prevention in the United States. Updated recommendations of the Advisory Committee on Immunization Practices (ACIP). MMWR Recomm Rep. 2000;49(RR-5):1–22; quiz CE1–CE7.
83. American Academy of Pediatrics. Poliovirus infections. In: Pickering LK, Baker CJ, Long SS, McMillan JA (eds). Red Book: 2006 Report of the Committee on Infectious Diseases. Elk Grove Village, IL: American Academy of Pediatrics, 2006; pp. 542–547.
84. Parashar UD, Alexander JP, Glass RI, et al. Prevention of rotavirus gastroenteritis among infants and children. Recommendations of the Advisory Committee on Immunization Practices (ACIP). MMWR Recomm Rep. 2006; 55(RR-12):1–13.
85. Araujo EC, Clemens SA, Oliveira CS, et al. Safety, immunogenicity, and protective efficacy of two doses of RIX4414 live attenuated human rotavirus vaccine in healthy infants. J Pediatr (Rio J). 2007;83(3):217–224.
86. Ruiz-Palacios GM, Perez-Schael I, Velazquez FR, et al. Safety and efficacy of an attenuated vaccine against severe rotavirus gastroenteritis. N Engl J Med. 2006;354(1): 11–22.
87. Clinical Review for STN 125265/0 Rotarix. 2008. Available from: http://www.fda.gov/downloads/BiologicsBloodVaccines/Vaccines/ApprovedProducts/UCM133580.pdf (accessed 25 May 2013).
88. Marin M, Guris D, Chaves SS, et al. Prevention of varicella: recommendations of the Advisory Committee on Immunization Practices (ACIP). MMWR Recomm Rep. 2007; 56(RR-4):1–40.
89. Advisory Committee on Immunization Practices. ACIP Provisional Recommendations for Use of Zoster Vaccine. 2008.
90. Diaz PS, Au D, Smith S, et al. Lack of transmission of the live attenuated varicella vaccine virus to immunocompromised children after immunization of their siblings. Pediatrics. 1991;87(2):166–170.
91. Fiore AE, Shay DK, Broder K, et al. Prevention and control of influenza: recommendations of the Advisory Committee on Immunization Practices (ACIP), 2008. MMWR Recomm Rep. 2008;57(RR-7):1–60.
92. Ali T, Scott N, Kallas W, et al. Detection of influenza antigen with rapid antibody-based tests after intranasal influenza vaccination (FluMist). Clin Infect Dis. 2004; 38(5):760–762.
93. Talbot TR, Crocker DD, Peters J, et al. Duration of virus shedding after trivalent intranasal live attenuated influenza vaccination in adults. Infect Control Hosp Epidemiol. 2005;26(5):494–500.
94. Cha TA, Kao K, Zhao J, et al. Genotypic stability of cold-adapted influenza virus vaccine in an efficacy clinical trial. J Clin Microbiol. 2000;38(2):839–845.
95. Buonagurio DA, O'Neill RE, Shutyak L, et al. Genetic and phenotypic stability of cold-adapted influenza viruses in a trivalent vaccine administered to children in a day care setting. Virology. 2006;347(2):296–306.
96. Edwards KM, Dupont WD, Westrich MK, et al. A randomized controlled trial of cold-adapted and inactivated vaccines for the prevention of influenza A disease. J Infect Dis. 1994;169(1):68–76.
97. Ohmit SE, Victor JC, Rotthoff JR, et al. Prevention of antigenically drifted influenza by inactivated and live attenuated vaccines. N Engl J Med. 2006;355(24):2513–2522.

98. Monto AS, Ohmit SE, Petrie JG, et al. Comparative efficacy of inactivated and live attenuated influenza vaccines. N Engl J Med. 2009;361(13):1260–1267.
99. Wang Z, Tobler S, Roayaei J, Eick A. Live attenuated or inactivated influenza vaccines and medical encounters for respiratory illnesses among US military personnel. JAMA. 2009;301(9):945–953.
100. Martin PJ, Counts GW Jr, Appelbaum FR, et al. Life expectancy in patients surviving more than 5 years after hematopoietic cell transplantation. J Clin Oncol. 2010; 28(6):1011–1016.

14

CHAPTER 14

Late pulmonary complications after allogeneic hematopietic stem cell transplantion: bronchiolitis obliterans syndrome (BOS) and organizing pneumonia (OP)

Lee Gazourian[1], *Gerald L Weinhouse*[1], *Joseph H Antin*[2,3], *and Vincent T Ho*[2,3]

[1]Division of Pulmonary Medicine, Brigham and Women's Hospital, Boston, MA, USA
[2]Division of Hematologic Malignancies, Dana-Farber Cancer Institute, Boston, MA, USA
[3]Harvard Medical School, Boston, MA, USA

Introduction

With improved supportive care, and better tolerated conditioning regimens, day 100 mortality and incidence of early transplant-related pulmonary toxicities have declined in recent years. However, chronic graft-versus-host disease (GVHD) and its associated pulmonary manifestations, especially bronchiolitis obliterans syndrome (BOS) and (cryptogenic) organizing pneumonia (COP or BOOP), remain major challenges facing long-term hematopoietic stem cell transplantation (HSCT) survivors, with often devastating impact on quality of life. While chronic GVHD (cGVHD) is reported in about 50% or more patients after HSCT, pulmonary manifestations are likely to be vastly underdiagnosed. In this chapter, we focus on the current understanding of BOS and COP as the most common late noninfectious pulmonary complications after allogeneic HSCT.

Bronchiolitis obliterans syndrome (BOS)

Airflow obstruction following allogeneic HSCT was first described in the early 1980s, and new-onset airflow obstruction after HSCT has been estimated to occur in up to 26% of transplant patients and 32% among patients with cGVHD [1–4]. BOS represents a severe form of airflow obstruction. It is a late noninfectious pulmonary complication of allogeneic HSCT, and the majority of cases present between 200 days and 3 years after HSCT; however, earlier and later presentations can occur [5, 6]. BOS is considered a form of cGVHD, and the prevalence is estimated to be between 5 and 10% of all allogeneic transplants [7, 8]. Once diagnosed, BOS patients have a very poor prognosis, with a 2-year mortality rate of approximately 55% [5, 9]. In addition, patients who present early after HSCT (<150 days) and demonstrate a rapid decline (>30% decline in forced expiratory volume

Blood and Marrow Transplantation Long-Term Management: Prevention and Complications, First Edition. Edited by Bipin N Savani.

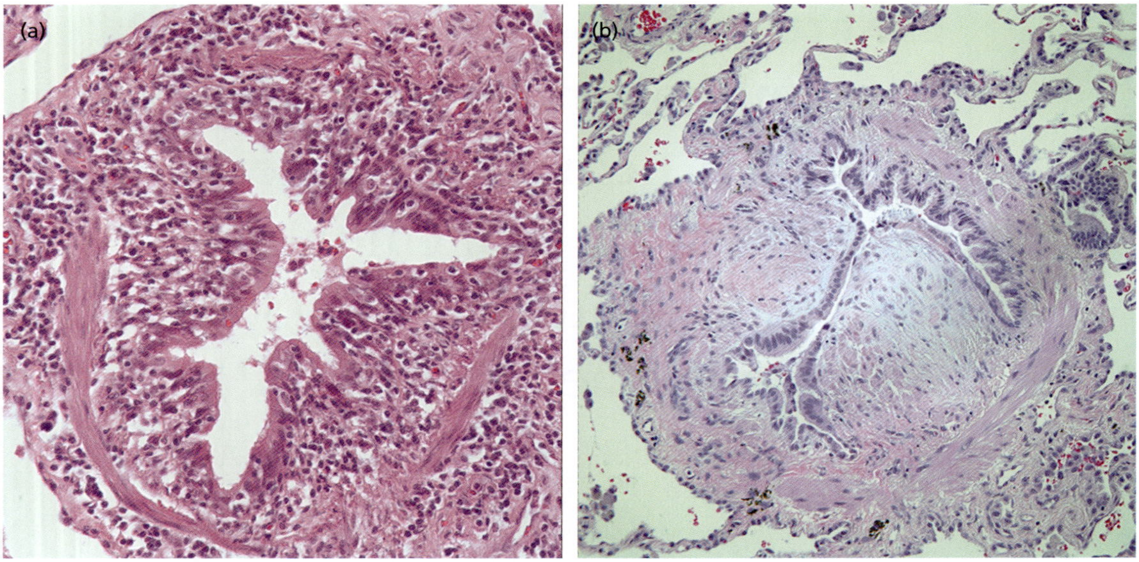

Figure 14.1 (a) Acute lymphocytic bronchiolitis; (b) bronchiolitis obliterans. Photo (c) Dr. Lester Kobzik.

in 1 s (FEV_1) from baseline) in pulmonary function have the worst prognosis [3, 5, 10, 11].

The etiology of BOS remains unknown, but it is suspected that BOS represents a form of donor alloreactivity against host antigens in the lungs. Pathologic studies have suggested that a lymphocytic bronchiolitis (Figure 14.1a) affecting both large and small airways may represent an early and reversible stage of BOS. In contrast, the fibrinous obliteration of the distal airways may represent the late and irreversible manifestation (Figure 14.1b) [12–14]. The pathologic findings of bronchiolitis obliterans (BO) in the HSCT population mirror those observed in BO associated with chronic lung transplant rejection [15].

The clinical factor most closely associated with the development of BOS is the presence of cGVHD at another site; it is rare for patients to have BOS without cGVHD affecting other organ systems [3, 7, 9, 10, 16–18]. Other risk factors reported to be associated with BOS include high risk underlying malignancy at transplant, busulfan-based myeloablative conditioning regimens, peripheral blood stem cell source, human leukocyte antigen mismatch and/or unrelated donors, male recipients with female donors, older patient and donor age, use of methotrexate for GVHD prophylaxis, acute GVHD, respiratory viral infections within the first 100 days after transplantation, history of pneumonitis, low immunoglobulin levels, and reduced pretransplant pulmonary function tests (PFTs) [3, 5–7, 9, 10, 16–20].

The clinical presentation of BOS is usually insidious and nonspecific and may include a dry cough, shortness of breath, or dyspnea on exertion, but up to 20% of patients are asymptomatic [10]. In the absence of routine spirometric screening, reports of disease prevalence likely underestimate the true burden of BOS, since symptomatic patients typically already have moderate to severe airflow obstruction [10]. Physical examination is rarely helpful in the diagnosis of BOS but may reveal hyperinflation, diffuse crackles, or wheeze. In the later stages of the disease a prolonged expiratory phase on auscultation may be noted [10].

In 2005 the National Institutes of Health (NIH) Consensus Criteria for the diagnosis of BOS was established and include [8]:

1 FEV_1/forced vital capacity (FVC) ratio <0.7 and forced expiratory volume in 1 s <75% predicted.

2 Evidence of air trapping or small airway thickening or bronchiectasis on high-resolution chest computed tomography (with inspiratory and expiratory cuts), residual volume >120%, or pathologic confirmation of constrictive bronchiolitis.

3 Absence of infection in the respiratory tract, documented with investigations directed by clinical symptoms, such as radiologic studies (radiographs or computed tomographic scans) or microbiologic cultures (sinus aspiration, upper respiratory tract viral screen, sputum culture, or bronchoalveolar lavage).
4 Organizing pneumonia not due to infections may represent a manifestation of either acute GVCH or cGVHD and is considered a common feature.

It is important to note the NIH consensus criteria were established as a means to standardize the diagnostic criteria for BOS, but they have limitations. To date, the sensitivity and specificity of pulmonary function testing and the diagnosis of BOS in the HSCT population are unknown. There are many pre- and posttransplant factors that can result in a restrictive pattern on pulmonary function testing which can influence their interpretability, including respiratory tract infections, prior exposure to chemotherapy and radiotherapy, pleural effusions, pulmonary fibrosis, steroid myopathy, and sclerodermoid skin manifestations of cGVHD [21–24]. Patients with combined restrictive and obstructive deficits may lead to a false normalization of the FEV_1/FVC ratio, and in these patients an elevated residual volume/total lung capacity may suggest the presence of air trapping and should raise suspicion for BOS. Chest radiographs and high-resolution computed tomography (HRCT) can be useful to identify pleural effusions and evidence of pulmonary fibrosis. Physical exam and maximal inspiratory pressure and maximal expiratory pressure on pulmonary function testing can be used to differentiate restrictive deficits that are the result of skin or fascial fibrosis and muscle weakness, respectively. In difficult cases, pressure–volume relationships using esophageal balloon manometry can be used to quantify components of chest wall and lung restriction.

The current recommendations from the American Society of Blood and Marrow Transplantation are for screening PFTs at baseline, 6 months, 1 year, and yearly thereafter. Experts in the field have advocated for more frequent screening (every 3 months) during the first 1–2 years after transplant, especially in patients with cGVHD affecting other organ systems [21, 25]. An additional approach proposed is to follow the FEV_1 decline over time compared with pretransplant values rather than a strict FEV_1 threshold [21]. Chien et al. [3] demonstrated that a decline in FEV_1 of greater than 5% per year with an FEV_1/FVC ratio of <0.8 has been shown to identify airflow obstruction after transplantation and is associated with a 2.3-fold increase in attributable mortality in patients with cGVHD.

Chest radiographs in patients with BOS are usually normal or may show hyperinflation [10, 26]. HRCT findings in BOS after HSCT include bronchiectasis, bronchial wall thickening, centri-lobular nodules, and mosaic attenuation. The mosaic attenuation represents air trapping best appreciated on expiratory imaging [27–31]. Quantitative HRCT measurements of lung attenuation and airway dilation may provide a more sensitive and specific means to identify patients with BOS, but prospective studies are needed before routine use can be recommended [32–34].

The initial evaluation for patients presenting with new onset airflow obstruction should include: PFTs with and without bronchodilator challenge, chest radiograph, complete blood count with differential and infectious disease evaluation, including sputum Gram stain and culture, viral respiratory panel, and a thorough evaluation for cGVHD affecting other organ systems. If initial evaluation is unrevealing and the airflow obstructive persists or progresses, then a high-resolution chest computed tomography with inspiratory and expiratory images should be considered. Based on respiratory symptoms and the pathologic findings of the HRCT scan, a further work-up by bronchoalveolar lavage (BAL) may be required to exclude an infectious etiology. Transbronchial biopsy for the diagnosis of BO is currently not recommended given its low sensitivity and poor predictive value [35]. Although, open lung biopsy or video-assisted thoracoscopic surgery (VATS) procedures remains the gold standard for the diagnosis of BO they are associated with significant morbidity and life-threatening complications, and are not recommended as part of the routine evaluation [36].

Unfortunately, there are currently no known effective measures to protect patients from the development of BOS. Given the association with respiratory infections early after transplantation, it is recommended that patients adhere to routine guidelines for preventing infectious complications including: (1) routine pre- and posttransplantation vaccinations, (2) performing frequent and thorough hand hygiene, (3) avoiding close contact with persons with respiratory illnesses, and (4) exercise careful hand hygiene when in crowded areas

[37]. In a small randomized controlled trial Vos et al. [38] demonstrated that prophylactic azithromycin (250 mg) three times a week after lung transplantation significantly reduced the incidence of BOS at 2 years from 44.2% to 12.5%. Further studies in the HSCT population would be needed to define the role of azithromycin as a preventative strategy. In light of the strong association between BOS and cGVHD, measures taken to prevent cGVHD might also lead to lower incidence of BOS. There are currently no standard prophylactic medications given to prevent cGVHD, as immune suppressive combinations such as tacrolimus and sirolimus, which, while effective at preventing acute GVHD, have largely failed to reduce the incidence of chronic GVHD [39]. Alternative measures to lower cGVHD, and therefore potentially BOS, might involve adding anti-thymocyte globulin (ATG) to the conditioning regimen, or preferential use of marrow instead of blood as stem cell source [40].

To date there have been no large randomized clinical trials evaluating specific treatments for BOS in the HSCT population. Current treatment approaches are based on small uncontrolled trials and expert opinions. In addition, treatment approaches have been adapted from experience treating BOS in the lung transplant population where 50% of patients develop BOS by 5.6 years posttransplantation [41].

Current consensus for the initial management of BOS consists of high-dose systemic corticosteroids with continuation or augmentation of immunosuppressive therapy (prednisone at 1 mg/kg daily) for 2–6 weeks followed by a taper over 3–9 months [35, 42, 43]. Retrospective data suggest that patients who respond to increased immunosuppression tend to do so in the first 3–9 months and prolonged therapy may increase the risk of complications without significant benefit [5, 44].

The use of inhaled corticosteroids with and without long-acting bronchodilator has been studied retrospectively and has been shown to improve symptoms as well as FEV_1 [45, 46]. One approach is the initiation of high-dose inhaled corticosteroids once early airflow obstruction has been identified with reassessment of PFTs in 2–4 weeks. If there is a continued decline in PFTs then the addition of systemic immunosuppression would be indicated [35]. A phase II clinical trial evaluating the efficacy of budesonide/formoterol in BOS has been completed and analysis of the results is ongoing.

Azithromycin, a macrolide antibiotic, has been shown to modulate cytokine production and polymorphonuclear cell function. It has been associated with improved FEV_1 and delayed progression of BOS after lung transplantation [47–50]. In a small observational study of eight patients with BOS after HSCT, azithromycin was associated with improvements in FEV_1 and FVC [51].

Montelukast, a leukotriene receptor antagonist, has been used in addition to inhaled corticosteroids and azithromycin in both lung transplant and HSCT. Studies to date in HSCT have been very small, but there are currently two ongoing phase II clinical trials evaluating montelukast. One active study is a phase II randomized controlled multicenter trial evaluating the efficacy of the combination of fluticasone, azithromycin, and montelukast in newly diagnosed BOS after HSCT population. The second study is a nonrandomized trial to look at the efficacy of 6 months of montelukast therapy compared with historical controls and the pretreatment rate of decline in FEV_1. Montelukast is a very well tolerated treatment and increasingly being utilized in the treatment of BOS. However, the evidence supporting its use in the HSCT population is currently limited to small case series [52].

For refractory BOS not responsive to conventional therapy, extracorporeal photopheresis (ECP) therapy is a well-tolerated option. Clinical data regarding the efficacy of ECP are limited to case series and small trials in patients with BOS and steroid-refractory cGVHD [53–56]. Limitations of ECP therapy include the time commitment and required vascular access. ECP involves extracorporeal exposure of peripheral blood mononuclear cells to photoactivated 8-methoxypsoralen via ultraviolet light exposure. It is believed that treatment selectively effects autoreactive T cells and may increase regulatory T cells [43]. Larger studies are needed to validate the efficacy of this treatment.

Other potential therapies being evaluated in BOS include imatinib mesylate, rituximab, inhaled cyclosporine, TNF-α inhibitors, low-dose IL-2, and bortezomib. However, while these agents may have activity in cGVHD, their specific use for the treatment of BOS remains investigational.

Advanced BOS often requires supportive care including supplemental oxygen and pulmonary rehabilitation. A recent retrospective study of patients with BOS following HSCT demonstrated that pulmonary rehabilitation improved 6-min walk distance, subjective symptoms of dyspnea, and exercise tolerance in patients with BOS and is recommended by the NIH consensus statement on chronic GVHD for the treatment of BOS [57]. Lung transplantation has been utilized to treat end-stage BOS with similar survival to the general lung transplant population and should be considered in patients with advanced lung disease without other significant co-morbidities [58–60].

Organizing pneumonia

Organizing pneumonia (OP) is a distinct clinicopathologic syndrome observed after a variety of pulmonary insults. Often, however, its cause remains unknown, and it is referred to as cryptogenic (COP). When OP is found in association with one of its many potential causes, it may be referred to as secondary OP. The term bronchiolitis obliterans organizing pneumonia (BOOP) has been used interchangeably with COP, but is often confused with bronchiolitis obliterans syndrome (BOS); as such, the use of the term BOOP should best be avoided.

OP is an inflammatory lung disease that bears little resemblance to other inflammatory conditions in the lungs such as asthma, usual interstitial pneumonitis (UIP), and BOS. It is not a progressive fibrotic process like UIP or BOS, and unlike BOS it is generally more responsive to steroid therapy. OP is a proliferative bronchiolitis triggered by alveolar-epithelial injury resulting in exposure and denudation of the epithelial basal laminae. Fibrinoid inflammatory cell clusters form, develop into fibro-inflammatory buds, and finally mature into buds characterized by the absence of many inflammatory cells or fibrin. Apoptotic activity is increased in the newly formed connective tissue, which stands in contrast with UIP. The cytokine profile suggests activation of macrophages and T-helper cells.

The histologic hallmark of OP is the finding of organized, polypoid granulation tissue within the distal airways (Masson bodies) and extending to the peripheral bronchioles and alveoli (Figure 14.2) [61]. Mild interstitial inflammation may be present in the bronchiolar walls with mononuclear cells and foamy macrophages. Concentric rings of fibroblasts and connective tissue (collagen bundles) characterize the buds. Importantly, lung architecture is preserved; there is no associated traction bronchiectasis or honeycombing.

The signs and symptoms of OP in HSCT patients are indistinguishable from those with OP in non-HSCT patients. Fever, dyspnea, and a nonproductive cough are the most common presenting symptoms. The

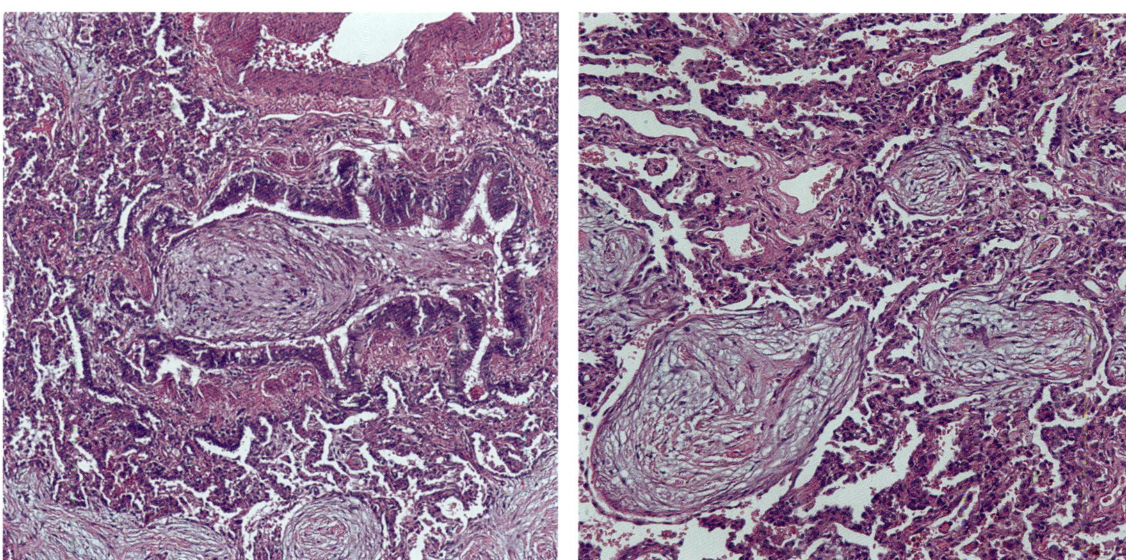

Figure 14.2 Cryptogenic organizing pneumonia. Photo (c) Dr. Lester Kobzik.

presentation is subacute, with symptoms being insidious at onset but slowly worsening over days to weeks with a median duration of symptoms of 13 days prior to diagnosis [62]. The median time to diagnosis following HSCT is 108 days, but it has been reported between 5 days and >2800 days after transplantation [62, 63].

Patients with OP typically have crackles heard on exam and imaging which reveals focal or multifocal peripheral, sometimes triangular, alveolar, or nodular ground glass infiltrates with air bronchograms. These infiltrates are often migratory, and it has been reported that OP in immunocompromised patients, including HSCT patients, have fewer areas of consolidation compared with immunocompetent patients, and are more likely to have ground glass and nodular infiltrates [64]. Given the abnormal infiltrative patterns on radiographic imaging, a thorough work-up to rule out an underlying pulmonary infectious process is necessary to establish the diagnosis of COP, especially in the immune-compromised host.

Restrictive physiology as demonstrated by a symmetric reduction in FVC and FEV_1 is the most common physiologic abnormality found by pulmonary function testing. The diffusion capacity is also decreased from baseline in approximately two-thirds of cases.

Bronchoscopy with BAL may provide information that supports the diagnosis of OP but cannot establish it. Transbronchial biopsies may also support a provisional diagnosis of OP but must be interpreted with caution owing to potential sampling error and the fact that the organizing pneumonia histology may be seen focally as part of other lung injuries but not necessarily represent the dominant histologic process. However, bronchoscopy may serve to exclude infectious or neoplastic processes, and a BAL cytologic analysis with an increase in lymphocytes characterized by a decrease in CD4/CD8 and an increase in neutrophils and eosinophils lends support to the diagnosis [65–67].

OP affects men and women equally, and the average age of patients at diagnosis in the general population is 50 years [68] and 30 years in the HSCT population [62]. OP is known to occur in response to respiratory infections, medications, radiation, environmental/inhalational exposure, and rheumatologic disorders. After HSCT, OP is most commonly associated with acute GVHD or cGVHD. Patients with acute GVHD involving skin or cGVHD involving the gut and oral cavity were more likely than controls to develop OP, and progressive GVHD was more likely to be associated with the development of OP than "quiescent" GVHD. Accordingly, the incidence of OP is somewhat dependent on the HSCT population studied. For example, in one study of all lung biopsies in HSCT patients at one institution over a 22-year period of time, the incidence of OP was 0.9%. However, Palmas et al. [69] reported an incidence of 1.7% in patients who received an allogeneic BMT and survived at least 3 months, and Patriarca et al. [70] reported an incidence of 10.3% among allogeneic BMT patients with unrelated donors.

Mild, asymptomatic OP may be managed by observation alone. The presence of symptoms or signs of disease progression, however, necessitate treatment. The majority of cases of OP respond to systemic corticosteroids; it is estimated that approximately 80% of patients with OP-complicating HSCT respond to treatment similar to the general population [69, 71, 72]. Prednisone begun at 0.5–1.0 mg/kg for 1–3 months followed by a slowly decreasing dose over a variable period of time ranging from 3 to 12 months has been recommended for more severe cases [68]. Patients with moderate OP may be considered for lower, shorter courses. Relapse may occur in 25–30% of cases, but those who relapse at prednisone doses of 20 mg daily or less have an excellent prognosis [68].

For those patients who cannot be treated with steroids or have limiting adverse effects, macrolides may be beneficial. Azithromycin 250 mg three times weekly and clarithromycin 250 mg twice daily have both been used with anecdotal success. Other immune suppressive agents, such as cyclosphosphamide at a dose of 100–125 mg daily and mycophenolate mofetil 1000 mg twice daily, may also be considered in individual circumstances.

OP has an excellent prognosis for most, with a mortality rate among the general population of approximately 5% [68]. The case fatality rate among patients with OP who have undergone HSCT is reported to be 16–19% [62, 71]. There is no specific prevention strategy recommended beyond those aimed at reducing the incidence of the associated causes.

Conclusion

Late-onset pulmonary complications following HSCT continue to represent a major clinical challenge to the management of the post-HSCT population. Unlike COP, effective therapies for the management of BOS have yet to be established. Clinical trials are currently ongoing and will hopefully provide more guidance into the management of this devastating complication of HSCT.

Acknowledgment

We would like to thank Dr Lester Kobzik for providing the histopathology images of BO and COP.

References

1. Ralph DD, Springmeyer SC, Sullivan KM, et al. Rapidly progressive air-flow obstruction in marrow transplant recipients. Possible association between obliterative bronchiolitis and chronic graft-versus-host disease. Am Rev Respir Dis. 1984;129(4):641–644. Epub 1984/04/01.
2. Roca J, Granena A, Rodriguez-Roisin R, et al. Fatal airway disease in an adult with chronic graft-versus-host disease. Thorax. 1982;37(1):77–78. Epub 1982/01/01.
3. Chien JW, Martin PJ, Gooley TA, et al. Airflow obstruction after myeloablative allogeneic hematopoietic stem cell transplantation. Am J Respir Crit Care Med. 2003;168(2):208–214. Epub 2003/03/22.
4. Link H, Ostendorf P, Wilms K, et al. Pulmonale Komplikationen nach allogener Knochenmarktransplantation [Pulmonary complications following allogeneic bone marrow transplantation]. Prax Klin Pneumol. 1983;37(Suppl 1): 1043–1047. Epub 1983/10/01. .
5. Dudek A. Bronchiolitis obliterans in chronic graft-versus-host disease: analysis of risk factors and treatment outcomes. Biol Blood Marrow Transplant. 2003;9(10):657–666.
6. Santo Tomas LH, Loberiza FR Jr, Klein JP, et al. Risk factors for bronchiolitis obliterans in allogeneic hematopoietic stem-cell transplantation for leukemia. Chest. 2005;128(1): 153–161. Epub 2005/07/09.
7. Au BK, Au MA, Chien JW. Bronchiolitis obliterans syndrome epidemiology after allogeneic hematopoietic cell transplantation. Biol Blood Marrow Transplant. 2011; 17(7):1072–1078. Epub 2010/12/04.
8. Filipovich AH, Weisdorf D, Pavletic S, et al. National Institutes of Health Consensus Development Project on criteria for clinical trials in chronic graft-versus-host disease: I. Diagnosis and staging working group report. Biol Blood Marrow Transplant. 2005;11(12):945–956. Epub 2005/12/13.
9. Clark JG, Schwartz DA, Flournoy N, et al. Risk factors for airflow obstruction in recipients of bone marrow transplants. Ann Intern Med. 1987;107(5):648–656. Epub 1987/11/01.
10. Clark JG, Crawford SW, Madtes DK, Sullivan KM. Obstructive lung disease after allogeneic marrow transplantation. Clinical presentation and course. Ann Intern Med. 1989; 111(5):368–376. Epub 1989/09/01.
11. Chien JW, Martin PJ, Flowers ME, et al. Implications of early airflow decline after myeloablative allogeneic stem cell transplantation. Bone Marrow Transplant. 2004;33(7):759–764. Epub 2004/02/18.
12. Yousem SA. The histological spectrum of pulmonary graft-versus-host disease in bone marrow transplant recipients. Hum Pathol. 1995;26(6):668–675. Epub 1995/06/01.
13. Trisolini R, Bandini G, Stanzani M, et al. Morphologic changes leading to bronchiolitis obliterans in a patient with delayed non-infectious lung disease after allogeneic bone marrow transplantation. Bone Marrow Transplant. 2001; 28(12):1167–1170. Epub 2002/01/23.
14. Yokoi T, Hirabayashi N, Ito M, et al. Broncho-bronchiolitis obliterans as a complication of bone marrow transplantation: a clinicopathological study of eight autopsy cases. Nagoya BMT Group. Virchows Arch. 1997;431(4):275–282. Epub 1997/11/22.
15. Estenne M, Maurer JR, Boehler A, et al. Bronchiolitis obliterans syndrome 2001: an update of the diagnostic criteria. J Heart Lung Transplant. 2002;21(3):297–310. Epub 2002/03/19.
16. Holland HK, Wingard JR, Beschorner WE, et al. Bronchiolitis obliterans in bone marrow transplantation and its relationship to chronic graft-v-host disease and low serum IgG. Blood. 1988;72(2):621–627. Epub 1988/08/01.
17. Nakaseko C, Ozawa S, Sakaida E, et al. Incidence, risk factors and outcomes of bronchiolitis obliterans after allogeneic stem cell transplantation. Int J Hematol. 2011;93(3):375–382. Epub 2011/03/23.
18. Nishio N, Yagasaki H, Takahashi Y, et al. Late-onset non-infectious pulmonary complications following allogeneic hematopoietic stem cell transplantation in children. Bone Marrow Transplant. 2009;44(5):303–308. Epub 2009/04/08.
19. Ringden O, Remberger M, Ruutu T, et al. Increased risk of chronic graft-versus-host disease, obstructive bronchiolitis, and alopecia with busulfan versus total body irradiation: long-term results of a randomized trial in allogeneic marrow recipients with leukemia. Nordic Bone Marrow Transplantation Group. Blood. 1999;93(7):2196–2201. Epub 1999/03/26.
20. Moghadam KG, Marghoob B, Alimoghadam K, et al. Bronchiolitis obliterans following hematopoietic stem cell transplantation. Hematology/oncology and stem cell therapy. 2010;3(2):100–101. Epub 2010/06/15.
21. Williams KM, Chien JW, Gladwin MT, Pavletic SZ. Bronchiolitis obliterans after allogeneic hematopoietic stem

cell transplantation. JAMA. 2009;302(3):306–314. Epub 2009/07/16.

22. Wilczynski SW, Erasmus JJ, Petros WP, et al. Delayed pulmonary toxicity syndrome following high-dose chemotherapy and bone marrow transplantation for breast cancer. Am J Respir Crit Care Med. 1998;157(2):565–573. Epub 1998/02/26.
23. Wolff D, Reichenberger F, Steiner B, et al. Progressive interstitial fibrosis of the lung in sclerodermoid chronic graft-versus-host disease. Bone Marrow Transplant. 2002;29(4): 357–360. Epub 2002/03/16.
24. Skert C, Patriarca F, Sperotto A, et al. Sclerodermatous chronic graft-versus-host disease after allogeneic hematopoietic stem cell transplantation: incidence, predictors and outcome. Haematologica. 2006;91(2):258–261. Epub 2006/02/08.
25. Majhail NS, Rizzo JD, Lee SJ, et al. Recommended screening and preventive practices for long-term survivors after hematopoietic cell transplantation. Biol Blood Marrow Transplant. 2012;18(3):348–371. Epub 2011/12/20.
26. Afessa B, Litzow MR, Tefferi A. Bronchiolitis obliterans and other late onset non-infectious pulmonary complications in hematopoietic stem cell transplantation. Bone Marrow Transplant. 2001;28(5):425–434. Epub 2001/10/11.
27. Gunn ML, Godwin JD, Kanne JP, et al. High-resolution CT findings of bronchiolitis obliterans syndrome after hematopoietic stem cell transplantation. J Thorac Imaging. 2008;23(4):244–250. Epub 2009/02/11.
28. Jung JI, Jung WS, Hahn ST, et al. Bronchiolitis obliterans after allogenic bone marrow transplantation: HRCT findings. Korean J Radiol. 2004;5(2):107–113. Epub 2004/07/06.
29. Ooi GC, Peh WC, Ip M. High-resolution computed tomography of bronchiolitis obliterans syndrome after bone marrow transplantation. Respiration. 1998;65(3):187–191. Epub 1998/07/22.
30. Padley SP, Adler B, Muller NL. High-resolution computed tomography of the chest: current indications. J Thorac Imaging. 1993;8(3):189–199. Epub 1993/01/01.
31. Sargent MA, Cairns RA, Murdoch MJ, et al. Obstructive lung disease in children after allogeneic bone marrow transplantation: evaluation with high-resolution CT. AJR Am J Roentgenol. 1995;164(3):693–696. Epub 1995/03/01.
32. Gazourian L, Coronata AMF, Rogers AJ, et al. Airway dilation in bronchiolitis obliterans after allogeneic hematopoietic stem cell transplantation. Respir Med. 2013;107(2): 276–283.
33. Knollmann FD, Kapell S, Lehmkuhl H, et al. Dynamic high-resolution electron-beam CT scanning for the diagnosis of bronchiolitis obliterans syndrome after lung transplantation. Chest. 2004;126(2):447–456. Epub 2004/08/11.
34. Knollmann FD, Ewert R, Wundrich T, et al. Bronchiolitis obliterans syndrome in lung transplant recipients: use of spirometrically gated CT. Radiology. 2002;225(3):655–662. Epub 2002/12/04.
35. Hildebrandt GC, Fazekas T, Lawitschka A, et al. Diagnosis and treatment of pulmonary chronic GVHD: report from the Consensus Conference on Clinical Practice in Chronic GVHD. Bone Marrow Transplant. 2011;46(10):1283–1295. Epub 2011/03/29.
36. White DA, Wong PW, Downey R. The utility of open lung biopsy in patients with hematologic malignancies. Am J Respir Crit Care Med. 2000;161(3 Pt 1):723–729. Epub 2000/03/11.
37. Tomblyn M, Chiller T, Einsele H, et al. Guidelines for preventing infectious complications among hematopoietic cell transplantation recipients: a global perspective. Biol Blood Marrow Transplant. 2009;15(10):1143–1238. Epub 2009/09/15.
38. Vos R, Vanaudenaerde BM, Verleden SE, et al. A randomised controlled trial of azithromycin to prevent chronic rejection after lung transplantation. Eur Respir J. 2011;37(1):164–172. Epub 2010/06/22.
39. Cutler C, Kim HT, Hochberg E, et al. Sirolimus and tacrolimus without methotrexate as graft-versus-host disease prophylaxis after matched related donor peripheral blood stem cell transplantation. Biol Blood Marrow Transplant. 2004;10(5):328–336. Epub 2004/04/28.
40. Socie G, Schmoor C, Bethge WA, et al. Chronic graft-versus-host disease: long-term results from a randomized trial on graft-versus-host disease prophylaxis with or without anti-T-cell globulin ATG-Fresenius. Blood. 2011;117(23):6375–6382. Epub 2011/04/07.
41. Trulock EP, Christie JD, Edwards LB, et al. Registry of the International Society for Heart and Lung Transplantation: Twenty-Fourth Official Adult Lung and Heart–Lung Transplantation Report – 2007. J Heart Lung Transplant. 2007;26(8):782–795. Epub 2007/08/19.
42. Pandya CM, Soubani AO. Bronchiolitis obliterans following hematopoietic stem cell transplantation: a clinical update. Clin Transplant. 2010;24(3):291–306. Epub 2009/10/24.
43. Sengsayadeth SM, Srivastava S, Jagasia M, Savani BN. Time to explore preventive and novel therapies for bronchiolitis obliterans syndrome after allogeneic hematopoietic stem cell transplantation. Biol Blood Marrow Transplant. 2012; 18(10):1479–1487. Epub 2012/03/28.
44. Sanchez J, Torres A, Serrano J, et al. Long-term follow-up of immunosuppressive treatment for obstructive airways disease after allogeneic bone marrow transplantation. Bone Marrow Transplant. 1997;20(5):403–408. Epub 1997/10/27.

45. Bashoura L, Gupta S, Jain A, et al. Inhaled corticosteroids stabilize constrictive bronchiolitis after hematopoietic stem cell transplantation. Bone Marrow Transplant. 2008;41(1):63–67. Epub 2007/10/16.
46. Bergeron A, Belle A, Chevret S, et al. Combined inhaled steroids and bronchodilatators in obstructive airway disease after allogeneic stem cell transplantation. Bone Marrow Transplant. 2007;39(9):547–553. Epub 2007/03/14.
47. Vos R, Vanaudenaerde BM, Ottevaere A, et al. Long-term azithromycin therapy for bronchiolitis obliterans syndrome: divide and conquer? J Heart Lung Transplant. 2010;29(12):1358–1368. Epub 2010/07/14.
48. Gerhardt SG, McDyer JF, Girgis RE, et al. Maintenance azithromycin therapy for bronchiolitis obliterans syndrome: results of a pilot study. Am J Respir Crit Care Med. 2003;168(1):121–125. Epub 2003/04/04.
49. Yates B, Murphy DM, Forrest IA, et al. Azithromycin reverses airflow obstruction in established bronchiolitis obliterans syndrome. Am J Respir Crit Care Med. 2005;172(6):772–775. Epub 2005/06/25.
50. Gottlieb J, Szangolies J, Koehnlein T, et al. Long-term azithromycin for bronchiolitis obliterans syndrome after lung transplantation. Transplantation. 2008;85(1):36–41. Epub 2008/01/15.
51. Khalid M, Al Saghir A, Saleemi S, et al. Azithromycin in bronchiolitis obliterans complicating bone marrow transplantation: a preliminary study. Eur Respir J. 2005;25(3):490–493. Epub 2005/03/02.
52. Or R, Gesundheit B, Resnick I, et al. Sparing effect by montelukast treatment for chronic graft versus host disease: a pilot study. Transplantation. 2007;83(5):577–581. Epub 2007/03/14.
53. Alcindor T, Gorgun G, Miller KB, et al. Immunomodulatory effects of extracorporeal photochemotherapy in patients with extensive chronic graft-versus-host disease. Blood. 2001;98(5):1622–1625. Epub 2001/08/25.
54. Oyan B, Koc Y, Emri S, Kansu E. Improvement of chronic pulmonary graft-vs-host disease manifesting as bronchiolitis obliterans organizing pneumonia following extracorporeal photopheresis. Med Oncol. 2006;23(1):125–129. Epub 2006/04/29.
55. Lucid CE, Savani BN, Engelhardt BG, et al. Extracorporeal photopheresis in patients with refractory bronchiolitis obliterans developing after allo-SCT. Bone Marrow Transplant. 2011;46(3):426–429. Epub 2010/06/29.
56. Greinix HT, van Besien K, Elmaagacli AH, et al. Progressive improvement in cutaneous and extracutaneous chronic graft-versus-host disease after a 24-week course of extracorporeal photopheresis – results of a crossover randomized study. Biol Blood Marrow Transplant. 2011;17(12):1775–1782. Epub 2011/05/31.
57. Tran J, Norder EE, Diaz PT, et al. Pulmonary rehabilitation for bronchiolitis obliterans syndrome after hematopoietic stem cell transplantation. Biol Blood Marrow Transplant. 2012;18(8):1250–1254. Epub 2012/02/04.
58. Boas SR, Noyes BE, Kurland G, et al. Pediatric lung transplantation for graft-versus-host disease following bone marrow transplantation. Chest. 1994;105(5):1584–1586. Epub 1994/05/01.
59. Calhoon JH. Lung transplantation in a patient with a prior bone marrow transplant. Chest. 1992;102(3):948.
60. Holm AM, Riise GC, Hansson L, et al. Lung transplantation for bronchiolitis obliterans syndrome after allo-SCT. Bone Marrow Transplant. 2012;Epub 2012/10/16.
61. Cordier JF. Cryptogenic organising pneumonia. Eur Respir J. 2006;28(2):422–446. Epub 2006/08/02.
62. Freudenberger TD, Madtes DK, Curtis JR, et al. Association between acute and chronic graft-versus-host disease and bronchiolitis obliterans organizing pneumonia in recipients of hematopoietic stem cell transplants. Blood. 2003;102(10):3822–3828. Epub 2003/07/19.
63. Yoshihara S, Yanik G, Cooke KR, Mineishi S. Bronchiolitis obliterans syndrome (BOS), bronchiolitis obliterans organizing pneumonia (BOOP), and other late-onset noninfectious pulmonary complications following allogeneic hematopoietic stem cell transplantation. Biol Blood Marrow Transplant. 2007;13(7):749–759. Epub 2007/06/21.
64. Lee KS, Kullnig P, Hartman TE, Muller NL. Cryptogenic organizing pneumonia: CT findings in 43 patients. AJR Am J Roentgenol. 1994;162(3):543–546. Epub 1994/03/01.
65. Mukae H, Kadota J, Kohno S, et al. Increase of activated T-cells in BAL fluid of Japanese patients with bronchiolitis obliterans organizing pneumonia and chronic eosinophilic pneumonia. Chest. 1995;108(1):123–128. Epub 1995/07/01.
66. Costabel U, Teschler H, Guzman J. Bronchiolitis obliterans organizing pneumonia (BOOP): the cytological and immunocytological profile of bronchoalveolar lavage. The Eur Respir J. 1992;5(7):791–797. Epub 1992/07/01.
67. Poletti V, Cazzato S, Minicuci N, et al. The diagnostic value of bronchoalveolar lavage and transbronchial lung biopsy in cryptogenic organizing pneumonia. Eur Respir J. 1996;9(12):2513–2516. Epub 1996/12/01.
68. Epler GR. Bronchiolitis obliterans organizing pneumonia, 25 years: a variety of causes, but what are the treatment options? Expert Rev Respir Med. 2011;5(3):353–361. Epub 2011/06/28.
69. Palmas A, Tefferi A, Myers JL, et al. Late-onset noninfectious pulmonary complications after allogeneic bone marrow transplantation. Br J Haematol. 1998;100(4):680–687. Epub 1998/04/08.
70. Patriarca F, Skert C, Sperotto A, et al. Incidence, outcome and risk factors of late-onset noninfectious pulmonary

complications after unrelated donor stem cell transplantation. Bone Marrow Transplant. 2004;33(7):751–758. Epub 2004/02/03.

71. Afessa B, Peters SG. Chronic lung disease after hematopoietic stem cell transplantation. Clin Chest Med. 2005; 26(4):571–586, vi. Epub 2005/11/03.

72. Vasu TS, Cavallazzi R, Hirani A, et al. Clinical and radiologic distinctions between secondary bronchiolitis obliterans organizing pneumonia and cryptogenic organizing pneumonia. Respir Care. 2009;54(8):1028–1032. Epub 2009/08/05.

15

CHAPTER 15

Post-transplantation bone disease: prevalence, monitoring, prevention, and management guidelines

Kathryn Dahir, Brandon Perry, and Shubhada Jagasia

Division of Diabetes, Endocrinology and Metabolism, Department of Medicine, Vanderbilt University Medical Center, Nashville, TN, USA

Stem cell transplantion-related bone loss

Bone is a dynamic, highly organized tissue composed of specialized cells, minerals, proteins, and water. Osteoblasts are the major bone-forming cells, whereas osteoclasts resorb bone. The mineral content of bone includes calcium, phosphorus, and magnesium. Bone growth is completed by early adulthood, at which time peak bone mass is reached. Bone remodeling is the cycle of breakdown and regeneration that continues throughout life. Net bone loss occurs when breakdown outpaces regeneration. Bone loss occurs with aging in both sexes but is notably accelerated in postmenopausal women due to loss of the protective effects of estrogen. Osteopenia and osteoporosis represent progressively more severe degrees of bone loss and microscopic structural disruption. Unchecked, bone loss increases the risk of fractures. Hip fractures, in particular, impart increased morbidity and mortality [1–4].

A number of factors contribute to fracture risk. The Fracture Risk Assessment Tool (FRAX®, http://www.shef.ac.uk/FRAX) endorsed by the World Health Organization incorporates several factors to estimate the 10-year risk of sustaining a fracture. The components of FRAX are age, sex, weight, height, a history of previous fracture, a parent with a history of hip fracture, current smoking, glucocorticoid use, rheumatoid arthritis, secondary osteoporosis, alcohol intake, and bone mineral density (BMD) of the femoral neck. Though FRAX is widely used in the nontransplant setting, it has not been well studied among the stem cell transplantation (SCT) population [5, 8, 9, 10].

Rapid bone loss occurs in the first 6–12 months after SCT. Use of immunosuppressing drugs, especially glucocorticoids, is likely the most significant contributor to early bone loss. Glucocorticoid use is an independent risk factor for bone loss and fractures in other populations. Up to 50% of individuals treated with glucocorticoids >3 months develop secondary osteoporosis, 50% of whom suffer a fracture [11, 12]. Glucocorticoids directly inhibit bone formation and indirectly enhance bone breakdown [13–21]. Glucocorticoid-associated bone loss is generally reversible with medication discontinuation [11, 12]. Calcineurin inhibitors may also contribute to bone loss, likely through direct effects on osteoclasts and T cells. However, incorporation of the calcineurin inhibitor tacrolimus allows lower glucocorticoid dosing and results in less bone loss [22].

Hypogonadism is common among SCT recipients and is associated with increased bone loss. Other risk factors for bone loss among SCT recipients include advanced

Blood and Marrow Transplantation Long-Term Management: Prevention and Complications, First Edition. Edited by Bipin N Savani.

age, direct damage to bone-forming stem cells from chemotherapy or irradiation, thyroid disease, kidney disease, secondary hyperparathyroidism, and immobility [13–21].

Prevalence

The reported prevalences of osteoporosis and osteopenia before transplant have been as high as 29% and 43%, respectively. The reported prevalence of bone loss leading to osteopenia or osteoporosis after transplant has been as high as 73%. Bone loss may be more severe after allogeneic SCT compared with autologous SCT, possibly due to the greater intensity of immunosuppression required in allogeneic SCT [13–21]. Fracture risk associated with SCT-related bone loss has not been well studied. One study has reported increased bone loss without increased risk of fracture [23]. Several other studies have reported significantly increased fracture risk among solid organ transplant recipients, who manifest similar patterns of bone loss and share similar risk factors, most notably glucocorticoid-intensive immunosuppressive therapy. In these individuals, reported fracture rates have ranged from 10 to 65%. Fracture risk is highest during the early posttransplant period of rapid bone loss and improves within 6–24 months following transplantation [24–29].

Monitoring

Bone mass is clinically assessed by evaluation of bone mineral density (BMD). The most widely used method is dual-energy X-ray absorptiometry (DXA). DXA allows precise measurement of BMD with minimal exposure to ionizing radiation. In adults, accepted sites of measurement include the femoral neck, total hip, and spine. The radius may be used if the hip or spine cannot be measured. DXA scores are reported in grams of mineral per square centimeter and then standardized against average scores from specific populations. The *Z*-score represents the standard deviation of BMD compared with an age-, gender-, and ethnicity-matched population. The *Z*-score is the preferred indicator of BMD in children, adolescents, premenopausal women, and men up to the age of 49 years. The *T*-score represents the standard deviation of BMD compared with a normal, young adult population and is the preferred indicator of BMD in postmenopausal women and men aged 50 years or older [19]. A *Z*-score greater than two standard deviations below normal has been associated with increased risk of secondary causes of bone loss, such as celiac disease, hyperparathyroidism, or alcohol abuse [30, 31].

The optimal approach to screening for bone disease in SCT recipients is not known. Some clinicians advocate pretransplant DXA, especially among individuals with significant risk factors for bone disease. Most clinicians recommend DXA within 1 year of transplantation and repeat DXA every 1–2 years, depending on clinical course and risk factor profile. Graft-versus-host disease and other conditions that require increased glucocorticoid exposure (≥5 mg prednisone daily for >3 months) should prompt annual screening [13–21].

Biochemical bone turnover markers (BTMs) may be useful in guiding treatment of osteoporosis in selected individuals. Bisphosphonates, estrogens, and calcitriol work primarily by decreasing bone breakdown and correspondingly decrease markers of bone breakdown. Two of the most reliable assays test for urinary collagen type 1 cross-linked N-telopeptide (NTX) and serum collagen type 1 cross-linked C-telopeptide (CTX). A decrease in either of these markers 6–12 months after initiating antiresorptive therapy is associated with a decreased fracture risk over the subsequent 2–3 years [32–36]. Serum CTX should decrease by at least 30%, and urinary NTX should decrease by at least 50%. Though BTMs have been used extensively in research, their precise roles in clinical practice have not been well defined. Some evidence suggests BTMs may improve patient adherence. In addition, some clinicians advocate using BTMs to guide duration of therapy [35, 36].

Prevention

Many experts recommend treating all SCT recipients for bone loss immediately after transplant, regardless of BMD. Bisphosphonates are the preferred first line agents for this purpose. Hormone replacement therapy (HRT) for carefully selected women helps prevent bone loss as well. All SCT recipients need adequate intake of vitamin D and calcium [13–21].

Adequate calcium and vitamin D are necessary to maintain bone health. Previously, the recommended daily intake of calcium has been 1200 mg daily for postmenopausal women and 1000 mg daily for men and premenopausal women. Recent studies have suggested an increased risk of coronary artery disease with higher calcium intake. Other studies have shown either a decrease or no significant change in coronary artery disease risk with calcium intake. Natural dietary sources of calcium, such as low-fat dairy products, may be safer than supplements. Further study is needed to determine optimal calcium intake. Vitamin D is discussed in the following section [60, 90–94].

Exercise and fall prevention help to maintain bone mass and prevent fractures. Exercise alone or in combination with occupational therapy has reduced falls by 25–50% in some studies [33, 37–42]. Small studies of resistance training, with or without bisphosphonate therapy, have shown improvements in lumbar spine BMD among lung transplant recipients and heart transplant recipients [39, 42]. Performing timely cataract surgery, if indicated, may reduce fall risk [43]. Treating vitamin D deficiency improves fall and fracture risks [42–44].

Therapeutic options

Bisphosphonates are the best-studied drugs for prevention of SCT-related bone loss and are generally the recommended first-line agents [13–22, 45–47]. Side effects are relatively uncommon but potentially severe. Oral bisphosphonates can cause severe inflammation of the esophagus, especially in the presence of impaired swallowing. Intravenous formulations are available for individuals who cannot tolerate the oral drugs [20]. Bisphosphonate-related osteonecrosis of the jaw (BRONJ) is a painful but rare complication most commonly associated with dental procedures after treatment with bisphosphonates. Multiple myeloma further increases the risk of BRONJ, especially with zoledronic acid; the risk is higher with long-term bisphosphonate therapy [48, 49]. Atypical femur fractures have been reported among some individuals treated with bisphosphonates. The risk appears to correlate with duration of therapy. The absolute risk appears to be low however, and should not preclude therapy for individuals at high risk for osteoporosis-related fractures [50–58]. Bisphosphonates should be avoided in patients with significant kidney disease [21].

Calcitriol and estrogen have shown some benefit in SCT-related bone loss. An activated form of vitamin D, calcitriol can cause severe hypercalcemia and requires careful monitoring of serum and urine calcium levels and kidney function [13, 59]. High doses of calcitriol may induce bone loss through osteoclast activation [58]. Women who experience ovarian insufficiency may benefit from HRT with estrogen and progestin [13, 59]. The selective estrogen receptor modulator raloxifene has not been studied in the SCT population [16]. Testosterone may provide some protection against bone loss in hypogonadal men, but replacement may not prevent fracture [60]. HRT in men and women carries significant health risks and should be administered with caution [13, 59]. Hypogonadism has been discussed in further detail in Chapter 18. Teriparatide has not been well studied in the transplant population [52, 59]. A history of irradiation of the bone is a contraindication to teriparatide owing to an increased risk of osteosarcoma observed in a rat model, though this correlation has not been observed in humans [61, 62]. Several studies of calcitonin in SCT and solid organ transplant recipients have demonstrated no significant benefit on bone loss [63–66]. Calcitonin may improve acute fracture-related pain but is ineffective for chronic pain [67, 68]. Denosumab has not been studied in the transplant population.

Management

- All SCT recipients should maintain adequate vitamin D intake, as discussed in the next section.
- Total daily calcium intake should not exceed 1200 mg. Dietary sources of calcium may confer less cardiovascular risk than supplements [34–39]. Some dietary sources of calcium are listed in Table 15.1.
- Measurement of 24-h urine calcium may help guide therapy.
- All SCT recipients should avoid smoking and alcohol abuse.
- Weight-bearing exercise, balance training, occupational therapy, vitamin D sufficiency, and timely cataract surgery may prevent falls and reduce fracture risk.
- Glucocorticoid use should be limited to the extent possible to minimize bone loss and fracture risk.
- A screening DXA should be completed within the first year after SCT. Some clinicians advocate pretransplant DXA, especially among individuals with significant risk factors for bone loss. The optimal frequency of DXA screening has not been defined. One approach is to rescreen every 1–2 years those individuals undergoing treatment for bone loss or on glucocorticoid therapy (≥5 mg prednisone daily for >3 months). Other individuals may be screened every 3–5 years [69].
- A *Z*-score greater than two standard deviations below normal should prompt consideration for evaluation of

Table 15.1 Dietary sources of calcium [89]

Food	Calcium per serving (mg)
Yogurt, plain, low fat, 8 ounces	415
Mozzarella, part skim, 1.5 ounces	333
Sardines, canned in oil, with bones, 3 ounces	325
Yogurt, fruit, low fat, 8 ounces	313–384
Cheddar cheese, 1.5 ounces	307
Milk, nonfat, 8 ounces[a]	299
Soymilk, calcium-fortified, 8 ounces	299
Milk, reduced-fat (2% milk fat), 8 ounces	293
Milk, buttermilk, lowfat, 8 ounces	284
Milk, whole (3.25% milk fat), 8 ounces	276
Orange juice, calcium-fortified, 6 ounces	261
Tofu, firm, made with calcium sulfate, ½ cup[b]	253
Salmon, pink, canned, solids with bone, 3 ounces	181
Cottage cheese, 1% milk fat, 1 cup	138
Tofu, soft, made with calcium sulfate, ½ cup[b]	138
Ready-to-eat cereal, calcium-fortified, 1 cup	100–1000
Frozen yogurt, vanilla, soft serve, ½ cup	103
Turnip greens, fresh, boiled, ½ cup	99
Kale, raw, chopped, 1 cup	100
Kale, fresh, cooked, 1 cup	94
Ice cream, vanilla, ½ cup	84

[a]Calcium content varies slightly by fat content; the more fat, the less calcium the food contains.
[b]Calcium content is for tofu processed with a calcium salt. Tofu processed with other salts does not provide significant amounts of calcium.

secondary causes of bone loss, such as celiac disease, parathyroidism, or alcohol abuse.

- The utility of FRAX in predicting fracture risk in SCT recipients is uncertain.
- Bisphosphonates are generally considered first-line medications for the treatment and prevention of bone loss. Some experts recommend treating all SCT recipients with bisphosphonates immediately after transplantation, regardless of pretransplant BMD.
- Choice of bisphosphonate, optimal dosing, and duration of therapy for prevention or treatment of SCT-related bone loss remain uncertain. Patient preference, drug tolerance, risk factors for adverse side effects, and cost should guide drug choice. US Food and Drug Administration (FDA)-approved dosing for prevention and treatment of osteoporosis are listed in Table 15.2 [70].
- Any anticipated dental procedures should be completed before starting bisphosphonate therapy to minimize the risk of BRONJ.
- Calcitriol may be used with caution if bisphosphonates are contraindicated or not tolerated.
- Sex HRT may be useful in carefully selected individuals. Teriparatide may be helpful but has not been well studied in the SCT recipients. Teriparatide is contraindicated in individuals who have received radiation therapy to the bone.
- The optimal duration of anti-osteoporosis therapy in SCT recipients is unknown. Some experts advocate a minimal duration of 1–2 years. Serial DXA and serial measurements of BTMs may provide some guidance [18].
- BTMs may promote medication adherence. BTMs should not be used to diagnose or refute bone disease [32–36].

Vitamin D deficiency

Vitamin D is a fat-soluble vitamin with many diverse functions. Vitamin D plays central roles in the maintenance of calcium and phosphorus levels and in the maintenance of bone health. Deficiency results in weakening of the bones, a condition known as osteomalacia. In adults, osteomalacia causes bone pain, increased risk of fracture, muscle weakness, and dental problems. Vitamin D deficiency is also associated with muscle pain and increased fall risk. Large studies among the elderly have linked vitamin D deficiency with an increased risk of fractures, and correcting vitamin D deficiency slows bone loss, decreases fall risk, and decreases fracture risk in this population [1, 42, 44, 71–73]. Nonskeletal functions of vitamin D include regulation of cell growth, immune function, and glucose tolerance. Deficiency has correlated with increased risks of tuberculosis, cardiovascular disease, autoimmune disease, diabetes, and a number of cancers [1, 72, 73].

Table 15.2 Selected FDA-approved anti-osteoporosis medications [30]

Drug	Route	Dose	Serious adverse effects
Bisphosphonates			
Alendronate	Oral	10 mg daily 70 mg weekly 5 mg once daily for treatment of steroid-induced osteoporosis 5 mg once daily or 35 mg once weekly for prevention of osteoporosis	Esophageal ulceration, osteonecrosis of the jaw
Risedronate	Oral	5 mg daily 35 mg weekly 75 mg on two consecutive days of the month 150 mg monthly	Esophageal ulceration, osteonecrosis of the jaw
Ibandronate	Oral	2.5 mg daily 150 mg once monthly	Esophageal ulceration, osteonecrosis of the jaw
	Intravenous	3 mg every 3 months	
Zoledronic acid	Intravenous	5 mg yearly 5 mg every 2 years for prevention of osteoporosis	Osteonecrosis of the jaw, acute renal failure, proteinuria
Parathyroid hormone			
Teriparatide	Subcutaneous	20 μg daily	Hypercalcemia; contraindicated in patients who have received radiation therapy to the bone
Estrogen			
Various preparations	Oral, transdermal patch; vaginal, cream	Dose depends on preparation	Thromboembolic events, stroke, breast cancer

The major sources of vitamin D derive from sun exposure and diet. Ultraviolet radiation converts a vitamin D precursor in the skin to its active form. Dietary sources of vitamin D are limited, but include fatty fish oils and eggs. In the USA, milk is often fortified with vitamin D. Dietary supplements are available in two different forms. Cholecalciferol, or vitamin D3, is derived from animal sources and is the form produced by the human body. Ergocalciferol, or vitamin D2, derives from plant sources. Ergocalciferol is less potent than cholecalciferol, and an ergocalciferol dose up to three times higher than cholecalciferol may be required to maintain sufficient levels [72, 73].

Vitamin D deficiency is common among SCT recipients for several reasons. Dietary deficiency is common. Prolonged hospitalization and aggressive sun protection contribute to inadequate sun exposure. Graft-versus-host disease, mucositis, pancreatic insufficiency, or bacterial overgrowth may cause poor absorption of vitamin D. Drugs commonly used to treat stem cell patients, especially glucocorticoids and other antirejection medications, also contribute to vitamin D deficiency [74–76]. Correcting vitamin D deficiency alone is not sufficient to prevent SCT-related bone loss [13–21]. Some studies have linked vitamin D deficiency with poor outcomes in certain leukemias [77, 78]. Studies in solid organ transplant recipients suggest that vitamin D may reduce the risk of rejection, likely by modulating immune function [79]. Though excessive vitamin D intake may cause adverse effects, such as hypercalcemia and increased risk of kidney stones, the doses recommended for supplementation have been well tolerated [73, 77, 80]. As SCT recipients enjoy longer survival, treating vitamin D deficiency may prevent future complications and improve outcomes.

Prevalence

The estimated prevalence of vitamin D deficiency is 40–100% among the elderly in many countries, including the USA. In other populations studied, the prevalence has ranged from 32 to 52% [73]. Among SCT patients, the reported prevalence of vitamin D deficiency has been as high as 70% before transplant and as high as 90% after transplant [59, 74–76, 81–83].

Monitoring

Screening for vitamin D deficiency is recommended for high-risk populations, including SCT patients. The optimal frequency of monitoring remains uncertain, however. The preferred method of screening for vitamin D deficiency is measurement of serum 25-hydroxyvitamin D (25(OH)D). 25(OH)D is the major circulating form of vitamin D and most accurately reflects vitamin D status. The optimal level of 25(OH)D has been the source of debate. The target 25(OH)D level recommended by most experts has ranged from 20 to 50 ng/mL. Though supplemental vitamin D has an excellent safety profile, there is some evidence that levels of 25(OH)D above 50 ng/mL may be associated with an increased risk of adverse outcomes, including hypercalcemia, kidney stones, and all-cause mortality [72, 73, 84].

Prevention

The recommended daily dietary intake of vitamin D has ranged from 400 to 600 international units for children and adults up to age 70 years, and 800 international units for adults over age 70 years. Individuals at higher risk for vitamin D deficiency may require 2000 international units per day or more to maintain sufficient levels. Dietary supplementation with either cholecalciferol or ergocalciferol is effective to maintain sufficient vitamin D levels [73, 84].

Management

- SCT patients should be routinely screened for vitamin D deficiency by measurement of serum 25(OH)D levels. The optimal frequency of monitoring remains unclear.
- Most individuals require 800–2000 international units of cholecalciferol per day. Higher doses of ergocalciferol may be required. Daily intake should be adjusted to maintain serum 25(OH)D levels of 20–50 ng/mL. Many experts recommend a minimal target 25(OH)D level of 30 ng/mL. Either cholecalciferol or ergocalciferol is acceptable, though higher doses of ergocalciferol are required.
- For vitamin D deficiency, one approach is to treat with ergocalciferol 50 000 units per week, for 4–8 weeks, while continuing daily supplementation. Vitamin D sufficiency should be confirmed after treatment by repeating measurement of 25(OH)D [73].

Osteonecrosis

Osteonecrosis, also known as avascular necrosis, refers to bone death caused by interruption of blood supply to the portion of bone involved. Osteonecrosis tends to affect areas of bone with limited blood supply, most commonly the femoral heads, and is often bilateral. The precise mechanisms involved remain poorly understood. Trauma, abnormal clotting, and abnormal lipid processing leading to occlusion of small vessels have all been implicated. Osteonecrosis may be asymptomatic early in the disease process and in cases with smaller areas of involvement. More advanced disease causes severe pain. Osteonecrosis of the femoral head often presents with groin pain worsened by weight-bearing. Untreated, osteonecrosis may progress to collapse and destruction of the bone involved, often leading to severe arthritis and joint dysfunction [84–88].

Prevalence

The reported prevalence of osteonecrosis after SCT has ranged from 3 to 19%. Osteonecrosis occurs more commonly after allogeneic versus autologous SCT. The risk of osteonecrosis is directly proportional to the dose and duration of glucocorticoid use. Other reported risk factors for osteonecrosis include the presence of graft-versus-host disease, male gender, total body irradiation, cigarette smoking, alcohol use, and exposure to multiple immunosuppressive medications. Age as a risk factor is unclear [84–88].

Prevention

As osteonecrosis is relatively uncommon, optimal preventive strategies are not well known. Modifiable risk factors include tobacco use, alcohol use, and exposure to immunosuppressing medications. Some evidence suggests that statin medications may decrease the risk of osteonecrosis [84–88].

Monitoring

Osteonecrosis should be suspected in patients with bone or joint pain, especially groin pain that worsens with weight bearing. Imaging studies are necessary to diagnose osteonecrosis. No laboratory studies are diagnostic. Magnetic resonance imaging (MRI) is the preferred imaging modality to evaluate for osteonecrosis. If MRI is contraindicated, radionuclide bone scan and computed tomography are acceptable but less-sensitive alternatives. Plain radiography may demonstrate advanced disease but does not detect early disease [85–89].

Management

- All patients should avoid tobacco and excessive alcohol use.
- Minimizing immunosuppressive therapy, especially glucocorticoids, may decrease the risk of osteonecrosis.
- Patients with suspected osteonecrosis should be evaluated with MRI unless contraindicated. Alternative imaging studies are radionuclide bone scan and computed tomography. Plain radiography is not helpful in early disease.
- Patients with osteonecrosis should be referred to an orthopedic surgeon. Mild cases may be managed conservatively with pain control, limitation of weight bearing, and immobility. More advanced cases require surgical intervention. Total hip arthroplasty is often the treatment of choice for severe osteonecrosis of the femoral head [89].

Conclusion

SCT presents a multifactorial threat to bone health, correlating with bone loss, vitamin D deficiency, and osteonecrosis. Bone loss is common, and glucocorticoid use is likely the most significant contributor. The associated fracture risk and the optimal screening and treatment strategies remain uncertain. Vitamin D deficiency is likewise commonly associated with SCT. Though vitamin D sufficiency alone does not prevent SCT-related bone loss, supplementation is convenient, well tolerated, and may provide a number of skeletal and nonskeletal health benefits. Osteonecrosis is a less common but potentially debilitating complication of SCT. Several risk factors contribute to vitamin D deficiency and osteonecrosis, including glucocorticoid use. Current guidelines for management of SCT-related bone disease are based on limited evidence and expert opinion. Most experts recommend a comprehensive approach that includes minimization of glucocorticoid use, timely evaluation of BMD, anti-osteoporosis medication therapy, vitamin D supplementation, and lifestyle modifications focusing on fall prevention, exercise, and avoiding substance abuse.

References

1. Shoback D, Sellmeyer D, Bikle D. Metabolic bone disease. In: Gardner D, Shoback D (eds). Greenspan's Basic and Clinical Endocrinology, 9th edn. New York: McGraw-Hill, 2011; pp. 277–284.
2. Harvey N, Dennison E, Cooper C, et al. Epidemiology of osteoporotic fractures. In: Rosen CJ, Compston JE, Lian JB (eds). Primer on the Metabolic Bone Diseases and Disorders of Mineral Metabolism, 7th edn. Washington, DC: American Society for Bone and Mineral Research, 2008; pp. 198–203.
3. Drake MT, Khosla S. Role of sex steroids in the pathogenesis of osteoporosis. In: Rosen CJ, Compston JE, Lian JB, et al. (eds). Primer on the Metabolic Bone Diseases and Disorders of Mineral Metabolism, 7th edn. Washington, DC: American Society for Bone and Mineral Research, 2008; pp. 208–213.
4. Chrischilles EA, Butler CD, Davis CS, Wallace RB. A model of lifetime osteoporosis impact. Arch Intern Med 1991;151:2026–2032.
5. Kanis JA, Borgstrom F, De Laet C, et al. Assessment of fracture risk. Osteoporos Int. 2005;16:581–589.
6. Kanis JA, Johnell O, Oden A, et al. Risk of hip fracture according to the World Health Organization criteria for osteopenia and osteoporosis. Bone. 2000;27:585–590.
7. Kanis JA, Oden A, Johnell O, et al. The burden of osteoporotic fractures: a method for setting intervention thresholds. Osteoporos Int. 2001;12:417–427.

8. Kanis JA, Johnell O, Oden A, et al. FRAX and the assessment of fracture probability in men and women from the UK. Osteoporos Int. 2008;19:385–397.
9. Ensrud KE, Lui LY, Taylor BC, et al. A comparison of prediction models for fractures in older women: is more better? Arch Intern Med. 2009;169:2087–2094.
10. Hippisley-Cox J, Coupland C. Predicting risk of osteoporotic fracture in men and women in England and Wales: prospective derivation and validation of QFractureScores. BMJ. 2009;339:b4229.
11. Canalis E, Mazziotti G, Giustina A, Bilezikian JP. Glucocorticoid-induced osteoporosis: pathophysiology and therapy. Osteoporos Int. 2007;18:1319–1328.
12. Van Staa TP, Leufkens HG, Abenhaim L, et al. Use of oral corticosteroids and risk of fractures. J Bone Miner Res. 2000;15:993–1000.
13. Cohen A, Shane E. Osteoporosis after solid organ and bone marrow transplantation. Osteoporos Int. 2003 14: 612–630.
14. Schulte CMS, Beelen DW. Bone loss following hematopoietic stem cell transplantation: a long-term follow-up. Blood. 2004 103(10):3635–3643.
15. Heidewig Hautmann A, Elad S, Lawitschka A, et al. Metabolic bone diseases in patients after allogeneic hematopoietic stem cell transplantation: report from the Consensus Conference on Clinical Practice in Chronic Graft-versus-Host Disease. Transpl Int. 2011;9(24):867–869.
16. Ebeling PR. Transplantation osteoporosis. In: Rosen CJ, Compston JE, Lian JB (eds). Primer on the Metabolic Bone Diseases and Disorders of Mineral Metabolism, 7th edn. Washington, DC: American Society for Bone and Mineral Research, 2008; pp. 279–285.
17. Wellbaecher KN. Mechanisms of osteoporosis after hematopoietic cell transplantation. Biol Blood Marrow Transplant. 2000;6(2A):165–174.
18. Ebeling PR. Approach to the patient with transplantation-related bone loss. J Clin Endocrinol Metab. 2009;94(5): 1483–1490.
19. Mattano LA Jr. Strategic approaches to osteoporosis in transplantation. Pediatr Transplant. 2004;8(Suppl 5):51–55.
20. McClune BL, Polgreen LE, Burmeister LA, et al. Screening, prevention and management of osteoporosis and bone loss in adult and pediatric hematopoietic cell transplant recipients. Bone Marrow Transplant. 2011;46:1–9.
21. Yao S, McCarthy PL, Dunford LM, et al. High prevalence of early-onset osteopenia/osteoporosis after allogeneic stem cell transplantation and improvement after bisphosphonate therapy. Bone Marrow Transplant. 2008;41:393–398.
22. Tauchmanova L, Selleri C, Esposito M, et al. Beneficial treatment with risedronate in long-term survivors after allogeneic-stem cell transplantation for hematological malignancies. Osteoporos Int. 2003;14:1013–1019.
23. Savani BN, Donobue T, Kozanas E, et al. Increased risk of bone loss without fracture risk in long-term survivors after allogeneic stem cell transplantation. Biol Blood Marrow Transplant. 2007;13(5):517–520.
24. Eastell R, Dickson ER, Hodgson SF, et al. Rates of vertebral bone loss before and after liver transplantation in women with primary biliary cirrhosis. Hepatology. 1991;14:296–300.
25. McDonald JA, Dunstan CR, Dilworth P, et al. Bone loss after liver transplantation. Hepatology. 1991;14:613–619.
26. Henderson NK, Sambrook PN, Kelly PJ, et al. Bone mineral loss and recovery after cardiac transplantation. Lancet. 1995;346:905.
27. Shane E, Rivas M, Staron RB, et al. Fracture after cardiac transplantation: a prospective longitudinal study. J Clin Endocrinol Metab. 1996;81:1740–1746.
28. Shane E, Rivas MC, Silverberg SJ, et al. Osteoporosis after cardiac transplantation. Am J Med. 1993;94:257–264.
29. Ramsey-Goldman R, Dunn JE, Dunlop DD, et al. Increased risk of fracture in patients receiving solid organ transplants. J Bone Miner Res. 1999;14:456–463.
30. Lewiecki EM, Watts NB, McClung MR, et al. Official positions of the International Society for Clinical Densitometry. J Clin Endocrinol Metab. 2004;89:3651–3655.
31. Fitzpatrick LA. Secondary causes of osteoporosis. Mayo Clin Proc. 2002;77:453–468.
32. Reginster JY, Sarkar S, Zegels B, et al. Reduction in P1NP, a marker of bone metabolism, with raloxifene treatment and its relationship with vertebral fracture risk. Bone. 2004;34: 344–351.
33. Eastell R, Hannon RA, Garnero P, et al. Relationship of early changes in bone resorption to the reduction in fracture risk with ridedronate: review of statistical analysis. J Bone Miner Res. 2007;22:1656–1660.
34. Bauer DC, Black DM, Garnero P, et al. Change in bone turnover and hip, non-spine, and vertebral fracture in alendronate-treated women: the Fracture Intervention Trial. J Bone Miner Res. 2004;19:1250–1258.
35. Rosen HN. Use of biochemical markers of bone turnover in osteoporosis. 2012. Available from: http://www.uptodate.com/contents/use-of-biochemical-markers-of-bone-turnover-in-osteoporosis (accessed 13 May 2013).
36. Szulc P, Delmas PD. Biochemical markers of bone turnover in osteoporosis. In: Rosen CJ, Compston JE, Lian JB, et al. (eds). Primer on the Metabolic Bone Diseases and Disorders of Mineral Metabolism, 7th edn. Washington, DC: American Society for Bone and Mineral Research, 2008; pp. 174–179.

37. Close J, Ellis M, Hooper R, et al. Prevention of falls in the elderly trial (PROFET): a randomized controlled trial. Lancet. 1999;353:93–97.
38. Province MA, Hadley EC, Hornbrook MC, et al. The effects of exercise on falls in elderly patients. A preplanned meta-analysis of the FICSIT Trials. Frailty and Injuries: Cooperative Studies of Intervention Techniques. JAMA. 1995;273:1341–1347.
39. Wolf SL, Barnhart HX, Kutner NG, et al. Reducing frailty and falls in older persons: an investigation of Tai Chi and computerized balance training. Atlanta FICSIT Group. Frailty and Injuries: Cooperative Studies of Intervention Techniques. J Am Geriatr Soc. 1996;44:489–497.
40. Mitchell MJ, Baz MA, Fulton MN, et al. Resistance training prevents vertebral osteoporosis in lung transplant recipients. Transplantation. 2003;76:557–562.
41. Braith RW, Magyari PM, Fulton MN, et al. Comparison of calcitonin versus calcitonin and resistance exercise as prophylaxis for osteoporosis in heart transplant recipients. Transplantation. 2006;81:1191–1195.
42. Bischoff-Ferrari H. Prevention of falls. In: Rosen CJ, Compston JE, Lian JB, et al. (eds). Primer on the Metabolic Bone Diseases and Disorders of Mineral Metabolism, 7th edn. Washington, DC: American Society for Bone and Mineral Research, 2008; pp. 222–225.
43. Harwood RH, Foss AJ, Osborn F, et al. Falls and health status in elderly women following first eye cataract surgery: a randomized controlled trial. Br J Ophthalmol. 2005;89:53–59.
44. Bischoff-Ferrari HA, Dawson-Hughes B, Willett CW, et al. Effect of vitamin D on falls: a meta-analysis. JAMA. 2004;291:1999–2006.
45. Tauchmanova L, Ricci P, Serio B, et al. Short-term zoledronic acid treatment increases bone mineral density and marrow clonogenic fibroblast progenitors after allogeneic stem cell transplantation. J Clin Endocrinol Metab. 2005;90:627–634.
46. Grigg AP, Shuttleworth P, Reynolds J, et al. Pamidronate reduces bone loss after allogeneic stem cell transplantation. J Clin Endocrinol Metab. 2006;91:3835–3843.
47. Rosen H. Bisphosphonates in the management of osteoporosis in postmenopausal women. 2012. Available from: http://www.uptodate.com/contents/bisphosphonates-in-the-management-of-osteoporosis-in-postmenopausal-women (accessed 13 May 2013).
48. Boonyapakorn T, Schirmer I, Reichart PA, et al. Bisphosphonate-induced osteonecrosis of the jaws: prospective study of 80 patients with multiple myeloma and other malignancies. Oral Oncol. 2008;44(9):857–869.
49. Zervas K, Verrou E, Teleioudis Z, et al. Incidence, risk factors and management of osteonecrosis of the jaw in patients with multiple myeloma: a single-centre experience in 303 patients. Br J Haematol. 2006;134(6):620–623.
50. Black DM, Kelly MP, Genant HK, et al. Bisphosphonates and fractures of the subtrochanteric or diaphyseal femur. NEJM. 2010;362(19):1761–1771.
51. Odvina CV, Levy S, Rao S, et al. Unusual mid-shaft fractures during long-term bisphosphonate therapy. Clin Endocrinol (Oxf). 2010;72:161–168.
52. Rizzoli R, Akesson K, Bouxsein M, et al. Subtrochanteric fractures after long-term treatment with bisphosphonates: a European Society on Clinical and Economic Aspects of Osteoporosis and Osteoarthritis, and International Osteoporosis Foundation Working Group Report. Osteoporos Int. 2011;22:373–390.
53. Meier RP, Perneger TV, Stern R, et al. Increasing occurrence of atypical femoral fractures associated with bisphosphonate use. Arch Intern Med. 2012;172:930–936.
54. Park-Wyllie LY, Mamdani MM, Juurlink DN, et al. Bisphosphonate use and the risk of subtrochanteric or femoral shaft fractures in older women. JAMA. 2011;305:783–789.
55. Kim SY, Schneeweiss S, Katz JN, et al. Oral bisphosphonates and risk of subtrochanteric or diaphyseal femur fractures in a population-based cohort. J Bone Miner Res. 2011;26:993–1001.
56. Schilcher J, Michaëlsson K, Aspenberg P. Bisphosphonate use and atypical fractures of the femoral shaft. N Engl J Med. 2011;364:1728–1737.
57. Shane E, Burr D, Ebeling PR, et al. Atypical subtrochanteric and diaphyseal femoral fractures: report of a task force of the American Society for Bone and Mineral Research. J Bone Miner Res. 2010;25:2267–2294.
58. Erben RG. Vitamin D analogs and bone. J Musculoskelet Neuronal Interact. 2001;2(1):59–69.
59. Moreira Kulak CA, Cochenski Borba VZ, Kulak J Jr, Ribeiro Custodio M. Osteoporosis after transplantation. Curr Osteopros Rep. 2012;10:48–55.
60. Bolland MJ, Grey A, Avenell A, et al. Calcium supplements with or without vitamin D and risk of cardiovascular events: reanalysis of the Women's Health Initiative limited access dataset and meta-analysis. BMJ. 2011;342:d2040.
61. Miller PD. Safety of parathyroid hormone for the treatment of osteoporosis. Curr Osteoporos Rep. 2008;6(1):12–16.
62. Andrews EB, Gilsenan AW, Midkiff K, et al. The US postmarketing surveillance study of adult osteosarcoma and teriparatide: Study design and findings from the first 7 years. J Bone Miner Res. 2012;27(12):2429–2437.
63. Valimake M, Kinnunen K, Volin L, et al. A prospective study of bone loss and turnover after allogeneic bone marrow transplantation: effect of calcium supplementation with or without calcitonin. Bone Marrow Transplant. 1999;23:355–361.

64. Garcia-Delgado I, Preito S, Fragnas LG, et al. Calcitonin, etidronate and calcidiol treatment in bone loss after cardiac transplantation. Calcif Tissue Int. 1997;60:155–159.
65. Cremer J, Struber M, Wagenbreth I, et al. Progression of steroid-associated osteoporosis after heart transplantation. Ann Thorac Surg. 1999;67:130–133.
66. Hay JE, Malinchoc M, Diskson ER. A controlled trial of calcitonin therapy for the prevention of post-liver transplantation atraumatic fractures in patients with primary biliary cirrhosis and primary sclerosing cholangitis. J Hepatol. 2001;34:299–305.
67. Reginster JY, Meurmans L, Deroisy R, et al. A 5-year controlled randomized study of prevention of postmenopausal trabecular bone loss with nasal salmon calcitonin and calcium. Eur J Clin Invest. 1994;24:565–569.
68. Overgaard K, Agnusdei D, Hansen MA, et al. Dose–response bioactivity and bioavailability of salmon calcitonin in premenopausal and postmenopausal women. J Clin Endocrinol Metab. 1991;72:344–349.
69. Shane E, Rosen HN. Osteoporosis after solid organ or stem cell transplantation. 2012. Available from: http://www.uptodate.com/contents/osteoporosis-after-solid-organ-or-stem-cell-transplantation (accessed 13 May 2013).
70. Lips P, van Schoor NM, Bravenhoer N. Vitamin D-related disorders. In: Rosen CJ, Compston JE, Lian JB, et al. (eds). Primer on the Metabolic Bone Diseases and Disorders of Mineral Metabolism, 7th edn. Washington, DC: American Society for Bone and Mineral Research, 2008; pp. 329–335.
71. Bischoff-Ferrari HA, Willett WC, Wong JB, et al. Fracture prevention with vitamin D supplementation: a meta-analysis of randomized controlled trials. JAMA. 2005;293: 2257–2264.
72. Holick M. Vitamin D deficiency. N Engl J Med. 2007; 357(3):266–281.
73. Rosenblatt J, Bissonnette A, Ahmad R, et al. Immunomodulatory effects of vitamin D: implications for GVHD. Bone Marrow Transplant. 2010;45(9):1463–1468.
74. Joseph RW, Alousi A, Konda B, et al. High incidence of vitamin D deficiency in patients undergoing allogeneic stem cell transplantation. Am J Hematol. 2011;86(11):954–956.
75. Sproat L, Bolwell B, Rybicki L, et al. Vitamin D level after allogeneic hematopoietic stem cell transplant. Biol Blood Marrow Transplant. 2011;17:1079–1083.
76. Gunasekaran U, Agarwal N, Jagasia M, Jagasia S. Endocrine complications in long-term survivors after allogeneic stem cell transplant. Semin Hematol. 2012; 49(1): 66–72.
77. Drake MT, Maurer MJ, Link BK, et al. Vitamin D insufficiency and prognosis in non-Hodgkin's lymphoma. J Clin Oncol. 2010;28(27):4191–4198.
78. Shanafelt TD, Drake MT, Maurer MJ. Vitamin D insufficiency and prognosis in chronic lymphocytic leukemia. Blood. 2010;117(5):1492–1498.
79. Jackson RD, LaCroix AZ, Gass M, et al. Calcium plus vitamin D supplementation and the risk of fractures. N Engl J Med. 2006; 354:669–683.
80. Holick MF, Binkley NC, Bischoff-Ferran HA, et al. Evaluation, treatment, and prevention of vitamin D deficiency: an Endocrine Society Clinical Practice Guideline. J Clin Endocrinol Metab. 2011;96(7):1911–1930.
81. Kreutz M, Eissner G, Hahn J, et al. Variations in 1α,25-dihydroxyvitamin D_3 and 25-hydroxyvitamin D_3 serum levels during allogeneic bone marrow transplantation. Bone Marrow Transplant. 2004;33(8):871–873.
82. Robien K, Strayer LG, Majhail N, et al. Vitamin D status among long-term survivors of hematopoietic cell transplantation. Bone Marrow Transplant. 2011;46:1472–1479.
83. Kananen K, Volin L, Laitinen K, et al. Prevention of bone loss after allogeneic stem cell transplantation by calcium, vitamin D, and sex hormone replacement with or without pamidronate. J Clin Endocrinol Metab. 2005;90(7): 3877–3885.
84. Campbell S, Sun CL, Kurlan S, et al. Predictors of avascular necrosis of bone in long-term survivors of hematopoietic cell transplantation. Cancer. 2009;115(18):4127–4135.
85. McAvoy S, Baker KS, Mulrooney D, et al. Corticosteroid dose as a risk factor for avascular necrosis of the bone after hematopoietic cell transplantation. Biol Blood Marrow Transplant. 2010;16:1231–1236.
86. Zadegan F, Raould A, Bizot P, et al. Osteonecrosis after allogeneic bone marrow transplantation. Clin Orthop Relat Res. 2008;466:287–293.
87. Jagasia S, Misfeldt A, Griffith M. Age and total-body irradiation in addition to corticosteroid dose are important risk factors for avascular necrosis of the bone. Biol Blood Marrow Transplant. 2010;16:1747–1751.
88. Jones LC. Osteonecrosis (avascular necrosis of bone). 2013. Available from: http://www.uptodate.com/contents/osteonecrosis-avascular-necrosis-of-bone (accessed 13 May 2013).
89. National Institutes of Health. Office of Dietary Supplements. Dietary supplement fact sheet: calcium. Available from: http://ods.od.nih.gov/factsheets/Calcium-HealthProfessional/ (accessed 24 May 2013).
90. Wang L, Manson JE, Song Y, Sesso HD. Systematic review: vitamin D and calcium supplementation in the prevention of cardiovascular events. Ann Intern Med. 2010; 152(5):315–323.
91. Reid IR, Bolland MJ, Grey A. Does calcium supplementation increase cardiovascular risk? Clin Endocrinol (Oxf). 2010; 73(6):689–695.

92. Guessous I, Bochud M, Bonny O, Burnier M. Calcium, vitamin D and cardiovascular disease. Kidney Blood Press Res. 2011;34(6):404–417.
93. LaCroix AZ, Kotchen J, Anderson G, et al. Calcium plus vitamin D supplementation and mortality in postmenopausal women: the Women's Health Initiative calcium–vitamin D randomized controlled trial. J Gerontol A Biol Sci Med Sci. 2009;64(5):559–567.
94. Wang L, Manson JE, Sesso HD. Calcium intake and risk of cardiovascular disease: a review of prospective studies and randomized clinical trials. Am J Cardiovasc Drugs. 2012;12(2):105–116.

16

CHAPTER 16
Ocular complications: prevalence, monitoring, prevention, and management guidelines

André Tichelli and Alicia Rovó
Hematology Division, Basel University Hospital, Basel, Switzerland

Introduction

The eye is one of the targets of late effects after allogeneic hematopoietic stem cell transplantation (HSCT). Most of the ocular complications after HSCT have been recognized for a long time and are well described. The majority concern the anterior ocular segment and include cataract formation and dry eye syndrome (Figure 16.1). Long-term complications of the posterior chamber occur with lower frequency and are less well known [1]. The two main ocular complications, cataract and dry eye syndrome, present different risk factors and their frequencies evolve differently over the decades. The resulting visual impairment caused by late ocular complications accounts for a significant chronic health condition after HSCT. Compared with their siblings, allogeneic receipts were more likely to report visual impairment [2]. Limitation of visual acuity in patients treated with HSCT is most often associated with cataract formation. Cataracts are associated with a fourfold risk of visual acuity [3]. Ocular graft-versus-host disease (GVHD) with dry eye syndrome and conjunctivitis can cause significant impairment in quality of life, leads to important visual loss, and decreases activity of daily living [4].

Cataract formation

Cataract was one of the first late effects reported in patients after allogeneic HSCT (Table 16.1). It soon became evident that cataract formation is closely related to total body irradiation (TBI) used as conditioning. The probability of developing cataract is dependent on the total radiation dose, the number of radiation fractions, and the dose rate used. In patients receiving single-dose TBI of 10 Gy or more, the probability of cataract formation at 10 years increases to around 80% or higher. Fractionation of the radiation dose has a sparing effect on the lens [5, 6]. Fractionation delays the appearance of cataract formation, reduces its severity, and leads to a lower incidence. The probability of cataract formation after fractionated TBI at 10 years ranges between 40 and 70%. Dose rate of radiation is also related with cataract formation. The 10-year probability for cataract formation and the probability for requiring cataract surgery were significantly increased in patients treated with a dose rate higher than 0.04 Gy/min [7, 8]. For patients conditioned without TBI, the probability of cataract formation is about 5–20% at 10 years. After TBI conditioning, cataract appears usually within 3–5 years, and most of the patients will need surgical repair.

Blood and Marrow Transplantation Long-Term Management: Prevention and Complications, First Edition. Edited by Bipin N Savani.

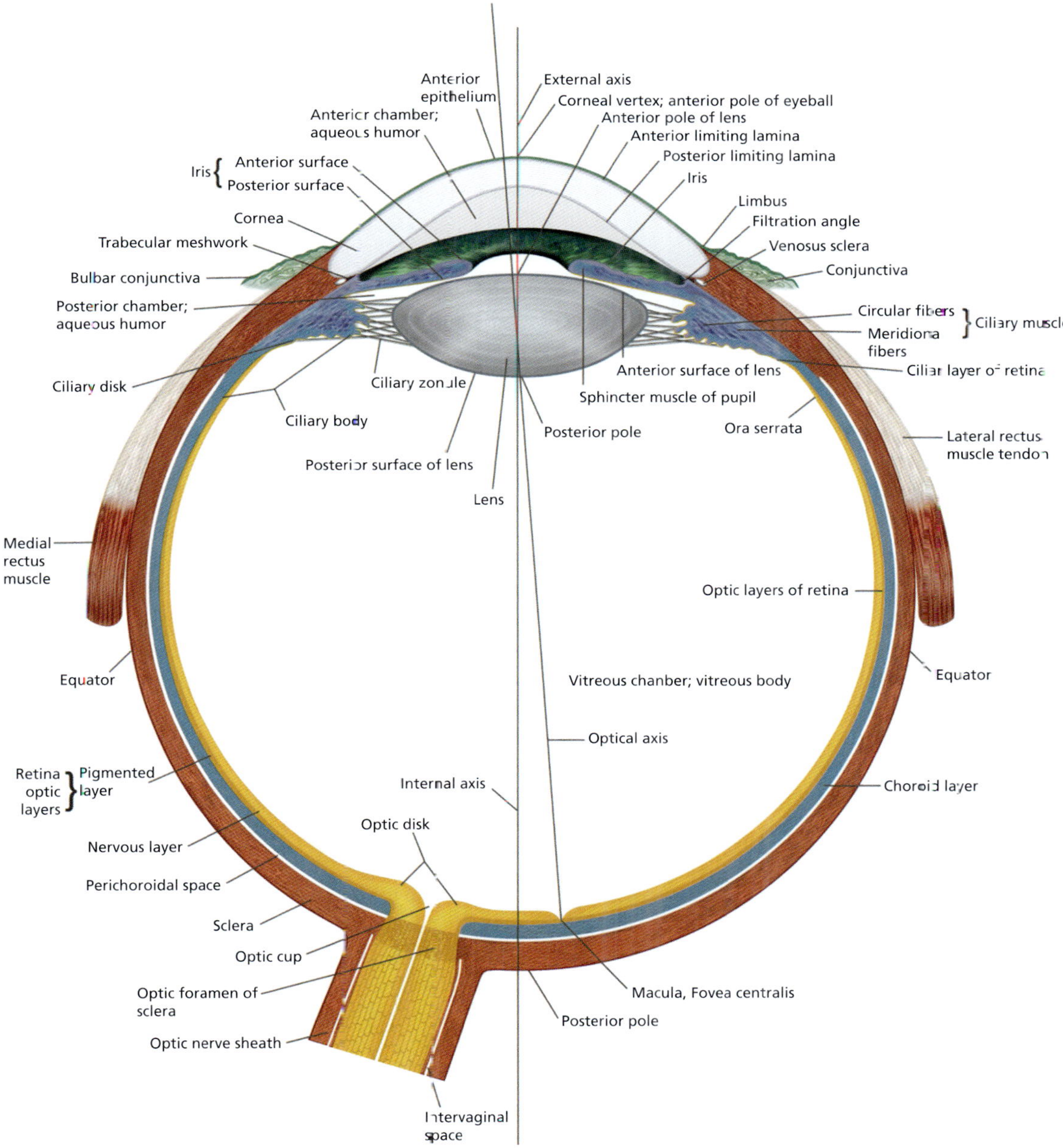

Figure 16.1 Anatomy of the human eye.

Table 16.1 Types of ocular complications after HSCT; screening; prevention and treatment of ocular events

Type of complication	Main risk factors	Screening	Prevention	Treatment
Cataract	• TBI • Single-dose TBI greater than fractionation of the dose • Higher dose rate of radiation therapy • Prolonged use of corticosteroids	• Split-lamp examination yearly • Visual acuity	• Conditioning without TBI • Avoid long-term treatment with corticosteroids	• Cataract operation • YAG-laser posterior capsulotomy in case of posterior capsular opacification after surgery
Dry eye syndrome	• GVHD • TBI • Some medicaments	• Ocular examination • Measurement of visual acuity at 6 and 12 months • In case of symptoms, thereafter yearly examinations	• Prevention of GVHD	• Topical lubricants • Topical anti-inflammatory drugs • Autologous serum eye drops • Systemic treatment of GVHD • Treatment of ocular superinfection
Microvascular retinopathy	• Allogeneic HSCT • TBI • Cyclosporine (?)	• Funduscopy • Measurement of visual acuity at 6 and 12 months	• Conditioning without TBI	• Reduction of cyclosporine dose • Most often self-limited process
CMV- or toxoplasmosis- retinitis	• Alemtuzumab-based conditioning	• Funduscopy • Measurement of visual acuity in case of symptoms		• Systemic treatment of CMV or toxoplasmosis treatment

Busulfan as a non-TBI-containing conditioning regimen has a significant lower risk of cataract formation. In an analysis of four randomized studies, the incidence of cataract was significantly higher for patients conditioned with cyclophosphamide and TBI compared with those treated with cyclophosphamide and busulfan [9]. With this regimen, cataract appears significantly later, and lens opacification is nonsevere and in most cases does not need cataract surgery. In a large meta-analysis including 3172 patients from 18 trials, patients conditioned with TBI and cyclophosphamide had significantly higher cataract rates (odds ratio 12.69; 95% confidence interval, 1.72–93.22; $p = 0.01$), interstitial pneumonitis, later growth or development problems than patients receiving busulfan and cyclophosphamide, but presented lower rates of liver veno-occlusive diseases and hemorrhagic cystitis [10].

Children are not spared from cataract formation. In a single-center cohort of 75 children aged between 2 and 18 years at HSCT, all 17 patients with single-dose TBI, 15 from 18 patients with fractionated TBI, and only 11 from 33 patients conditioned with busulfan developed cataract. In contrast to the patients conditioned with TBI, none of the patients receiving busulfan needed surgical repair [11]. In children, visual development is not completed until around the age of 8–10 years. Therefore, cataract formation could play a relevant role in children during their amblyogenic period. This has to be considered in the treatment decision, *a fortiori* that children rarely report spontaneously on gradual visual loss [12].

In patients not receiving TBI, the main risk factors for cataract formation are older age, use of corticosteroids, and allogeneic compared with autologous transplantation. An additive effect of use of cyclosporine to steroids on cataract formation has been reported after renal transplantation [13]. GVHD per se and the graft source used for HSCT (bone marrow versus peripheral blood) do not appear to affect the risk of cataract [14]. Indeed, the lens does not become a target of GVHD, since it has no vascularization. The higher rate of cataract in allogeneic transplanted recipients described in some studies is most probably due to the increased use of corticosteroids to treat chronic GVHD. Approximately 45% of recipients of HSCT treated with corticosteroids for a period of more than 3 months develop cataracts at 10 years. In patients receiving TBI, the influence of steroids on cataract formation is controversial. In these patients, the strong cataractogenic effect of the radiation therapy could mask the impact of corticosteroids. Some authors report on the influence of steroids on cataract formation in patients receiving fractionated, but non-single-dose TBI [15].

During the last decade, changes introduced in practice regarding conditioning regimen changed the pattern of cataract formation after HSCT over time. While TBI was universally used for more than two decades, nowadays the protocols using high doses of TBI tend to be restricted to specific indications. According to unpublished data from the European Group for Blood and Marrow Transplantation (EBMT) database, the number of recipients of allogeneic HSCT that received TBI for conditioning between 1980 and 1990 was 6963 of 8448 (82%), and between 2005 and 2009 the figure was 14 230 of 37 273 (38%). Therefore, cataract, which was an almost obligatory late complication after HSCT, has been decreasing in frequency over the last decade. In a group of 620 patients, transplanted between 1997 and 2007 and conditioned without TBI, only eight patients presented with steroid-induced cataract [16]. Likewise, in a prospective study of 101 consecutive patients who were treated with allogeneic HSCT between 2004 and 2007 and conditioned mainly with a nonmyeloablative regimen, no cataract was observed [4]. Therefore, cataract, which was a frequent late ocular complication in the early transplantation era, has greatly decreased in frequency and now has a lower clinical impact in patients treated with HSCT.

Prevention and management

The best option to prevent the clinical impact of cataract formation is to opt for a non-TBI-associated conditioning regimen. In those cases where a radiation regimen is needed, the following lens-sparing options are available: reduction of the total dose of TBI; use of fractionated radiation therapy; use of a low dose rate of radiation. Lens shielding during TBI has been used to decrease the incidence and severity of cataract formation. However, eye shielding during TBI could theoretically increase the risk of relapse in the eye or in the central nervous system (CNS). In a retrospective analysis of 188 children treated with TBI, 139 had eye shielding and 49 did not. The prevalence of cataract was 90% without eye shielding and 31% with. Two of the patients with eye shielding and none of the group without eye shielding had CNS relapse of the acute leukemia [17]. However, despite the study's lack of statistical significance, the reduced number of patients, and the low complication rate expected in respect of a local relapse do not allow a definitive conclusion on the risk of eye or CNS relapse due to the eye shielding.

Cataracts are effectively treated surgically. Cataract extraction can be performed safely even when ocular sicca is present. Surgery is indicated if vision is impaired and the impairment is interfering with daily life activities. In patients treated with TBI it is usually performed 4–6 years after HSCT [18]. Since children do not always notice a gradual visual loss, regular eye examination and early surgery of cataract is often indicated to correct reduced vision and to prevent the development of amblyopia [19]. Posterior capsular opacification, also called after-cataract or secondary cataract, is the most frequent complication of cataract surgery. Following cataract surgery, between 40 and 90% of all recipients develop posterior capsular opacification. This complication leads to a progressive visual impairment after surgery, and is caused mainly by remnant lens epithelial cell proliferation, collagen deposition, and lens fiber generation [20]. Posterior capsule opacification has also been reported following cataract surgery of HSCT recipients. Some of these patients will need YAG-laser posterior capsulotomy at 1–6 years after first surgery [21]. In most cases, visual acuity after laser therapy successfully improves without any sequelae.

Dry eye syndrome and ocular graft-versus-host disease

Dry eye syndrome belongs to the most common ocular complication after allogeneic HSCT (Table 16.1). It occurs in 40–75% of all patients. Dry eye syndrome is responsible for a number of secondary manifestations of the ocular surface, such as punctuate keratitis, persistent epithelial defects, corneal keratinization, and, in the extreme case, ulceration and perforation of the cornea. In many cases dry eye syndrome is part of a more general sicca syndrome after HSCT, including xerostomia, genital skin complications, and dryness of the skin. In its most extensive forms it clinically resembles Sjögren syndrome. Dry eye syndrome and its consecutive keratoconjunctivitis sicca syndrome are closely related to GVHD. Ocular GVHD develops in 40–60% of patients after allogeneic HSCT [4].

The development of ocular GVHD is strongly associated with systemic GVHD. In most cases, other manifestations of chronic GVHD involving the skin and the mucosa accompany the ocular disease; however, single ocular complications may occur [4]. A severe form of ocular GVHD, presenting as a Sjögren-type syndrome, was first described after HSCT in 1977 [22]. However, unlike spontaneous Sjögren syndrome, none of the transplanted patients developed autoantibodies. Dry eye syndrome also seems to be associated with the source of stem cells used for HSCT. Hence, the severity of dry eye syndrome is significantly increased in patients who received mobilized peripheral blood progenitor cells, compared with patients treated with bone marrow or umbilical cord blood [23]. However, irrespective of the source of stem cells, chronic GVHD remains an independent risk factor. For unexplained reasons, dry eye syndrome appeared with some delay in patients receiving peripheral blood progenitor cells. One explanation could be that patients receiving peripheral blood progenitor cells were treated earlier and with more intensive immunosuppression, and that this immunosuppressive treatment was tapered later. A correlation between the severity of ocular GVHD and the severity of chronic GVHD has been reported [24, 25]. Therefore, severe ocular GVHD manifestations are related to a poor prognosis.

Dry eye syndrome may also appear independently of GVHD. In a retrospective study of the EBMT, the probability of developing keratoconjunctivitis sicca at 15 years after allogeneic HSCT was 38% for patients with and 10% for patients without chronic GVHD [26]. In patients with autologous HSCT, however, dry eye syndrome is usually not observed [27]. Factors other than GVHD associated with dry eye syndrome are female patients, older age at transplantation, the use of radiation therapy, chemotherapy, and lid and lacrimal gland dysfunction.

Ocular GVHD is the consequence of the direct attack of eye structures by donor lymphocytes. The T-cell-mediated process affects mainly the conjunctival tissue of the eye. The conjunctiva is a major target of ocular GVHD. In acute GVHD, fibrinoid material with cellular debris and inflammatory cells are found in the conjunctival tissue. The conjunctival inflammatory cells are found in a significantly higher proportion in GVHD-related dry eyes, and are more frequent in severe dry eyes compared with mild dry eyes. The increase of inflammatory cell numbers and of inflammatory cytokine production confirm that inflammation is involved in the pathogenesis of GVHD-related dry eye [28]. Ocular surface alterations after allogeneic HSCT have been evaluated in a prospective study and compared with age-matched healthy controls. Decreased corneal sensitivity, meibomian gland dysfunction and increased tear evaporation were found in transplanted recipients, with and without GVHD, but not in the healthy controls [29]. Hence, the dry eye syndrome seems to be the consequence of decreased tear production and increased evaporation rate of tears. Physiologically, the meibomian glands (a special kind of sebaceous gland of the rim of the eyelids) produce a lipid film that covers the ocular surface and prevents tear evaporation. Therefore, a meibomian gland dysfunction may be responsible for the higher evaporation tear rate by failure of lipid material production. In chronic GVHD there is more of a fibrotic process, with inflammatory destruction of the conjunctiva and the lacrimal glands, resulting in tear deficiency and often a damaged ocular surface [30].

The diagnosis of ocular GVHD is based on clinical findings. Up to now, no pathognomonic diagnostic features have been identified for the diagnosis of ocular chronic GVHD [12]. Ocular chronic GVHD can affect every layer of the eye and lead to a number of abnormalities of the eye: lacrimal gland dysfunction and lacrimal duct obstruction; meibomian gland obstruction; conjunctive inflammation with hyperemia, serosanguineous exudates, and pseudomembranous conjunctivitis; scleritis; affection of the cornea; complications of the vitreous and the choroids. The lenses are not a direct target of the GVHD, but cataract may appear as a consequence of chronic corticosteroid therapy used to treat GVHD [11]. The severity of the ocular chronic GVHD depends on the involvement of the different ocular tissues and the extent of the tear film dysfunction. Clinical ocular manifestations can be worsened by infections of the eye. However, after remission of the GVHD, keratoconjunctivitis sicca generally persists, and tear function does not normalize.

A first clinical staging of conjunctival GVHD was proposed in 1984: stage 1, conjunctival hyperemia; stage 2, conjunctival hyperemia with chemotic response or serosanguineous exudate; stage 3, pseudomembranous conjunctivitis; stage 4, pseudomembranous conjunctivitis plus corneal epithelial slough [24]. These grading criteria concern mainly patients with acute GVHD. Therefore, a clinical grading for conjunctival chronic GVHD was proposed which was based on the degree of cicatrization: grade 1, conjunctival hyperemia occurring on the bulbar or palpebral conjunctiva in at least one eye; grade 2, palpebral conjunctival fibrovascular changes occurring along the superior border of the upper eyelid or the lower border of the tarsal plate of the lower eyelid, with or without conjunctival epithelial sloughing, involving <25% of the total surface area on at least one eyelid; grade 3, palpebral conjunctival fibrovascular changes occurring along the superior border of the upper eyelid, or the lower border of the tarsal plate of the lower eyelid, involving 25–75% of the total surface area in at least one eyelid; grade 4, involves >75% of the total surface area with or without a cicatricial entropion in at least one eyelid [31]. More recently, the participants of the German–Austrian–Swiss Consensus Conference on Clinical Practice on Chronic GVHD proposed a novel approach of clinical staging representing the complete spectrum of the disease. They agreed that the staging system should include the overall extent of chronic GVHD, addressing tissue involvement, inflammatory activity, and the presence or not of complications and functional impairment (Table 16.2) [12].

Table 16.2 Staging and documentation for criteria for ocular chronic GVHD according to the German–Austrian–Swiss Consensus Conference on Clinical Practice in Chronic GVHD [12]

Involvement of different ocular tissues	(a) Extent of lacrimal gland dysfunction (including Schirmer test results) (b) Involvement of the lids (e.g., blepharitis, meibomian gland dysfunction, and erythema) (c) Involvement of the conjunctiva (e.g., cicatricial conjunctivitis) (d) Involvement of the cornea (e.g., keratitis and epithelial defects)
Inflammatory activity (e.g., redness of the lid margins, hyperemia of the conjunctiva)	(a) No inflammation (b) Mild inflammation (c) Moderate inflammation (d) Severe inflammation
Presence of sight-threatening complications/ functional impairment	(a) Complications (e.g., corneal perforation) (b) Functional impairment (e.g., reduced visual acuity) (c) Secondary glaucoma

Late effects after reduced-intensity conditioning (RIC) have not yet been systematically investigated. RIC provides similar donor engraftment, increases the probability of relapse, decreases early transplant-related mortality, but does not affect overall survival. From present knowledge, we can hypothesize about the type and extent of late effects expected in long-term survivors treated with RIC. Indeed, most of the late effects of allogeneic HSCT are related either to the consequences of GVHD and its treatment or to the toxicity of the transplant preparative regimen. According to this hypothesis, dry eye syndrome and ocular GVHD should not be decreased after RIC. This hypothesis seems to be confirmed by a study of 101 patients treated with allogeneic HSCT who had received nonmyeloablative conditioning. These patients conditioned with RIC had a similar rate of dry eye syndrome and ocular GVHD to those receiving myeloablative treatment including TBI and cyclophosphamide [4].

Prevention and management

There are no real measures to prevent dry eye syndrome and ocular GVHD, except the use of prophylactic immunosuppressive treatment after allogeneic HSCT. Secondary complications of dry eye syndrome, such as punctuate keratitis, persistent epithelial defects, corneal keratinization, ulceration, and perforation of the cornea, can be prevented by early detection and treatment of ocular GVHD as well as the treatment of infectious complications of the eye. Therefore, clinical evaluation of visual acuity with special attention to sicca syndrome is recommend at least 6 months, 1 year, and yearly thereafter for all recipients of allogeneic HSCT. When patients experience visual symptoms, they should undergo ocular examination immediately [32]. Regular control of visual acuity and search for early manifestation of dry eye syndrome is of particular importance in young children, since they often do not express spontaneously their visual impairment.

Treatment of dry eye syndrome and of ocular GVHD consists mainly of the use of topical and systemic drugs. Topical treatment plays a major role, and includes primarily lubricants and anti-inflammatory agents. Artificial tears for eye lubrication with preservative-free medications are preferred, since preservative-containing eye drops are cytotoxic for the ocular surface, particularly when frequent application is needed over long periods of time. During nighttime, a lubricating ointment may provide more relief than artificial tears, because these products will stay on the eyes and, therefore, provide longer periods of relief. During daytime they are not indicated since they blur the vision [12].

Eye drops that include anti-inflammatory agents are often used when lubricants are not sufficient. Topical agents such as prednisolone acetate 1%, cyclosporine, mycophenolate, or retinoic acid may be of benefit in treating mild to moderate conjunctivitis in the setting of chronic GVHD [30]. Topical corticosteroid or cyclosporine is the most commonly used for the treatment of ocular inflammation. Higher ocular drug concentration can be achieved with topical agents, compared with systemic administration of the drugs. Used in dry eye accompanied by systemic GVHD, this topical treatment can reduce the need for systemic immunosuppressive therapy and, therefore, decrease side effects [31]. Topical cyclosporine formulations 0.05% and 0.1% are safe and effective in the treatment of moderate to severe dry eye disease [33]. This treatment has been shown to improve symptoms and corneal sensitivity, and to decrease tear evaporation rate and degree of inflammation [34, 35]. Actually, there is an ongoing prospective randomized study on the use of cyclosporine eye drops in preventing GVHD disease of the eye in patients who have undergone HSCT for hematological cancer or bone marrow failure disorder (ClinicalTrials.gov identifier: NCT00755040). However, topical treatments have to be used with caution, since they can produce adverse ocular complications, such as corticosteroid-induced glaucoma, cataracts, infectious keratitis, and corneal thinning [34]. Therefore, the ocular treatment has to be supervised by ophthalmologists.

Autologous serum eye drops are useful in severe dry eye syndrome related to various diseases. In the setting of HSCT, the use of autologous serum eye drops has shown some efficacy in cases series and case–control studies. An improvement was noted in a small study of 14 patients: a response was observed in all patients within 4 weeks, and this response could be maintained in 7 of the 14 patients [36]. The mechanism through which autologous serum eye drops improve dry eye after allogeneic HSCT remains to be elucidated. Autologous tear drops contain some epidermal growth factors, vitamins, and cytokines and substances which can provide a therapeutic effect for ocular surface epithelium. However, the risk of contamination by microorganisms and subsequent infection is of concern. Contaminated products have been reported in up to 28% of the preparations [37]. Contraindications for autologous serum eye drops are the risk for bacterial and viral infections.

In severe ocular GVHD and in patients with GVHD of other organs, systemic immunosuppressive treatment has to be used. However, there are no studies on the efficacy of systemic treatment in ocular GVHD.

Ocular complications of the posterior segment

Complications of the posterior chamber can be divided into retinal microvascular changes, optic disk edema, hemorrhagic complications, and infectious retinitis (Table 16.1). Most of them occur in the early phase after transplantations. Fungal infections typically are observed within 120 days of HSCT, while herpes zoster, cytomegalovirus (CMV), and toxoplasmic retinitis occur later. Ischemic retinopathy with cotton-wool spots and optic-disk edema has been described in 13 of 127 (10%) patients following HSCT. Secondary changes included retinal hemorrhages and lipid deposits [38]. This type of microvascular retinopathy has been observed mainly in HSCT patients conditioned with TBI and receiving cyclosporine as GVHD prophylaxis. In most cases, retinal lesions, including optical disc edema without signs of cerebral edem, may appear within 6 months and 2 years, and they resolve with withdrawal or reduction of immunosuppressive therapy. This ocular complication has mainly been observed after allogeneic HSCT; however, it has been described after autologous transplantation as well [39]. An atypical pattern of retinopathy after allogeneic HSCT has on rare occasions been reported. In contrast to classical microvascular retinopathy, the dominant feature was microvascular incompetence characterized by microaneurysms, hard exudates, and retinal edema appearing much later, up to 62 months after transplantation [40]. Cotton-wool exudates were not seen in these patients. The significance of the atypical microvascular retinopathy is uncertain. The retinal changes are usually discovered as part of routine review, without any loss of visual acuity. It is difficult to determine a relationship between these retinal complications and GVHD. In a series of 397 patients, 51 of them developed posterior segment complications. Chronic GVHD was the only significant factor associated with the development of microvascular retinopathy [41]. However, other studies failed to find a correlation between this retinopathy and GVHD. The uncomplicated natural course with spontaneous resolution of most of these events would argue against a pathogenetic role of GVHD [38].

Single cases of central serous chorioretinopathy [42] and posterior scleritis with choriodal detachment [43, 44] have been reported. These ocular complications that occurred rather early after HSCT resolved after initiation of immunosuppressive treatment applied for GVHD. Because of the temporal association between the onset of visual symptoms and GVHD, and the correlation of improvement with the immunosuppressive treatment, GVHD is presumed to have a causal role in the development of this rare posterior chamber eye complication.

CMV infection of the retina is a well-recognized complication in patients with acquired immune deficiency syndrome, but is rarely seen after HSCT. During a 14-year period, 10 of 5721 patients developed CMV retinitis at a median time of 251 days after HSCT [45]. In most cases, patients presented with the ocular symptoms of decreased vision and floaters (Table 16.1). However, an increased incidence of CMV retinitis has been reported in patients receiving unrelated nonmyeloablative HSCT with alemtuzumab-based conditioning. Four of seventeen patients with alemtuzumbab and none of the patients conditioned without alemtuzumab developed CMV retinitis. All four patients reported ocular symptoms and three of the four patients had bilateral retinitis [46]. Dilated funduscopic examination is essential for evaluation of patients with reduced visual acuity and for screening of asymptomatic patients [47].

References

1. Anderson NG, Regillo C. Ocular manifestations of graft versus host disease. Curr Opin Ophthalmol. 2004;15(6): 503–507.
2. Sun CL, Francisco L, Kawashima T, et al. Prevalence and predictors of chronic health conditions after hematopoietic cell transplantation: a report from the Bone Marrow Transplant Survivor Study. Blood. 2010;116(17) 3129–3139.
3. Allan EJ, Flowers ME, Lin MP, et al. Visual acuity and anterior segment findings in chronic graft-versus-host disease. Cornea. 2011;30(12):1392–1397.
4. Westeneng AC, Hettinga Y, Lokhorst H, et al. Ocular graft-versus-host disease after allogeneic stem cell transplantation. Cornea. 2010;29(7):758–763.
5. Deeg HJ, Flournoy N, Sullivan KM, et al. Cataracts after total body irradiation and marrow transplantation: a sparing effect of dose fractionation. Int J Radiat Oncol Biol Phys. 1984;10(7):957–964.
6. Tichelli A, Gratwohl A, Egger T, et al. Cataract formation after bone marrow transplantation. Ann Intern Med. 1993; 119(12):1175–1180.
7. Belkacemi Y, Labopin M, Vernant JP, et al. Cataracts after total body irradiation and bone marrow transplantation in patients with acute leukemia in complete remission: a study of the European Group for Blood and Marrow Transplantation. Int J Radiat Oncol Biol Phys. 1998;41(3):659–668.
8. van Kempen-Harteveld ML, Belkacemi Y, Kal HB, et al. Dose–effect relationship for cataract induction after single-dose total body irradiation and bone marrow transplantation for acute leukemia. Int J Radiat Oncol Biol Phys. 2002;52(5):1367–1374.
9. Socie G, Clift RA, Blaise D, et al. Busulfan plus cyclophosphamide compared with total-body irradiation plus cyclophosphamide before marrow transplantation for myeloid leukemia: long-term follow-up of 4 randomized studies. Blood. 2001;98(13):3569–3574.
10. Xu SX, Tang XH, Xu HQ, et al. Total body irradiation plus cyclophosphamide versus busulphan with cyclophosphamide as conditioning regimen for patients with leukemia undergoing allogeneic stem cell transplantation: a meta-analysis. Leuk Lymphoma. 2010;51(1):50–60.
11. Fahnehjelm KT, Törnquist AL, Olsson M, Winiarski J. Visual outcome and cataract development after allogeneic stem-cell transplantation in children. Acta Ophthalmol Scand. 2007;85(7):724–733.
12. Dietrich-Ntoukas T, Cursiefen C, Westekemper H, et al. Diagnosis and treatment of ocular chronic graft-versus-host disease: report from the German–Austrian–Swiss Consensus Conference on Clinical Practice in Chronic GVHD. Cornea. 2012;31(3):299–310.

13. Nakamura T, Sasaki H, Nagai K, et al. Influence of cyclosporin on steroid-induced cataracts after renal transplantation. Jpn J Ophthalmol. 2003;47(3):254–259.
14. Friedrichs B, Tichelli A, Bacigalupo A, et al. Long-term outcome and late effects in patients transplanted with mobilised blood or bone marrow: a randomised trial. Lancet Oncol. 2010;11(4):331–338.
15. Dunn JP, Jabs DA, Wingard J, et al. Bone marrow transplantation and cataract development. Arch Ophthalmol. 1993; 111(10):1367–1373.
16. Tabbara KF, Al-Ghamdi A, Al-Mohareb F, et al. Ocular findings after allogeneic hematopoietic stem cell transplantation. Ophthalmology. 2009;116(9):1624–1629.
17. van Kempen-Harteveld ML, van Weel-Sipman MH, Emmens C, et al. Eye shielding during total body irradiation for bone marrow transplantation in children transplanted for a hematological disorder: risks and benefits. Bone Marrow Transplant. 2003;31(12):1151–1156.
18. Calissendorff BM, Bolme P. Cataract development and outcome of surgery in bone marrow transplanted children. Br J Ophthalmol. 1993;77(1):36–38.
19. Holmstrom G, Borgstrom B, Calissendorff B. Cataract in children after bone marrow transplantation: relation to conditioning regimen. Acta Ophthalmol Scand. 2002;80(2): 211–215.
20. Awasthi N, Guo S, Wagner BJ. Posterior capsular opacification: a problem reduced but not yet eradicated. Arch Ophthalmol. 2009;127(4):555–562.
21. Najima Y, Kakihana K, Ohashi K, et al. Incidence, risk factors, and clinical outcomes of cataracts following hematopoietic stem cell transplantation. Am J Hematol. 2011; 86(6):508–510.
22. Gratwohl AA, Moutsopoulos HM, Chused TM, et al. Sjögren-type syndrome after allogeneic bone-marrow transplantation. Ann Intern Med. 1977;87(6):703–706.
23. Uchino M, Ogawa Y, Uchino Y, et al. Comparison of stem cell sources in the severity of dry eye after allogeneic haematopoietic stem cell transplantation. Br J Ophthalmol. 2012;96(1):34–37.
24. Jabs DA, Wingard J, Green WR, et al. The eye in bone marrow transplantation. III. Conjunctival graft-vs-host disease. Arch Ophthalmol. 1989;107(9):1343–1348.
25. Mencucci R, Rossi FC, Bosi A, et al. Ophthalmological aspects in allogenic bone marrow transplantation: Sjögren-like syndrome in graft-versus-host disease. Eur J Ophthalmol. 1997;7(1):13–18.
26. Tichelli A, Duell T, Weiss M, et al. Late-onset keratoconjunctivitis sicca syndrome after bone marrow transplantation: incidence and risk factors. European Group for Blood and Marrow Transplantation (EBMT) Working Party on Late Effects. Bone Marrow Transplant. 1996;17(6):1105–1111.
27. Ogawa Y, Okamoto S, Wakui M, et al. Dry eye after haematopoietic stem cell transplantation. Br J Ophthalmol. 1999; 83(10):1125–1130.
28. Riemens A, Stoyanova E, Rothova A, Kuiper J. Cytokines in tear fluid of patients with ocular graft-versus-host disease after allogeneic stem cell transplantation. Mol Vis. 2012; 18:797–802.
29. Wang Y, Ogawa Y, Dogru M, et al. Baseline profiles of ocular surface and tear dynamics after allogeneic hematopoietic stem cell transplantation in patients with or without chronic GVHD-related dry eye. Bone Marrow Transplant. 2010; 45(6):1077–1083.
30. Riemens A, te Boome L, Imhof S, et al. Current insights into ocular graft-versus-host disease. Curr Opin Ophthalmol. 2010;21(6):485–494.
31. Robinson MR, Lee SS, Rubin BI, et al. Topical corticosteroid therapy for cicatricial conjunctivitis associated with chronic graft-versus-host disease. Bone Marrow Transplant. 2004; 33(10):1031–1035.
32. Majhail NS, Rizzo JD, Lee SJ, et al. Recommended screening and preventive practices for long-term survivors after hematopoietic cell transplantation. Bone Marrow Transplant. 2012;47(3):337–341.
33. Sall K, Stevenson OD, Mundorf TK, Reis BL. Two multicenter, randomized studies of the efficacy and safety of cyclosporine ophthalmic emulsion in moderate to severe dry eye disease. CsA Phase 3 Study Group. Ophthalmology. 2000;107(4):631–639.
34. McGhee CN, Dean S, Danesh-Meyer H. Locally administered ocular corticosteroids: benefits and risks. Drug Saf. 2002;25(1):33–55.
35. Wang Y, Ogawa Y, Dogru M, et al. Ocular surface and tear functions after topical cyclosporine treatment in dry eye patients with chronic graft-versus-host disease. Bone Marrow Transplant. 2008;41(3):293–302.
36. Ogawa Y, Okamoto S, Mori T, et al. Autologous serum eye drops for the treatment of severe dry eye in patients with chronic graft-versus-host disease. Bone Marrow Transplant. 2003;31(7):579–583.
37. Leite SC, de Castro RS, Alves M, et al. Risk factors and characteristics of ocular complications, and efficacy of autologous serum tears after haematopoietic progenitor cell transplantation. Bone Marrow Transplant. 2006;38(3): 223–227.
38. Bernauer W, Gratwohl A, Keller A, Daicker B. Microvasculopathy in the ocular fundus after bone marrow transplantation. Ann Intern Med. 1991;115(12):925–930.
39. Johnson DW, Cagnoni PJ, Schossau TM, et al. Optic disc and retinal microvasculopathy after high-dose chemotherapy and autologous hematopoietic progenitor cell support. Bone Marrow Transplant. 1999;24(7):785–792.

40. Bylsma GW, Hall AJ, Szer J, West R. Atypical retinal microvasculopathy after bone marrow transplantation. Clin Experiment Ophthalmol. 2001;29(4):225–229.
41. Coskuncan NM, Jabs DA, Dunn JP, et al. The eye in bone marrow transplantation. VI. Retinal complications. Arch Ophthalmol. 1994;112(3):372–379.
42. Cheng LL, Kwok AK, Wat NM, et al. Graft-vs-host-disease-associated conjunctival chemosis and central serous chorioretinopathy after bone marrow transplant. Am J Ophthalmol. 2002;134(2):293–295.
43. Kim RY, Anderlini P, Naderi AA, et al. Scleritis as the initial clinical manifestation of graft-versus-host disease after allogenic bone marrow transplantation. Am J Ophthalmol. 2002;133(6):843–845.
44. Strouthidis NG, Francis PJ, Stanford MR, et al. Posterior segment complications of graft versus host disease after bone marrow transplantation. Br J Ophthalmol. 2003;87(11):1421–1423.
45. Crippa F, Corey L, Chuang EL, et al. Virological, clinical, and ophthalmologic features of cytomegalovirus retinitis after hematopoietic stem cell transplantation. Clin Infect Dis. 2001;32(2):214–219.
46. Song WK, Min YH, Kim YR, Lee SC. Cytomegalovirus retinitis after hematopoietic stem cell transplantation with alemtuzumab. Ophthalmology. 2008;115(10):1766–1770.
47. Cesaro S, Boaro MP, Pillon M, et al. Immune reconstitution complicated by CMV retinitis in a pediatric patient who underwent haploidentical CD34$^+$-selected hematopoietic stem cell transplant for acute lymphoblastic leukemia. Int J Hematol. 2008;88(2):145–148.

17

CHAPTER 17

Oral complications in hematopoietic stem cell transplantation survivorship

Sharon Elad[1], *Corey Cutler*[2], *and Nathaniel Treister*[3]

[1]Division of Oral Medicine, Eastman Institute for Oral Health, University of Rochester Medical Center, Rochester, NY, USA
[2]Harvard Medical School, Department of Medical Oncology, Dana-Farber Cancer Institute, Boston, MA, USA
[3]Harvard School of Dental Medicine, Division of Oral Medicine and Dentistry, Dana-Farber/Brigham and Women's Cancer Center, Boston, MA, USA

Introduction

Hematopoietic cell transplantation (HCT) survivors are at risk for developing a wide range of oral complications that can contribute to both morbidity and mortality (Table 17.1). Survivors of allogeneic HCT are at highest risk, with the primary factor being chronic graft-versus-host disease (cGVHD), although oral complications may arise due to other HCT-related factors. Oral function is essential for many aspects of normal daily activities, and any compromise can profoundly impact quality of life, overall health, and psychosocial well-being. This chapter provides an overview of the main oral complications in HCT survivorship with an emphasis on epidemiology, diagnosis, management, and long-term considerations.

Epidemiology

The most significant risk factor for developing oral complications is cGVHD. It is estimated that 40–70% of patients will develop cGVHD, with at least half developing oral involvement of the mucosa or salivary glands [1]. The onset of complications can be months to years after HCT. In addition to cGVHD, other factors, including late effects of the conditioning regimen, long-term immunosuppression, and medications, can contribute further to oral complications. Therefore, the at-risk population is large.

As the life expectancy of pediatric patients undergoing hematopoietic cell transplantation (HSCT) has increased, there has been greater emphasis on late complications of transplantation, including those affecting the head and neck. It has become increasingly evident that HSCT conditioning can have a significant impact on growth and development years after the transplant. Children are affected by cGVHD less frequently and often less severely than adults, but the differences become minimal with increasing age. Overall, oral cGVHD is estimated to affect approximately 20% of the pediatric population post-allogeneic-HSCT [2–5].

Oral mucosal complications

Non-infectious oral mucosal complications

Oral mucosal cGVHD

cGVHD is a common complication following allogeneic-HSCT, and the oral cavity is one of the most frequently affected sites. The oral manifestations of cGVHD include

Blood and Marrow Transplantation Long-Term Management: Prevention and Complications, First Edition. Edited by Bipin N Savani.

Table 17.1 Common long-term oral complications in patients post-HSCT

Tissue affected	Oral complication
Salivary gland	Xerostomia
	Mucoceles
	Sialoadenitis
Dental and periodontal	Dental decay
	Desquamative gingivitis
	Periodontitis
	Drug-induced gingival overgrowth
Musculoskeletal	Sclerodermatous cGVHD
	Developmental abnormalities of jaws and teeth
Mucosal	Mucosal cGVHD
	Oral candidiasis
	Herpetic reactivation
	Atrophy
	Reactive inflammatory lesions
Malignancy	Posttransplant lymphoproliferative disorder
	Squamous cell carcinoma
Neurosensory	Taste disorder

lichenoid lesions, erythema, and ulcerations (Figure 17.1a). The lichenoid lesions appear as striations, plaques, papules, or patches. The erythema is the "redness" of the oral mucosa, typically in association with lichenoid changes. Ulcerations appear smooth and yellow and are usually seen centrally in the context of surrounding white and red features [6, 7]. Superficial mucoceles frequently affect the palate or vestibule and are discussed in the "Salivary gland complications" section. With respect to diagnosis, according to the National Institutes of Health (NIH) consensus criteria the "lichenoid" manifestation is considered a diagnostic criterion, whereas erythema and ulcerations are considered distinctive manifestations that are not sufficient for the diagnosis of oral cGVHD [8]. The NIH criteria also delineated the format for clinical evaluation using the NIH assessment instruments (Figure 17.2).

The buccal and labial mucosa and the tongue are most frequently affected, although other mucosal surfaces may be involved. The ulcerative and erythematous lesions are particularly associated with sensitivity to acidic and spicy foods and drinks; however, symptoms can vary greatly, and even cases of mild lichenoid changes can be clinically significant [9]. Of note, even in more severe cases, there may be minimal or in some cases no discomfort at rest [10].

When the oral mucosa is refractory to systemic therapies, or when the oral mucosa is the only site of cGVHD involvement, the use of topical immunomodulatory agents can be highly effective in reducing signs and symptoms. Topical therapy with high-potency corticosteroids and tacrolimus in various formulations (e.g., gel, ointment, solution) has been well described [11, 12] (Table 17.2). Some patients may also benefit from palliative therapy with topical anesthetics and various over-the-counter products for management of pain, in particular prior to meals or tooth brushing.

Use of a children's toothpaste (free of sodium lauryl sulfate and strong flavoring) effectively minimizes sensitivity during tooth brushing. A consultation with a dietician may assist the patient in maintaining adequate oral intake when there is significantly impaired function.

Mucosal atrophy

Mucosal atrophy is an often subtle finding that may be evident in patients with a history of oral cGVHD or longstanding anemia in which the mucosa appears thinned and more fragile appearing. This change is most evident on the tongue dorsum, which may present with a smooth, depapillated surface.

Fibrovascular polyp

This lesion has also been reported as "pyogenic granuloma" and has been described in patients post-HSCT, in most cases in association with cGVHD and calcineurin inhibitor therapy [13]. Lesions are composed of fibrovascular tissue and present as an elevated pinkish–reddish mass that is typically lobulated with surface ulceration [14]. Diagnosis requires biopsy, and management is surgical excision and removal of any obvious localized factors (e.g., plaque/calculus, sharp edges of teeth).

Verruciform xanthoma

Verruciform xanthoma is a rare benign oral mucosal lesion that has been described in association with oral cGVHD and is characterized histopathologically by

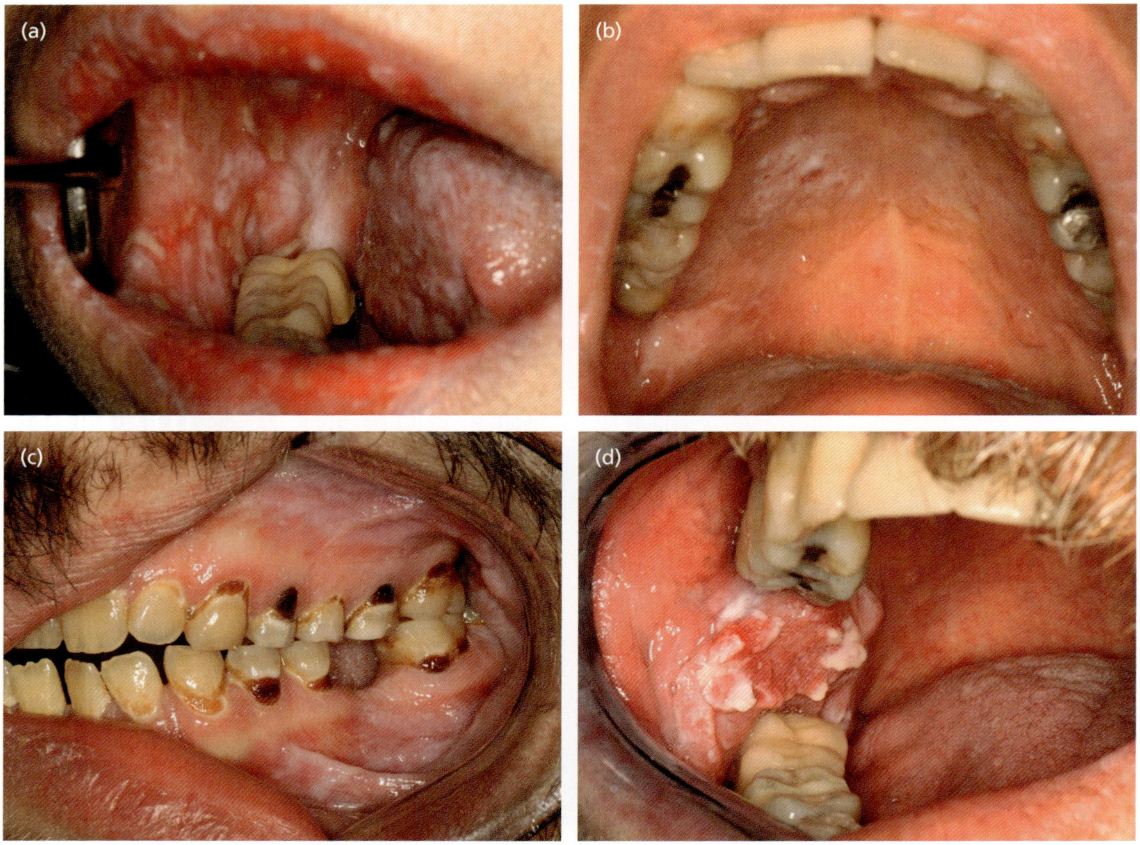

Figure 17.1 Oral cGVHD and associated complications. (a) Mucosal cGVHD of the buccal mucosa with prominent white reticular/hyperkeratotic changes, erythema, and multiple ulcerations; (b) multiple superficial mucoceles of the soft and hard palate; (c) typical pattern of cGVHD-associated dental decay affecting the cervical margins; (d) squamous cell carcinoma of the right buccal mucosa in a patient with a history of oral cGVHD.

papillary epithelial hyperplasia and the presence of foamy macrophages in connective tissue papillae [15]. The clinical appearance is highly variable and may present as a well-defined raised or flat, pebbly textured lesion that can be easily mistaken for malignancy. Diagnosis requires biopsy and management is simple surgical excision.

Infectious oral mucosal complications

On account of long-term immunosuppression and the use of intraoral topical corticosteroids, oral mucosal infections are common, with the most frequent being oral candidiasis and herpes simplex virus (HSV) reactivation.

Oral candidiasis

Oral candidiasis is the most prevalent oral fungal infection in cancer patients and is common in patients post-HSCT (Figure 17.3a) [16]. Symptoms range from none to severe burning and sensitivity, and may be accompanied by an unpleasant taste. Pseudomembranous candidiasis is the most common form appearing as white curd-like papules and plaques throughout the oral cavity. Erythematous candidiasis is more frequent in association with dentures or following antibiotic therapy and the appearance may be subtle compared with the pseudomembranous form. Angular cheilitis is another form of oral candidiasis characterized by erythema and

(a)

0	1	2	3
No symptoms	Mild symptoms with disease signs, but *not* limiting oral intake significantly	Moderate symptoms with disease signs, with *partial* limitation of oral intake	Severe symptoms with disease signs, with *major* limitation of oral intake

(b)

Mucosal change	No evidence of cGVHD		Mild		Moderate		Severe	
Erythema	None	0	Mild erythema or moderate erythema (<25%)	1	Moderate (≥25%) or Severe erythema (<25%)	2	Severe erythema (≥25%)	3
Lichenoid	None	0	Hyperkeratotic changes(<25%)	1	Hyperkeratotic changes(25–50%)	2	Hyperkeratotic changes (≥50%)	3
Ulcers	None	0	None	0	Ulcers involving (≤20%)	3	Severe ulcerations (≥20%)	6
Mucoceles*	None	0	1–5 mucoceles	1	6–10 scattered mucoceles	2	Over 10 mucoceles	3
			*Mucoceles scored for lower labial and soft palate only				**Total score for all mucosal changes**	

(c)

Symptoms Please rate how severe the following symptoms have been in the <u>last seven days.</u> Please fill in the circle below from 0 (symptom has not been present) to 10 (the symptom was as bad as you can imagine it could be) for each item.	**Not Present** 0	1	2	3	4	5	6	7	8	9	**As Bad As You Can Imagine** 10
Your **mouth dryness** as its WORST?	O	O	O	O	O	O	O	O	O	O	O
Your **mouth pain** at its WORST?	O	O	O	O	O	O	O	O	O	O	O
Your **mouth sensitivity** at its WORST?	O	O	O	O	O	O	O	O	O	O	O

Figure 17.2 Oral cGVHD assessment instruments (http://www.asbmt.org). (a) Organ scoring of cGVHD: patients are scored based on the functional impact of oral cGVHD, which is one of nine target organs that can be scored resulting in a definition of mild chronic, moderate, or severe chronic GVHD [8]. (b) Clinician oral cGVHD activity assessment scale. The combined score of the four oral manifestations ranges between 0 and 15, with a higher score reflecting more extensive oral cGVHD activity [53]. (c) The patient self-report oral cGVHD activity assessment scale includes three questions that assess the severity of oral chronic GVHD symptoms using an 11-point scale (dryness: worst mouth dryness; pain: worst mouth pain at rest; sensitivity: worst mouth pain with eating/drinking) [53].

cracking that affects the commissures and may extend to the perioral skin (Figure 17.3b).

Oral candidiasis is caused by overgrowth of *Candida*, which is a normal inhabitant of the oral flora in the majority of the healthy population. Microbiologically, the most common *Candida* species associated with oral candidiasis are *C. albicans*, *C. glabrata*, *C. tropicalis*, and *C. krusei*. Laboratory colonization does not necessarily imply that an active oral infection is present; therefore, culture is of limited clinical utility and clinical signs are vital for diagnosis. The predisposing factors can be categorized as local (e.g., salivary gland hypofunction, use

Table 17.2 Management of oral cGVHD and its sequelae [6, 7, 38]

Pharmacologic treatment	Other considerations
Oral mucosal cGVHD	
Mouthwashes • Dexamethasone 0.5 mg/5 mL (0.01%) • Clobetasol 0.1 mg/5 mL (0.05%) • Budesonide 3 mg/10 mL (0.03%) • Tacrolimus 0.5 mg/5 mL (0.01%) Gels • Fluocinonide 0.05% • Clobetasol 0.05% Injectable solution (intralesional) • Triamcinolone (40 mg/mL) Ointment (for lips) • Tacrolimus 0.1%	Antifungal prophylaxis to prevent oral candidiasis is often required. Diet adjustments may be needed to minimize mucosal irritation.
Salivary gland cGVHD	
Xerostomia Sialogogue therapy • Pilocarpine • Cevimeline	Additional means to reduce xerostomia include salivary stimulants (gum/candy), and oral moisturizing agents.
Dental caries Topical fluoride therapy Remineralization therapy	Additional means to prevent dental caries include good oral hygiene, sugar-free diet, and frequent dental check-ups.
Sclerotic cGVHD	
Intralesional steroid therapy (see above)	Additional means to slow down the progression include physical therapy and surgery to disrupt mucosal bands.

of topical corticosteroids) and systemic (e.g., immunosuppression, use of antibiotics).

Oral candidiasis is managed with topical and systemic anti-fungal medications. In most cases, topical polyene (e.g., nystatin suspension) or azole (e.g., clotrimazole troches) therapy is effective. When topical antifungal therapy is ineffective, or if dosing compliance is a concern, systemic fluconazole should be initiated.

Herpes virus reactivation

HSV reactivation can be encountered in patients post-HSCT, particularly in patients with cGVHD on long-term immunosuppressive therapy [17, 18]. Crop-like and coalescent ulcerations can present extraorally on the lips and perioral skin, as well as intraorally where both keratinized and nonkeratinized surface can be affected (Figure 17.3c). Occasionally it is an oral manifestation of a systemic HSV reactivation and fever may be present. Despite suppressive acyclovir prophylaxis, breakthrough infections can develop. In the context of oral mucosal cGVHD, there should be high suspicion for HSV when new ulcers develop that are disproportionately painful, especially if ulcers are on keratinized mucosa or if there has been an increase in systemic immunosuppressive therapy or tapering or inconsistent dosing of acyclovir. Diagnosis should be confirmed by viral culture/polymerase chain reaction or cytopathology.

The management of HSV reactivation is with systemic therapy with acyclovir, famciclovir, or valacyclovir [19]. In case of breakthrough recrudescence, the prophylactic acyclovir dose should be increased or another agent should be substituted. If resistance is suspected, culture and acyclovir susceptibility testing is recommended.

Sporadic reports of cytomegalovirus-associated nonspecific oral ulcers have been described in patients post-HSCT [20]. This apparently infrequent complication remains poorly characterized and its clinical significance is unclear.

Salivary gland complications

Although likely underrecognized and underdiagnosed owing to its often subtle and somewhat nonspecific clinical features, salivary gland hypofunction is common in survivors of HCT, with the primary causes being cGVHD [21] and total body irradiation. Saliva plays a critical role in daily oral function, including taste, chewing and swallowing, speech, dental health, and prevention of oral infection [22]. Dysfunction characterized by altered composition and reduced output results in complications ranging from xerostomia and difficulty eating and swallowing to accelerated dental decay and early tooth loss (see "Dental and periodontal complications" section). Diagnosis is typically made by history and examination, with characteristic features including dry mouth and difficulty speaking and eating, dry-appearing/shiny mucosa,

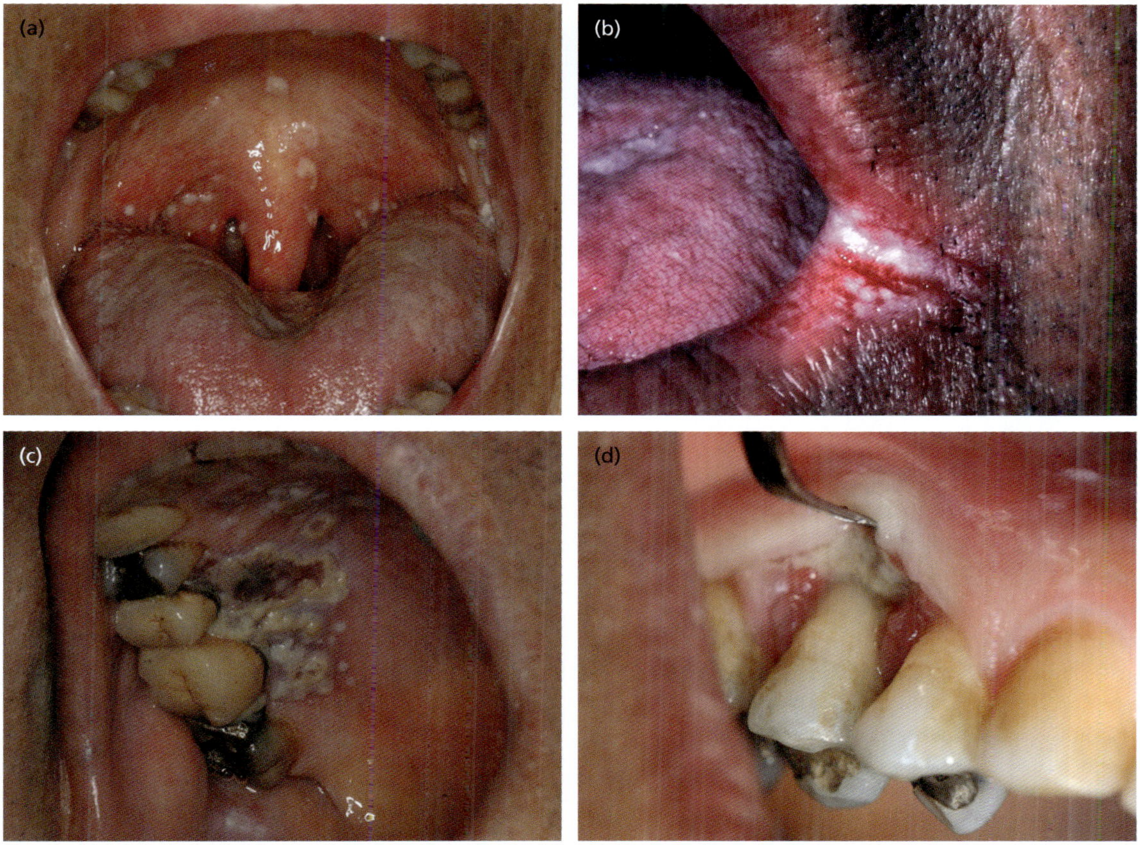

Figure 17.3 Oral infections post-HSCT: (a) pseudomembranous oral candidiasis of the soft palate and tongue; (b) angular cheilitis with characteristic erythema and cracking of the corners of the mouth; (c) HSV reactivation with multiple coalescing vesicular ulcerations; (d) bisphosphonate-related osteonecrosis of the jaw with characteristic exposed necrotic bone and secondary soft tissue infection with swelling and purulence.

thick/sticky saliva with lack of pooling, and the presence of tooth demineralization and decay (Figure 17.1c).

Superficial mucoceles are small (<0.5 cm) clear saliva-filled mucosal vesicles that arise from inflamed minor salivary glands (in particular of the soft palate and labial mucosa), typically in association with signs of oral mucosal cGVHD (Figure 17.1b) [23]. These lesions are typically painless but described by patients as an "annoyance" as they frequently erupt in clusters during meals and can persist for hours or days before resolving spontaneously. Sialoadenitis is a poorly characterized condition in which patients develop recurrent pain and swelling of the salivary glands, typically in association with long-standing cGVHD and xerostomia symptoms. Patients with sialoadenitis symptoms should be evaluated for the presence of sialoiths (salivary stones).

The etiology of salivary gland complications can be broadly categorized as being conditioning related, cGVHD related, or medication related. Conditioning regimens with and without total body irradiation have been proposed as a cause of late salivary gland hypofunction, even in the absence of cGVHD; however, findings have been inconsistent [24–28]. Despite being a well-characterized target of cGVHD, salivary gland involvement is frequently underrecognized as clinical findings can be equivocal and dry mouth symptoms may persist from the time of transplant due to conditioning-related changes. Finally, medications are believed to be the most frequent cause of salivary gland hypofunction in the general population, and survivors of HCT are frequently prescribed multiple prescription medications that may result in xerostomia and dysgeusia [29].

Management of salivary gland complications is primarily driven by symptoms (Table 17.2). Patients with salivary gland hypofunction should be instructed to drink water and avoid dehydrating beverages such as coffee, tea, and alcohol. Patients may also benefit from regular use of sugar-free gum/candy, which helps stimulate salivary flow, as well as over-the-counter dry mouth products, including rinses and gels. Prescription sialogogue therapy with pilocarpine or cevimeline can increase salivary flow and is generally safe and well tolerated in this patient population [30–32]. While systemic immunosuppressive therapy does not typically result in significant improvement in xerostomia symptoms, some patients with concurrent oral mucosal cGVHD appear to benefit from intensive topical steroid therapy (see “Oral Mucosal Complications” section), which may be due to an effect on minor salivary gland function. Superficial mucoceles are typically transient and minimally symptomatic and, therefore, do not require specific therapy. In severe cases that interfere with eating and swallowing, topical steroid regimens may lessen the number and frequency of lesions (Table 17.2).

Dental and periodontal complications

Dental caries

Extensive dental decay has been reported in patients with cGVHD [33]. The typical pattern of caries affects numerous teeth at the cervical and interproximal aspects, and can progress to the pulp tissue rapidly, often within 1–2 years of HSCT (Figure 17.1c). Early changes include whitish decalcification lesions and incisal edge chipping due to the demineralized and weakened enamel.

Several factors contribute to the onset of dental decay, including modifications in salivary secretion, changes in the oral flora, dietary alterations, and compromised oral care due to symptomatic cGVHD. Reduced and altered salivary flow is the main reason for the increased risk for dental decay. With impaired salivary function there is lack of washing effect, insufficient buffering capacity, reduced immune-protection, and reduced availability of elements necessary for remineralization. These changes along with chronic immunosupporession may lead to changes in the oral flora, promoting a more cariogenic environment [24, 34]. Changes in the diet due to symptomatic oral cGVHD may contribute to a more sugary and soft oral intake that tends to adhere to the oral surfaces, which in turn increases the risk for dental decay. Additionally in the presence of symptomatic oral cGVHD, oral hygiene may be compromised and inefficient, and patients may lack motivation due to impaired quality of life.

Prevention and management of dental caries requires several approaches (Table 17.2). Patients should be routinely screened for dental caries every 6 months. The frequency of bitewing radiographs should be determined based on risk assessment, starting with every 6 months and increasing the intervals if the dentition is stable. Fluoride applications can help prevent decay and can be applied at home using prescription-strength gel and paste, or in-office using varnish, gels, and foams. The intensity of fluoride therapy should be determined by patient risk and dental caries history. In addition to fluoride, various products based on calcium phosphate or casein protein have been suggested to promote remineralization in at-risk patients. Reinforcement of good oral hygiene practice is crucial for the successful prevention of dental decay and periodontal disease. Basic oral care includes brushing and flossing daily, and in particular after meals. Patients should be counseled about their diet and the importance of reduced sugar intake. Dental caries requires restorative management with appropriate materials, and careful follow-up for recurrent and new areas of decay.

Desquamative gingivitis

Typical gingival manifestations of cGVHD include lichenoid changes that may present with areas of desquamation and painful erosions [7]. Gingival involvement is typically seen in the context of more extensive oral changes (see “Oral mucosal complications” section). Plaque and calculus exacerbate this condition; therefore, maintaining good oral hygiene is an essential component of management [35].

Periodontitis

Periodontitis is a common disease in the global adult population, and it has been suggested that, owing to the compromised immune status of patients post-HSCT, they may be at an increased risk for more severe periodontitis. Sporadic case reports have described severe gingival recession and aggressive periodontitis; however, a lack of long-term studies makes it impossible to conclude whether or not a trend for increased chronic adult periodontitis exists [36, 37]. In patients with sclerodermatous cGVHD, the loss of elasticity may result in focal and potentially severe gingival recession at the vestibular frenula attachments [38].

Drug-induced gingival overgrowth

Gingival overgrowth is associated with several medications that are used in patients post-HSCT. This condition is primarily associated with calcineurin inhibitors, and in particular cyclosporine, although other associated medications (e.g., calcium channel blockers) may also be prescribed for management of HSCT-associated complications [39]. Clinical features can range from bulbous interdental papillae to extensive growth covering the teeth. The color and texture are normal in the absence of secondary inflammation. Poor oral hygiene is a significant risk factor.

Dose reduction or conversion from cyclosporine to tacrolimus can be effective in reversing gingival hyperplasia without the need to discontinue the medication. Optimal oral hygiene is a critical component of management, and conservative periodontal treatment may minimize the need for surgical intervention [40].

Musculoskeletal disturbances

Musculoskeletal complications affecting the oral cavity are relatively infrequent in survivors of HCT, but when present can be associated with significant morbidity. These can be broadly categorized as developmental abnormalities affecting the teeth and maxillofacial bones (limited to children), and functional disturbances secondary to cGVHD-mediated sclerotic changes.

Exposure to chemotherapy and/or radiation therapy to the head and neck region in children undergoing treatment for cancer can have an adverse impact on normal growth and development of teeth and surrounding structures [41–45]. Treatment at a younger age is associated with a greater potential for long-term effects. Abnormal findings include microdontia (small-sized teeth) and missing teeth or hypodontia (failure of the teeth to develop), as well as hypoplasia of the mandible and reduced vertical dimension of the maxillofacial complex. Management may require multidisciplinary specialized care.

Limited mouth opening and reduced oral function can develop secondary to cGVHD as a result of two distinct processes. Patients with advanced sclerodermatous cGVHD of the skin and fascia may develop perioral involvement and progressively limited mobility from an "outside in" mechanism; this is typically a very late complication. Painful myospasm may develop in areas of advanced sclerosis. Patients with long-standing oral mucosal cGVHD are at risk for developing fibrosis and band formation of the posterior buccal mucosa, similarly leading to restricted mouth opening. Home oral care can be challenging, placing these patients at very high risk for dental caries, especially in the presence of salivary gland cGVHD and other risk factors. Management is primarily intensive physical therapy and management of symptoms (Table 17.2).

Malignancy

One of the most serious and potentially life-threatening oral complications in HCT survivors is secondary malignancy. The two malignancies of primary concern that can present intraorally are posttransplant lymphoproliferative disease and squamous cell carcinoma (SCC). Posttransplant lymphoproliferative disease is typically a very early post-HCT event that may present as a painful solitary mucosal mass or ulceration [46].

Nearly 50% of solid tumors that arise post-allogeneic-HCT are oral SCCs, and a history of cGVHD is associated with increased risk [47]. Patients with a history of Fanconi anemia and dyskeratosis congenita are at significantly increased risk regardless of the presence of cGVHD and must be screened routinely. Mucosal abnormalities that should prompt biopsy include focal masses, atypical plaque-like lesions, and nonhealing ulcers with associated induration (Figure 17.1d). Signs of malignancy may be challenging to discern in patients with long-standing oral cGVHD changes. Depending on the location and stage, oral SCC may be treated with surgery, chemotherapy, and/or radiation therapy. Limited data suggest that long-term outcomes may be inferior in HCT patients compared with non-HCT patients [48].

Medication-related oral complications

Certain medications that are routinely used in the post-HCT setting can be associated with specific and unique oral complications. These can be categorized as immunosuppressive agents used for the prevention and management of GVHD, and antiresorptive therapy (primarily with aminobisphosphonates) in patients with multiple myeloma. A number of other medications can be associated with oral complications, in particular xerostomia; however, none of these are specifically related to HCT and will not be mentioned further.

Immunosuppressive therapy with calcineurin inhibitors (cyclosporine and tacrolimus) and mammalian target of rapamycin inhibitors (sirolimus) are infrequently associated with oral mucosal lesions. Calcineurin inhibitor-associated fibrovascular polyps are discussed in the "Oral mucosal complications" section. Sirolimus therapy is associated with the development of painful aphthous-like ulcerations that primarily affect the nonkeratinized oral mucosa. The natural history and course of these lesions remains poorly characterized; however, they appear to be responsive to topical and intralesional corticosteroid therapy [49, 50].

Osteonecrosis of the jaw is a well-defined complication of antiresorptive therapy with intravenous bisphosphonates (IVBP) [51]. In HSCT survivorship, the at-risk population is primarily patients with multiple myeloma due to the use of long-term IVBP therapy, but also patients with steroid-induced osteoporosis [52]. Primary risk factors include the cumulative dose of IVBP, oral health status, and a history of recent dental extractions. Lesions typically present as areas of exposed necrotic bone with variable localized infection of the surrounding soft tissue (Figure 17.3d). Management is directed towards elimination of infection and control of symptoms, and when feasible removal of mobile necrotic bone sequestra.

Conclusions

Oral complications after transplantation are common, with numerous potential issues arising in this single organ system. As early recognition of oral complications is essential to ensure the best possible outcomes, screening efforts should be performed routinely. Common complications should be recognized and managed by transplantation physicians, although oral medicine specialist referral is often required for recalcitrant issues, or for complex and uncommon diagnoses. Reinforcement of the importance of good oral hygiene practice and routine visits to the dentist is an essential component of oral health maintenance. With this team approach, optimal patient outcome can be assured.

References

1. Hull KM, Kerridge I, Schifter M. Long-term oral complications of allogeneic haematopoietic SCT. Bone Marrow Transplant. 2011;47:265–270.
2. Klingebiel T, Schlegel PG. GVHD: overview on pathophysiology, incidence, clinical and biological features. Bone Marrow Transplant. 1998;21(Suppl 2):S45–S49.
3. Yumura-Yagi K, Inoue M, Sakata N, et al. Chronic graft-versus-host disease in children and adolescents after bone marrow transplantation from HLA-matched donors. Int J Hematol. 2000;71:278–282.
4. Nicolatou-Galitis O, Kitra V, Van Vliet-Constantinidou C, et al. The oral manifestations of chronic graft-versus-host disease (cGVHD) in paediatric allogeneic bone marrow transplant recipients. J Oral Pathol Med. 2001;30: 148–153.
5. Treister NS, Woo SB, O'Holleran EW, et al. Oral chronic graft-versus-host disease in pediatric patients after hematopoietic stem cell transplantation. Biol Blood Marrow Transplant. 2005;11:721–731.
6. Meier JK, Wolff D, Pavletic S, et al. Oral chronic graft-versus-host disease: report from the International Consensus Conference on Clinical Practice in cGVHD. Clin Oral Investig. 2011;15:127–139.
7. Schubert MM, Correa ME. Oral graft-versus-host disease. Dent Clin North Am. 2008;52:79–109, viii–ix.
8. Filipovich AH, Weisdorf D, Pavletic S, et al. National Institutes of Health Consensus Development Project on Criteria for Clinical Trials in Chronic Graft-versus-Host Disease: I. Diagnosis and Staging Working Group report. Biol Blood Marrow Transplant. 2005;11:945–956.
9. Wolff D, Gerbitz A, Ayuk F, et al. Consensus conference on clinical practice in chronic graft-versus-host disease (GVHD): first-line and topical treatment of chronic GVHD. Biol Blood Marrow Transplant. 2010;16:1611–1628.
10. Treister NS, Cook EF Jr, Antin J, et al. Clinical evaluation of oral chronic graft-versus-host disease. Biol Blood Marrow Transplant. 2008;14:110–115.
11. Couriel D, Carpenter PA, Cutler C, et al. Ancillary therapy and supportive care of chronic graft-versus-host disease: National Institutes of Health consensus Development Project on Criteria for Clinical Trials in Chronic Graft-versus-Host Disease: V. Ancillary Therapy and Supportive Care Working Group report. Biol Blood Marrow Transplant. 2006;12:375–396.
12. Elad S, Zeevi I, Finke J, et al. Improvement in oral chronic graft-versus-host disease with the administration of effervescent tablets of topical budesonide – an open, randomized, multicenter study. Biol Blood Marrow Transplant. 2011; 18:134–140.

13. Lee L, Miller PA, Maxymiw WG, et al. Intraoral pyogenic granuloma after allogeneic bone marrow transplant. Report of three cases. Oral Surg Oral Med Oral Pathol. 1994;78: 607–610.
14. Al-Mohaya M, Treister N, Al-Khadra O, et al. Calcineurin inhibitor-associated oral inflammatory polyps after transplantation. J Oral Pathol Med. 2007;36:570–574.
15. Shahrabi Farahani S, Treister NS, Khan Z, Woo SB. Oral verruciform xanthoma associated with chronic graft-versus-host disease: a report of five cases and a review of the literature. Head Neck Pathol. 2011;5:193–198.
16. Lalla RV, Latortue MC, Hong CH, et al. A systematic review of oral fungal infections in patients receiving cancer therapy. Support Care Cancer. 2010;18:985–992.
17. Schubert MM, Peterson DE, Flournoy N, et al. Oral and pharyngeal herpes simplex virus infection after allogeneic bone marrow transplantation: analysis of factors associated with infection. Oral Surg Oral Med Oral Pathol. 1990; 70:286–293.
18. Palmason S, Marty FM, Treister NS. How do we manage oral infections in allogeneic stem cell transplantation and other severely immunocompromised patients? Oral Maxillofac Surg Clin North Am. 2011;23:579–599, vii.
19. Elad S, Zadik Y, Hewson I, et al. A systematic review of viral infections associated with oral involvement in cancer patients: a spotlight on *Herpesviridea*. Support Care Cancer. 2010;18:993–1006.
20. Lloid ME, Schubert MM, Myerson D, et al. Cytomegalovirus infection of the tongue following marrow transplantation. Bone Marrow Transplant. 1994;14:99–104.
21. Imanguli MM, Atkinson JC, Mitchell SA, et al. Salivary gland involvement in chronic graft-versus-host disease: prevalence, clinical significance, and recommendations for evaluation. Biol Blood Marrow Transplant. 2010;16:1362–1369.
22. Kaufman E, Lamster IB. The diagnostic applications of saliva – a review. Crit Rev Oral Biol Med. 2002;13: 197–212.
23. Campana F, Sibaud V, Chauvel A, et al. Recurrent superficial mucoceles associated with lichenoid disorders. J Oral Maxillofac Surg. 2006;64:1830–1833.
24. Jones LR, Toth BB, Keene HJ. Effects of total body irradiation on salivary gland function and caries-associated oral microflora in bone marrow transplant patients. Oral Surg Oral Med Oral Pathol. 1992;73:670–676.
25. Chaushu G, Itzkovitz-Chaushu S, Yefenof E, et al. A longitudinal follow-up of salivary secretion in bone marrow transplant patients. Oral Surg Oral Med Oral Pathol Oral Radiol Endod. 1995;79:164–169.
26. Dahllof G, Bagesund M, Remberger M, Ringden O. Risk factors for salivary dysfunction in children 1 year after bone marrow transplantation. Oral Oncol. 1997;33:327–331.
27. Garming-Legert K, Remberger M, Ringden O, et al. Long-term salivary function after conditioning with busulfan, fractionated or single-dose TBI. Oral Dis. 2011;17: 670–676.
28. Garming Legert K, Remberger M, Ringden O, et al. Salivary secretion in children after fractionated or single-dose TBI. Bone Marrow Transplant. 2012;47:404–410.
29. Moore PA, Guggenheimer J. Medication-induced hyposalivation: etiology, diagnosis, and treatment. Compend Contin Educ Dent. 2008;29:50–55.
30. Singhal S, Powles R, Treleaven J, et al. Pilocarpine hydrochloride for symptomatic relief of xerostomia due to chronic graft-versus-host disease or total-body irradiation after bone-marrow transplantation for hematologic malignancies. Leuk Lymphoma. 1997;24:539–543.
31. Nagler RM, Nagler A. Pilocarpine hydrochloride relieves xerostomia in chronic graft-versus-host disease: a sialometrical study. Bone Marrow Transplant. 1999;23:1007–1011.
32. Carpenter PA, Schubert MM, Flowers ME. Cevimeline reduced mouth dryness and increased salivary flow in patients with xerostomia complicating chronic graft-versus-host disease. Biol Blood Marrow Transplant. 2006;12: 792–794.
33. Castellarin P, Stevenson K, Biasotto M, et al. Extensive dental caries in patients with oral chronic graft-versus-host disease. Biol Blood Marrow Transplant. 2012;18:1573–1579.
34. Dens F, Boogaerts M, Boute P, et al. Caries-related salivary microorganisms and salivary flow rate in bone marrow recipients. Oral Surg Oral Med Oral Pathol Oral Radiol Endod. 1996;81:38–43.
35. Lo Russo L, Fedele S, Guiglia R, et al. Diagnostic pathways and clinical significance of desquamative gingivitis. J Periodontol. 2008;79:4–24.
36. Acikgoz A, Ozden FO, Fisgin T, et al. Oral and dental findings in Fanconi's anemia. Pediatr Hematol Oncol. 2005;22: 531–539.
37. da Fonseca MA, Murdoch-Kinch CA. Severe gingival recession and early loss of teeth in a child with chronic graft versus host disease: a case report. Spec Care Dentist. 2007; 27:59–63.
38. Treister N, Duncan C, Cutler C, Lehmann L. How we treat oral chronic graft-versus-host disease. Blood. 2012;120: 3407–3418.
39. Bondon-Guitton E, Bagheri H, Montastruc JL. Drug-induced gingival overgrowth: a study in the French Pharmacovigilance Database. J Clin Periodontol. 2012;39: 513–518.
40. Aimetti M, Romano F, Peccolo DC, Debernardi C. Non-surgical periodontal therapy of shallow gingival recession defects: evaluation of the restorative capacity of marginal gingiva after 12 months. J Periodontol. 2005;76:256–261.

41. Goho C. Chemoradiation therapy: effect on dental development. Pediatr Dent. 1993;15:6–12.
42. Kaste SC, Goodman P, Leisenring W, et al. Impact of radiation and chemotherapy on risk of dental abnormalities: a report from the Childhood Cancer Survivor Study. Cancer. 2009;115:5817–5827.
43. van der Pas-van Voskuilen IG, Veerkamp JS, Raber-Durlacher JE, et al. Long-term adverse effects of hematopoietic stem cell transplantation on dental development in children. Support Care Cancer. 2009;17:1169–1175.
44. Vesterbacka M, Ringden O, Remberger M, et al. Disturbances in dental development and craniofacial growth in children treated with hematopoietic stem cell transplantation. Orthod Craniofac Res. 2012;15:21–29.
45. Pedersen LB, Clausen N, Schroder H, et al. Microdontia and hypodontia of premolars and permanent molars in childhood cancer survivors after chemotherapy. Int J Paediatr Dent. 2012;22:239–243.
46. Elad S, Meyerowitz C, Shapira MY, et al. Oral posttransplantation lymphoproliferative disorder: an uncommon site for an uncommon disorder. Oral Surg Oral Med Oral Pathol Oral Radiol Endod. 2008;105:59–64.
47. Curtis RE, Metayer C, Rizzo JD, et al. Impact of chronic GVHD therapy on the development of squamous-cell cancers after hematopoietic stem-cell transplantation: an international case–control study. Blood. 2005;105: 3802–3811.
48. Mawardi H, Elad S, Correa ME, et al. Oral epithelial dysplasia and squamous cell carcinoma following allogeneic hematopoietic stem cell transplantation: clinical presentation and treatment outcomes. Bone Marrow Transplant. 2011;46:884–891.
49. Chuang P, Langone AJ. Clobetasol ameliorates aphthous ulceration in renal transplant patients on sirolimus. Am J Transplant. 2007;7:714–717.
50. de Oliveira MA, Martins EMF, Wang Q, et al. Clinical presentation and management of mTOR inhibitor-associated stomatitis. Oral Oncol. 2011;47:998–1003.
51. Ruggiero SL, Dodson TB, Assael LA, et al. American Association of Oral and Maxillofacial Surgeons position paper on bisphosphonate-related osteonecrosis of the jaws – 2009 update. J Oral Maxillofac Surg. 2009;67:2–12.
52. Hautmann AH, Elad S, Lawitschka A, et al. Metabolic bone diseases in patients after allogeneic hematopoietic stem cell transplantation: report from the Consensus Conference on Clinical Practice in Chronic Graft-versus-Host Disease. Transpl Int. 2011;24:867–879.
53. Pavletic SZ, Martin P, Lee SJ, et al. Measuring therapeutic response in chronic graft-versus-host disease: National Institutes of Health Consensus Development Project on Criteria for Clinical Trials in Chronic Graft-versus-Host Disease: IV. Response Criteria Working Group report. Biol Blood Marrow Transplant. 2006;12: 252–266.

18

CHAPTER 18

Sexual dysfunction in long-term survivors: monitoring and management

Andrea L Utz and Shubhada Jagasia

Division of Diabetes, Endocrinology, and Metabolism, Vanderbilt University Medical Center, Nashville, TN, USA

Introduction

The increased use and success of stem cell transplantation has led to increasing numbers of long-term survivors. Endocrine and reproductive complications of stem cell transplantation and its sequelae are common; however, predictors for long-term dysfunction have not been clearly established. Thus, in most cases, it is prudent to discuss the potential for gonadal dysfunction and to consider interventions that may preserve fertility, such as storage of gametes or embryos, if possible, prior to the initiation of toxic therapies. This chapter will focus on reproductive, gonadal steroid, and sexual function in men following stem cell transplantation.

By definition, male hypogonadism is inadequate testosterone and/or spermatozoa production. Impairments at the level of the hypothalamus, pituitary, and/or testes can lead to hypogonadism. In the majority of men who have undergone stem cell transplantation, hypogonadism is due to dysfunction at the level of the testes due to chemotherapeutic or radiation damage to Sertoli or Leydig cells of the testes. However, brain radiation may rarely impair hypothalamic or pituitary function, and a number of drugs can also negatively affect the function of the hypothalamus and pituitary with respect to the gonadal axis (Box 18.1).

Many chemotherapeutics have direct testicular toxicity, with alkylating agents being the most detrimental. Effects within the testicle are subdivided into effects on the germinal epithelium containing Sertoli cells, which produce gametes, and/or on Leydig cells, which are the source of testosterone. The germinal epithelium is most sensitive to the toxic effects of chemotherapeutics and radiation, and thus fertility may be impaired while testosterone function often remains intact or recovers after an initial decline in function following induction and transplantation.

Chemotherapeutic and radiation effects on gonadal function

The factors that primarily influence risk of hypogonadism include gender, age at treatment, underlying malignancy, type and dose of chemotherapeutic, location and dose of radiation, and time since treatment [1]. In individuals who undergo stem cell transplantation, effects on gonadal function are a result of conditioning regimens prior to transplant, as well as previous therapies, for patients with an underlying malignancy Some data also suggest that graft-versus-host disease (GVHD) may contribute to infertility [2]. In addition to chemotherapeutics

Blood and Marrow Transplantation Long-Term Management: Prevention and Complications, First Edition. Edited by Bipin N Savani.

Box 18.1 Common causes of male hypogonadism in the stem cell transplant population

- Testicular toxicity caused by chemotherapeutics
- Testicular damage induced by testicular radiation
- Hypothalamic/pituitary damage due to radiation
- Chronic illness
- Underlying malignancy
- Glucocorticoids
- Opiates
- Hyperprolactinemia; generally drug induced (dopamine antagonists, including antipsychotics, metoclopramide, some selective serotonin reuptake inhibitors)

and radiation, the underlying malignancy type appears to predict baseline sperm production. In some studies, men with lymphoma have been reported to have impaired semen parameters prior to treatment initiation [3].

In the treatment of lymphoma, the initial chemotherapeutic choice has an impact on gonadal function. Alkylating agents are the primary cause of gonadal dysfunction, with procarbazine and cyclophosphamide producing the most toxicity [1], and there is an increased risk of gonadal damage with increasing doses of these agents. A threshold dose has not been determined under which gonadal function is likely to remain intact; however, azoospermia is present in the majority of postpubertal men exposed to greater than 300 mg/kg of cyclophosphamide [4]. ABVD (adriamycin, bleomycin, vinblastine, dacarbazine) and EBVP (epirubicin, bleomycin, vinblastine, and prednisone) regimens do not include alkylating agents and generally do not produce long-term azoospermia. Common chemotherapeutic regimens for leukemia are less likely to produce persistent gonadal damage than regimens used for lymphoma [5].

Myeloablative conditioning regimens with alkylating agents frequently produce infertility, with higher dose and number of alkylating agents and the addition of total body irradiation (TBI) increasing the risk. Estimates of azoospermia following stem cell transplantation range between 48 and 85% [6]. A study of 64 men who underwent bone marrow transplantation showed recovery of spermatogenesis in 90% treated with cyclophosphamide alone, 50% treated with cyclophosphamide and busulfan or thiotepa, and only 17% of those who received cyclophosphamide and radiation [7]. In a study of 47 men who received busulfan and cyclophosphamide 120 mg/kg, evaluated at least 2 years after transplantation, 21 of 26 who had semen analyses had detectable sperm, of which 11 had counts over 20 million/mL. There are no available data that nonmyeloablative conditioning preserves fertility in men. A study of 32 men who received nonmyeloablative conditioning with alemtuzumab, fludarabine, and melphalan prior to stem cell transplantation for hematologic malignancies also showed a decline in germ cell and Leydig cell function [8]; however, further study is necessary to determine whether less-toxic conditioning regimens improve gonadal function in a larger population.

Pelvic radiation increases the risk of gonadal dysfunction. Radiation doses as low as 20 cGy have been shown to lower sperm count, but doses less than 70 cGy generally do not produce azoospermia. Pelvic radiation doses greater than 120 cGy have a significant risk of azoospermia [4]. Chronic GVHD appeared to be associated with an increased risk of azoospermia [2]. It is important to realize that some men with early azoospermia recover sperm production over time, with some men recovering spermatogenesis up to 10 years after transplant, and there is no clear correlation between age at transplant and likelihood of recovery [7].

While it is most common that gonadal dysfunction is due to direct testicular toxicity, in some cases previous cranial irradiation may contribute to hypogonadism by damaging the hypothalamus and/or pituitary. Hypothalamic and/or pituitary dysfunction following cranial radiation may occur within the early months after high-dose radiation or onset may be delayed for 10 years or more in those who receive lower radiation doses [9].

Addressing fertility in the stem cell transplant population

Although difficult to determine fertility rates in the stem cell population, one group performed a surveillance questionnaire study, including 37 362 transplant recipients, and found that 232 (0.6%) of transplanted women and partners of transplanted men had conceived a pregnancy. The birth rate in the transplant population was estimated to be only 14% of that in the general population [10]. As fertility rates are low and it is currently impossible to predict long-term outcome with respect to fertility preservation, sperm banking with cryopreservation is the most well-established means to preserve fertility in men who may be rendered infertile by cancer therapies. A follow-up study of 112 men who underwent stem cell transplantation for hematologic malignancy indicated that 79 (71%) were offered sperm storage and 42 banked sperm. Eighteen of 25 who attempted conception were successful with children born a median of 8 years (range 1–22 years) after stem cell transplantation [11].

In men who will undergo radiation therapy, testicular shielding should be considered. The use of gonadotropin-releasing hormone analogs in men, to suppress Leydig and Sertoli function during cancer therapy, have not been shown to have a beneficial effect [12]. Pre-pubertal boys who will undergo cancer therapy are a special challenge as they do not produce mature sperm. Although experimental techniques of testicular tissue cryopreservation have been proposed, it is not currently a recommended option as reliable sperm production has not been obtained [1].

The assessment of male fertility is most accurately determined with a semen analysis. The World Health Organization 2010 guidelines provide sperm quantity, motility, and morphology parameters that predict spontaneous pregnancy within a 12-month period [13]. It is generally recommended that at least two semen analyses be performed, separated by several weeks, prior to diagnosing inadequate sperm production. Samples should be analyzed within an hour of ejaculation and at least 48 h after last ejaculation. Other serum markers have been used, as surrogates in assessing germ cell viability and function, including follicle-stimulating hormone (FSH) and inhibin B levels. FSH levels rise and inhibin B levels fall with declining Sertoli cell function. However, at present, measurement of these levels is not recommended as studies have shown variability in predicting sperm quantity and quality [5].

The use of assisted reproduction techniques decreases the number of viable sperm needed for conception, as the use of intracytoplasmic sperm injection allows use of only one sperm per ovum for *in vitro* fertilization (IVF). Intrauterine insemination of a larger quantity of sperm can also be attempted to avoid IVF; however, conception rates are generally lower than that with IVF [12]. Children conceived from individuals who underwent chemotherapy or radiation as children do not show an increased risk of congenital malformation or genetic disease. However, there are minimal data to determine genetic disruption in gametes from individuals with relatively recent chemotherapeutic or radiation exposure, and contraception is strongly recommended during and for at least 3 months following treatment [1]. In men who do not produce adequate sperm for conception, do not have the financial resources for assisted reproductive technologies, or are concerned about potential genetic alterations, donor sperm or embryo or adoption can be considered.

Diagnosing testosterone deficiency

Guidelines for testing for hypogonadism following stem cell transplantation have not been established. It is expected in the early weeks to months after transplantation that the hypothalamic–pituitary–gonadal axis will be suppressed merely due to critical illness. Additionally, many medications, including opiates and glucocorticoids, will suppress testosterone production, primarily via suppression of the hypothalamic and pituitary signals. The time course of recovery from this suppression after stem cell transplant has not been established, and if suppressive medications are continued then it is expected that testosterone levels will remain low. One group recommends assessment of testosterone levels at 3, 6, 12, and 24 months posttransplant, with testosterone replacement if decreased bone density or hypogonadal symptoms are present. In men desiring fertility, they also recommend annual semen analyses at 1 year posttransplant for 5 years and then biennially [2].

In one small study of men following allogeneic bone marrow transplantation for hematologic malignancies, testosterone levels were measured over the first 12 months. The majority of the men received cyclophosphamide and TBI, with a small percentage receiving busulphan and no radiation. The nadir testosterone occurred at 6 weeks and returned to near baseline by 6 months (Figure 18.1). As the major decline in bone density occurs within the first 6 months, it is possible that testosterone deficiency may contribute in some degree to the early bone loss [14]. However, hypogonadism is not the sole contributor to early bone density loss, as a follow-up

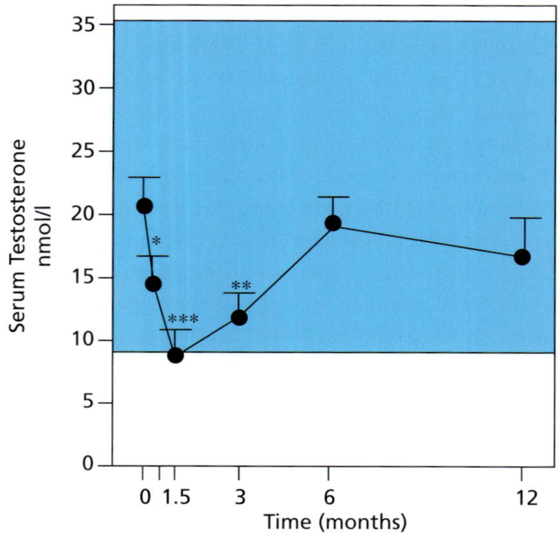

Figure 18.1 Serum concentration of testosterone (mean and standard error of the mean) in male patients following allogeneic bone marrow transplant * $p < 0.05$, ** $p < 0.01$, *** $p < 0.001$ for differences from baseline. Shaded area represents the normal range [14]. Reprinted by permission from Macmillan Publishers Ltd: *Bone Marrow Transplantation* 23(4)355–361 copyright 1999.

Box 18.2 Symptoms and signs of hypogonadism in men [16]

More specific:

- Incomplete or delayed sexual development, eunuchoidism
- Reduced sexual desire (libido) and activity
- Decreased spontaneous erections
- Breast discomfort, gynecomastia
- Loss of body (axillary and pubic) hair, reduced shaving
- Very small or shrinking testes
- Inability to father children, low or zero sperm count
- Height loss, low trauma fracture, low bone mineral density
- Hot flushes, sweats

Less specific:

- Decreased energy, motivation, initiative, and self-confidence
- Feeling sad or blue, depressed mood, dysthymia
- Poor concentration and memory
- Sleep disturbance, increased sleepiness
- Mild anemia (normochromic, normocytic)
- Reduced muscle bulk and strength
- Increased body fat, body mass index
- Diminished physical or work performance

study that evaluated treatment with calcium, vitamin D, and early gonadal steroid replacement did not completely mitigate posttransplant bone density decline [15].

The symptoms of testosterone deficiency are often vague and may be attributed to chronic illness or its treatment. Box 18.2 lists the common signs and symptoms that are associated with hypogonadism. Some signs, such as eunuchoid body habitus, occur in men who develop hypogonadism prior to puberty. At present, there are no established guidelines for treating low testosterone deficiency in the post-stem-cell-transplant population. Future studies to determine whether early testosterone replacement is beneficial and safe are warranted. If testosterone therapy is initiated, it is important to remember that gonadal function, particularly testosterone production, may improve over time and discontinuation of testosterone replacement therapy can be considered.

Screening for testosterone deficiency routinely involves measurement of a random total testosterone level, although early morning values are preferable. The normal range for total testosterone has not clearly been established; however, values greater than 350 ng/dL are generally considered normal, values less than 150 ng/dL are usually low, and values between 150 and 350 ng/dL are borderline. Owing to variation in laboratory methods for testosterone measurement, it is recommended that practitioners use reference ranges established by local laboratories to interpret results. In men with testosterone levels less than 350 ng/dL, further testing is indicated. Even in an individual with a random testosterone less than 150 ng/dL, it is important to perform additional testing to confirm persistently low levels prior to the initiation of testosterone replacement. There is normal circadian variation in testosterone production; therefore, measurement in the morning prior to 9 a.m., is recommended, as reference ranges have been established based on levels from morning blood samples from young, healthy men. As acute illness is likely to suppress testosterone production, measurement when the man is relatively well will provide the most accurate assessment.

Total testosterone assessment does not provide the complete assessment of a man's testosterone status.

Testosterone circulates systemically bound to sex-hormone-binding globulin and albumin. The portion of testosterone not bound to binding proteins is considered the "active" testosterone and most representative of testosterone status. In men with borderline testosterone levels, particularly those who may have conditions that affect binding-protein concentrations, determination of the free testosterone level is recommended. Assessing the unbound fraction of testosterone is biochemically complicated. The gold standard assay is assessment of free testosterone by equilibrium dialysis; however, this is an expensive assay and not practical for routine use. Immunoassays that provide a "direct" free testosterone measurement are commonly used but are generally felt to provide inaccurate values and should not be routinely used. A compromise between quality and cost is the assessment of the calculated free testosterone level – this is determined by measuring total testosterone, sex-hormone-binding globulin, and albumin and calculation of a free testosterone level. Many chemistry laboratories perform the calculation and present the data as a calculated free testosterone level, and online calculators are also available.

After it has been established that a man has a persistently low testosterone level, it is then appropriate to assess gonadotropin status by measurement of luteinizing hormone (LH) and FSH. It is important to measure these values prior to initiating testosterone to establish whether the primary pathology is at the level of the testicle or at the level of the hypothalamus and/or pituitary. If the LH level is elevated, the testosterone deficiency is due to dysfunction at the level of the testicle. If the LH level is not elevated, then a hypothalamic and/or pituitary disorder is the cause of the low testosterone. Once a man has initiated testosterone treatment, LH and FSH levels will be suppressed, no matter whether the primary problem is testicular or hypothalamic/pituitary, thus underscoring the need to assess gonadotropin levels prior to testosterone initiation.

If testosterone levels are low and the LH not elevated, this indicates secondary or hypogonadotropic hypogonadism. Causes of secondary hypogonadism include hypothalamic or pituitary radiation, tumors, inflammation, or infiltration. Opiate and glucocorticoid medications are common causes of hypogonadotropic hypogonadism. Hyperprolactinemia can also cause secondary hypogonadism, and medications that commonly cause hyperprolactinemia include antipsychotics, metoclopramide, opiates, and some selective serotonin reuptake inhibitors. Pituitary imaging, generally with magnetic resonance imaging, is recommended if there are symptoms of pituitary mass lesion (headache or vision impairment), severely low testosterone level (total testosterone less than 150 ng/dL), hyperprolactinemia, or biochemical evidence of other pituitary hormone deficiency [16].

Testosterone replacement therapies

The benefits of testosterone replacement include improved energy, muscle bulk and strength, increased bone density, increased libido and erectile function, and increased red blood cell production [17]. It is reasonable to consider testosterone replacement therapy in men with symptoms of hypogonadism and low testosterone levels. Absolute contraindications for testosterone treatment include active prostate or breast cancer. It is appropriate to assess for prostate cancer with digital rectal exam and prostate-specific antigen (PSA) prior to initiation of therapy. Other contraindications include hematocrit >50%, severe benign prostatic hypertrophy symptoms, or poorly controlled heart failure [16].

The US Food and Drug Adminstration (FDA)-approved testosterone replacement therapies include testosterone gels, patch, intramuscular injection, buccal tablet, and implantable pellets. Table 18.1 lists US FDA approved testosterone replacement therapies and recommended dosing regimens. The goal is to produce a testosterone level in the low to mid-normal range. Intramuscular testosterone injections are generally given every 7–14 days, with a peak expected within 48 h of the injection and subsequent decline in the level over the dosing interval. The dose of the testosterone injection should be adjusted to produce a mid-normal testosterone level at the midpoint between injections or low-normal at the nadir, prior to the subsequent injection. As testosterone levels naturally decline and with increasing risk of prostate disorders with age, it is appropriate to target a lower testosterone replacement level in older men.

According to Endocrine Society consensus guidelines, safety monitoring includes prostate assessment with digital rectal exam and PSA prior to initiation and at 3 and 6 months after initiation of testosterone in men over

Table 18.1 FDA-approved testosterone formulations for male hypogonadism

Testosterone formulations	Trade names	Common formulations	Usual doses	Considerations
Gel	Androgel	1% 12.5 mg/1.25 g	50–100 mg/day	Variable absorption
		1.62% 20.25 mg/1.25 g	40.5–81 mg/day	Potential transfer to others
	Testim	1% 50 mg/5 g	50–100 mg/day	Skin irritation
	Fortesta	10 mg/0.5 g	40–70 mg/day	
	Axiron	30 mg/1.5 mL	60–120 mg/day	
Patch	Androderm	2 mg, 4 mg	2–8 mg/day	Skin irritation
Intramuscular depot injections			100–200 mg q2wk or 50–100 mg qwk	Wide fluctuations of testosterone levels over dosing cycle
enanthate	Delatestryl	200 mg/mL		Injection pain
cypionate	Depo-testosterone	100 or 200 mg/mL		
Buccal tablets	Striant	30 mg per tablet	30 mg bid	Gum irritation
Implantable pellets	Testopel	75 mg per pellet	300–450 mg q3–6mo	Infection
				Implantation pain

bid: twice daily; qwk: every week; q2wk: every 2 weeks; q3–6mo: every 3–6 months.

40 and then according to age, race, and risk-related guidelines. Abnormalities on prostate exam, absolute PSA-level-based risk factors, and rate of rise of PSA should be assessed [16]. Testosterone treatment can increase hematocrit, and monitoring for erythrocytosis is recommended. Other side effects of testosterone include worsening of obstructive sleep apnea, gynecomastia and/or breast tenderness, and acne. In men desiring fertility, testosterone treatment can lower sperm production.

In men with secondary hypogonadism, alternative treatment with human chorionic gonadotropin, and in some cases combined with human menopausal gonadotropin or FSH, may restore testosterone levels and adequate sperm production. However, it is important to realize that these therapies are unlikely to stimulate normal testosterone or sperm production in men with a testicular insult due to chemotherapeutics or radiation.

When stem cell transplants are performed in boys prior to puberty, monitoring for appropriate timing of pubertal milestone attainment is required. Testicular toxicity may decrease testosterone production; however, in the majority of boys a compensatory increase in LH allows adequate testosterone production to promote normal pubertal progression. In those who receive high-dose testicular radiation or high-dose alkylating agents, testicular Leydig cell damage may develop and prevent pubertal progression. In those who receive high-dose cranial radiation, usually >30 Gy, secondary hypogonadism due to hypothalamic or pituitary injury may prevent pubertal progression. In both situations, appropriately timed testosterone supplementation will allow adequate development of secondary sexual characteristics [18].

Effects of stem cell transplantation on libido and sexual function

Decreased sexual activity and satisfaction are common in men and women after stem cell transplantation. Sexual function involves a complex interplay of many systems, including hormonal, neurologic, vascular, psychological, and interpersonal relations. Sexual symptoms include decreased interest, erectile dysfunction, anejaculation, retrograde ejaculation, or anorgasmia. Stem cell transplantation therapies can have an effect on many aspects which may lead to impaired sexual function [19, 20].

In a prospective study of patients who underwent myeloablative conditioning and stem cell transplantation, there was a decline in sexual activity and function in the first 6 months after transplant. Men had recovered to pretreatment sexual activity levels by 1 year (Figure 18.2) and function by 2 years after transplant. However, even at 5 years after transplant there was a significant decrement in sexual activity and function compared with normal control men, with 46% of men reporting sexual problems. There appeared to be an increased risk of sexual dysfunction in older men, those with pretransplant psychologic issues, and chronic GVHD [21]. A longitudinal study of patients undergoing bone marrow transplantation showed men to have decreased interest in sexual activity pretransplant. By year 1 after transplant men had increased concern about physical attractiveness and decreased sexual function [22].

There are multiple ways by which the underlying malignancy, treatment with chemotherapy or radiation, and GVHD may contribute to sexual dysfunction. Fatigue and depression may impair libido; decreased semen production is likely to cause a decrease in testicular size, which may alter body image; low testosterone contributes to fatigue, decreased libido, and erectile dysfunction; pelvic radiation or GVHD can induce scarring and atherosclerosis within the pelvic and penile vasculature [23]; autonomic neuropathy induced by chemotherapeutics may impair sexual function; and chronic GVHD can cause penile skin sensitivity. Commonly used medications, including those to treat depression, pain, and nausea, can have a negative effect on libido and sexual function. Corticosteroids frequently used for chronic GVHD suppress hypothalamic, pituitary, and gonadal function. Additionally, corticosteroids cause body adipose and muscle changes that may affect body image and affect mood and sleep [24].

Psychological factors likely play a significant role in determining return of sexual function after stem cell transplantation, with body image changes, fatigue, and depression being common findings. Interpersonal relationship and intimacy issues, functional concerns, and uncertainty with respect to fertility complicate the situation [24]. It has been shown that sexual function at 1 year is a strong predictor of function at 5 years; thus, addressing the issue early in the course after transplant may have a beneficial effect on subsequent outcome [21]. Behavioral therapies that focus on overcoming avoidance of sexual activity and gradual return to sexual activity have been successful. Meeting with a professional skilled in couples and intimacy counseling may also be beneficial [24].

In men with testosterone deficiency, replacement testosterone may be of benefit; however, there is no clear benefit of testosterone treatment on libido in the absence of testosterone deficiency. The effect of a decline in testosterone production, even if levels remain within the normal range, has not been well studied. Some investigators have defined an intermediate state of testosterone deficiency, with low normal levels of testosterone and moderately elevated LH levels, as Leydig cell insufficiency. A small trial of monthly testosterone injections and sildenafil in men early after transplant, at 2–24 months, appeared to show benefit with respect to sexual function [25]. As Leydig cell function frequently recovers during this time period, it is unclear that persistent treatment is necessary, and the long-term risks and benefits of testosterone in men who are not truly testosterone deficient remains to be determined.

It is important to determine whether decreased erectile function is the underlying source of decreased libido, as treatments and techniques to improve erectile function may improve desire. In a study of posttransplant patients, approximately half of patients reported that their healthcare providers did not discuss issues related to sexual functioning. However, in those patients who did report discussing sexual issues with their providers, fewer sexual problems were reported during long-term follow-up [22]. Means to address sexual function in cancer survivors are currently under investigation but have not yet been well validated. For the practicing clinician, tools that effectively and expediently address these sensitive issues are necessary. The Brief Sexual Function Inventory addresses sexual drive, erection, ejaculation, perception of sexual problems, and overall satisfaction [26]. This tool can provide a basis for addressing the primary issues that patients experience with respect to sexual function.

Treatment of erectile dysfunction

Erectile dysfunction is a common complaint in the general population and is particularly prevalent in men with psychiatric disorders, cardiovascular disease, obesity, diabetes mellitus, hyperlipidemia, and smokers. Erectile dysfunction is often due to a combination of factors, including impaired vasculature, neuronal signaling,

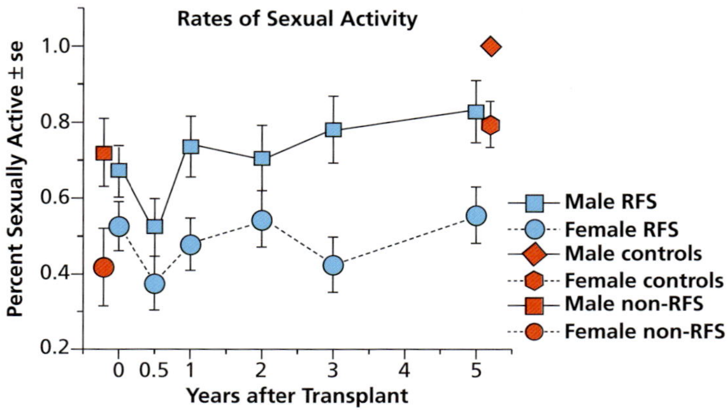

Figure 18.2 Percentage of males and females who were sexually active, among responding relapse-free-survivors (RFS) from before transplantation ($n = 109$) to 5 years after transplantation ($n = 80$). Rates are also plotted for non-RFS patients before transplantation ($n = 49$) and controls at 5 years ($n = 77$). Both men and women declined in rates of being sexually active from before transplantation to 6 months afterward ($p = 0.05$). On average, men improved by 1 year compared with 6-month levels ($p = 0.02$); women improved by 2 years ($p = 0.03$), but both remained below their respective controls at 5 years [21]. Republished with permission of American Society of Hematology, from Sexual function changes during the 5 years after high-dose treatment and hematopoietic cell transplantation for malignancy, with case-matched controls at 5 years Syrjala KL, et al. *Blood* 111:991 copyright 2008; permission conveyed through Copyright Clearance Center, Inc.

structural abnormalities, hormonal abnormalities, drug effects, psychiatric disorders, and interpersonal relationships. Drugs most associated with erectile dysfunction include antidepressants, antipsychotics, antihypertensives (beta blockers and thiazides), antihistamines, antiandrogens, alcohol, and opiates [27].

The first-line oral therapies for erectile dysfunction are phosphodiesterase 5 inhibitors (PDE5Is) – see Table 18.2. PDEI5s differ based on onset and duration of action, with sildenafil and vardenafil lasting 5 h and tadalafil up to 24–36 h. Medication costs vary and they are frequently not covered by insurance, which may play a role in medication choice. The medications are generally taken on an as needed basis, but low-dose tadalafil has been approved for daily use. Low doses are recommended in the setting of significant renal or hepatic dysfunction or when using potent inhibitors of CYP3A4 (ketoconazole, itraconazole, erythromycin, clarithromycin, protease inhibitors). PDE5Is are contraindicated in those using nitrates, and alpha blockers are relatively contraindicated due to a risk of hypotension. PDEI5s are relatively contraindicated in the setting of unstable angina and poorly controlled hypertension. Vardenafil should be avoided in the setting of long QTc. PDE5I side effects include headache, congestion, myalgias, dyspepsia, vision disturbances, hypotension, and hearing loss [27].

An alternative to systemic treatment for erectile dysfunction is intracavernous or intraurethral delivery of prostaglandin E1 (PGE1). PGE1 is either injected directly into the corpora cavernosa or inserted into the urethra, and called medicated urethral system for erection. With injection therapy, onset of action is rapid, within 5–20 min, and success rates are high at greater than 70%. Men with an increased risk of priapism (leukemia, multiple myeloma, sickle cell, thrombocythemia, polycythemia, hypercoaguable) and those taking monoamine oxidase inhibitors should not use PGE1. Injections can be given to men taking anticoagulants but injection site pressure is necessary. Other side effects include pain, hematoma, and penile fibrosis. Hypotension has been reported in intraurethral PGE1 use [27].

Mechanical treatments are also available for treatment of erectile dysfunction. Vacuum-assisted erection devices increase cavernosal blood flow and occlusive rings applied after tumescence slow venous drainage. Ejaculation is prevented with vacuum devices and their use is contraindicated in individuals with bleeding disorders or anticoagulant use. Penile prostheses are less commonly used,

Table 18.2 Treatment of erectile dysfunction

Treatment	Trade name	Usual dose	Considerations
Medications			
Phosphodiesterase-5 inhibitors			Should not be used with nitrates
sildenafil	Viagra	25–100 mg prn	Effective 4–5 h
tadalafil	Cialis	5–20 mg prn	Effective 24–36 h
		2.5–5 mg daily	
vardenafil	Levitra	5–20 mg prn	Effective 4–5 h
	Staxyn	10 mg prn	
Prostaglandin E1 (alprostadil)	MUSE	125–1000 µg prn	Intraurethral insertion
	Caverject, Edex	1–40 µg prn	Intracavernosal injection
Mechanical treatments			
Vacuum-assisted devices			Impairs ejaculation
Penile prostheses			Invasive

prn: as needed.

but implantable malleable rods or inflatable prostheses are available options.

Summary

Following hematopoietic stem cell transplantation, there is a significant risk of decreased gonadal and sexual function in men, with the type and dose of pretransplant and conditioning chemotherapy and radiation as the primary predictors of testicular dysfunction. Sperm production and subsequent fertility are frequently reduced after transplant, and it is appropriate to discuss sperm banking prior to treatment and to consider assisted reproductive treatments after transplant. While testosterone levels and sexual function frequently improve by 6–12 months after transplantation, long-term deficits may persist. Moreover, medications frequently used in this population may suppress testosterone production and affect sexual interest and function. Testing for testosterone deficiency is appropriate during the long-term follow-up of these patients, and testosterone replacement should be considered in those with persistent testosterone deficiency owing to its potential beneficial effects on libido, bone density, body composition, red blood cell production, and energy. Efforts to minimize medications that can affect libido and sexual function and initiation of medications or interventions that restore erectile dysfunction may significantly improve quality of life in the stem cell transplant population.

References

1. Leader A, Lishner M, Michaeli J, Revel A. Fertility considerations and preservation in haemato-oncology patients undergoing treatment. Br J Haematol. 2011;153:291–308.
2. Grigg AP, McLanchlan R, Zajac J, Szer J. Reproductive status in long-term bone marrow transplant survivors receiving busulfan-cyclophosphamide (120 mg/kg). Bone Marrow Transplant. 2000;26:1089–1095.
3. Sieniawski M, Reineke T, Josting A, et al. Assessment of male fertility in patient with Hodgkin's lymphoma treated in the German Hodgkin Study Group (GHSG) clinical trials. Ann Oncol. 2008;19:1795–1801.
4. Howell SJ, Shalet SM. Spermatogenesis after cancer treatment: damage and recovery. J Natl Cancer Inst Monogr 2005;2005(34):12–17.
5. Nakayama K, Milbourne A, Schover LR, et al. Gonadal failure after treatment of hematologic malignancies: from recognition to management for health-care providers. Nat Clin Pract Oncol. 2008;5:78–89.
6. Dvorak CC, Gracia CR, Sanders JE, et al. NCI, NHLBI/PBMTC First International Conference on Late Effects after

Pediatric Hematopoietic Cell Transplantation: Endocrine Challenges – Thyroid Dysfunction, Growth Impairment, Bone Health, & Reproductive Risks. Biol Blood Marrow Transplant. 2011;17:1725–1738.

7. Anserini P, Chiodi S, Spinelli S, et al. Semen analysis following allogeneic bone marrow transplantation. Additional data for evidence-based counseling. Bone Marrow Transplant. 2002;30:447–451.
8. Kyriacou C, Kottaridis PD, Eliahoo J, et al. Gonadal function post-transplant germ cell damage and Leydig cell insufficiency in recipients of nonmyeloablative transplantation for haematological malignancies. Bone Marrow Transplant. 2003;31:45–50.
9. Darzy KH. Radiation-induced hypopituitarism after cancer therapy: who, how and when to test. Nat Clin Pract Endocrinol Metab. 2008;5:88–99.
10. Salooja N, Szydlo RM, Socie G, et al. Pregnancy outcomes after peripheral blood or bone marrow transplantation: a retrospective survey. Lancet. 2001;358:271–276.
11. Babb A, Farah N, Lyons C, et al. Uptake and outcome of assisted reproductive techniques in long-term survivors of SCT. Bone Marrow Transplant. 2012;47:568–573.
12. Schover LR. Reproductive complications and sexual dysfunction in cancer survivors. In: Ganz PA (ed.). Cancer Survivorship Today and Tomorrow. New York: Springer, 2007; pp. 251–271.
13. World Health Organization, Department of Reproductive Health and Research. WHO Laboratory Manual for the Examination and Processing of Human Semen. Fifth edition. Geneva: World Health Organization, 2010.
14. Valimaki MJ, Kinnunen K, Volin L, et al. A prospective study of bone loss and turnover after allogeneic bone marrow transplantation: effect of calcium supplementation with or without calcitonin. Bone Marrow Transplant. 1999;23: 355–361.
15. Kananen K, Volin L, Laitinen K, et al. Prevention of bone loss after allogeneic stem cell transplantation by calcium, vitamin D, and sex hormone replacement with or without pamidronate. J Clin Endocrinol Metab. 2005;90: 3877–3885.
16. Bhasin S, Cunningham GR, Hayes FJ, et al. Testosterone therapy in men with androgen deficiency syndromes: an endocrine society clinical practice guideline. J Clin Endocrinol Metab. 2010;95:2536–2559.
17. Snyder PJ, Peachey H, Berlin JA, et al. Effects of testosterone replacement in hypogonadal men. J Clin Endocrinol Metab. 2000;85:2670–2677.
18. Cohen A, Bekassy AN, Gaiero A, et al. Endocrinological late complications after hematopoietic SCT in children. Bone Marrow Transplant. 2008;41:S43–S48.
19. Thygesen KH, Schjodt I, Jarden M. The impact of hematopoietic stem cell transplantation on sexuality: a systematic review of the literature. Bone Marrow Transplant. 2012; 47:716–724.
20. Syrjala KL, Martin P, Deeg J, Boeckh M. Medical and psychosocial issues in transplant survivors. In: Ganz PA (ed.). Cancer Survivorship Today and Tomorrow. New York: Springer, 2007; pp. 188–214.
21. Syrjala KL, Kurland BF, Abrams JR, et al. Sexual function changes during the 5 years after high-dose treatment and hematopoietic cell transplantation for malignancy, with case-matched controls at 5 years. Blood. 2008;111:989–996.
22. Humphreys CT, Tallman B, Altmaier EM, Barnette V. Sexual functioning in patients undergoing bone marrow transplantation: a longitudinal study. Bone Marrow Transplant. 2007;39:491–496.
23. Chatterjee R, Andrews HO, McGarrigle HH, et al. Cavernosal arterial insufficiency is a major component of erectile dysfunction in some recipients of high-dose chemotherapy/ chemo-radiotherapy for haematological malignancies. Bone Marrow Transplant. 2000;25:1185–1189.
24. Yi JC, Syrjala KL. Sexuality after hematopoietic stem cell transplantation. Cancer J. 2009;15:57–64.
25. Chatterjee R, Kottaridis PD, McGarrigle HH, Linch DC. Management of erectile dysfunction by combination therapy with testosterone and sildenafil in recipients of high-dose therapy for haematological malignancies. Bone Marrow Transplanat. 2002;29:607–610.
26. O'Leary MP, Fowler FJ, Lenderking WR, et al. A brief male sexual function inventory for urology. Urology. 1995;46: 697–706.
27. Albersen M, Mwamukonda KB, Shindel AW, Lue TF. Evaluation and treatment of erectile dysfunction. Med Clin North Am. 2011;95:201–212.

19

CHAPTER 19

Fertility issues, contraception, and pregnancy outcome in long-term survivors

Alicia Rovó[1], *Nina Salooja*[2], *Carl P Schwarze*[3], *Joerg P Halter*[1], *and André Tichelli*[1]

[1]Hematology Department, University Hospital of Basel, Basel, Switzerland
[2]Department of Medicine, Imperial College London, Hammersmith Hospital, London, UK
[3]University Children's Hospital, Tübingen, Germany

Introduction

Late side effects of hemopoietic stem cell transplantation (HSCT) can impact adversely on health in several ways. Some late complications may directly influence outcome after HSCT by increasing mortality rate and significantly impairing the physical health of long-term survivors. However, not all late effects are life threatening. In this respect, infertility holds a unique position in the care of long-term survivors of HSCT. While endocrine dysfunction is frequently symptomatic, infertility itself is not. Fertility problems may nonetheless impair the quality of life of the transplant recipient and also of their life partner if they wish to conceive a child [1]. Infertility is associated with significant psychological distress and levels of depression up to twice that of the normal population. Indeed, long-term survivors and their respective partners consider reproductive health issues and the possibility to parent a child of great importance. In contrast to other late effects, most of the preventive measures to overcome infertility after HSCT have to be considered, planned, and undertaken before HSCT.

This chapter will focus on the magnitude of risk and risk factors for infertility in female and male survivors treated with HSCT. Furthermore, we will discuss the issues of pregnancy after HSCT, pretransplant counseling, and the potential for preventive practice.

Female fertility after HSCT

Infertility is common in women following HSCT, usually as a result of the chemoradiotherapy given as pretransplant conditioning. Underlying disease and its treatment prior to transplant can also play a role. In addition to germ cells, tissues relevant to the maintenance of female fertility include the hormone-producing cells of the hypothalamic–pituitary axis and ovary, the uterus, and the reproductive tract. All of these can be adversely affected by radiation and/or chemotherapy.

A female's fertility potential is related to the number of oocytes present in the ovary. Primordial germ cells divide by mitosis in fetal life to form oogonia. These become surrounded by somatic cells to form primordial follicles, and as the germ cell enters early prophase they become known as the primary oocytes. Maximum numbers close to 6.8 million are reached approximately 5 months after conception, and no new oocytes will be

Blood and Marrow Transplantation Long-Term Management: Prevention and Complications, First Edition. Edited by Bipin N Savani.

made subsequently either in childhood or adult life. Instead, numbers decrease as a result of physiological programmed cell death (PCD) and by the age of 7 there are fewer than 300 000 oocytes remaining [2]. Additional gametes are lost after the menarche by menstruation. When a critically low number of oocytes remain, ovulation ceases and low levels of estrogen occur associated with menopausal symptoms. Anything which causes a reduction in the total number of oocytes will predispose to a premature menopause.

Several molecules are involved in germ-line PCD. Signal transducers and protein kinases activate inducers of apoptosis such as "Bax" from the Bcl-2 family. These in turn activate effector molecules such as caspase proteins which lead to cell degeneration. Much of our understanding of these pathways comes from studies in mice and rats. Bax-deficient mice, for example, have an extended ovarian lifespan due to the reduction in oocyte PCD [3]. The apoptotic pathway in the ovary is susceptible to upregulation by external stimuli such as radiation and chemotherapy. This explains why they can induce irreversible damage to oocytes even though the latter are mitotically inactive. Mice mutant for caspase-2 have not only been demonstrated to have an increased number of primordial follicles, but are almost completely resistant to cell death caused by doxorubicin [4].

Effects of chemoradiatiotherapy on female gonadal function

The radiation dose at which 50% human oocytes are lost (LD50) has been estimated as less than 2 Gy [5]. The significance of this depends on the age of the patient, because the latter parameter is linked to the total number of oocytes remaining in the ovary after treatment has been given. Using this estimated LD50 and a mathematical model for follicle decline, the effective sterilizing dose to the ovary has been estimated to be 20.3 Gy at birth, 18.4 Gy at 10 years, 16.5 Gy at 20 years and 14.3 Gy at 30 years [6].

The majority of children and adolescents conditioned with total body irradiation (TBI) for HSCT will develop ovarian failure. However, it was shown that about 50% of young girls transplanted before the age of 10 years with regimens containing fractionated TBI enter puberty spontaneously and experience menarche despite increased luteinizing hormone (LH)/follicle-stimulating hormone (FSH) levels [7, 8]. It must be expected, though, that these patients develop premature ovarian failure at a later point in time. Treatment with chemotherapy and radiotherapy has an additive gonadotoxic effect. Consequently, even lower radiation doses will cause gonadal failure when given in combination with chemotherapy.

Analysis of an eligible subgroup of 3390 survivors of the Childhood Cancer Survivor Study identified 215 (6.3%) with acute ovarian failure after cancer treatment as indicated by cessation of menstruation. Of these patients, 75% had received abdominal–pelvic radiation. Exposure of ovaries to more than 10 Gy radiation, older age at treatment, and use of alkylating agents or procarbazine were significant risk factors for the development of ovarian failure, as was an underlying diagnosis of Hodgkin lymphoma. Another report from the Childhood Cancer Survivor Study investigated fertility retrospectively in 5149 female participants and compared this with 1441 female siblings [9]. The incidence of pregnancy was significantly reduced in survivors compared with sibling controls (relative risk, RR 0.81). In multivariate analysis, risk factors for infertility included an ovarian–uterine radiation dose >5 Gy, treatment with cyclophosphamide or lomustine, and alkylating agent exposure. In addition to direct radiation to the pelvis or abdomen, these potentially sterilizing doses of radiation can be achieved or exceeded by TBI and craniospinal radiation. Abdominal radiation also has the potential to damage the uterus. Following high-dose direct abdominal radiation, irreversible changes to the uterus can occur, particularly in relation to blood flow and distensibility. Following the lower doses given with TBI in the context of HSCT, reduction in size and vascularity also occurs but may be at least partly mitigated by hormone replacement therapy. If TBI is given during childhood, however, before the uterus has fully developed, the risk of uterine compromise is greater. In a study which included 12 women who had received TBI in childhood there was a reduction in uterine volume to 40% of adult size despite the use of sex steroid replacement [10].

The likelihood of infertility following chemotherapy depends on the drug and cumulative dose to which the patient is exposed as well as patient age. Different classes of drugs vary in their ability to cause infertility, but the highest risk of ovarian failure occurs with alkylating agents (odds ratio 3.98 compared with nonexposed patient) and platinum derivatives (RR 1.7 compared with nonexposed patient) [11]. Two of the most commonly used agents for conditioning of myeloablative allografts are cyclophosphamide and busulphan. The gonadal toxicity induced by busulphan was first noted more than 50 years ago with cumulative doses of 150–400 mg associated with acute amenorrhea [12]. Similarly, for cyclophosphamide, cumulative doses have been shown to cause gonadal failure. In a study from the 1990s which looked at patients receiving cyclophosphamide at a dose of 100 mg/day for breast cancer, cumulative doses of cyclophosphamide greater than 11 g led to cessation of menstruation in most women over the age of 30, while cumulative doses of 5.2 g were sufficient to cause amenorrhea in 13 of 13 women over the age of 40 [13]. In the setting of conditioning for HSCT, cyclophosphamide can be used alone or else in combination with busulphan (BUCY) or TBI. When used alone, cyclophosphamide is compatible with recovery of gonadal function, particularly in younger women. In a single-center study, ovarian recovery occurred in all 26 women under the age of 26 receiving this regimen but in only 5 of 16 women over this age [14]. When cyclophosphamide is combined with TBI, ovarian failure is the norm, although resumption of menses in this setting has been described. The pretransplant conditioning regimen BUCY incorporating 16 mg/kg busulphan together with cyclophosphamide 200 mg/kg appears to be a particularly gonadotoxic regimen. Of 73 women receiving this regimen in Seattle, only one had recovery of ovarian function [15].

Management of gonadal failure and fertility issues in female recipients of HSCT

There are several clinical and laboratory indicators of gonadal failure in women. Clinical indicators include failure to go through puberty, absent menstruation (primary or secondary), and menopausal symptoms. Laboratory indicators include elevated serum FSH and LH, low level of anti-Müllerian hormone and reduced or absent antral follicles on ultrasound. Two FSH levels in the menopausal range measured at least 1 month apart and associated with amenorrhea/oligomenorrhea and low estradiol levels is strongly suggestive of ovarian failure.

In female patients, hypergonadotropic hypogonadism is almost always the rule, with elevated FSH and LH [16, 17] However, germ cell damage might not be detected by determination of basal serum LH/FSH levels until patients have reached the pubertal age range of >8 years. The gonadotropin-releasing-hormone test is able identify prepubertal females at risk as it results in an exaggerated response with abnormally high LH and FSH serum levels [7]. In the majority of transplanted girls, puberty will not occur spontaneously and sex-hormone replacement therapy will be required. In prepubertal girls, though rare, there is still a chance for recovery with achievement of spontaneous menarche. In this group, determination of LH/FSH is recommended from the age of 8 years. Induction of puberty should not be delayed after the age of 13 years. Precocious puberty is a rare event and necessitates treatment with gonadotropin-releasing hormone-agonists. Pubertal development in females with spontaneous puberty must be carefully monitored, including documentation of breast stage development, increase of height velocity during pubertal growth, and rising serum levels of estradiol [17]. It must be noted that the time interval from breast stage B2 (Tanner staging of puberty) [18] to peak height velocity is only 1 year (standard deviation SD ±0.77) [19]. However, other factors influencing growth, such as malnutrition, chronic GVHD and its treatment (steroids), damage to the growth plate (cranio-spinal radiation), and additional endocrine deficiencies (hypothyroidism, growth hormone deficiency), must also be considered.

In adult female patients, up to 90% require sex-hormone replacement therapy after HSCT. This replacement therapy can be interrupted every 1–2 years to evaluate spontaneous recovery [8, 20]. Normal clinical and laboratory parameters do not confirm fertility, however, and the only way of demonstrating definite fertility is pregnancy. Even where gonadal recovery and pregnancy occur, it is important that the patient is aware that their ovarian reserve will have been reduced by chemoradiotherapy and that a premature menopause remains probable.

Female patients without definitive evidence of gonadal failure after HSCT should be advised to use contraception if they wish to avoid pregnancy. Currently there are limited guidelines to assist clinicians in managing the contraceptive needs in this special population. After reviewing the evidence regarding the safety and efficacy of available methods of contraception for women who have been diagnosed with cancer, the Society of Family Planning recommends that women of childbearing age who are being treated for cancer avoid combined hormonal contraception (containing both estrogen and progesterone) when possible because they increase the risk of venous thromboembolism. Women who develop osteopenia or osteoporosis following chemotherapy should avoid the progesterone-only contraceptive injection [21]. Specific information on the ideal contraceptive choices for female recipients of HSCT is lacking, however.

Male fertility after HSCT

In the male, the Leydig cells are less vulnerable to chemotherapy and radiotherapy than are the Sertoli cells and germ cells; typically, serum LH levels are in the normal range for age, while serum FSH levels are increased as a reflection of this. The risk of Leydig cell dysfunction after radiotherapy is inversely related to age and directly correlated with the radiation dose to the testes: patients receiving doses of <12 Gy will usually not require testosterone replacement therapy, but doses of >20 Gy will cause Leydig cell failure in most prepubertal males and doses >30 Gy in most pubertal boys and young adults [7, 22]. Sperm concentration does not decrease immediately after cytotoxic treatment. During the first 4–8 weeks after chemotherapy has been administered, sperm counts may remain normal. Following a testicular radiation dose of 0.35–0.5 Gy, the nadir sperm count occurs after 4–6 months. The reason for this is that spermatogenic stem cells are more sensitive to chemotherapy and radiation than later stage germ cells, which will continue to mature into spermatozoids. Recovery of spermatogenesis therefore depends on the degree of destruction of the early sperm stem cells [23].

Absence of spermatozoa from semen is a frequent finding in male long-term survivors of HSCT as a result of chemoradiotherapy given before transplant as treatment or conditioning [24]. Azoospermia is less frequent in patients conditioned with busulphan and cyclophosphamide (50%) and uncommon in those treated with cyclophosphamide alone (10%) [25].

TBI used as part of the conditioning regimen has been shown to play a central role in subsequent infertility [26–28]. Radiotherapy to the testes with doses of 0.1 Gy will cause damage to the spermatogonia, 2–3 Gy to spermatocytes, and 4–6 Gy to spermatozoa. In the serum, FSH levels are increased and on clinical examination testicular volumes are typically below 10 mL [29, 30]. However, with increased follow-up, male recipients surviving more than 10 years, younger than 25 years at HSCT, and apparently without chronic GVHD have a reasonable likelihood of spermatogenesis, even those patients receiving conditioning with standard dose TBI [27]. Recovery of normal spermatogenesis as defined by World Health Organization guidelines remains unlikely, however [31].

It is possible that the strong impact of TBI on infertility masks other potential risk factors. Data showing a relationship between sperm recovery and GVHD are scarce, though in previous single-center studies such an association has been implicated [25, 27, 32]. A recent publication from the European Group for Blood and Marrow Transplantation (EBMT) reported sperm analyses from 224 males who had undergone allogeneic HSCT [28]. In that study, the median time between transplantation and sperm analysis was 63 months (8–275). They found that 69% of the recipients were azoospermic, and the rate of azoospermia in patients conditioned with TBI was 81%. In multivariate analysis, conditioning with TBI (RR 7.1; 95% confidence interval (CI) 3.4–14.8) and age >25 years at transplantation (RR 2.4; 95% CI 1.09–5.2) were significantly associated with a higher risk for azoospermia. In patients not conditioned with TBI, ongoing chronic GVHD was the main adverse factor for sperm recovery (RR 3.11; 95% CI, 1.02–9.47; $P = 0.045$). Therefore, independently of TBI, age greater than 25 years at HSCT and ongoing chronic GVHD can contribute to infertility in these patients after HSCT. The mechanism by which GVHD may lead to azoospermia remains unclear. In an animal model, injury to Leydig cells is associated with an intratesticular inflammatory response. Alloreactive donor T cells have been shown to infiltrate the testis during acute GVHD, resulting in an impairment of testosterone-producing cells. This experiment did not show evidence of a direct T cell infiltration of seminiferous tubules, but rather indicates an indirect effect of GVHD on spermatogenesis, leading to a loss of Leydig cell function [33]. Systemic inflammatory factors associated with ongoing chronic GVHD could also have an impact on sperm production. The authors of the latter study introduced a scoring system based on these risk factors to predict the probability of azoospermia in male long-term survivors (Figure 19.1).

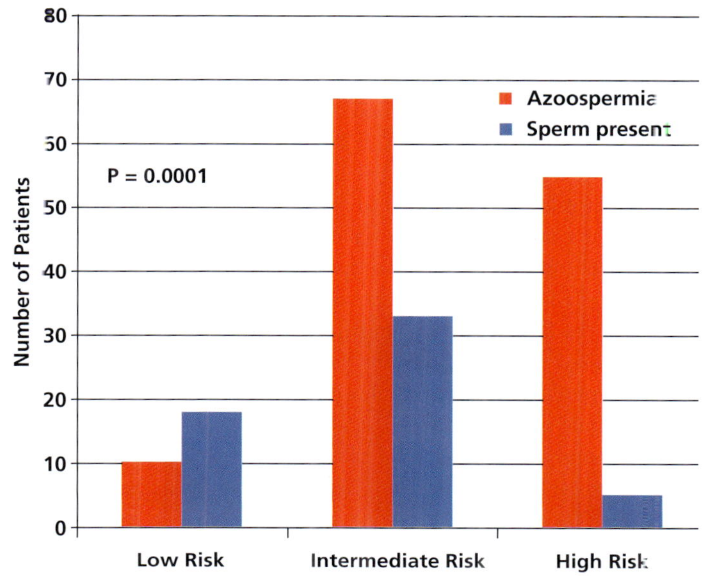

Score	0–1	1.5–3	3.5–4.5
Number of patients	28	100	60
Sperm present	18	33	5
Azoospermia	10	67	55
Percentage with azoospermia	36%	67%	92%

Figure 19.1 Risk of azoospermia according to score. TBI counted for 2 points, age more than 25 years at HSCT and ongoing chronic GVHD at time of sperm analysis (SFA) for 1 point, and time interval between HSCT and SFA shorter than 8 years for 0.5 points. A higher risk score is related with increased probability of azoospermia. Adapted from Rovó et al. Haematologica 2013 [28].

Management of gonadal failure and fertility issues in male recipients of HSCT

In most cases boys will enter puberty spontaneously; if the pubertal growth spurt is blunted, determination of testosterone is recommended. In prepubertal boys the determination of LH/FSH is recommended from the age of 9 years; induction of puberty, if necessary, should not be delayed beyond the age of 14 years. Even when pubertal development occurs spontaneously, close monitoring of testosterone levels is recommended to ensure that levels increase appropriately and that a normal pubertal height velocity and peak height velocity are achieved. If pubertal development does not progress normally, testosterone replacement therapy must be considered and others causes of growth failure must be evaluated.

Sex-hormone replacement will not be necessary in most adult male patients following HSCT despite spermatogenesis being reduced or absent. Usually the serum FSH levels are increased, but LH levels are normal [34]. Owing to the high probability of infertility after HSCT, the question of semen cryopreservation should be addressed before treatment commences [35, 36]. Paradoxically, the potential for recovery of spermatogenesis in some patients also necessitates the need for counseling in relation to contraception. Periodic analysis of sperm should be undertaken to evaluate this, particularly in patients who have received less gonadotoxic regimens. Even if sperm counts are low post-transplant or there is poor sperm motility, paternity may still be possible using assisted reproductive techniques [33].

Pregnancy outcome after HSCT

The definitive proof of recovered fertility would be successful pregnancy in females or fatherhood in males. A number of pregnancies following HSCT have been described [37, 38]. The true magnitude of fertility recovery following HSCT will always be difficult to determine, mainly because of the lack of complete data on pre- and posttransplant fertility status, but also because the patients' wishes in relationship to parenthood are frequently not known. The Bone Marrow Transplant Survivor Study used a mailed survey to assess the magnitude of compromise in reproductive function following transplant and to investigate pregnancy outcome. Data were presented on 619 women and partners of men treated with autologous ($n = 241$) or allogeneic ($n = 378$) HSCT between 21 and 45 years of age, and surviving 2 years or more. The median transplant to follow-up time was 7.7 years. Thirty-four patients reported 54 pregnancies after HSCT, of which 46 resulted in live birth; 26 partners of male patients reported 40 pregnancies and 8 female patients had 14 pregnancies. Infertility was associated with older age at HSCT (≥30 years), female sex, and TBI. Miscarriage or stillbirth did not occur more frequently than a comparative group of age-matched siblings [37]. These results are contrary to previous reported data in which an increase in spontaneous abortions and miscarriages, pre-term delivery, and low birth-weight babies occurred. Notably, the rate of congenital anomalies, developmental delay, and malignant disease were not higher than expected [38].

The largest single-center data evaluating pregnancies after HSCT comes from Seattle. Of 708 post-pubertal women receiving HSCT, 32 subsequently became pregnant, 25 of whom had received cyclophosphamide-only conditioning. Seven pregnancies were observed after TBI, but there were none following BUCY conditioning [15]. In a large multicenter cohort of 36 362 transplanted patients from the Late Effects Working Party of the EBMT, 229 centers reported on 312 conceptions in 113 patients and 119 partners of patients [38]. The largest percentage of pregnancies occurred in patients transplanted for severe aplastic anemia (47 out of 385, 12.2%). There was only one pregnancy after BUCY conditioning in a patient transplanted for thalassemia and conditioned with a lower dose of busulphan than traditionally used. A European study including seven pediatric centers evaluated fertility a median of 6 years (range 3–12) after HSCT and found that use of busulphan in conditioning was the major treatment-related risk factor for female patients with an odds ratio for infertility of 47.4 (95% CI 5.4–418.1) [39]. Successful pregnancy after conditioning with BUCY has been described in isolated reports, but the numbers are low [40–42].

A Report of the Center for International Blood and Marrow Transplant Research described 178 pregnancies of HSCT recipients transplanted between 2002 and 2007. There were 83 pregnancies (with 85% live birth) in female recipients and 95 pregnancies (86% live birth), with most pregnancies occurring 5–10 years after HSCT [43].

A survey from the EBMT [28] reported on fatherhood and cryopreservation of sperm in male patients who had undergone allogeneic HSCT. Participating centers provided the number of children parented by male patients before and after HSCT, the number of adopted children, methods used for conception (assisted reproductive techniques versus natural), and the availability of cryopreserved sperm collected before HSCT. Following transplant, 29/211 (14%) patients with a median age at HSCT of 21 years (2–55 years) became fathers (total number of children: 44). The median time interval between HSCT and the birth of the first child was 7.2 years (range: 1–21.6 years). Among the patients who fathered a child, 11 occurred with natural conception and 11 involved use of cryopreserved sperm. From the same cohort, additional information on wishes for paternity has recently been published [51]. That study demonstrated that the wish to father a child after HSCT is associated with paternity status before transplantation and the age of the patients at HSCT. The majority of patients expressing a wish to have a child after HSCT (78%) did not have children before HSCT and were young (<25 years). Irrespective of the high expectancy to father a child in this population, they did not have a higher rate of fatherhood (15%) compared with those patients who fathered a child before HSCT. Hence, the discrepancy between the wish to father a child and the lower rate of fatherhood is likely explained by the high degree of infertility in this cohort after transplantation (69% azoospermia).

A recent single-center questionnaire survey investigated the uptake and outcome of assisted reproductive techniques and pretransplant counseling in patients surviving a minimum of 2 years after allogeneic HSCT [44]. Of 434 patients, 212 (112 male) responded with a median transplant follow-up time of 11 years (range 2–29 years). Uptake of gamete and embryo storage was high when offered, and stored material was used frequently. Pregnancies in partners of male patients were often successful, and there was no evidence that the success rate of assisted reproductive technology in female recipients of HSCT was inferior to that of nontransplant patients. Not all patients were counseled about infertility, and of those that were, not all were offered fertility-preserving options. Ongoing physician education will be necessary to maintain and further improve the pretransplant counseling process and maximize invitations to store gametes and embryos in line with guidelines.

Preventive measures and counseling

In patients of child-bearing age it is important to use the least gonadotoxic regimen as conditioning and also in the initial treatment of the underlying disease. If potentially sterilizing treatment cannot be avoided then ovarian shielding during administration of TBI may be possible for some patients. However, longer follow-up of such patients will be required to establish whether normal pregnancy and delivery can occur without increasing the risk of leukemia relapse [45]. For patients receiving treatment likely to render them infertile, it is important that available assisted reproductive techniques are discussed (Figure 19.2). Cryopreservation of sperm for men and of embryos for women for use after transplant would be the

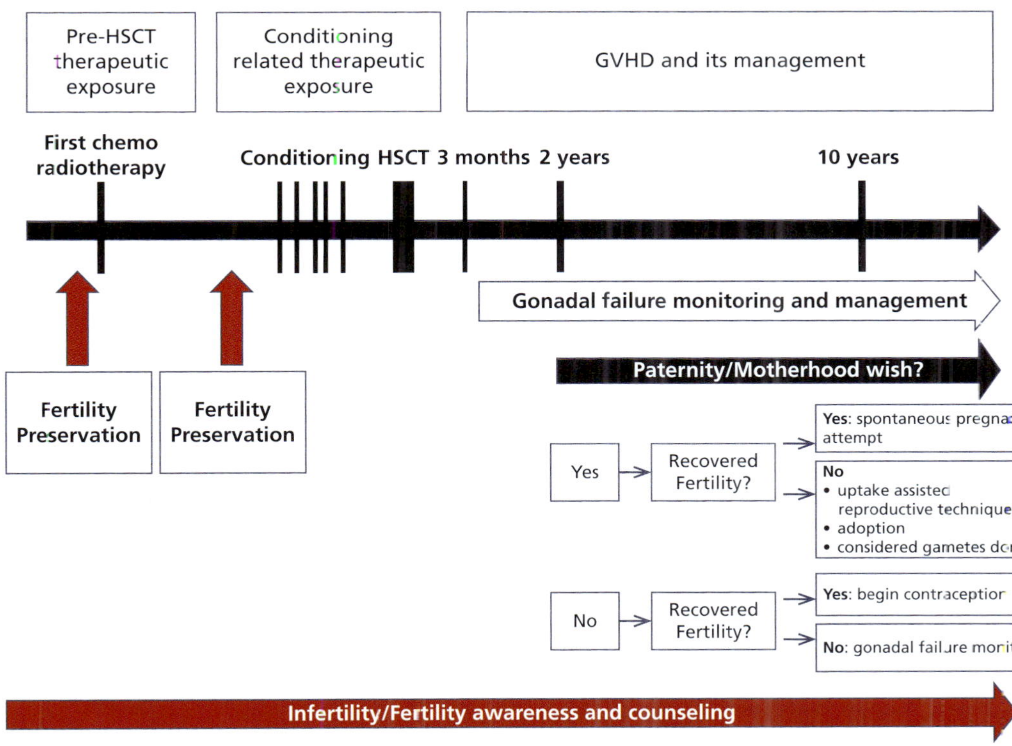

Figure 19.2 Fertility preventive measures and counseling in HSCT. The graphic represents a timeline from first therapy preceding HSCT to long follow-up after transplantation. Factors influencing the appearance of infertility are shown at the top of the graphic. The most effective option to circumvent infertility after HSCT is fertility preservation; thus, the arrows indicate the optimal timing for fertility preservation intervention as well as monitoring of gonadal failure and its management. The main issues to address regarding paternity wishes/contraception after HSCT are also summarized. A general recommendation is to delay spontaneous or assisted pregnancy for at least 2 years after HSCT. Consideration should be given to personalized pre- and posttransplantation fertility counseling conducted by a multidisciplinary team.

preferred options as there have been many successful pregnancies worldwide using these techniques.

Embryo cryopreservation requires that the patient receives hormones timed to her menstrual cycle to stimulate development of eggs which can then be collected and fertilized *in vitro*. This would usually require a delay in treatment of the underlying disease of several weeks and a committed male partner is necessary. For women who lack a partner, one further option is to freeze unfertilized eggs. This still requires a delay in treatment and is not yet considered standard treatment. Initially, oocyte banking was hampered by poor oocyte survival, and low fertilization and pregnancy rates. Recently, however, there have been more encouraging reports of the outcomes of oocyte freezing [46], and worldwide thousands of children have been born using frozen oocytes. Where treatment cannot be delayed it may be possible to obtain ovarian tissue laparoscopically for freezing. This is currently experimental with few successful pregnancies occurring after tissue has been transplanted. Nonetheless, orthotopic reimplantation of ovarian tissue has led to the birth of healthy babies providing proof of concept of this treatment [47]. Ovarian tissue banking is therefore a promising technique and notably provides the opportunity for preserving gonadal function not only in adults but also in prepubertal females undergoing treatment [48]. An additional concern regarding the reimplantation of frozen ovarian cortical strips is the potential to reintroduce malignant cells. In situations where there is a significant worry about ovarian involvement of the underlying disease, cryopreservation of ovarian tissue should be avoided.

In male recipients, cryopreservation of spermatozoa can preserve sperm viability and allows insemination after HSCT. Sperm cryopreservation should be encouraged and offered to all men at risk of infertility, and this should be done at the earliest possible time point. In adolescent boys this method is underutilized partly due to inconsistencies in fertility counseling and unclear guidelines regarding who should bank sperm. In this younger population, production of semen may be possible by masturbation, by penile vibratory stimulation, or rectal-electro stimulation under anesthetic or retrieved by testicular or epididymal aspiration. In prepubertal boys, testicular tissue can theoretically be harvested and cryopreserved with a view to reimplanting germ cells at a later date. Alternatively, spermatogonia can be matured *in vitro* for use in cycles of *in vitro* fertilization [20, 49].

Finally, a general recommendation is to delay spontaneous or assisted pregnancy for at least 2 years after HSCT, as this is the period of highest risk of relapse after HSCT [50].

References

1. Duffy C, Allen S. Medical and psychosocial aspects of fertility after cancer. Cancer J. 2009;15:27–33.
2. Matova N, Cooley L. Comparative aspects of animal oogenesis. Dev Biol. 2001;231:291–320.
3. Perez GI, Robles R, Knudson CM, et al. Prolongation of ovarian lifespan into advanced chronological age by Bax-deficiency. Nat Genet. 1999;21:200–203.
4. Bergeron L, Perez GI, Macdonald G, et al. Defects in regulation of apoptosis in caspase-2-deficient mice. Genes Dev. 1998;12:1304–1314.
5. Wallace WH, Thomson AB. Preservation of fertility in children treated for cancer. Arch Dis Child. 2003;88:493–496.
6. Wallace WH, Thomson AB, Saran F, Kelsey TW. Predicting age of ovarian failure after radiation to a field that includes the ovaries. Int J Radiat Oncol Biol Phys. 2005;62:738–744.
7. Sklar C. Reproductive physiology and treatment-related loss of sex hormone production. Med Pediatr Oncol. 1999; 33:2–8.
8. Socie G, Salooja N, Cohen A, et al. Nonmalignant late effects after allogeneic stem cell transplantation. Blood. 2003;101: 3373–3385.
9. Green DM, Kawashima T, Stovall M, et al. Fertility of female survivors of childhood cancer: a report from the childhood cancer survivor study. J Clin Oncol. 2009;27:2677–2685.
10. Holm K, Nysom K, Brocks V, et al. Ultrasound B-mode changes in the uterus and ovaries and Doppler changes in the uterus after total body irradiation and allogeneic bone marrow transplantation in childhood. Bone Marrow Transplant. 1999;23:259–263.
11. Meirow D. Reproduction post-chemotherapy in young cancer patients. Mol Cell Endocrinol. 2000;169:123–131.
12. Galton DA, Till M, Wiltshaw E. Busulfan (1, 4-dimethanesulfonyloxybutane, myleran); summary of clinical results. Ann N Y Acad Sci. 1958;68:967–973.
13. Koyama H, Wada T, Nishizawa Y, et al. Cyclophosphamide-induced ovarian failure and its therapeutic significance in patients with breast cancer. Cancer. 1977;39:1403–1409.
14. Sanders JE, Buckner CD, Amos D, et al. Ovarian function following marrow transplantation for aplastic anemia or leukemia. J Clin Oncol. 1988;6:813–818.

15. Sanders JE, Hawley J, Levy W, et al. Pregnancies following high-dose cyclophosphamide with or without high-dose busulfan or total-body irradiation and bone marrow transplantation. Blood. 1996;87:3045–3052.
16. Brennan BM, Shalet SM. Endocrine late effects after bone marrow transplant. Br J Haematol. 2002;118:58–66
17. Cohen A, Bekassy AN, Gaiero A, et al. Endocrinological late complications after hematopoietic SCT in children. Bone Marrow Transplant. 2008;41(Suppl 2):S43–S48.
18. Sloand E. Pediatric and adolescent breast health. Lippincotts Prim Care Pract. 1998;2:170–175.
19. Marshall WA, Tanner JM. Variations in pattern of pubertal changes in girls. Arch Dis Child. 1969;44:291–303.
20. Wallace WH, Anderson RA, Irvine DS. Fertility preservation for young patients with cancer: who is at risk and what can be offered? Lancet Oncol. 2005;6:209–218.
21. Patel A, Schwarz B. Cancer and contraception. Release date May 2012. SFP Guideline #20121. Contraception. 2012;86: 191–198.
22. Tichelli A, Rovo A, Passweg J, et al. Late complications after hematopoietic stem cell transplantation. Expert Rev Hematol. 2009;2:583–601.
23. Trottmann M, Becker AJ, Stadler T, et al. Semen quality in men with malignant diseases before and after therapy and the role of cryopreservation. Eur Urol. 2007;52:355–367.
24. Jacob A, Barker H, Goodman A, Holmes J. Recovery of spermatogenesis following bone marrow transplantation. Bone Marrow Transplant. 1998;22:277–279.
25. Anserini P, Chiodi S, Spinelli S, et al. Semen analysis following allogeneic bone marrow transplantation. Additional data for evidence-based counselling. Bone Marrow Transplant. 2002;30:447–451.
26. Savani BN, Kozanas E, Shenoy A, Barrett AJ. Recovery of spermatogenesis after total-body irradiation. Blood. 2006; 108:4292–4293.
27. Rovó A, Tichelli A, Passweg JR, et al. Spermatogenesis in long-term survivors after allogeneic hematopoietic stem cell transplantation is associated with age, time interval since transplantation, and apparently absence of chronic GvHD. Blood. 2006;108:1100–1105.
28. Rovó A, Aljurf M, Chiodi S, et al. Ongoing graft-versus-host disease is a risk factor for azoospermia afterallogeneic hematopoietic stem cell transplantation. A survey of the late effect working party of the European Group for Blood and Marrow Transplantation. Haematologica. 2013;98: 339–345.
29. Howell SJ, Shalet SM. Effect of cancer therapy on pituitary–testicular axis. Int J Androl. 2002;25:269–276.
30. Relander T, Cavallin-Stahl E, Garwicz S, et al. Gonadal and sexual function in men treated for childhood cancer. Med Pediatr Oncol. 2000;35:52–63.
31. World Health Organization. WHO Laboratory Manual for the Examination and Processing of Human Semen. Fifth edition. 2010; Geneva, World Health Organization.
32. Grigg AP, McLachlan R, Zaja J, Szer J. Reproductive status in long-term bone marrow transplant survivors receiving busulfan-cyclophosphamide (120 mg/kg). Bone Marrow Transplant. 2000;26:1089–1095.
33. Wagner AM, Beier K, Christen E, et al. Leydig cell injury as a consequence of an acute graft-versus-host reaction. Blood. 2005;105:2988–2990.
34. Mertens AC, Ramsay NK, Kouris S, Neglia JP. Patterns of gonadal dysfunction following bone marrow transplantation. Bone Marrow Transplant. 1998;22:345–350.
35. Schover LR, Brey K, Lichtin A, et al. Oncologists' attitudes and practices regarding banking sperm before cancer treatment. J Clin Oncol. 2002;20:1890–1897.
36. Schover LR, Brey K, Lichtin A, et al. Knowledge and experience regarding cancer, infertility, and sperm banking in younger male survivors. J Clin Oncol. 2002;20: 1880–1889.
37. Carter A, Robison LL, Francisco L, et al. Prevalence of conception and pregnancy outcomes after hematopoietic cell transplantation: report from the Bone Marrow Transplant Survivor Study. Bone Marrow Transplant. 2006;37: 1023–1029.
38. Salooja N, Szydlo RM, Socie G, et al. Pregnancy outcomes after peripheral blood or bone marrow transplantation: a retrospective survey. Lancet. 2001;358:271–276.
39. Borgmann-Staudt A, Rendtorff R, Reinmuth S, et al. Fertility after allogeneic haematopoietic stem cell transplantation in childhood and adolescence. Bone Marrow Transplant. 2012; 47:271–276.
40. Matias K, Matias C, Teixeira H, et al. Successful pregnancy following busulfan and cyclophosphamide conditioning and allogeneic bone marrow transplantation for chronic myeloid leukemia. Biol Blood Marrow Transplant. 2008; 14:944–945.
41. Atkinson HG, Apperley JF, Dawson K, et al. Successful pregnancy after allogeneic bone marrow transplantation for chronic myeloid leukaemia. Lancet. 1994;344:199.
42. Shah AJ. Successful pregnancy after busulfan/cytoxan conditioning regimen for AML. J Pediatr Hematol Oncol 2011;33:e180–e181.
43. Loren AW, Chow E, Jacobsohn DA, et al. Pregnancy after hematopoietic cell transplantation: a report from the Late Effects Working Committee of the Center for International Blood and Marrow Transplant Research (CIBMTR). Biol Blood Marrow Transplant. 2011;17:157–166.
44. Babb A, Farah N, Lyons C, et al. Uptake and outcome of assisted reproductive techniques in long-term survivors of SCT. Bone Marrow Transplant. 2012;47:568–573.

45. Nakagawa K, Kanda Y, Yamashita H, et al. Preservation of ovarian function by ovarian shielding when undergoing total body irradiation for hematopoietic stem cell transplantation: a report of two successful cases. Bone Marrow Transplant. 2006;37:583–587.
46. The Practice Committees of the American Society for Reproductive Medicine, Society for Assisted Reproductive Technology. Mature oocyte cryopreservation: a guideline. Fertil Steril. 2013;99:37–43.
47. Donnez J, Squifflet J, Jadoul P, et al. Pregnancy and live birth after autotransplantation of frozen-thawed ovarian tissue in a patient with metastatic disease undergoing chemotherapy and hematopoietic stem cell transplantation. Fertil Steril. 2011;95:1787–4.
48. The Practice Committees of the American Society for Reproductive Medicine, Society for Assisted Reproductive Technology. Ovarian tissue and oocyte cryopreservation. Fertil Steril. 2008;90:S241–S246.
49. Keros V, Hultenby K, Borgstrom B, et al. Methods of cryopreservation of testicular tissue with viable spermatogonia in pre-pubertal boys undergoing gonadotoxic cancer treatment. Hum Reprod. 2007;22:1384–1395.
50. Majhail NS, Rizzo JD, Lee SJ, et al. Recommended screening and preventive practices for long-term survivors after hematopoietic cell transplantation. Bone Marrow Transplant. 2012;47:337–341.
51. Rovó A, Aljurf M, Chiodi S, et al. Paternity wishes in long-term survivors after allogeneic hematopoietic SCT. A study of the Late Effects Working Party of the EBMT. Bone Marrow Transplant. 2013; doi: 10.1038/bmt.2012.255. [Epub ahead of print].

20

CHAPTER 20

Follow-up of children after hematopoietic stem cell transplantation: growth and development

Kristina K Hardy[1], *David A Jacobsohn*[2], *and Evelio Perez-Albuerne*[2]

[1]Department of Psychiatry & Behavioral Science, George Washington University, Neuropsychology Division, Children's National Medical Center, Washington, DC, USA
[2]Division of Blood and Marrow Transplantation, Children's National Medical Center, Center for Cancer and Blood Disorders, Washington, DC, USA

Introduction

This chapter focuses on growth and cognitive issues of children undergoing hematopoietic stem cell transplantation (HSCT). The chapter is split into two sections: the first on growth and the second on neurocognitive development.

Part I: Growth

Most pediatric patients undergoing HSCT have not completed their growth. Even in patients who have completed linear growth, HSCT can have long-term effects on other growth processes, such as bone mineralization and body composition. This part will discuss the effects of HSCT on linear growth, final adult height, weight, body composition (lean body mass and fat mass), and bone mineral density (BMD). The effect of patient factors, disease, transplant conditioning, and posttransplant complications on the risk of developing and the magnitude of problems with growth will be examined. Post-HSCT surveillance for these problems and treatment strategies will also be reviewed.

The *Z*-score is commonly used to report values of growth parameters relative to the population age-specific normal distribution. The *Z*-score, also referred to as a standard deviation score, normal score, or standard score, represents the number of standard deviations (SDs) above (if positive) or below (if negative) the population mean of the value of the parameter. For example, a height *Z*-score of −1 indicates a height of one SD below the age-specific mean population height, and a height *Z*-score of +2 indicates a height two SDs above the age-specific mean population height.

Linear growth

The principal site of linear growth is the epiphyseal growth plate (EGP), a cartilaginous area in the long bones where chondrocyte proliferation, deposition of extracellular matrix, chondrocyte apoptosis, osteoblast invasion, and mineralization occur in a programmed

Blood and Marrow Transplantation Long-Term Management: Prevention and Complications, First Edition. Edited by Bipin N Savani.

sequence to lengthen bones [1]. Growth hormone (GH) – mostly through the action of insulin-like growth factor (IGF)-1, but also directly – triiodothyronine (T3), sex hormones, leptin, and other signaling molecules influence growth rate and ultimate closure of the EGP [2, 3]. Decreased linear growth after transplant through direct effects on the EGP has been reported after total body irradiation (TBI) in children [4] and after cyclophosphamide administration in rats [5, 6]. Transplant also affects signaling molecules that influence the EGP. It is clear that many posttransplant patients with poor linear growth have abnormalities in some of these signaling molecules, particularly IGF-1, but in many studies the correlation between low IGF-1 levels and poor linear growth has not been strong. The relative influence of direct damage to the EGP versus damage to the hormone systems that regulate growth is not clear.

There are multiple factors that affect height after transplant, and these factors operate at different time points before, during, or after the transplant. The outcome measure of height or height velocity can be measured shortly after the transplant (1 year or less), at later time points, or the outcome measure can be final adult height. Based on standard growth curves for the US population at age 18 years [7], mean height for men is 176.8 cm, with a standard deviation of 6.7 cm; and mean height for women is 163.7 cm, with a standard deviation of 6.1 cm. The absolute magnitude of a *Z*-score unit at other ages can be calculated by recalling that the 95th percentile of a normal distribution has a *Z*-score of +1.64.

Factors that operate prior to transplant may include congenital underlying conditions treated with HSCT that are associated with decreased height. Studies that examine the effect of transplant on height in these populations are available for thalassemia [8–11], Hurler syndrome [12], and severe immunodeficiency syndromes [13]. The reported *Z*-score magnitude of this effect was −0.32 to −1.99 for thalassemia, −0.1 to −3.2 for Hurler syndrome, and −1.7 to −1.8 for immunodeficiency. For thalassemia and Hurler syndrome patients, those older at the time of transplant had the most negative *Z*-scores. The majority of children with malignant disease are healthy prior to diagnosis, and have a normal height distribution. Studies (in which most patients had leukemia) that measured heights at diagnosis and prior to HSCT showed decreases in height *Z*-scores of −0.02 to −0.5 [14–16].

Most studies have reported low height *Z*-scores immediately after HSCT, with the height at 1 year after HSCT ranging from a *Z*-score of −0.27 to −0.63 [14, 15]. In some reports that also measured pre-transplant height *Z*-scores, there was no significant difference [14]. When heights were measured more than 1 year after transplant, some studies reported *Z*-scores that were improved compared with the immediate posttransplant period, although still below pre-HSCT values [17]. Final height was also lower in several studies [18–25].

In most studies that examined the question, *Z*-scores at later time points or final adult height were significantly lower in patients who received TBI as part of their transplant conditioning [16, 17, 20–22, 26–32]. Exposure to cranial irradiation either before or at the time of transplant was an independent risk factor for poor linear growth and final height in several reports [31, 33, 34]. Other factors associated with poor posttransplant height were a younger age at transplant [21, 26, 29, 33], and significant or prolonged posttransplant complications (including graft-versus-host-disease (GVHD)) [13].

Patients whose indication for transplant was associated with decreased pre-HSCT height can undergo significant catch up growth if they do not have serious or prolonged complications after HSCT and were treated with a nonradiation-containing conditioning regimen. Patients in these groups who were transplanted at a younger age started from a height closer to normal, and also had more improvement in height posttransplant. Patients with thalassemia, all transplanted with nonradiation-containing conditioning regimens, showed improvement in posttransplant height *Z*-scores to values in the range of −0.56 to −0.1 if they were transplanted at age <7 years [9–11]. In a group of patients who mostly had various forms of immunodeficiency and (with one exception) received conditioning containing busulfan and cyclophosphamide, height *Z*-scores improved from −1.7 before HSCT to +0.5 four years after HSCT [13]. In contrast, successfully transplanted patients with Hurler syndrome had height *Z*-scores that continued to decrease [12], likely reflecting the continued effect of enzyme deficiency in tissues not converted to donor genotype with the HSCT.

Some post-HSCT patients had significantly decreased spontaneous or stimulated GH secretion, or IGF-1 levels [22, 24, 27, 28, 30, 31, 35–41]. TBI or especially cranial irradiation was a risk factor for the problem [22, 30, 31, 34]. Despite this association, multiple studies found that the correlation between low IGF-1 levels and decreased height Z-scores was not strong. There were many patients with decreased growth and normal IGF-1 levels, as well as patients with low IGF-1 levels but normal or near the best in the group linear growth [27, 28]. One study [13], which demonstrated catch-up growth in a group of immunodeficiency patients post-HSCT, showed increased IGF-1 levels post-HSCT. Other signaling molecules that affect growth were not examined in sufficient patients to draw meaningful conclusions.

Low IGF-1 levels represent a possible therapeutic target for treatment with exogenous GH. When post-HSCT patients with low Z-scores and IGF-1 levels were treated with GH, several studies reported improvements in growth velocity [27, 31, 35–39] and in final height Z-score compared with earlier Z-scores [36]. The fraction of patients who responded to GH therapy (mostly assessed by change in growth velocity) was variable, ranging from about 50 to 95%. Even responders did not improve growth velocity as much as patients with isolated GH deficiency typically improve with exogenous GH, suggesting that other factors also contributed to poor growth. Improvement with exogenous GH did not seem to differ based on prior radiation exposure. A subset of thalassemia patients who did not respond (no increase in IGF-1 levels and no improvement in height Z-score) to GH had more pathologic liver damage and higher serum ferritin levels than responders did [35].

Body composition

Body composition refers to the mass in various body compartments. Although models with up to four compartments exist, the models used in the studies described below use two compartments: fat mass and fat-free mass. All determinations of body mass in live patients are estimates and can be performed using a variety of techniques, including displacement (e.g., air displacement plethysmography, hydrometry), anthropometry (e.g., skin fold measurements), or radiographic techniques (e.g., dual-energy X-ray absorptiometry (DEXA), CT, magnetic resonance imagining (MRI)). The body mass index (BMI, equal to mass divided by height squared) is an easily calculated value that is often used as a proxy for fat mass. Use as a proxy assumes that the fat-free mass is the same as population normal values, which can be a false assumption in a number of situations, including in post-HSCT patients (see later). The signaling system most studied in association with body composition is insulin and insulin response.

Although it is likely that pre-existing conditions affect body composition prior to pediatric HSCT, there appear to be no published reports describing those populations. As expected because of the nutritional disruption that almost always accompanies HSCT, BMI is decreased shortly after HSCT, as are fat mass and fat-free mass [42]. Some studies reported patients more than 1 year after transplant return to a normal BMI [43–45], while others showed progressive decreases in BMI even as late as 10 years after HSCT [42, 46]. Reported risk factors for decreased BMI include chronic GVHD, older age, T-cell-depleted graft, low pre-transplant BMI [42], and cranial irradiation [44].

Post-HSCT patients with a normal BMI can show a decreased fat-free mass and increased fat mass that add up to a normal total mass. This condition is termed "sarcopenic obesity" and is associated with an increased risk of cardiovascular and metabolic problems in adults [47]. An increased (>0.5) waist circumference to height ratio is associated with abdominal adiposity, which is frequently seen in this condition. This body composition pattern has been reported in post-HSCT patients [43, 44]. Some studies found decreased fat-free mass and normal fat mass [42]. It does not appear that studies linking post-HSCT BMI or body compositions to health outcomes have been published in the literature, but extrapolation from adult studies suggests that these patients may be at increased risk for cardiovascular events. Increased basal insulin levels and decreased insulin responsiveness have been reported in post-HSCT patients, possibly due to the increase in fat mass despite a normal total mass [43, 45, 46, 48, 49].

Bone mineral density

In cohort studies, BMD is highest in late adolescence and young adulthood, and it declines at least slowly thereafter. Those observations have led to the hypothesis that individuals who have low BMD as a young adult will continue to have low BMD as they age, and will therefore be at higher risk for complications of osteoporosis eventually. Low BMD in a pediatric post-HSCT patient may not cause any immediate problems, but it creates a risk of serious health consequences later. BMD is most commonly measured using single photon absorptiometry, dual photon absorptiometry, or DEXA.

The studies discussed below all used DEXA to measure BMD.

Pediatric patients transplanted for malignant disease have low post-HSCT BMD, with *Z*-scores reported from −0.5 to −0.86 [50–52]. Factors associated with low BMD in some studies, but not in others, included exposure to radiation (TBI or craniospinal irradiation), male gender, low fat mass, and younger age at time of HSCT. The presence of GVHD and steroid treatment were not associated with low BMD in these studies [50–53].

In patients with thalassemia major, BMD values were low in patients post-HSCT, but were either similar to or better than BMD values in thalassemia patients receiving chronic transfusion who did not undergo HSCT [54, 55]. Delayed puberty was a risk factor for low BMD in this population.

Post-HSCT patients with low BMD were found to have lower 25-hydroxy-vitamin D levels than post-HSCT patients with BMD *Z*-score greater than −1 [56]. However, it does not appear that a controlled interventional study for low BMD in post-HSCT patients using vitamin D has been reported in the literature. There is one retrospective study comparing chronic GVHD patients on corticosteroids that received bisphosphonate therapy versus those that did not, suggesting that bisphosphonate therapy leads to improvement in BMD [57]. All patients in that study received vitamin D and calcium supplementation.

Summary and recommendations

Many pediatric patients who receive HSCT will have poor linear growth and reduced final adult height after HSCT. Height should be routinely measured and plotted on growth charts during follow-up, and patients with decreased height velocity >1 year after transplant should be evaluated for GH deficiency (including a stimulation test). Patients with deficient GH response (especially those still several years from the onset of puberty) should be referred to pediatric endocrinologists for a discussion of GH therapy. Endocrinologists, patients, and families should be advised that the response to exogenous GH (both fraction of patients responding and magnitude of response) will likely be less than the response seen in patients with isolated GH deficiency.

Patient weights and BMI should also be measured and plotted. Patients with low BMI should be evaluated for nutritional deficiencies. Unfortunately, there do not seem to be any specific interventions for sarcopenic obesity or low fat-free mass whose effectiveness has been documented in the literature. The role of routine body composition measurements is therefore not clear.

Patients should have their BMD measured (preferably by DEXA) after HSCT. Although there are no published studies supporting vitamin D and calcium supplementation in the pediatric post-HSCT group, supplementation is reasonable based on data from the general population. Bisphosphonates may be considered in specific patients, especially those with extremely low BMD and on corticosteroids.

Further information on growth and body composition after HSCT can be found in several recent review articles [58–61].

Part II: Cognitive development and learning

In comparison with knowledge about medical sequelae following HSCT in pediatric populations, relatively little is known about the quality of survivors' cognition and learning. In this part, we will review the extant literature with the following objectives: (1) identifying medical and psychosocial factors associated with transplant which may increase risk for cognitive changes over time, (2) discussing issues with research methodology that complicate our understanding of outcomes in this population, (3) characterizing global patterns of neurocognitive functioning in children receiving HSCT, and (4) describing the areas in need of additional research. Of note, the focus will be generally limited to late-onset neurocognitive changes rather than acute effects on mental status or cognition occurring in connection with a transient illness or drug-associated side effect.

HSCT-related factors that may affect cognitive development

Survivors of HSCT are hypothesized to be vulnerable to declines in cognitive and academic functioning over time, primarily as a consequence of their exposure to agents with known or suspected neurotoxicity. Although conditioning protocols can vary considerably according to diagnosis, a number of children are treated with agents known to increase risk for cognitive decline, such as high-dose chemotherapy and TBI. Neurocognitive outcomes in children treated with some of these agents have been extensively studied, particularly in samples of children treated for acute lymphoblastic leukemia (ALL). Survivors of ALL most frequently demonstrate intellectual functioning within normal limits, but treatment with intrathecal methotrexate and TBI has been associated with increased risk for deficits in processing speed, visual motor function, attention, working memory, and executive function [62–67]. These domains are considered "higher order" functions, largely of the prefrontal cortex, and are typically recruited for complex information processing. Because the areas of the brain responsible for higher order processes continue to develop throughout childhood and adolescence, they are thought to be particularly vulnerable to therapeutic agents that may disrupt the process of myelination [68]. Quantitative MRI studies have generally supported this theory, showing that reduced white matter volumes are correlated with poorer scores on measures of intellectual, academic, and attention functioning [63, 69] in survivors of ALL.

Although less is known about the possibility of neurocognitive late effects associated with other agents (or multi-agent combinations) used in pre-transplant conditioning or for the prevention or treatment of GVHD, the use of high-dose cytotoxic therapies is thought to be a risk factor for cognitive changes over time. It is relatively rare that chronic GVHD affects the central nervous system in children, but the possibility that neurocognitive functioning is also impacted in such cases has been posited in the literature for both pediatric and adult transplant recipients [70, 71]. In addition, long-term use of corticosteroids has been associated with changes in declarative memory and executive functioning in several samples, though the persistence of these changes following discontinuation of therapy is not yet well studied.

Finally, psychosocial factors may also account for cognitive changes in HSCT recipients, at least in the short term. A number of studies have documented that children experience heightened symptoms of anxiety, depression, and traumatic stress beginning in the pre-transplant phase and continuing through the first year following transplant (see also Phipps et al. [72]). Psychiatric symptoms such as these are known to impact neurocognitive functioning, particularly on tasks involving sustained attention, memory, and psychomotor speed. Because HSCT may be associated with lengthy hospital stays and limitations on activities (e.g., school attendance, participation in social and extracurricular activities), it is also possible that these disruptions in the developmental tasks of childhood may also contribute to changes in learning over time [73].

Methodological issues in transplant research with neurocognitive outcomes

In reviewing the relatively scant literature that includes neurocognitive outcomes in samples of HSCT patients, it is critical to note several methodological limitations that frequently characterize published findings and make it more difficult to draw conclusions across patient groups and treatment variables. These issues can be broadly classified into concerns with the study design, the size and composition of the study sample, and the selection and analysis of neurocognitive outcome measures. Collectively, it is likely that these issues account for much of the variability in findings across studies to date.

In terms of study design, although early publications often consisted of small-sample, retrospective reports, more recent studies describe prospective, longitudinal research. However, control groups have been included less often, though some studies have compared HSCT recipients with their healthy siblings (e.g., [74–76]). Samples also are typically quite varied in terms of diagnosis (especially malignant versus nonmalignant disease), type of transplant (autologous versus allogeneic), age at transplant, pre-transplant conditioning regimen, and so on. Even so, there are very little data available about cognitive functioning in certain subgroups of HSCT recipients. This is particularly true for those who have been transplanted with nonmalignant hematological disorders and some genetic or immunological conditions, as they typically are represented in very small numbers that preclude subgroup analysis.

Although long-term survival has increased, morbidity and mortality remain high for some subgroups of HSCT recipients; therefore, several longitudinal studies have small sample sizes and/or high rates of attrition [74, 77, 78]. Even when samples are restricted to children who are at least 1 year posttransplant, it is not uncommon for follow-up evaluations to capture only 30–50% of the original cohort (e.g., [74, 77]). It is important to note that, while attrition is often due to participant mortality over time, several reports documented relatively high rates of refusal or noncompliance (e.g., [78]). Because of this, it is difficult to draw conclusions from studies free from participation bias. Moreover, these studies often have limited statistical power to detect host and treatment variables (e.g., age, sex, socioeconomic status, and the use of total body or cranial radiation) that may moderate cognitive outcomes. Variability in findings may also be attributable to changes in treatment protocols over time, such that outcomes associated with older treatment regimens may no longer apply to children who are treated under modern therapeutic protocols [79]. Indeed, earlier studies tend to report higher rates of neurocognitive decline among young transplant recipients [75, 80], whereas more recent publications document few, if any, cognitive late effects [81, 82].

As has often been the case when evaluating neurocognitive functioning in samples of medically ill children, outcomes have been largely limited to global measures of intellectual functioning (i.e., intellectual quotient (IQ)) or academics. Given that any changes in these domains are thought to be mediated by declines in more specific neuropsychological processes, the relative lack of data measuring processing speed, sustained attention, working memory, and executive functioning limits our ability to characterize a neurocognitive "phenotype" in HSCT recipients with changes in learning over time. Because there are relatively few studies that have evaluated functioning more than 3 years post-HSCT, reliance on global measures of functioning may also mask subtle or emerging changes in neurocognition that may be impairing, even in children whose global intellectual functioning is within normal limits [74, 83].

Finally, the use of many traditional neuropsychological measures in repeated assessments over time can be associated with both practice effects and regression to the mean. In longitudinal studies, assessment of neurocognitive functioning is also complicated by the necessity of using age-appropriate measures. Thus, many participants are evaluated with different assessment tools at different time points in the same study. This leads to a quandary for researchers, who are forced to choose whether to collapse standardized scores for a single domain (e.g., verbal skills) across measures (e.g., [78]), allowing data for all participants and timepoints to be used, or to analyze only scores for participants that have been obtained from administration of the same measure (e.g., [84]).

Neurocognitive functioning following HSCT

A number of recent, larger sample (i.e., $n > 50$) prospective studies of cognitive outcomes in pediatric HSCT recipients reflect relatively stable intellectual functioning from pre-transplant to 1, 2, or 3 years posttransplant [78, 81, 84–87]. Generally speaking, patients transplanted for a variety of malignant and nonmalignant disorders appear to have cognitive functioning within normal limits prior to, and up to 3 years posttransplant. In the largest longitudinal trial to date ($n = 158$), Phipps et al. [78] described a mixed-diagnosis cohort of HSCT recipients evaluated prior to transplant, and 1, 3, and 5 years post HSCT. IQ scores for the sample were somewhat lower than normative samples (standard score mean of 93.7), though the change in slope of scores over time did not significantly differ from pre-transplant to 5 years posttransplant. Moreover, academic achievement scores were also stable for the sample across reading, spelling, and mathematics subject areas. These findings were largely consistent with similar studies of smaller, prospective samples evaluated over 2 years posttransplant [84, 85].

Although the preponderance of evidence indicates that transplant survivors experience few changes in global functioning over time, some specific neurocognitive processes may be more vulnerable to change, however. Both Shah et al. [74] and Smedler et al. [75], for example, described difficulties with visual–motor functioning over time in HSCT recipients. Shah et al. [74]. further described HSCT survivors' declines in verbal and nonverbal reasoning, as well as verbal memory, the latter occurring in participants evaluated 5 years posttransplant. In contrast, other investigators have reported that HSCT survivors demonstrated improved perceptual functioning over time, both compared with their siblings [82] and with their own pre-transplant scores [78].

Despite the variability in findings noted above, some factors have emerged as consistent predictors for post-HSCT neurocognitive decline or stability across studies. Not surprisingly, patients' pre-transplant cognitive functioning is often a critical predictor of later functioning [84, 88, 89]. In relatively large, prospective, longitudinal studies, global intellectual functioning measured during the pre-transplant workup significantly predicted IQ scores at later assessments conducted 1, 2, or 3 years following HSCT [78, 84].

Demographic factors have also significantly predicted neurocognitive outcomes in HSCT recipients. Specifically, a number of studies report that children who are younger at diagnosis and treatment (especially those <3 years of age) are at greater risk for declines in neurocognitive functioning over time [75, 81, 85, 90–92]. Consistent with existing data from healthy children, the socioeconomic status (SES) of patients has also been significantly associated with cognitive outcomes, such that children with lower SES are more likely to have poorer functioning [78]. Finally, maternal depression has also emerged as a predictor of neurocognitive decline in HSCT recipients [86].

Use of TBI as a conditioning agent has been associated with significant cognitive declines in some studies [75, 80], but with only very modest or nonsignificant changes in others [77, 81, 82, 91]. Cranial radiation has been more consistently linked with neurocognitive changes over time when it has been given prior to the transplant process [74, 77, 81, 93, 94], but not when it was used as part of pre-transplant conditioning [90]. Consistent with prior literature, cranial radiation is associated with more significant problems in younger children, particularly with regard to the impact on fine motor functioning [81, 94].

Children receiving HSCT also may present with medical conditions that have affected their neurodevelopment over a span of time prior to transplant. For example, patients with neurodevelopmental conditions (e.g., leukodystrophies) may have developmental delays as part of the phenotype of their disorder, many of which are likely to persist even following successful transplantation. Although the majority of such conditions have not yet been well studied, Prasad et al. [89] examined outcomes from a relatively large sample of children ($n = 159$) receiving HSCT for a variety of inherited metabolic disorders, such as mucopolysaccharidosis types I and III (Hurler's and Krabbe's disease, respectively). In general, those children with lower functioning prior to transplant continued to show difficulties during the posttransplant period; however, many children exhibited stabilization of developmental declines following transplant and were subsequently able to make some gains in functioning. The authors noted that children with diagnoses associated with progressive delays who were transplanted in early infancy tended to have better developmental outcomes than those who had already acquired significant cognitive delay at the time of transplant, a finding that supported prior results from small-sample studies [95, 96]. In particular, transplantation of infants with Krabbe's disease prior to the onset of symptoms has been associated with better cognitive outcomes than when HSCT occurs after symptoms are manifest.

Another subgroup of children increasingly receiving HSCT are those with severe combined immune deficiency (SCID). Two recent reports have been published describing HSCT recipients with SCID; in both, patients with SCID demonstrated intellectual functioning that was slightly below normal limits at least 1 year post-transplant [76, 97]. Lin et al. [97] noted that children in their study did make gains in skills over time, just at a slower rate than would be expected. In addition, Titman et al. [76] found that, whereas age at transplantation and conditioning regiment were not associated with poorer outcomes, children with adenosine deaminase-deficient SCID and consanguinity exhibited worse functioning.

Studies of long-term survivorship are rare, and thus little is known about the stability or change in cognitive functioning in adults who received HSCT as children or adolescents. In the largest study to date, Sanders et al. [98] examined quality of life outcomes in 214 adult survivors of childhood hematopoietic cell transplantation compared with 197 sibling controls. Neurocognitive functioning was evaluated indirectly, through self-reported questionnaire measures. Although no differences were found between survivors and siblings for everyday memory functioning, survivors reported a significantly greater number of neurobehavioral symptoms particularly with regard to expressive and receptive language skills. Consistent with some of the findings from prospective studies described above, a number of demographic and medical factors were associated with the scope and severity of self-reported neurocognitive symptoms. Specifically, survivors who were transplanted at <13 years of age and those who received more therapy (including cranial radiation) prior to transplant were more likely to report memory difficulties. Both females and individuals who received more pre-transplant therapies (e.g., second remission or relapse therapy) were more likely to report greater neurobehavioral symptoms. Of interest, there were no differences in reported cognition or memory as a function of diagnosis, conditioning regimen, chronic GVHD, or donor type.

Areas in need of further research

As described, much of the recent literature indicates that HSCT recipients generally show few lasting changes in global cognition over time. There remain gaps in our knowledge that should be addressed by future researchers so that families and physicians considering HSCT can be fully informed about potential risks associated with certain disease and treatment groups. Of critical importance is the need for prospective research with samples of children that are increasingly receiving HSCT, including children with sickle-cell disease, immunodeficiencies, and a host of other metabolic and genetic disorders. Given that specific neurocognitive processes (e.g., working memory, attention, processing speed) are increasingly identified as areas vulnerable to decline in the presence of disease or cytotoxic treatment in children, it will also be important to include a broader range of neurocognitive outcomes than the global measures of intelligence and academic functioning that have been frequently reported [83]. Finally, children undergoing HSCT are at increased risk for psychiatric morbidity, including anxiety and depression, both prior to and up to a year following the procedure (see also Ref. [99]). Both anxiety and depression also can impact neurocognitive functioning [100, 101], though the extent to which psychological factors may be associated with variability in neurocognitive outcomes is not well documented in this population [79]. For children who do experience declines in the quality of their thinking and learning, more information is needed as to timing and trajectory of neurocognitive decline relative to survivors' baseline functioning, as well as the disease, treatment, and sociodemographic predictors of change over time.

Conclusions

Existing literature evaluating cognitive sequelae of HSCT is sparse and characterized by relatively small, medically heterogeneous samples that often lack baseline data, prospective design, or longitudinal follow-up. Still, the preponderance of the evidence indicates that the majority of HSCT recipients experience few, if any, neurocognitive consequences associated with transplant, at least with regard to global intellectual functioning. Some notable exceptions that have been reported frequently in the literature include children who are younger at the time of transplant and those who receive cranial radiation prior to HSCT. In addition, children who are lower functioning at time of transplant, particularly those with disease- or treatment-related cognitive dysfunction, are more likely to have poorer cognitive outcomes over time. Although TBI was once regarded as a risk factor for neurocognitive late effects, the majority of well-designed, longitudinal studies have not supported this. Despite the generally positive prognosis, future research is needed to better characterize the onset, severity, and course of neurocognitive difficulties in affected individuals. Finally, it is important to continue to study HSCT preparative regimens (i.e., reduced-intensity conditioning) that may be associated with reducing toxicities, including neurocognitive.

References

1. Burdan F, Szumilo J, Korobowicz A, et al. Morphology and physiology of the epiphyseal growth plate. Folia Histochem Cytobiol. 2009;47(1):5–16. Epub 2009/05/08.
2. Gat-Yablonski G, Yackobovitch-Gavan M, Phillip M. Nutrition and bone growth in pediatrics. Pediatr Clin North Am. 2011;58(5):1117–1140, ix. Epub 2011/10/11.
3. Siebler T, Robson H, Shalet SM, Williams GR. Glucocorticoids, thyroid hormone and growth hormone interactions: implications for the growth plate. Horm Res. 2001;56(Suppl 1):7–12. Epub 2002/01/12.
4. Miyazaki O, Nishimura G, Okamoto R, et al. Induction of systemic bone changes by preconditioning total body irradiation for bone marrow transplantation. Pediatr Radiol. 2009;39(1):23–29. Epub 2008/10/28.
5. Xian CJ, Cool JC, van Gangelen J, et al. Effects of etoposide and cyclophosphamide acute chemotherapy on growth plate and metaphyseal bone in rats. Cancer Biol Ther. 2007;6(2):170–177. Epub 2007/01/16.
6. Zilberman O, Narsman M, Forsberg CM, Sven L. Effects of cyclophosphamide on the femoral epiphyseal growth plate in young Sprague-Dawley rats. Acta Odontol Scand. 2002;60(4):208–212. Epub 2002/09/12.
7. Hamill PV, Drizd TA, Johnson CL, et al. Physical growth: National Center for Health Statistics percentiles. Am J Clin Nutr. 1979;32(3):607–629. Epub 1979/03/01.
8. De Simone M, Olioso P, Di Bartolomeo P, et al. Growth and endocrine function following bone marrow transplantation for thalassemia. Bone Marrow Transplant. 1995;15(2):227–233. Epub 1995/02/01.
9. De Simone M, Verrotti A, Iughetti L, et al. Final height of thalassemic patients who underwent bone marrow transplantation during childhood. Bone Marrow Transplant. 2001;28(2):201–205. Epub 2001/08/18.

10. Li CK, Chik KW, Wong GW, et al. Growth and endocrine function following bone marrow transplantation for thalassemia major. Pediatr Hematol Oncol. 2004;21(5):411–419. Epub 2004/06/19.
11. Khoshniat M, Ghavamzadeh A, Larijani B, et al. Effect on growth parameters of bone marrow transplantation with a chemotherapy-only conditioning regimen. Transplant Proc. 2003;35(8):3085–3088. Epub 2003/12/31.
12. Polgreen LE, Tolar J, Plog M, et al. Growth and endocrine function in patients with Hurler syndrome after hematopoietic stem cell transplantation. Bone Marrow Transplant. 2008;41(12):1005–1011. Epub 2008/02/19.
13. Adan L, de Lanversin ML, Thalassinos C, et al. Growth after bone marrow transplantation in young children conditioned with chemotherapy alone. Bone Marrow Transplant. 1997;19(3):253–256. Epub 1997/02/01.
14. Afify Z, Shaw PJ, Clavano-Harding A, Cowell CT. Growth and endocrine function in children with acute myeloid leukaemia after bone marrow transplantation using busulfan/cyclophosphamide. Bone Marrow Transplant. 2000;25(10):1087–1092. Epub 2000/06/01.
15. Arvidson J, Lonnerholm G, Tuvemo T, et al. Prepubertal growth and growth hormone secretion in children after treatment for hematological malignancies, including autologous bone marrow transplantation. Pediatr Hematol Oncol. 2000;17(4):285–297. Epub 2000/06/09.
16. Hovi L, Saarinen-Pihkala UM, Vettenranta K, et al. Growth in children with poor-risk neuroblastoma after regimens with or without total body irradiation in preparation for autologous bone marrow transplantation. Bone Marrow Transplant. 1999;24(10):1131–1136. Epub 1999/12/01.
17. Cohen A, Duell T, Socie G, et al. Nutritional status and growth after bone marrow transplantation (BMT) during childhood: EBMT Late-Effects Working Party retrospective data. European Group for Blood and Marrow Transplantation. Bone Marrow Transplant. 1999;23(10):1043–1047. Epub 1999/06/18.
18. Bernard F, Bordigoni P, Simeoni MC et al. Height growth during adolescence and final height after haematopoietic SCT for childhood acute leukaemia: the impact of a conditioning regimen with BU or TBI. Bone Marrow Transplant. 2009;43(8):637–642. Epub 2008/11/18.
19. Chemaitilly W, Boulad F, Heller G, et al. Final height in pediatric patients after hyperfractionated total body irradiation and stem cell transplantation. Bone Marrow Transplant. 2007;40(1):29–35. Epub 2007/05/01.
20. Clement-De Boers A, Oostdijk W, Van Weel-Sipman MH, et al. Final height and hormonal function after bone marrow transplantation in children. J Pediatr. 1996; 129(4):544–550. Epub 1996/10/01.
21. Cohen A, Rovelli A, Bakker B, et al. Final height of patients who underwent bone marrow transplantation for hematological disorders during childhood: a study by the Working Party for Late Effects-EBMT. Blood. 1999;93(12):4109–4115. Epub 1999/06/11.
22. Cohen A, Rovelli A, Van-Lint MT, et al. Final height of patients who underwent bone marrow transplantation during childhood. Arch Dis Child. 1996;74(5):437–440. Epub 1996/05/01.
23. Couto-Silva AC, Trivin C, Esperou H, et al. Final height and gonad function after total body irradiation during childhood. Bone Marrow Transplant. 2006;38(6):427–432. Epub 2006/08/01.
24. Sanders JE, Guthrie KA, Hoffmeister PA, et al. Final adult height of patients who received hematopoietic cell transplantation in childhood. Blood. 2005;105(3):1348–1354. Epub 2004/09/30.
25. Shinagawa T, Tomita Y, Ishiguro H, et al. Final height and growth hormone secretion after bone marrow transplantation in children. Endocr J. 2001;48(2):133–138. Epub 2001/07/18.
26. Bakker B, Massa GG, Oostdijk W, et al. Pubertal development and growth after total-body irradiation and bone marrow transplantation for haematological malignancies. Eur J Pediatr. 2000;159(1–2):31–37. Epub 2000/02/01.
27. Brauner R, Adan L, Souberbielle JC, et al. Contribution of growth hormone deficiency to the growth failure that follows bone marrow transplantation. J Pediatr. 1997; 130(5):785–792. Epub 1997/05/01.
28. Brauner R, Fontoura M, Zucker JM, et al. Growth and growth hormone secretion after bone marrow transplantation. Arch Dis Child. 1993;68(4):458–463. Epub 1993/04/01.
29. Couto-Silva AC, Trivin C, Esperou H, et al. Bone markers after total body irradiation in childhood. Bone Marrow Transplant. 2010;45(3):437–441. Epub 2009/08/18.
30. Couto-Silva AC, Trivin C, Esperou H, et al. Changes in height, weight and plasma leptin after bone marrow transplantation. Bone Marrow Transplant. 2000;26(11):1205–1210. Epub 2001/01/10.
31. Giorgiani G, Bozzola M, Locatelli F, et al. Role of busulfan and total body irradiation on growth of prepubertal children receiving bone marrow transplantation and results of treatment with recombinant human growth hormone. Blood. 1995;86(2):825–831. Epub 1995/07/15.
32. Liesner RJ, Leiper AD, Hann IM, Chessells JM. Late effects of intensive treatment for acute myeloid leukemia and myelodysplasia in childhood. J Clin Oncol. 1994 12(5):916–924. Epub 1994/05/01.
33. Frisk P, Arvidson J, Gustafsson J, Lonnerholm G. Pubertal development and final height after autologous bone marrow transplantation for acute lymphoblastic leukemia.

Bone Marrow Transplant. 2004;33(2):205–210. Epub 2003/11/25.

34. Huma Z, Boulad F, Black P, et al. Growth in children after bone marrow transplantation for acute leukemia. Blood. 1995;86(2):819–824. Epub 1995/07/15.
35. De Simone M, Di Bartolomeo P, Olioso P, et al. Growth after recombinant human growth hormone (rhGH) treatment in transplanted thalassemic patients. Bone Marrow Transplant. 1997;20(7):567–573. Epub 1997/10/23.
36. Isfan F, Kanold J, Merlin E, et al. Growth hormone treatment impact on growth rate and final height of patients who received HSCT with TBI or/and cranial irradiation in childhood: a report from the French Leukaemia Long-Term Follow-Up Study (LEA). Bone Marrow Transplant. 2012;47(5):684–693. Epub 2011/07/05.
37. Olshan JS, Willi SM, Gruccio D, Moshang T Jr. Growth hormone function and treatment following bone marrow transplant for neuroblastoma. Bone Marrow Transplant. 1993;12(4):381–385. Epub 1993/10/01.
38. Papadimitriou A, Urena M, Hamill G, et al. Growth hormone treatment of growth failure secondary to total body irradiation and bone marrow transplantation. Arch Dis Child. 1991;66(6):689–692. Epub 1991/06/01.
39. Polgreen LE, Plog M, Schwender JD, et al. Short-term growth hormone treatment in children with Hurler syndrome after hematopoietic cell transplantation. Bone Marrow Transplant. 2009;44(5):279–285. Epub 2009/03/03.
40. Bakker B, Oostdijk W, Bresters D, et al. Disturbances of growth and endocrine function after busulphan-based conditioning for haematopoietic stem cell transplantation during infancy and childhood. Bone Marrow Transplant. 2004;33(10):1049–1056. Epub 2004/03/30.
41. Sanders JE, Pritchard S, Mahoney P, et al. Growth and development following marrow transplantation for leukemia. Blood. 1986;68(5):1129–1135. Epub 1986/11/01.
42. Inaba H, Yang J, Kaste SC, et al. Longitudinal changes in body mass and composition in survivors of childhood hematologic malignancies after allogeneic hematopoietic stem-cell transplantation. J Clin Oncol. 2012;30(32):3991–3997. Epub 2012/10/04.
43. Neville KA, Cohn RJ, Steinbeck KS, et al. Hyperinsulinemia, impaired glucose tolerance, and diabetes mellitus in survivors of childhood cancer: prevalence and risk factors. J Clin Endocrinol Metab. 2006;91(11):4401–4407. Epub 2006/09/07.
44. Nysom K, Holm K, Michaelsen KF, et al. Degree of fatness after allogeneic BMT for childhood leukaemia or lymphoma. Bone Marrow Transplant. 2001;27(8):817–820. Epub 2001/07/31.
45. Shalitin S, Phillip M, Stein J, et al. Endocrine dysfunction and parameters of the metabolic syndrome after bone marrow transplantation during childhood and adolescence. Bone Marrow Transplant. 2006;37(12):1109–1117. Epub 2006/05/16.
46. Tomita Y, Ishiguro H, Yasuda Y, et al. High incidence of fatty liver and insulin resistance in long-term adult survivors of childhood SCT. Bone Marrow Transplant. 2011;46(3):416–425. Epub 2010/06/22.
47. Prado CM, Wells JC, Smith SR, et al. Sarcopenic obesity: a critical appraisal of the current evidence. Clin Nutr. 2012;31(5):583–601. Epub 2012/07/20.
48. Frisk P, Rossner SM, Norgren S, et al. Glucose metabolism and body composition in young adults treated with TBI during childhood. Bone Marrow Transplant. 2011;46(10):1303–1308. Epub 2010/12/15.
49. Taskinen M, Saarinen-Pihkala UM, Hovi L, Lipsanen-Nyman M. Impaired glucose tolerance and dyslipidaemia as late effects after bone-marrow transplantation in childhood. Lancet. 2000;356(9234):993–997. Epub 2000/10/21.
50. Bhatia S, Ramsay NK, Weisdorf D, et al. Bone mineral density in patients undergoing bone marrow transplantation for myeloid malignancies. Bone Marrow Transplant. 1998;22(1):87–90. Epub 1998/07/25.
51. Kaste SC, Shidler TJ, Tong X, et al. Bone mineral density and osteonecrosis in survivors of childhood allogeneic bone marrow transplantation. Bone Marrow Transplant. 2004;33(4):435–441. Epub 2004/01/13.
52. Nysom K, Holm K, Michaelsen KF, et al. Bone mass after allogeneic BMT for childhood leukaemia or lymphoma. Bone Marrow Transplant. 2000;25(2):191–196. Epub 2000/02/16.
53. Ruble K, Hayat MJ, Stewart KJ, Chen AR. Bone mineral density after bone marrow transplantation in childhood: measurement and associations. Biol Blood Marrow Transplant. 2010;16(10):1451–1457. Epub 2010/04/27.
54. Bielinski BK, Darbyshire PJ, Mathers L, et al. Impact of disordered puberty on bone density in beta-thalassaemia major. Br J Haematol. 2003;120(2):353–358. Epub 2003/01/25.
55. Leung TF, Hung EC, Lam CW, et al. Bone mineral density in children with thalassaemia major: determining factors and effects of bone marrow transplantation. Bone Marrow Transplant. 2005;36(4):331–336. Epub 2005/06/22.
56. Frisk P, Arvidson J, Ljunggren O, Gustafsson J. Decreased bone mineral density in young adults treated with SCT in childhood: the role of 25-hydroxyvitamin D. Bone Marrow Transplant. 2012;47(5):657–662. Epub 2011/07/19.
57. Carpenter PA, Hoffmeister P, Chesnut CH III, et al. Bisphosphonate therapy for reduced bone mineral density in children with chronic graft-versus-host disease. Biol Blood Marrow Transplant. 2007;13(6):683–690. Epub 2007/05/29.

58. Ranke MB, Schwarze CP, Dopfer R, et al. Late effects after stem cell transplantation (SCT) in children – growth and hormones. Bone Marrow Transplant. 2005;35(Suppl 1): S77–S81. Epub 2005/04/07.
59. Rogers PC, Meacham LR, Oeffinger KC, et al. Obesity in pediatric oncology. Pediatr Blood Cancer. 2005;45(7):881–891. Epub 2005/07/22.
60. Sanders JE. Growth and development after hematopoietic cell transplant in children. Bone Marrow Transplant. 2008;41(2):223–227. Epub 2007/10/09.
61. Shalet SM, Brennan BM. Growth and growth hormone status after a bone marrow transplant. Horm Res. 2002; 58(Suppl 1):86–90. Epub 2002/10/10.
62. Campbell LK, Scaduto M, Sharp W, et al. A meta-analysis of the neurocognitive sequelae of treatment for childhood acute lymphocytic leukemia. Pediatr Blood Cancer. 2007; 49(1):65–73. Epub 2006/04/22.
63. Carey ME, Haut MW, Reminger SL, et al. Reduced frontal white matter volume in long-term childhood leukemia survivors: a voxel-based morphometry study. AJNR Am J Neuroradiol. 2008;29(4):792–797. Epub 2008/01/11.
64. Mennes M, Stiers P, Vandenbussche E, et al. Attention and information processing in survivors of childhood acute lymphoblastic leukemia treated with chemotherapy only. Pediatr Blood Cancer. 2005;44(5):478–486. Epub 2005/05/27.
65. Peterson CC, Johnson CE, Ramirez LY, et al. A meta-analysis of the neuropsychological sequelae of chemotherapy-only treatment for pediatric acute lymphoblastic leukemia. Pediatr Blood Cancer. 2008;51(1):99–104. Epub 2008/03/07.
66. Ashford J, Schoffstall C, Reddick WE, et al. Attention and working memory abilities in children treated for acute lymphoblastic leukemia. Cancer. 2010;116(19):4638–4645. Epub 2010/06/24.
67. Jain N, Brouwers P, Okcu MF, et al. Sex-specific attention problems in long-term survivors of pediatric acute lymphoblastic leukemia. Cancer. 2009;115(18):4238–4245. Epub 2009/06/19.
68. Khong PL, Leung LH, Fung AS, et al. White matter anisotropy in post-treatment childhood cancer survivors: preliminary evidence of association with neurocognitive function. J Clin Oncol. 2006;24(6):884–890. Epub 2006/02/18.
69. Reddick WE, Shan ZY, Glass JO, et al. Smaller white-matter volumes are associated with larger deficits in attention and learning among long-term survivors of acute lymphoblastic leukemia. Cancer. 2006;106(4):941–949. Epub 2006/01/18.
70. Grauer O, Wolff D, Bertz H, et al. Neurological manifestations of chronic graft-versus-host disease after allogeneic haematopoietic stem cell transplantation: report from the Consensus Conference on Clinical Practice in chronic graft-versus-host disease. Brain. 2010;133(10):2852–2865. Epub 2010/09/18.
71. Sostak P, Padovan CS, Yousry TA, et al. Prospective evaluation of neurological complications after allogeneic bone marrow transplantation. Neurology. 2003;60(5):842–848. Epub 2003/03/12.
72. Phipps S, Dunavant M, Lensing S, Rai SN. Acute health-related quality of life in children undergoing stem cell transplant: II. Medical and demographic determinants. Bone Marrow Transplant. 2002;29(5):435–442. Epub 2002/03/29.
73. Shah AJ, Rosser T, Goodarzian F. Neurologic sequealae of hematopoietic stem cell transplantation (HSCT). In: Demirer T, (ed). New Advances in Stem Cell Transplantation. Rijeka: InTech, 2012; pp. 517–532.
74. Shah AJ, Epport K, Azen C, et al. Progressive declines in neurocognitive function among survivors of hematopoietic stem cell transplantation for pediatric hematologic malignancies. J Pediatr Hematol Oncol. 2008;30(6):411–418. Epub 2008/06/06.
75. Smedler AC, Ringden K, Bergman H, Bolme P. Sensory-motor and cognitive functioning in children who have undergone bone marrow transplantation. Acta Paediatr Scand. 1990;79(6–7):613–621. Epub 1990/06/01.
76. Titman P, Pink E, Skucek E, et al. Cognitive and behavioral abnormalities in children after hematopoietic stem cell transplantation for severe congenital immunodeficiencies. Blood. 2008;112(9):3907–3913. Epub 2008/07/23.
77. Kramer JH, Crittenden MR, DeSantes K, Cowan MJ. Cognitive and adaptive behavior 1 and 3 years following bone marrow transplantation. Bone Marrow Transplant. 1997;19(6):607–613. Epub 1997/03/02.
78. Phipps S, Rai SN, Leung WH, et al. Cognitive and academic consequences of stem-cell transplantation in children. J Clin Oncol. 2008;26(12):2027–2033. Epub 2008/04/19.
79. Tremolada M, Bonichini S, Pillon M, et al. Quality of life and psychosocial sequelae in children undergoing hematopoietic stem-cell transplantation: a review. Pediatr Transplant. 2009;13(8):955–970. Epub 2009/06/12.
80. McGuire T, Sanders JE, Hill JD, et al. Neuropsychological function in children given total-body irradiation for marrow transplantation. Exp Hematol. 1991;19:578 (abstract).
81. Phipps S, Dunavant M, Srivastava DK, et al Cognitive and academic functioning in survivors of pediatric bone marrow transplantation. J Clin Oncol. 2000;18(5):1004–1011. Epub 2000/03/01.
82. Barrera M, Atenafu E. Cognitive, educational, psychosocial adjustment and quality of life of children who survive

hematopoietic SCT and their siblings. Bone Marrow Transplant. 2008;42(1):15–21. Epub 2008/04/01.
83. Bingen K, Schroedl RL, Anderson L, et al. A multimethod assessment of psychosocial functioning and late effects in survivors of childhood cancer and hematopoietic cell transplant. J Pediatr Hematol Oncol. 2012;34(1):22–28. Epub 2011/11/16.
84. Kupst MJ, Penati B, Debban B, et al. Cognitive and psychosocial functioning of pediatric hematopoietic stem cell transplant patients: a prospective longitudinal study. Bone Marrow Transplant. 2002;30(9):609–617. Epub 2002/10/31.
85. Simms S, Kazak AE, Golomb V, et al. Cognitive, behavioral, and social outcome in survivors of childhood stem cell transplantation. J Pediatr Hematol Oncol. 2002;24(2):115–119. Epub 2002/05/07.
86. Barrera M, Atenafu E, Andrews GS, Saunders F. Factors related to changes in cognitive, educational and visual motor integration in children who undergo hematopoietic stem cell transplant. J Pediatr Psychol. 2008;33(5):536–546. Epub 2007/10/27.
87. Arvidson J, Larsson B, Lonnerholm G. A long-term follow-up study of psychosocial functioning after autologous bone marrow transplantation in childhood. Psychooncology. 1999;8(2):123–134. Epub 1999/05/21.
88. Phipps S, Brenner M, Heslop H, et al. Psychological effects of bone marrow transplantation on children and adolescents: preliminary report of a longitudinal study. Bone Marrow Transplant. 1995;15(6):829–835. Epub 1995/06/01.
89. Prasad VK, Mendizabal A, Parikh SH, et al. Unrelated donor umbilical cord blood transplantation for inherited metabolic disorders in 159 pediatric patients from a single center: influence of cellular composition of the graft on transplantation outcomes. Blood. 2008;112(7):2979–2989. Epub 2008/07/01.
90. Kramer JH, Crittenden MR, Halberg FE, et al. A prospective study of cognitive functioning following low-dose cranial radiation for bone marrow transplantation. Pediatrics. 1992;90(3):447–450. Epub 1992/09/01.
91. Chou RH, Wong GB, Kramer JH, et al. Toxicities of total-body irradiation for pediatric bone marrow transplantation. Int J Radiat Oncol Biol Phys. 1996;34(4):843–851. Epub 1996/03/01.
92. Levy JM, Tello T, Giller R, et al. Late effects of total body irradiation and hematopoietic stem cell transplant in children under 3 years of age. Pediatr Blood Cancer. 2012;(4):700–704. Epub 2012/08/01.
93. Smedler AC, Nilsson C, Bolme P. Total body irradiation: a neuropsychological risk factor in pediatric bone marrow transplant recipients. Acta Paediatr. 1995;84(3):325–330. Epub 1995/03/01.
94. Cool VA. Long-term neuropsychological risks in pediatric bone marrow transplant: what do we know? Bone Marrow Transplant. 1996;18(Suppl 3):S45–S49. Epub 1996/12/01.
95. Escolar ML, Poe MD, Provenzale JM, et al. Transplantation of umbilical-cord blood in babies with infantile Krabbe's disease. N Engl J Med. 2005;352(20):2069–2081. Epub 2005/05/20.
96. Staba SL, Escolar ML, Poe M, et al. Cord-blood transplants from unrelated donors in patients with Hurler's syndrome. N Engl J Med. 2004;350(19):1960–1969. Epub 2004/05/07.
97. Lin M, Epport K, Azen C, et al. Long-term neurocognitive function of pediatric patients with severe combined immune deficiency (SCID): pre- and post-hematopoietic stem cell transplant (HSCT). J Clin Immunol. 2009;29(2):231–237. Epub 2008/09/23.
98. Sanders JE, Hoffmeister PA, Storer BE, et al. The quality of life of adult survivors of childhood hematopoietic cell transplant. Bone Marrow Transplant. 2010;45(4):746–754. Epub 2009/09/01.
99. Packman W, Weber S, Wallace J, Bugescu N. Psychological effects of hematopoietic SCT on pediatric patients, siblings and parents: a review. Bone Marrow Transplant. 2010;45(7):1134–1146. Epub 2010/04/13.
100. Bishop SJ. Neurocognitive mechanisms of anxiety: an integrative account. Trends Cogn Sci. 2007;11(7):307–316. Epub 2007/06/08.
101. Mayberg S. Visions, values, and our future. Behav Healthc Tomorrow. 1997;6(6):47–48. Epub 1997/11/03.

CHAPTER 21

Posttransplant diabetes mellitus: monitoring, prevention, and management guidelines

Prathima Jasti, Shichun Bao, and Shubhada Jagasia
Division of Diabetes, Endocrinology, and Metabolism, Department of Medicine, Vanderbilt University Medical Center, Nashville, TN, USA

Introduction

Hematopoietic stem cell transplant (HSCT) has evolved as a curative therapy over the past few decades, for hematologic and lymphoid malignancies as well as non-malignant conditions. With advances in the science of transplantation, the life expectancy of transplant patients is increasing. Overall survival at 5 years for those who were disease-free for 2 years or more after allogeneic stem cell transplant was found to be 89%, with much longer survival for those who received autologous transplant [1]. As the number of long-term survivors of HSCT increase, there is growing recognition of cardiovascular and metabolic complications [2]. Exposure to chemotherapy before and during the transplantation period, as well as prolonged immunosuppressive therapy, increases the risk of chronic health conditions. Posttransplant diabetes mellitus (PTDM) is a major long-term complication of HSCT that can affect the graft status and overall prognosis of a transplant patient. Diabetes is a cardiovascular risk equivalent similar to peripheral vascular disease, cerebrovascular accident, abdominal aortic aneurysm, and chronic kidney disease with absolute risk of subsequent cardiovascular events of more than 20% over 10 years. Early identification and management of diabetes in these patients is therefore important among all members of the multifaceted teams that follow these patients. This chapter elaborates the pathogenesis and the diagnostic and therapeutic strategies of PTDM.

Epidemiology

Prevalence

Major epidemiological studies on long-term survivors report prevalence of PTDM from 7 to 17%, with higher rates in the first 1–2 years after transplantation [3]. Continued immunosuppressive treatment is associated with higher prevalence of diabetes. The bone marrow transplant survivor study is a large epidemiological retrospective study of HSCT survivors and healthy sibling controls reporting the long-term complications and functional status 2 years after transplant through a well-validated patient questionnaire. This study showed a prevalence of new-onset diabetes after transplant of 7.6% in 1089 HSCT survivors followed for a mean of 8.6 years, excluding those who were on continued immunosuppression. There was no significant increase in the risk of diabetes in recipients of autologous transplant compared with siblings, yet the odds ratio for diabetes in

Blood and Marrow Transplantation Long-Term Management: Prevention and Complications, First Edition. Edited by Bipin N Savani.

allogeneic transplant recipients was 3.65 compared with age, sex, and body mass index (BMI) matched sibling controls [2]. Recent investigation on a mixed cohort of adult and pediatric HSCT transplant recipients showed that 32% of patients with diabetes in the early posttransplantation period had persistent disease at the 2-year anniversary [4]. In addition to overt diabetes, impaired glucose tolerance (IGT) was also reported at higher rates, especially in survivors of allogeneic transplantation. In a study on adult and pediatric leukemia survivors, IGT was reported in 26% of transplant survivors, in contrast to 8% in non-transplanted controls and none in healthy controls [5].

Risk factors

In addition to traditional risk factors for type 2 diabetes like older age, obesity, minority ethnicity, metabolic syndrome, family history of diabetes, and history of smoking, there are some factors unique to the transplant status. The major risk factors attributed to PTDM are allogeneic transplant, exposure to total body irradiation (TBI), nonwhite race, older age at transplant as well as at follow up, and higher BMI. Baker et al. reported a 3.42-fold increased risk of diabetes associated with exposure to TBI and over twofold increased risk with nonwhite ethnicity [2]. Smaller studies in childhood survivors of bone marrow transplant also showed increased risk of diabetes as well as insulin resistance with TBI [6, 7]. Majhail et al. showed that cumulative prednisone dose of 0.25 mg/kg daily is a risk factor for diabetes in this population [4]. In a recent prospective study on 84 patients, our group showed that elevated pre-transplantation c-peptide level (>3.6 ng/mL) is a risk factor for PTDM in the immediate posttransplant period as well as an independent predictor of overall survival [8]. Chronic graft versus host disease (cGVHD) has been shown to increase risk of insulin resistance [5], but major studies failed to show association with diabetes [2, 9]. This indicates that increased risk of diabetes with cGVHD is possibly due to effect of immunosuppressants used rather than the disease itself. Role of donor type (related versus unrelated) is also controversial. Several studies in the solid organ transplant population confirmed that higher pre-transplantation insulin levels, elevated random blood glucose, and impaired fasting glucose (IFG) levels are associated with development of PTDM, but data in the HSCT group are lacking [10].

Pathogenesis

Pathogenesis of posttransplant diabetes shares features of both type 1 and type 2 diabetes with insulin deficiency and insulin resistance, respectively. The main defect is likely relative insulin deficiency as seen in type 2 diabetes due to mismatch between insulin production and insulin requirement. Factors such as inflammation and medications used in transplant patients seem to accelerate the rate of development of relative insulin deficiency.

Pathogenesis of type 2 diabetes

The normal pancreatic β cell compensates for decrease in insulin action by increasing insulin synthesis and vice versa [11]. Deviation from this relation occurs when β cell function is inadequate for a specific degree of insulin sensitivity and results in IGT and subsequently type 2 diabetes. Thus, β cell dysfunction is the crucial mechanism in the pathogenesis of type 2 diabetes. In addition, sustained hyperglycemia can cause inflammation and worsen β cell function and insulin resistance, commonly referred to as glucose toxicity [12]. Type 2 diabetes is characterized by a combination of resistance to insulin action in the skeletal muscle, adipose tissue and liver, and pancreatic β cell dysfunction.

Inflammation and role of T regulatory cells

Inflammatory and immunologic mechanisms involved in allogeneic HSCT play a key role in the development of insulin resistance and diabetes mellitus. T regulatory cells (Tregs), which are the immunosuppressive subset of $CD4^+$ T cells, are implicated in the prevention of autoimmune diseases and inhibition of autoimmune responses. Recently, Tregs ($CD4^+$ $CD25^+$ T lymphocytes) have been associated with improvements in adipose tissue inflammation, whereas conventional T cells ($CD8^+$ effector T cells) promote release of inflammatory cytokines from adipose tissue macrophages [13]. After allo-stem cell transplant (allo-SCT), patients with fewer Tregs may be more prone to insulin resistance and PTDM as well as poor overall survival [8]. Increased gut homing and decreased skin homing of Tregs have been demonstrated in early PTDM, which could be implicated in underlying insulin resistance [14]. CD26 is a membrane-associated glycoprotein with intrinsic dipeptidyl peptide IV (DPP IV) activity, expressed on $CD4^+$ T lymphocytes and implicated in the regulation of T cell migration and cytokine activation. The principal action of DPP IV is degradation of incretin hormones, namely glucagon-like peptide (GLP-1) and glucose-dependant insulinotropic polypeptide. The incretin hormones, secreted from the gut after an oral glucose load have favorable effects on carbohydrate metabolism like stimulation of insulin secretion, delaying gastric emptying as well as promoting β cell regeneration and preventing β cell apoptosis [15]. Previous studies in mice showed that inhibiting the activity of DPP IV enzyme helps improvement of diabetes by increasing regulatory T cells and also GLP-1 levels [16, 17].

Immunosuppressants

Corticosteroids are commonly used for myeloablation and for treatment of GVHD owing to their anti-inflammatory effects. Steroid-induced hyperglycemia is caused by both decreased β-cell insulin production and insulin resistance; that is, reduced effectiveness of insulin in suppressing hepatic glucose production and in increasing glucose uptake in muscle and fatty tissue (Figure 21.1). Insulin resistance is mediated through post-insulin-receptor effects on skeletal muscle cells [18].

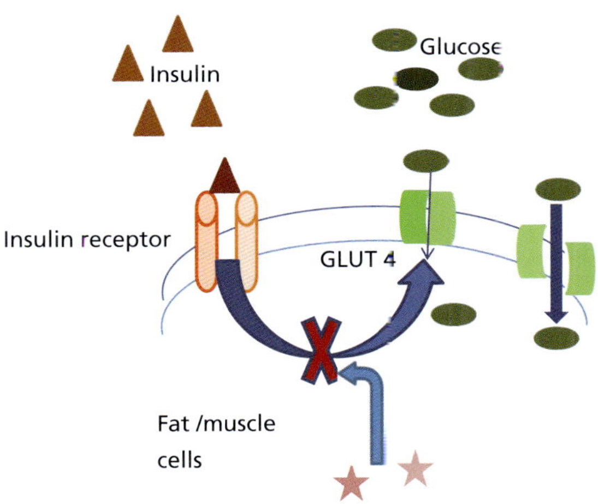

Figure 21.1 Effect of glucocorticoids on insulin action. Glucocorticoids inhibit peripheral glucose uptake through the glucose transporter (GLUT 4), whose action is mediated by insulin. This leads to insulin resistance in fat and muscle cells. Redrawn from: http://dtc.ucsf.edu/types-of-diabetes/type1/understanding-type-1-diabetes/how-the-body-processes-sugar/blood-sugar-other-hormones/.

Systemic absorption of local steroids like budesonide and beclomethasone can be increased in patients with altered mucosal integrity as a result of GVHD [19]. Tacrolimus (prograf) and cyclosporine inhibit the T cell activator protein calcineurin, thereby suppressing T cell activation and cytokine gene expression. Tacrolimus has a more deleterious effect on glucose metabolism than cyclosporine. Both these agents cause morphological and functional abnormalities in pancreatic islet cells, resulting in decreased insulin synthesis and secretion. Effects of tacrolimus are dose dependent and also reversible [20]. Mycophenolate mofetil inhibits purine synthesis, whereas sirolimus is a macrolide antibiotic that inhibits the protein kinase mammalian target of rapamycin (mTOR). Risk of PTDM with mycophenolate and sirolimus is inconclusive. Animal studies demonstrated islet cell dysfunction when sirolimus is used alone or in conjunction with calcineurin inhibitors [20].

Screening and diagnosis

Improved life expectancy after transplantation places this group of patients at risk of microvascular complications from diabetes, and early diagnosis is therefore beneficial in preventing long-term complications. Consensus guidelines [21] for solid organ transplant recipients recommend using American Diabetes Association (ADA)–World Health Organization (WHO) criteria for diagnosis of diabetes, as shown in Table 21.1. In the absence of unequivocal hyperglycemia, tests should be confirmed with venous plasma glucose on another day. The revised ADA criteria define IFG as fasting plasma glucose (FPG)

Table 21.1 WHO and ADA criteria for diagnosis of diabetes (from Ref. [48])

Criteria
Random plasma glucose[a] ≥200 mg/dL (11.1 mM) with symptoms of diabetes (polyuria, polydipsia, unexplained weight loss)
OR
Fasting plasma glucose[b] ≥126 mg/dL (7.0 mM)
OR
2 h postprandial glucose after 75 g oral glucose tolerance test (OGTT) ≥200 mg/dL

[a]Random glucose is measured at anytime with no meal relation.
[b]Fasting glucose is measured after 8 h of caloric restriction.

of 100–125 mg/dL and IGT as 2-h postprandial glucose of 140–199 mg/dL [22]. Even though ADA revised the diagnostic criteria in 2009 to include hemoglobin A1C ≥ 6.5%, its use in the transplant population can cause spurious results due to anemia and repeated blood transfusions. Fructosamine is another less commonly used biomarker of glycemia, which measures glycated serum albumin. It gives an estimate of short-term glycemic control in the past 2–4 weeks and is not affected by hemoglobinopathies, red cell turnover, or recent blood transfusions [23].

Screening for diabetes should be an integral part of initial pre-transplantation evaluation. A detailed history regarding symptoms of diabetes, previous history of pre-diabetes, steroid-induced diabetes or gestational diabetes, smoking, obesity, hyperlipidemia, and family history of diabetes or cardiovascular disease should be obtained. FPG should be measured and followed periodically to identify individuals with IFG so that appropriate intervention to reduce their future risk of diabetes can be undertaken [21]. All patients should be counseled regarding the risk of PTDM and the importance of lifestyle modifications to prevent weight gain.

Monitoring

Some patients may have resolution of hyperglycemia when tapered off of corticosteroids but will continue to have a lifelong increased risk of developing diabetes, for which they should be monitored annually. Solid organ transplant guidelines recommend measurement of random glucose at regular intervals when immunosuppressant drug levels are measured. In addition, the expert panel on renal transplant population recommends measurement of FPG every week for the first 4 weeks after transplant, then once every 3 months up to 1 year and then yearly [21]. The OGTT should be done in individuals with normal FPG but suspected IGT. Since HSCT patients share many features of the solid organ transplant population, these guidelines can be adopted in recipients of SCT, until specific guidelines are created for this population.

Patients who develop diabetes should undergo annual screening for microalbuminuria, dilated eye exam, and foot evaluation, owing to their increased risk of nephropathy, retinopathy, and neuropathy, respectively [22]. A yearly fasting lipid panel and regular monitoring of blood pressure should follow the general guidelines for diabetes patients [22]. Hemoglobin A1C should be monitored at least twice yearly or every 3 months if changes in medication are made. Caveats to this testing should be considered when interpreting the results, as mentioned in the "Screening and diagnosis" section.

Prevention

The transplant population is predisposed to insulin resistance, hypertension, and hyperlipidemia that together with hyperglycemia compose the metabolic syndrome and promote atherosclerosis and cardiovascular events. It is therefore prudent for physicians to emphasize the importance of early screening and measures to prevent hyperglycemia in this population.

The main steps of PTDM prevention include identification of patients at risk before transplantation and controlling modifiable risk factors pre- and posttransplantation. Patients with metabolic risk factors including obesity, dyslipidemia, hypertension, and pre-diabetes should be counseled on lifestyle modification, which is the most effective preventive therapy, as shown in several diabetes prevention studies [24–26] and should be considered the first-line treatment. Changes in lifestyle, including diet modification, weight loss, and regular exercise, slow the progression to diabetes. The beneficial effects appear to continue after the original intervention. Regular reinforcement of these benefits is important for successful compliance. Metformin therapy can be considered in individuals with pre-diabetes who have other risk factors for diabetes prior to HSCT, but is usually discontinued after HSCT, owing to compromised renal function, increased risk of lactic acidosis, and interaction with cyclosporine. Patients who smoke should be encouraged to stop smoking. Patients who drink alcohol excessively should be encouraged to limit alcohol consumption to one drink a day for females and two drinks a day for males per ADA guidelines [22]. Blood pressure and lipids (especially low-density lipoprotein) should be controlled to the recommended target levels of 130/80 mmHg and 100 mg/dL, respectively [22].

The two immunosuppressive agents most responsible for PTDM are glucocorticoids and tacrolimus. Thus, in affected patients, the dose of those agents should be decreased as soon as possible [27].

Management

Prevention of PTDM, early detection, and appropriate treatment of patients with new-onset diabetes are key considerations in the management of transplant recipients as this can ameliorate the long-term complications. Several large trials have shown that intensive glycemic control in type 1 and type 2 diabetics has significant benefits in preventing long-term complications, including retinopathy, nephropathy, and cardiovascular events, especially when treated early in the course of the disease [28, 29]. Since patients with PTDM are also at similar risk of long-term complications, management guidelines and glycemic targets can be based on ADA guidelines for general diabetics. There are no comparative trials on oral agents or insulin used to treat patients with PTDM. As a result, treatment decisions should be based on individual patient age, life expectancy, safety, efficacy, and tolerability. In the immediate posttransplant period, insulin therapy is the safest option given the risk of acute decompensation, renal or hepatic insufficiency, variability in appetite and oral intake, and alterations in steroid and anti-rejection medications. Oral agents can be considered in the long-term management. Comprehensive cardiovascular risk reduction should be the major focus of management. Adjustment of the immunosuppressive regimen should be strongly considered in consultation with the transplant physician, and this decision should be made after carefully weighing the risks of hyperglycemia and rejection. Lowering corticosteroid dose and switching tacrolimus to cyclosporine in renal transplant patients has shown beneficial effect on glucose metabolism [30].

Therapeutic lifestyle modification

The international consensus guidelines on solid organ transplant recipients recommend a stepwise approach to manage new-onset diabetes after transplant, beginning with lifestyle modification and then adding oral hypoglycemic agents or insulin in case of worsening hyperglycemia [20]. But in reality, dietary restriction is difficult in transplant patients who may be already malnourished due to prior chemotherapy as well as gastrointestinal GVHD. Some of these patients also have restricted exercise capacity due to steroid myopathy or anemia. Nevertheless, referral to a dietician and diabetes educator specialized in diabetes is recommended to emphasize the importance of appropriate diet, weight control, and education on self-monitoring of blood glucose. Hematocrit of patients should be kept in mind when choosing a glucose meter as only some of them have higher sensitivities at lower hematocrit values [31]. Avoidance of simple carbohydrates and moderate intensity exercise of at least 150 min per week is encouraged.

Insulin

We consider use of insulin as the safest and most effective approach for achieving rapid glycemic control in patients with PTDM who are on high-dose corticosteroids or have profound hyperglycemia [3]. Insulin has no known interactions with drugs used in transplant patients. A patient-centered approach should be adopted while choosing an insulin regimen, with consideration given to literacy level and complexity. Once-daily basal insulin, with either insulin glargine or detemir, helps reduce fasting hyperglycemia. Bolus or meal-time doses with short-acting insulins like regular, lispro, aspart, or glulisine are used for postprandial hyperglycemia, which is often encountered because of insulin resistance in these patients. Owing to variable oral intake and renal dysfunction causing decreased insulin clearance and risk of hypoglycemia, meal-time insulin can be dosed based on carbohydrate intake or taken at the end of the meal, if intake is variable based on nausea or decreased appetite. Premixed insulin is a suboptimal alternative in patients who cannot deal with multiple daily injections, as it poses a risk of wider blood glucose fluctuations and difficulty in titration due to variable peak and duration of action. Patients on short-term high-dose corticosteroids benefit from short-acting insulin alone.

Oral hypoglycemic agents

No large comparative studies have confirmed the safety of oral hypoglycemic agents in transplant patients. Though metformin and sulfonylureas are the first-line oral agents in the treatment of type 2 diabetes, their use in PTDM is cautioned owing to frequently encountered renal and hepatic impairment. Metformin carries risk of lactic acidosis due to frequent intravenous contrast administration for imaging purposes and interaction with cyclosporine [3]. Second-generation sulfonylureas like glimepiride and glipizide have been shown to be associated with less risk of severe hypoglycemia when compared with glibenclamide [32]. Hypoglycemia risk with sulfonylureas is further increased in the case of GVHD of gut leading to limited oral intake. The meglitinide analogues (repaglinide and nateglinide) are non-sulfonylurea insulin secretagogues which are administered with meals and are a safer alternative in this situation owing to shorter duration of action and absence of interaction with immunosuppressants. Since epidemiological and clinical studies showed postprandial glucose as an independent risk factor for cardiovascular disease [33], lowering this with meglitinides will have favorable long-term effects. Evidence exists that repaglinide has less weight gain and hypoglycemia effect than glyburide does [34]. Animal studies have shown that rosiglitazone (thiazolidinedione) protects against the pancreatic β cell death induced by cyclosporine [35]. Small clinical studies also confirmed an insulin sensitizing effect in the transplant population with only mild edema as a side effect and no weight gain [36]. But owing to the adverse effect of liver toxicity, weight gain, and controversial effect on cardiovascular events [37], we do not recommend using these agents in PTDM.

The newer classes of drugs which act through the incretin hormones, secreted by intestine, are glucagon-like peptide-1 (GLP-1) agonists and dipeptidyl peptidase-4 (DPP-4) inhibitors. GLP-1 is rapidly degraded by the enzyme DPP-4, and hence DPP-4 inhibitors prolong the action of incretin hormones. Randomized control studies showed similar reduction in hemoglobin A1C with GLP-1 agonists when compared with insulin glargine in poorly controlled type 2 diabetes mellitus [38]. GLP-1 agonists may cause decreased absorption of immunosuppressive agents due to delayed gastric emptying, and hence their levels need to be more frequently monitored [3]. These agents are contraindicated in patients with low glomerular filtration rate. Use of DPP-4 inhibitors in the renal transplant population with new-onset diabetes has shown significant decrease in hemoglobin A1C levels without altering levels of tacrolimus, sirolimus, or glomerular filtration rate and no major side effects [39]. Confirmation of their safety and efficacy in larger populations is needed.

Bile acid binding resins (colestipol, colesevelam) have only a modest effect on lowering blood glucose and are limited by gastrointestinal side effects and interference with absorption of drugs, including cyclosporine. Alpha-glucosidase inhibitors, which mainly reduce postprandial hyperglycemia by decreasing glucose absorption in the gastrointestinal tract, are also associated with bloating and gastrointestinal intolerance, especially in those with gut GVHD. We recommend against the use of both these classes of medications in PTDM. A summary of oral agents used in treating diabetes is given in Table 21.2.

Combination oral therapy can also be used, but caution is advised to avoid hypoglycemia. The most commonly used combination is metformin and sulfonylurea.

Glycemic targets

Hemoglobin A1C goal for most nonpregnant adults is <7%, with less stringent levels for those at high risk of hypoglycemia, limited life expectancy, or extensive co-morbid conditions. Fasting blood glucose of 70–130 mg/dL and postprandial glucose (1–2 h after meal) of <180 mg/dL without significant hypoglycemia are most desirable. These guidelines are based on standards of medical care in diabetes published by the ADA [22].

Hypoglycemia is a major limiting factor for the control of diabetes. When severe, this can lead to major adverse events, including seizures, coma, and death. Education regarding the signs and symptoms of hypoglycemia, like palpitations, diaphoresis, dizziness, confusion, and tremor, should be an essential part of management of diabetes. Treatment with glucose (15–20 g) is the usual approach for a conscious individual, whereas glucagon injection by a family member is needed if the patient is unable to treat themselves. Self-monitoring of glucose and appropriate balance of insulin use, carbohydrate intake, and exercise are necessary for preventing hypoglycemia. Patients should be encouraged to carry a carbohydrate source at all times and also to check their glucose prior to driving or operating heavy machinery.

Other associated co-morbidities

Diabetes complications observed in nontransplant patients with diabetes are also observed in PTDM [40]. Therefore, routine care recommended for nontransplant patients to prevent microvascular and macrovascular complications should also be applied to PTDM patients.

Table 21.2 Summary of major oral hypoglycemic drugs (adapted from Refs [12, 21])

Class of drugs	Mechanism of action	Advantages	Disadvantages	Special considerations
Biguanides (metformin)	• Inhibition of hepatic glucose production • Decreased intestinal glucose absorption	• No weight gain • No hypoglycemia	• Gastrointestinal side effects • Lactic acidosis (rare) • Vitamin B12 defeciency	• Contraindicated in renal failure • Risk of lactic acidosis increased with frequent intravenous contrast administration
Sulfonylureas (glyburide, glipizide, glimepiride)	• Closure of K_{ATP} channels on β cell membrane and stimulation of insulin secretion	• Rapid reduction of fasting glucose • Low cost	• Weight gain • Increased risk of hypoglycemia	• Increased risk of hypoglycemia in liver and kidney dysfunction
Thiazolidinediones (pioglitazone, rosiglitazone)	• Activation of nuclear transcription factor PPAR-γ, increasing peripheral insulin sensitivity	• No hypoglycemia • Lowering of triglycerides, increases high-density lipoprotein	• Slow onset of action • Weight gain • Edema • Osteoporosis • Heart failure	• Controversial risk of cardiovascular adverse events • Have anti-inflammatory properties by reducing circulating concentrations of cytokines
Meglitinides (repaglinide, nateglinide)	• Closure of K_{ATP} channels on β cell membrane and stimulation of insulin secretion	• Short duration of action • Less risk of hypoglycemia	• Weight gain • Need for multiple doses	• Useful in reducing postprandial hyperglycemia
GLP-1 agonists (exenatide, liraglutide)	• Glucose-dependent increase in insulin secretion and decrease in glucagon secretion • Delay in gastric emptying	• Weight reduction by increasing satiety	• Gastrointestinal side effects, pancreatitis; medullary thyroid tumors in animals • High cost • Only available in injectable form	• May decrease absorption of immunosuppressive drugs • May worsen symptoms in patients with GVHD of gut
DPP-4 inhibitors (sitagliptan, saxagliptan, linagliptan)	• Inhibition of degradation of GLP-1, hence increasing insulin secretion	• No hypoglycemia	• Pancreatitis • Long-term efficacy not known	• Small studies in transplant population show beneficial effects

GLP-1: glucagon-like peptide-1; DPP-4: dipeptidyl peptidase-4.

Transplant recipients who develop PTDM have an increased risk for metabolic syndrome and cardiovascular diseases [3]. The most significant consequences of PTDM include decreased patient survival and decreased allograft survival [41, 42], an increased risk of infectious complications, and morbid cardiovascular events.

A cohort analysis based on an HSCT survivor study showed a 2.06-fold higher prevalence of hypertension compared with a group of siblings, matched for gender, sex, race, and BMI [2]. An allogeneic group had a higher risk of new-onset dyslipidemia (relative risk: 2.31) and hypertension (relative risk: 2.5) compared with an autologous group [43]. A cross-sectional study of 86 adult allogeneic HSCT patients showed a 49% prevalence of metabolic syndrome, which was a 2.2-fold increase compared with age- and sex-matched controls [44]. An Italian cohort study on 85 HSCT survivors in complete remission at 5 years demonstrated 34% prevalence of metabolic syndrome compared with 15% in the general population [45]. Metabolic syndrome places HSCT patients at increased risk of cardiovascular complications. The risk of premature death resulting from cardiac complications in HSCT patients was 2.3-fold higher than the US general population [46]. Therefore, dyslipidemia and hypertension should be treated as strictly as in non-transplant diabetes as per guidelines [22]. Detailed management of dyslipidemia in PTDM will be discussed in Chapter 25.

Multiple acute rejection episodes have also been demonstrated to be a risk factor for cardiovascular complications [47]. Thus, individual tailoring of immunosuppressive therapy is important with the aim of controlling PTDM and reducing cardiovascular diseases.

Summary and recommendations

• Increase in life expectancy of HSCT recipients has led to higher prevalence of chronic health conditions.
• Prevalence of PTDM ranges from 7 to 17% in several epidemiological studies.
• Risk factors specific for PTDM include allogeneic transplant, age at transplant, treatment with TBI, prednisone dose of greater than 0.25 mg/(kg day), BMI, and nonwhite race.
• Pathogenesis of PTDM involves relative loss of β cell function and increased insulin resistance from effect of immunosuppressive agents and inflammation.
• Prevention and early treatment of PTDM is a crucial step in the reduction of cardiovascular mortality associated with this condition.
• Diagnosis is based on ADA criteria for the general population, with either random plasma glucose ≥200 mg/dL or FPG ≥126 mg/dL or hemoglobin A1C ≥6.5%, confirmed by repeat venous blood sample in the case of absence of unequivocal response.
• Regular monitoring of FPG helps in early identification of new-onset diabetes.
• Insulin is the preferred treatment in the short term, and oral hypoglycemic agents can be used in long term.
• Choice of hypoglycemic agents depends on the individual patient's age, renal and hepatic function, presence of cGVHD, oral intake, and tolerability.
• Lowering steroid dose and switching from tacrolimus to cyclosporine is highly beneficial.
• Yearly monitoring for microvascular complications of diabetes is recommended.
• In addition to overt diabetes, HSCT recipients are also at higher risk of developing metabolic syndrome and IGT. Treatment of these conditions by lifestyle modification is beneficial in preventing or delaying the onset of diabetes.

References

1. Baker KS, Armenian S, Bhatia S. Long-term consequences of hematopoietic stem cell transplantation: current state of the science. Biol Blood Marrow Transplant. 2010;16: S90–S96.
2. Baker KS, Ness KK, Steinberger J, et al. Diabetes, hypertension, and cardiovascular events in survivors of hematopoietic cell transplantation: a report from the bone marrow transplantation survivor study. Blood. 2007;109: 1765–1772.
3. Griffith ML, Jagasia M, Jagasia SM. Diabetes mellitus after hematopoietic stem cell transplantation. Endocr Pract. 2010;16:699–706.
4. Majhail NS, Challa TR, Mulrooney DA, et al. Hypertension and diabetes mellitus in adult and pediatric survivors of allogeneic hematopoietic cell transplantation. Biol Blood Marrow Transplant. 2009;15:1100–1107.
5. Taskinen M, Saarinen-Pihkala UM, Hovi L, Lipsanen-Nyman M. Impaired glucose tolerance and dyslipidaemia as late effects after bone-marrow transplantation in childhood. Lancet. 2000;356:993–997.
6. Traggiai C, Stanhope R, Nussey S, Leiper AD. Diabetes mellitus after bone marrow transplantation during childhood. Med Pediatr Oncol. 2003;40:128–129.
7. Lorini R, Cortona L, Scaramuzza A, et al. Hyperinsulinemia in children and adolescents after bone marrow transplantation. Bone Marrow Transplant. 1995;15:873–877.
8. Griffith ML, Jagasia MH, Misfeldt AA, et al. Pretransplantation C-peptide level predicts early posttransplantation diabetes mellitus and has an impact on survival after allogeneic stem cell transplantation. Biol Blood Marrow Transplant. 2011;17:86–92.
9. Baker KS, Gurney JG, Ness KK, et al. Late effects in survivors of chronic myeloid leukemia treated with hematopoietic cell transplantation: results from the Bone Marrow Transplant Survivor Study. Blood. 2004;104:1898–1906.
10. Shehab-Eldin W, Shoker A. Predictors of new onset of diabetes after transplantation in stable renal recipients. Nephron Clin Pract. 2008;110:c1–c9.
11. Bergman RN. Lilly lecture 1989. Toward physiological understanding of glucose tolerance. Minimal-model approach. Diabetes. 1989;38:1512–1527.
12. Stumvoll M, Goldstein BJ, van Haeften TW. Type 2 diabetes: principles of pathogenesis and therapy. Lancet. 2005;365: 1333–1346.

13. Nishimura S, Manabe I, Nagasaki M, et al. CD8+ effector T cells contribute to macrophage recruitment and adipose tissue inflammation in obesity. Nat Med. 2009;15:914–920.
14. Engelhardt BG, Jagasia SM, Crowe JE Jr, et al. Predicting posttransplantation diabetes mellitus by regulatory T-cell phenotype: implications for metabolic intervention to modulate alloreactivity. Blood. 2012;119:2417–2421.
15. Drucker DJ. The biology of incretin hormones. Cell Metab. 2006;3:153–165.
16. Kim SJ, Nian C, McIntosh CH. Sitagliptin (MK0431) inhibition of dipeptidyl peptidase IV decreases nonobese diabetic mouse CD4+ T-cell migration through incretin-dependent and -independent pathways. Diabetes. 2010; 59:1739–1750.
17. Tian L, Gao J, Hao J, et al. Reversal of new-onset diabetes through modulating inflammation and stimulating beta-cell replication in nonobese diabetic mice by a dipeptidyl peptidase IV inhibitor. Endocrinology. 2010;151:3049–3060.
18. Rizza RA, Mandarino LJ, Gerich JE. Cortisol-induced insulin resistance in man: impaired suppression of glucose production and stimulation of glucose utilization due to a postreceptor detect of insulin action. J Clin Endocrinol Metab. 1982;54:131–138.
19. Dilger K, Halter J, Bertz H, et al. Pharmacokinetics and pharmacodynamic action of budesonide after buccal administration in healthy subjects and patients with oral chronic graft-versus-host disease. Biol Blood Marrow Transplant. 2009;15:336–343.
20. Subramanian S, Trence DL. Immunosuppressive agents: effects on glucose and lipid metabolism. Endocrinol Metab Clin North Am. 2007;36:891–905, vii.
21. Davidson J, Wilkinson A, Dantal J, et al. New-onset diabetes after transplantation: 2003 international consensus guidelines. Proceedings of an international expert panel meeting. Barcelona, Spain, 19 February 2003. Transplantation. 2003; 75:SS3–SS24.
22. American Diabetes Association. Standards of medical care in diabetes – 2012. Diabetes Care. 2012;35(Suppl 1): S11–S63.
23. True MW. Circulating biomarkers of glycemia in diabetes management and implications for personalized medicine. J Diabetes Sci Technol. 2009;3:743–747.
24. Pan XR, Li GW, Hu YH, et al. Effects of diet and exercise in preventing NIDDM in people with impaired glucose tolerance. The Da Qing IGT and Diabetes Study. Diabetes Care. 1997;20:537–544.
25. Tuomilehto J, Lindstrom J, Eriksson JG, et al. Prevention of type 2 diabetes mellitus by changes in lifestyle among subjects with impaired glucose tolerance. N Engl J Med. 2001;344:1343–1350.
26. Knowler WC, Barrett-Connor E, Fowler SE, et al. Reduction in the incidence of type 2 diabetes with lifestyle intervention or metformin. N Engl J Med. 2002;346:393–403.
27. Duclos A, Flechner LM, Faiman C, Flechner SM. Post-transplant diabetes mellitus: risk reduction strategies in the elderly. Drugs Aging. 2006;23:781–793.
28. UK Prospective Diabetes Study (UKPDS) Group. Intensive blood-glucose control with sulphonylureas or insulin compared with conventional treatment and risk of complications in patients with type 2 diabetes (UKPDS 33). Lancet. 1998;352:837–853.
29. Nathan DM, Cleary PA, Backlund JY, et al. Intensive diabetes treatment and cardiovascular disease in patients with type 1 diabetes. N Engl J Med. 2005;353:2643–2653.
30. Wyzgal J, Oldakowska-Jedynak U, Paczek L, et al. Posttransplantation diabetus mellitus under calcineurin inhibitor. Transplant Proc. 2003;35:2216–2218.
31. Tang Z, Lee JH, Louie RF, Kost GJ. Effects of different hematocrit levels on glucose measurements with handheld meters for point-of-care testing. Arch Pathol Lab Med. 2000;124:1135–1140.
32. Holstein A, Plaschke A, Egberts EH. Lower incidence of severe hypoglycaemia in patients with type 2 diabetes treated with glimepiride versus glibenclamide Diabetes Metab Res Rev. 2001;17:467–473.
33. Bonora E, Muggeo M. Postprandial blood glucose as a risk factor for cardiovascular disease in type II diabetes: the epidemiological evidence. Diabetologia. 2001;44:2107–2114.
34. Marbury T, Huang WC, Strange P, Lebovitz H. Repaglinide versus glyburide: a one-year comparison trial. Diabetes Res Clin Pract. 1999;43:155–166.
35. Kim JW, Yang JH, Park HS, et al. Rosiglitazone protects the pancreatic beta-cell death induced by cyclosporine A. Biochem Biophys Res Commun. 2009;390:763–768.
36. Villanueva G, Baldwin D. Rosiglitazone therapy of post-transplant diabetes mellitus. Transplantation. 2005;80: 1402–1405.
37. Scheen AJ. Outcomes and lessons from the PROactive study. Diabetes Res Clin Pract. 2012;98:175–186.
38. Heine RJ, Van Gaal LF, Johns D, et al. Exenatide versus insulin glargine in patients with suboptimally controlled type 2 diabetes: a randomized trial Ann Intern Med 2005;143:559–569.
39. Lane JT, Odegaard DE, Haire CE, et al. Sitagliptin therapy in kidney transplant recipients with new-onset diabetes after transplantation. Transplantation. 2011;92:e56–e57.
40. Burroughs TE, Swindle J, Takemoto S, et al. Diabetic complications associated with new-onset diabetes mellitus in renal transplant recipients. Transplantation. 2007;83: 1027–1034.

41. Miles AM, Sumrani N, Horowitz R, et al. Diabetes mellitus after renal transplantation: as deleterious as non-transplant-associated diabetes? Transplantation. 1998;65:380–384.
42. Jindal RM, Hjelmesaeth J. Impact and management of posttransplant diabetes mellitus. Transplantation. 2000;70: SS58–SS63.
43. Majhail NS, Flowers ME, Ness KK, et al. High prevalence of metabolic syndrome after allogeneic hematopoietic cell transplantation. Bone Marrow Transplant. 2009;43:49–54.
44. Tichelli A, Bucher C, Rovo A, et al. Premature cardiovascular disease after allogeneic hematopoietic stem-cell transplantation. Blood. 2007;110:3463–3471.
45. Annaloro C, Usardi P, Airaghi L, et al. Prevalence of metabolic syndrome in long-term survivors of hematopoietic stem cell transplantation. Bone Marrow Transplant. 2008; 41:797–804.
46. Bhatia S, Francisco L, Carter A, et al. Late mortality after allogeneic hematopoietic cell transplantation and functional status of long-term survivors: report from the Bone Marrow Transplant Survivor Study. Blood. 2007;110: 3784–3792.
47. Fellstrom B. Risk factors for and management of post-transplantation cardiovascular disease. Biodrugs. 2001;15: 261–278.
48. Expert Committee on the Diagnosis and Classification of Diabetes Mellitus. Report of the Expert Committee on the Diagnosis and Classification of Diabetes Mellitus. Diabetes Care. 2003;26(Suppl 1):S5–S20.

CHAPTER 22

Thyroid disease: monitoring and management guidelines

M Kathleen Figaro[1], *Cheryl A Fassler*[2], *Shubhada Jagasia*[1], *and Vipul T Lakhani*[1]

[1]Division of Diabetes, Endocrinology & Metabolism, Vanderbilt University Medical Center, Nashville, TN, USA

[2]University of Tennessee Health Science Center/Baptist Hospital, Nashville, TN, USA

Background

Hematopoietic allogeneic stem-cell transplantation (allo-HCT) has become an increasingly common treatment option for a variety of hematologic diseases over the past few decades. Survival following transplantation has increased steadily, leading to an increased focus on long-term complications. Studies suggest that, owing to systemic complications, total body irradiation (TBI), and various drugs in the conditioning regimen, thyroid gland abnormalities are more common in allo-HCT recipients than in the general population [1–4]. Several factors are associated with increased risk of thyroid abnormalities after allo-HCT. These include age, thyroid autoimmunity status of the donor and recipient, history of TBI, the primary hematological disease, and the pre-transplantation chemotherapy regimen. In assessing a patient's individual risk, the background prevalence of functional and anatomical thyroid disease should be considered in addition to the rates of thyroid abnormalities in allo-HCT recipients.

Epidemiological data on the US population shows the background prevalence of elevated thyroid stimulating hormone (TSH) levels (normal range, 0.3–5.1 mIU/L) to be 9.5%, while the prevalence of suppressed TSH is 2.2%. Up to 5% of women and 3% of men have subclinical hypothyroidism [5]. The percentage of US residents with high serum TSH concentration (4.5 mIU/L) is below 5% until age 40. The rate then increases rapidly so that those over the age of 70 have a prevalence of over 14%. The prevalence of low TSH is actually highest in populations without thyroid disease risk factors at ages 20–39 years and again after age 79 years. In the US population, the prevalence of thyroid nodules varies depending on what technique is used to identify the nodules. Up to 5% of patients have a nodule by palpation and up to 67% have a nodule by high-resolution ultrasound [6, 7]. The prevalence is low in children and increases with age. Thyroid disease is more prevalent in women than in men in all age groups [8].

By contrast, one study suggests some form of thyroid dysfunction occurs in up to 47.5% of patients, both children and adults, after TBI associated with allo-HCT [9]. Short-term changes after HCT in thyroid function can sometimes reflect euthyroid sick syndrome rather than true hypothyroidism [1, 10]. Acute complications such as graft versus host disease (GVHD) or sepsis may affect the hypothalamic–pituitary–thyroid axis. Steroid use in allo-HCT depresses total triiodothyronine (T3) and thyroxine (T4), decreases T4 to T3 conversion, and lowers TSH within the limits of normal, likely through inhibition of thyroid-releasing hormone secretion from the

Blood and Marrow Transplantation Long-Term Management: Prevention and Complications, First Edition. Edited by Bipin N Savani.

hypothalamus [11]. Androgens, given for post-allo-HCT hypogonadism typically lower thyroxine-binding globulin, along with total T4 and T3 [12].

In addition, medications used in this population of patients that can alter thyroid function testing include tyrosine kinase inhibitors, lenolidomide [13], mitotane, 5-fluorouracil, and L-asparaginase [14, 15]. Anatomical abnormalities of the thyroid can be observed during surveillance imaging for the primary malignancy post-transplant [16]. Computerized tomography (CT) or ^{18}F-fluorodeoxyglucose (^{18}FDG) positron emission tomography (PET) imaging may reveal thyroid abnormalities or nodules, which require further investigation. The primary clinical focus is determining the presence of malignancy in any thyroid nodules incidentally found. In this population, positive PET uptake, especially if it is focal, is more likely to indicate malignancy [17]. Therefore, thyroid function tests and any incident thyroid nodules must be interpreted in the context of the clinical history, physical exam, and current medications of each patient undergoing allo-HCT. Table 22.1 provides a brief outline of thyroid manifestations to be aware of in patients undergoing stem-cell transplantation.

Hypothyroidism

The most frequent functional thyroid abnormality in long-term allo-HCT survivors is subclinical hypothyroidism with mild TSH elevation (e.g., <10 mIU/L). The

Table 22.1 Thyroid manifestations in stem cell transplant recipients

Thyroid abnormality	Risk/causes	Testing	Treatment	Follow-up
Hypothyroidism	• Adoptive autoimmunity from donor • TBI • Medications • Preparatory regimens • GVHD	• TSH and fT4 prior to allo-HCT, 3 months post HCT, yearly TSH thereafter • Novel symptoms	• Thyroid hormone	• Monitor thyroid tests annually for development of hyperthyroidism or inadequate replacement
Hyperthyroidism	• Adoptive autoimmunity from donor • Underlying autoimmune thyroid disease in recipient • Thyroiditis • Genetic predisposition to thyroid diseases on basis of HLA type and family history • Autoimmune thyroiditis and GVHD • Disturbed immune reconstitution post allo-HCT	• TSH and fT4 prior to allo-HCT, 3 months post HCT, yearly TSH thereafter • Novel symptoms	• Depends on cause: – beta-blockers – observation in cases of mild disease – thionamides – I-131 – thyroidectomy	• Monitor thyroid tests for development of hypothyroidism
Thyroid nodules and cancer	• Family history • Radiation	• TSH • Ultrasound • Nuclear uptake/scan • FNAB	• Observation • Thyroidectomy • Radioiodine ablation	• Thyroglobulin • Ultrasound • Functional imaging
Pregnancy related hypothyroidism	• Adoptive autoimmunity from donor • TBI • Medications • Preparatory regimens	• TSH and fT4 levels	• Hormone replacement to maintain TSH ≤2.5 mIU/L	• Prior to and in every trimester of the pregnancy

FNAB: fine-needle aspiration biopsy; fT4: free thyroxine; HLA: human leukocyte antigen.

acute phase is characterized by reduction of serum thyroxine levels and inhibition of thyrotropin secretion [18]. Hypothyroidism often presents at 6–12 months following allo-HCT [19] with an incidence of 5–25% [19, 20]. Rarely, overt hypothyroidism occurs; there is apparently a greater risk at the extremes of age [1, 21]. The frequency of hypothyroidism within the first year has been found to be between 5 and 20% and appears to increase with duration of follow-up posttransplantation [19, 20].

Signs and symptoms

Hypothyroidism often presents 6–12 months following allo-HCT [19] with an incidence of 5–25% [19, 20]. Hypothyroidism is sometimes difficult to identify after allo-HCT because its symptoms can be similar to symptoms or side effects of allo-HCT. The symptoms include fatigue, slow mentation, constipation, hair and skin changes, weight gain, and changes in menses. In addition, chronic hypothyroidism is linked to unfavorable changes in lipid profiles and increased cardiovascular risk [22].

Risks

Several aspects of the underlying disease necessitating allo-HCT or its treatment increase the susceptibility to hypothyroidism. These include the use of TBI, the conditioning regimen, usually the combination of busulfan and cyclophosphamide, use of tyrosine kinase inhibitor agents, sequelae of transplantation (T cell depletion, GVHD, viral infection or reactivation), adoptive transfer from the donor and immune reconstitution post-HCT [9, 23]. Allo-HCT recipients who survive for more than 1 year and who receive either a TBI-based myeloablative or reduced-intensity conditioning regimen incur similar risks for hypothyroidism after 3 years of follow-up. Increased age at time of transplant is associated with higher risk of hypothyroidism [21]. However, TBI remains the main risk factor for hypothyroidism after allo-HCT [3, 24].

A family of multi-target tyrosine kinase inhibitors currently used as anticancer and conditioning agents prior to all-HCT can induce hypothyroidism. The mechanism of the thyroid abnormalities seen is thought to be a destructive thyroiditis, sometimes preceded by subclinical or clinical hyperthyroidism [25]. Examples include sunitinib, which can induce hypothyroidism in 53–85% of patients [26], and sorafenib, which may also produce a thyroiditis-induced hypothyroidism [27].

Preexisting autoimmune thyroid disease, with positive thyroid antibodies, increases the likely need for replacement therapy and development of clinically significant hypothyroidism. Therefore, these titers can be checked initially to guide the frequency of follow-up testing and possible treatment for hypothyroidism. However, those without autoimmune thyroid disease prior to transplant are also at risk of subclinical hypothyroidism coincident with allo-HCT.

Evaluation and management

Testing for TSH and free thyroxine (fT4) allows adequate assessment and follow-up of the pituitary–thyroid axis in the majority of patients with hypothyroidism. Thyroid antibodies are helpful in determining thyroid autoimmunity. For mild elevations of TSH (e.g., <10 mIU/L), repeat testing in 2–3 months prior to starting thyroid replacement is appropriate, especially if thyroid antibodies are negative, because hypothyroidism may be transient and self-limited. When used to confirm suspected thyroid disease, TSH has a high sensitivity (98%) and specificity (92%). Our recommendations for screening after allo-HCT include checking TSH and fT4 prior to and at 3 months post allo-HCT and annually thereafter. This frequency may be altered based on symptoms or signs.

Treatment with thyroid hormone replacement should be initiated in cases of overt primary or central hypothyroidism. Therapeutic total replacement dosing is approximately 1.6 μg of levothyroxine per kilogram of body weight. A lower initial dose may be used when TSH is only mildly elevated, in the elderly population, or in those with coronary artery disease. Clinical benefits begin in 3–5 days, but a given dose will take 6–8 weeks to equilibrate. The TSH and fT4 levels should be checked 6–8 weeks after a dose adjustment. TSH goals are usually in the 1–2 mIU/L range. Nomograms of TSH levels in the US population suggest that the majority of persons without known thyroid disease have a TSH near 1.2 mIU/L [5]. Initiation of agents that alter thyroid-binding globulin, such as estrogen, testosterone, or glucocorticoids, should prompt follow-up TSH testing in 6–8 weeks.

The utility of thyroid function testing has sufficient yield to have been recommended in the pediatric cancer population post allo-bone marrow transplant [28]. The utility of long-term testing in adults has not been evaluated specifically but is likely of sufficient yield in this population because of the increasing rates of hypothyroidism with age. A potential benefit of treating subclinical hypothyroidism is the prevention of progression to overt hypothyroidism. However, this potential benefit has not been studied in allo-HCT patients.

Approximately 10% of hypothyroid patients, most with continued symptoms of hypothyroidism, are dissatisfied with the outcome of levothyroxine replacement when compared with a euthyroid population [29]. Combination drugs containing T4 and T3, such as liotrix, are available, but there is no evidence of additional benefits over T4 alone. Although some patients may prefer using T4 and T3 together, several recent studies have indicated that they do not have better measurable outcomes than patients who use T4 alone [30]. Furthermore, combined T4 and T3 supplementation versus T4 supplementation alone has not been studied in the bone marrow transplant population.

Hyperthyroidism

Hyperthyroidism is less common than hypothyroidism among allo-HCT recipients but has been documented. It appears that hyperthyroidism can be an early complication of allo-HCT, with an incidence of 12% within 3 months of the transplant [31]. Hyperthyroidism can also occur as a later complication of allo-HCT, with a 15% occurrence rate 12–18 months posttransplant [9]. Perz et al. noted a 10.3% frequency of subclinical thyrotoxicosis but only a 3.1% rate of overt thyrotoxicosis following allo-HCT [32].

Signs and symptoms

Symptoms of hyperthyroidism include hand tremor, palpitations, weight loss, excessive sweating, heat intolerance, frequent bowel movements, irritability, and muscle weakness, as well as thyroid tenderness and pain, but patients may also be relatively asymptomatic [32]. Clinicians may assign the symptoms of hyperthyroidism to other conditions, such as the underlying disorder for which the allo-HCT was performed or as a treatment side effect. For example, weight loss and diarrhea are common symptoms of GVHD, and thyrotoxicosis symptoms may be mistaken for sepsis. Physical examination findings may include tachycardia, neck tenderness and thyroid enlargement, or painless, normal-sized thyroid. The development of thyrotoxic periodic paralysis is a rare presenting symptom; the case reported by Au and colleagues was 22 months post allo-HCT [33]. Six months later, the same patient, a Chinese man, also developed unilateral proptosis and diplopia, consistent with Graves' disease [34].

Risks

The presence of autoimmune thyroid disease in the donor increases the risk of the development of hyperthyroidism in the allo-HCT recipient. Several case reports document transfer of autoimmune thyroiditis from donor to recipient [35–38]. The use of iodinated contrast in allo-HCT patients who have underlying autonomous thyroid nodules is an additional risk factor [25].

Causes of hyperthyroidism

Graves' disease has been reported following allo-HCT, as late as 3 years post-transplant in a patient with chronic GVHD [34, 39]. It has been documented in siblings who have participated as donor and recipient of allo-HCT [2]. The disease is postulated to be caused by a passive transfer of a pathogenic clone of lymphocytes from donor to recipient via bone marrow cells [36].

Several possible mechanisms for the development of hyperthyroidism post allo-HCT have been described. These include adoptive autoimmunity, thyroiditis related to viral infection, genetic predisposition to thyroid disease based on human leukocyte antigen (HLA) type, and family history of thyroid disease. In addition, development of autoimmune thyroiditis as part of GVHD or the possibility that the recipient of the allo-HCT transplant has their own persistent intrathyroidal lymphocyte population that produces autoantibodies have been described. Disturbed immune reconstitution following allo-HCT, in which the hyperthyroidism is clinically mild and transient, has been described [23]. A combination of toxic factors and a dysregulated immune process may also cause posttransplant hyperthyroidism [32].

There is also an association between the development of autoimmune thyroiditis and irradiation of the thyroid gland or GVHD. This may result in transient hyperthyroidism followed by hypothyroidism [31]. Perz et al. [32] presented several patients who developed overt thyrotoxicosis and had all received alemtuzumab to deplete

T-cells. They posited a possible link between the drug and an immune phenomenon post allo-HCT. All three patients had the allele HLA-B 0801. This allele may also predispose to autoimmune hyperthyroidism after allo-HCT.

Evaluation and treatment

Thyroid function tests including TSH and fT4 at baseline, in the first 3 months post allo-HCT, and then on a yearly basis are adequate to identify most patients with post-allo-HCT hyperthyroidism, in both the early and late stages. If patients develop symptoms referable to hyperthyroidism, more frequent testing will be necessary. When thyroid tests indicate hyperthyroidism, thyroid autoantibodies should be measured. Thyroid uptake with I-123 helps establish a diagnosis. An elevated 24-h radioactive iodine uptake (RAIU) confirms endogenous hyperthyroidism. RAIU can distinguish between increased thyroid hormone synthesis, which is associated with elevated uptake, and thyroiditis, which is associated with low uptake [6]. During the hyperthyroid phase of subacute thyroiditis, Doppler thyroid flow will be reduced and RAIU will be less than 1%. However, in the setting of iodinated contrast from prior CT scans, I-123 uptakes may be difficult to interpret and might be falsely low [40].

Treatment of hyperthyroidism consists of treatment of symptoms with beta-blockers as well as treatment of the underlying cause. Three major treatments, anti-thyroid drugs (ATDs), radioactive iodine therapy, and surgery, have been used to treat endogenous or Graves' hyperthyroidism. However, many cases of hyperthyroidism soon after allo-HCT are due to thyroiditis and can be followed with observation alone or with use of beta-blockers to moderate symptoms. These individuals are at risk for the later development of hypothyroidism, and periodic thyroid function tests are indicated.

Thyroid nodules in allo-HCT patients

Thyroid nodules can be discovered upon palpation or incidentally during other imaging procedures. Determining whether the nodules are symptomatic or malignant is the aim of the evaluation. In patients receiving TBI and allo-HCT, a recent retrospective study demonstrated the occurrence of thyroid carcinoma was significantly higher than in the general population [8].

Signs and symptoms

Most thyroid nodules are without symptoms. A small number of patients complain of pain at the site of the nodule that can be referred to the ear or jaw. If the nodule is large, it can compress the esophagus or trachea and cause difficulty swallowing or stridor. Less commonly, patients may complain of hoarseness or difficulty speaking because of compression of the larynx. A rapidly enlarging mass is concerning in patients with known history of malignancy. Rapidly enlarging neck masses could represent the thyroid or pathological cervical lymphadenopathy [4]. Often, this leads to a diagnostic ultrasound of the thyroid gland and cervical lymph nodes.

Risks

Female gender, age <10 years at HCT, and chronic GVHD increase the risk of secondary thyroid cancer after allo-HCT [4]. In particular, the risk of thyroid tumors after TBI is elevated and dose related [41]. The period between irradiation and presentation of thyroid cancer may be many years. However, the observed-to-expected ratio of thyroid tumors is 5.79, suggesting an increased risk [42]. Secondary thyroid malignancies after allo-HCT for malignant disorders occur at an incidence of 0.2% in children and at 5.75-fold above expected rates for age-matched population controls [43].

Age at allo-HCT and occurrence of thyroid cancer are strongly related [44]. However, large-scale data surrounding thyroid cancer after TBI is limited. In a long-term follow-up of children who had undergone allo-HCT, the cumulative incidence of nodule occurrence increased with increasing time from diagnosis. The 10-year cumulative incidence of benign and malignant thyroid nodules was 16% and 8%, respectively [3]. The lifetime risk for developing a palpable thyroid nodule in the general population, by contrast, is estimated to be 5–10%.

Evaluation and management

Life-long thyroid function monitoring, with screening for nodules of the thyroid using ultrasound, is likely useful for survivors treated with TBI and allo-HCT. However, the interval at which these scans should be done in adult survivors is not currently known.

Malignancy should be considered in patients who have a rapidly enlarging thyroid mass, personal history of external beam radiation exposure as a child, exposure to ionizing radiation, family history of thyroid cancer, concerning ultrasound characteristics, or who have focal thyroid abnormality on ^{18}FDG-PET imaging [6].

Evaluation of thyroid nodules requires the ability to distinguish benign lesions from malignancy in a highly reliable and cost-effective manner. This includes TSH measurement to assess whether there is hyper- or hypothyroidism and ultrasound of the thyroid. Ultrasound is the imaging test of choice and should be performed in those nodules found incidentally by other imaging modalities, including CT and magnetic resonance imaging [6]. Sonographic signs of the thyroid nodule that confer an increased risk for malignancy include increased intranodular vascularity, large size, and the presence of microcalcifications, irregular borders, and hypoechogenicity. This should be followed by fine-needle aspiration biopsy (FNAB) when suspicious signs are found on the sonogram. However, if the TSH is suppressed, a thyroid scan should be performed prior to FNAB. A nodule found to be hyperfunctioning on scan has a very low risk of malignancy and thus should not be biopsied.

Ultrasonography-guided FNAB provides sensitivity higher than 80% and specificity higher than 90% [45]. Follow-up and management of cytologically benign lesions involves periodic sonograms to assess stability in the size of the nodule. Timing of follow-up sonogram is individualized based on clinical history, physical exam, and clinical suspicion and ultrasound features. If sequential sonograms reveal an increase in nodule size, repeat ultrasonography-guided FNAB may be appropriate. Malignant or suspicious cytological results should prompt total thyroidectomy by a surgeon skilled in thyroid cancer surgery. For atypia of undetermined significance found on FNAB, management options include repeat FNAB in 3–6 months and, if again atypical, thyroidectomy. An alternative is direct surgical consultation for thyroidectomy if there is increased suspicion for malignancy. The need for remnant ablation with radioiodine is determined by the stage of thyroid cancer and suspicion for recurrence or persistent disease [6]. The treatment of thyroid cancer should be coordinated with an endocrinologist, thyroid surgeon, and the oncologist in cases of advanced disease.

Statement regarding thyroid disorder and pregnancy post HCT

Many women, though premenopausal, are hypogonadal post allo-HCT. Estrogen supplementation can increase levels of thyroid-binding globulin and may translate to an increase in the dose of thyroid hormone. Repeat testing and appropriate adjustments in the dose should be performed, especially if pregnancy is being considered. Pre-conception testing to maintain TSH ≤2.5 mIU/L should be pursued, and such goals should also be achieved by testing in every trimester during pregnancy [46]. Patients should be encouraged to separate their thyroid hormone from their prenatal vitamins by several hours, to prevent problems associated with malabsorption of thyroid hormone due to the iron and calcium content in prenatal vitamins.

There are data supporting thyroid hormone replacement in women with positive thyroid antibodies, since this may improve fertility and prevent first-trimester miscarriages. Maternal and fetal complications associated with abnormal thyroid hormone levels during pregnancy can include abnormalities in weight gain in the mother and/or fetus, maternal blood pressure, and timing of delivery.

Conclusions

Allo-HCT survivors are at an increased risk for thyroid abnormalities many years after the procedure. Clinicians will do well to follow patients long term in order to monitor the ongoing risk of thyroid-related complications. It is also important to consider how pre-transplant risk factors interact with allo-HCT-related exposures to increase the risk of these complications. In addition, post-HCT pregnancy requires special vigilance for hypothyroidism and the attendant complications to pregnancy. Finally, patients may enjoy greater quality of life when their thyroid function is optimized in the peri- and post-allo-HCT period.

References

1. Ishiguro H, Yasuda Y, Tomita Y, et al. Long-term follow-up of thyroid function in patients who received bone marrow

transplantation during childhood and adolescence. J Clin Endocrinol Metab. 2004;89:5981–5986.

2. Savani BN, Griffith ML, Jagasia S, Lee SJ. How I treat late effects in adults after allogeneic stem cell transplantation. Blood. 2011;117:3002–3009.
3. Vivanco M, Dalle JH, Alberti C, et al. Malignant and benign thyroid nodules after total body irradiation preceding hematopoietic cell transplantation during childhood. Eur J Endocrinol. 2012;167:225–233.
4. Cohen A, Rovelli A, Merlo DF, et al. Risk for secondary thyroid carcinoma after hematopoietic stem-cell transplantation: an EBMT Late Effects Working Party Study. J Clin Oncol. 2007;25:2449–2454.
5. Hollowell JG, Staehling NW, Flanders WD, et al. Serum TSH, T_4, and thyroid antibodies in the United States population (1988 to 1994): National Health and Nutrition Examination Survey (NHANES III). J Clin Endocrinol Metab. 2002;87:489–499.
6. Cooper DS, Doherty GM, Haugen BR, et al. Revised American Thyroid Association management guidelines for patients with thyroid nodules and differentiated thyroid cancer. Thyroid. 2009;19:1167–1214.
7. Tan GH, Gharib H. Thyroid incidentalomas: management approaches to nonpalpable nodules discovered incidentally on thyroid imaging. Ann Intern Med. 1997;126:226–231.
8. Canaris GJ, Manowitz NR, Mayor G, Ridgway EC. The Colorado thyroid disease prevalence study. Arch Intern Med. 2000;160:526–534.
9. Tauchmanova L, Selleri C, Rosa GD, et al. High prevalence of endocrine dysfunction in long-term survivors after allogeneic bone marrow transplantation for hematologic diseases. Cancer. 2002;95:1076–1084.
10. Matsumoto M, Ishiguro H, Tomita Y, et al. Changes in thyroid function after bone marrow transplant in young patients. Pediatr Int. 2004;46:291–295.
11. Haugen BR. Drugs that suppress TSH or cause central hypothyroidism. Baillieres Best Pract Res Clin Endocrinol Metab. 2009;23:793–800.
12. Tahboub R, Arafah BM. Sex steroids and the thyroid. Baillieres Best Pract Res Clin Endocrinol Metab. 2009;23:769–780.
13. Figaro MK, Clayton W Jr, Usoh C, et al. Thyroid abnormalities in patients treated with lenalidomide for hematological malignancies: results of a retrospective case review. Am J Hematol. 2011;86:467–470.
14. Djurica SN, Plecas V, Milojevic Z, et al. Direct effects of cytostatic therapy on the functional state of the thyroid gland and TBG in serum of patients. Exp Clin Endocrinol. 1990;96:57–63.
15. Ferster A, Glinoer D, Van Vliet G, Otten J. Thyroid function during L-asparaginase therapy in children with acute lymphoblastic leukemia: difference between induction and late intensification. Am J Pediatr Hematol Oncol. 1992;14:192–196.
16. Kang KW, Kim SK, Kang HS, et al. Prevalence and risk of cancer of focal thyroid incidentaloma identified by 18F-fluorodeoxyglucose positron emission tomography for metastasis evaluation and cancer screening in healthy subjects. J Clin Endocrinol Metab. 2003;88:4100–4104.
17. Are C, Hsu JF, Schoder H, et al. FDG-PET detected thyroid incidentalomas: need for further investigation? Ann Surg Oncol. 2007;14:239–247.
18. Hershman JM, Eriksen E, Kaufman N, Champlin RE. Thyroid function tests in patients undergoing bone marrow transplantation. Bone Marrow Transplant. 1990;6:49–51.
19. Al-Fiar FZ, Colwill R, Lipton JH, et al. Abnormal thyroid stimulating hormone (TSH) levels in adults following allogeneic bone marrow transplants. Bone Marrow Transplant. 1997;19:1019–1022.
20. Sklar CA, Kim TH, Ramsay NK. Thyroid dysfunction among long-term survivors of bone marrow transplantation. Am J Med. 1982;73:688–694.
21. Al-Hazzouri A, Cao Q, Burns LJ, et al. Similar risks for hypothyroidism after allogeneic hematopoietic cell transplantation using TBI-based myeloablative and reduced-intensity conditioning regimens. Bone Marrow Transplant. 2009;43:949–951.
22. Ochs N, Auer R, Bauer DC, et al. Meta-analysis: subclinical thyroid dysfunction and the risk for coronary heart disease and mortality. Ann Intern Med. 2008;148:832–845.
23. Sherer Y, Shoenfeld Y. Autoimmune diseases and autoimmunity post-bone marrow transplantation. Bone Marrow Transplant. 1998;22:873–881.
24. Chow EJ, Liu W, Srivastava K, et al. Differential effects of radiotherapy on growth and endocrine function among acute leukemia survivors: a childhood cancer survivor study report. Pediatr Blood Cancer. 2013; 60:110–115.
25. Hamnvik OP, Larsen PR, Marqusee E. Thyroid dysfunction from antineoplastic agents. J Natl Cancer Inst. 2011;103:1572–1587.
26. Torino F, Corsello SM, Longo R, et al. Hypothyroidism related to tyrosine kinase inhibitors: an emerging toxic effect of targeted therapy. Nat Rev Clin Oncol. 2009;6:219–228.
27. Iavarone M, Perrino M, Vigano M, et al. Sorafenib-induced destructive thyroiditis. Thyroid. 2010;20:1043–1044.
28. Landier W, Armenian SH, Lee J, et al. Yield of screening for long-term complications using the children's oncology group long-term follow-up guidelines. J Clin Oncol. 2012;30:4401–4408.
29. Wiersinga WM. Do we need still more trials on T4 and T3 combination therapy in hypothyroidism? Eur J Endocrinol. 2009;161:955–959.

30. Grozinsky-Glasberg S, Fraser A, Nahshoni E, et al. Thyroxine–triiodothyronine combination therapy versus thyroxine monotherapy for clinical hypothyroidism: meta-analysis of randomized controlled trials. J Clin Endocrinol Metab. 2006;91:2592–2599.
31. Kami M, Tanaka Y, Chiba S, et al. Thyroid function after bone marrow transplantation: possible association between immune-mediated thyrotoxicosis and hypothyroidism. Transplantation. 2001;71:406–411.
32. Perz JB, Marin D, Szydlo RM, et al. Incidence of hyperthyroidism after unrelated donor allogeneic stem cell transplantation. Leuk Res. 2007;31:1433–1436.
33. Au WY, Lie AK, Kung AW, et al. Thyrotoxic periodic paralysis after allogeneic haematopoietic stem cell transplantation. Br J Haematol. 2005;129:160–161.
34. Hon C, Yau K, Chan EY, et al. Graves' ophthalmopathy after allogeneic stem cell transplantation. Ann Hematol. 2006;85:887–888.
35. Kishimoto Y, Yamamoto Y, Ito T, et al. Transfer of autoimmune thyroiditis and resolution of palmoplantar pustular psoriasis following allogeneic bone marrow transplantation. Bone Marrow Transplant. 1997;19:1041–1043.
36. Holland FJ, McConnon JK, Volpe R, Saunders EF. Concordant Graves' disease after bone marrow transplantation: implications for pathogenesis. J Clin Endocrinol Metab. 1991;72:837–840.
37. Berisso GA, van Lint MT, Bacigalupo A, Marmont AM. Adoptive autoimmune hyperthyroidism following allogeneic stem cell transplantation from an HLA-identical sibling with Graves' disease. Bone Marrow Transplant. 1999;23: 1091–1092.
38. Sklar C, Boulad F, Small T, Kernan N. Endocrine complications of pediatric stem cell transplantation. Front Biosci. 2001;6:G17–G22.
39. Mulligan SP, Joshua DE, Joasoo A, Kronenberg H. Autoimmune hyperthyroidism associated with chronic graft-versus-host disease. Transplantation. 1987;44:463–464.
40. Surks MI, Ortiz E, Daniels GH, et al. Subclinical thyroid disease: scientific review and guidelines for diagnosis and management. JAMA. 2004;291:228–238.
41. Sklar C, Whitton J, Mertens A, et al. Abnormalities of the thyroid in survivors of Hodgkin's disease: data from the Childhood Cancer Survivor Study. J Clin Endocrinol Metab. 2000;85:3227–3232.
42. Rizzo JD, Curtis RE, Socie G, et al. Solid cancers after allogeneic hematopoietic cell transplantation. Blood. 2009;113: 1175–1183.
43. Majhail NS, Brazauskas R, Rizzo JD, et al. Secondary solid cancers after allogeneic hematopoietic cell transplantation using busulfan–cyclophosphamide conditioning. Blood. 2011;117:316–322.
44. Socie G, Curtis RE, Deeg HJ, et al. New malignant diseases after allogeneic marrow transplantation for childhood acute leukemia. J Clin Oncol. 2000;18:348–357.
45. Kundel A, Zarnegar R, Kato M, et al. Comparison of microarray analysis of fine needle aspirates and tissue specimen in thyroid nodule diagnosis. Diagn Mol Pathol. 2010;19:9–14.
46. De Groot L, Abalovich M, Alexander EK, et al. Management of thyroid dysfunction during pregnancy and postpartum: an Endocrine Society clinical practice guideline. J Clin Endocrinol Metab. 2012;97:2543–2565.

23

CHAPTER 23

Special issues related to female long-term survivors

Melissa A Merideth[1], *Kristin Clay Chabarria*[2], *Tajana Klepac Pulanic*[3,4], *and Pamela Stratton*[5]

[1]Medical Genetics Branch, National Human Genome Research Institute, National Institutes of Health, Bethesda, MD, USA
[2]Louisiana State University Health Science Center School of Medicine, New Orleans, LA, USA
[3]University of Zagreb School of Medicine, Zagreb, Croatia
[4]Community Health Center East, Zagreb, Croatia
[5]Program in Reproductive and Adult Endocrinology, Eunice Kennedy Shriver National Institute of Child Health and Human Development, National Institutes of Health, Bethesda, MD, USA

Introduction

Recent advances in bone marrow transplantation techniques and management of patients have led to increased numbers of annual transplants, as well as improved long-term prognosis for these patients. With survivorship increasing, patients have shifted their care from large academic medical centers to community private practices closer to home. There is a general paucity of evidence-based data available to these providers about the management of gynecologic issues posttransplant. This chapter seeks to present major issues to address in long-term posttransplant gynecologic care by summarizing existing data regarding risk evaluation, screening, management, and treatment. We will highlight areas of future research, and supplement current guidelines with clinical observations noted in caring for this population. Routine gynecologic care enables early detection and treatment of gynecologic complications, thus reducing their long-term morbidity and mortality, as well as helping to improve quality of life for women after transplantation.

Genital graft-versus-host disease

Incidence and risk factors

Female genital tract graft-versus-host disease (GVHD) affects the vulva and the vagina, and is reported to affect at least one-quarter of female allogeneic hematopoietic stem cell transplant (allo-HSCT) survivors [1, 2]. While acute female genital GVHD in the first 100 days after transplant occurs in 11–17%, more commonly it occurs later as chronic GVHD (cGVHD) with rates about 20% [1, 3]. Prevalence rates of vulvovaginal GVHD are likely underestimated due to underdiagnosis. Women after HSCT are not typically questioned about gynecologic issues by transplant teams, nor are they routinely examined by gynecologists at regular intervals. Usually, they are referred for gynecologic examination only when they report symptoms. Importantly, patients may be less likely to self-report gynecologic symptoms unless directly asked, leaving many cases of genital cGVHD unrecognized until major complications occur.

The most consistently reported independent risk factor for genital GVHD is stem cell source; peripheral

Blood and Marrow Transplantation Long-Term Management: Prevention and Complications, First Edition. Edited by Bipin N Savani.

blood stem cell transplantation is associated with a higher risk for development of cGVHD than bone marrow transplantation (BMT) [2, 4]. Studies have failed to demonstrate an association between the presence of genital tract infections, pretransplant conditioning regimens, or GVHD prophylaxis, donor sex, or age of recipient or donor with the development of genital tract cGVHD [1, 2]. Interestingly, neither extent of cGVHD in other organ systems nor site of organ involvement appears to correlate with severity of genital GVHD. However, vaginal synechiae, the most severe form of genital GVHD, is associated with the sclerotic form of skin cGVHD, a more severe expression of cutaneous cGVHD [3]. As with other GVHD sites, genital cGVHD may be initiated or flare in the setting of tapering immunosuppression, after donor lymphocyte infusion, and with intercurrent infections [1].

Table 23.1 Modified severity scoring for chronic genital GVHD

Grade I (Minimal)*

- Generalized erythema and edema
- Reticulated leukokeratosis
- Erythematous patches on mucosal surfaces of the vulva
- Erythema and tenderness on light pressure over opening(s) of Skene's and/or Bartholin's ducts

Grade II (Moderate)*

- Erosions over any part of the vulva or vagina
- Fissures in vulvar folds – interlabial sulcus; fourchette

Grade III (Severe)*

- Agglutination of clitoral hood
- Labial resorption
- Introital stenosis
- Vaginal synechiae
- Hematocolpos/hematometra or complete vaginal closure
- Fasciitis of levator sling

*any of the following

Adapted from [3]: Stratton P, Turner ML, Childs R, et al. Vulvovaginal chronic graft-versus-host disease with allogeneic hematopoietic stem cell transplantation. *Obstet Gynecol.* 2007 Nov;110(5):1041–1049.

Clinical evaluation

Initial symptoms of genital GVHD may include dryness, burning, itching, dysuria, pain to touch, and dyspareunia [3, 5, 6]. The most common complaints are vulvar burning and pain, which occur when urine touches the vulva. Corresponding vulvar signs include erythema and eroded or fissured vulvar mucosa. Pelvic and vaginal symptoms may persist a few days after intercourse as the mucosa may be fragile, easily damaged, and take several days to heal. It is important to distinguish introital from deep dyspareunia. Introital pain occurs in patients with inflammation of the openings of the vestibular glands (Bartholin's, Skene's), with vulvar erosions or fissures and with labial fusion. Deep dyspareunia occurs in patients with vaginal scarring or shortening, a later and more severe finding in vulvovaginal GVHD.

When presenting with genital cGVHD, most patients have coexisting cGVHD in other organs, especially skin and oral mucosa [1–3, 7]. However, genital cGVHD may be an isolated manifestation in rare instances [1, 8]. Although vulvar disease typically precedes vaginal disease [9], treatment of vulvar disease alone will not prevent development of vaginal disease. Vaginal synechiae can appear as fine cobwebs, arcuate or purse-string narrowing, or dense scars. The dense, sclerotic changes may pull the vaginal walls together to completely obliterate, or shorten and narrow, the vaginal canal to about 5 cm long and one finger-breadth wide. Sclerotic vaginal changes resulting in vaginal stenosis have three consequences: (1) inability to perform cervical cytology screening, (2) complaints of amenorrhea or cyclic pain due to hematocolpos or hematometra arising from trapped menstruation or hormonal contraceptive-use-associated withdrawal bleeding and (3) difficulty with intercourse [1, 7, 8, 10–13]. Severity scoring of genital cGVHD, described by multiple authors [1–3, 14], is summarized in Table 23.1 [15].

Examination begins with careful inspection of the vulva, perineum, and perianal area to note any erythema, reticulated (lace-like) leukokeratosis, fissures, erosions, labial changes, and lesions. The vestibular gland openings and vulvar skin are palpated with a cotton-tipped applicator (q-tip) for tenderness. The vaginal examination starts with a gentle digital examination (using water as a lubricant) to evaluate for the above-described synechiae. After gentle digital exam confirms a patent vagina, a speculum exam can be done, taking care to minimize stretching of any noted tender synechiae.

Other common vulvar or vaginal conditions with symptoms of pain and irritation are considered in the assessment of genital tract complaints after transplant. Mild genital cGVHD mimics genital tract atrophy from ovarian failure caused by prior chemotherapy or transplant conditioning regimens, but physical findings are different. The vulva and vagina of patients with ovarian insufficiency show pallor and atrophy, whereas those with genital cGVHD may have erythema, fissures, erosions, and scarring which are not characteristics of menopause. The leukoplakia of human papillomavirus-associated neoplasia is a flat plaque and is associated with pruritis but differs from vulvar GVHD, which is reticulated. Acute genital GVHD may be distinguished from a chemotherapy-induced drug reaction of intertriginous skin [16]. During or shortly after chemotherapy, these skin changes appear as erythema progressing to painful erosions in the axilla, groin, and vulva. Burning before and during urination in women who have marked hematuria suggests *BK polyomavirus*-associated *hemorrhagic cystitis*. Hematuria is not a characteristic feature in genital GVHD. Patients with vulvovaginal lichen planus present with chronic genital symptoms, including burning, pruritus, dyspareunia, and vaginal discharge. Findings include painful vulvar introital erosions edged by a reticulate white border, mimicking genital GVHD. Vaginal lesions can also be found. Unchecked and untreated, the condition can also lead to vaginal stenosis [17, 18].

Treatment and prevention

The treatment is tailored to the clinical features. Erythema, erosions, and fissures are treated with topical immunosuppressive medication. Options for treatment include first-line steroids of varying potencies or calcineurin inhibitors (i.e., cyclosporine, 0.1% tacrolimus ointment). For extensive vulvar disease, superpotent steroid ointment such as clobetasol propionate is applied in a very thin layer to affected areas every night at bedtime until improvement, usually for 4–5 weeks, and then tapered to a maintenance dose of two or three times a week. If less potent topical glucocorticoid (or calcineurin inhibitor) treatment such as hydrocortisone cream is used, a twice a day regimen is used until improved, followed by tapering to daily application before decreasing to a maintenance dose of two or three times a week.

Topical steroid therapy for genital GVHD is effective in most cases. Usually, within 6–8 weeks of starting clobetasol ointment, the vulvar erosions and fissures heal, and vulvar pain resolves. If the patient experiences irritation or lack of improvement with the prescribed regimen, other topical agents like cyclosporine or tacrolimus can be used [2, 19]. Calcineurin is a cytoplasmic enzyme important in T lymphocyte activation; these calcineurin inhibitors decrease the local T-cell-mediated immunoresponse. After active genital cGVHD is treated, tapering the dosage over time to twice weekly application for maintenance therapy is recommended [20]. Recurrence of genital cGVHD has been reported after abruptly discontinuing any topical immunosuppressive regimen [2, 5].

Treatment of vaginal scarring addresses the density and extent of architectural changes. Cobweb and other newly formed scars may be gently lysed manually during vaginal examination. Patients with mild and moderate adhesions may be medically managed by using dilators lubricated with a pea-sized amount of clobetasol ointment (or other topical immunosuppressive agent) and one-half inch of estrogen cream two or three times a week until the vaginal scarring is lysed. Using dilators of increasing diameters enables an increase in vaginal caliber and depth. A slow-release ultralow dose estradiol vaginal ring (2 mg; 75 µg/24 h) can be used for those with less narrowing and mechanically keeps open the upper vagina, requiring replacement every 3 months [3]. In some patients using the ring, new vaginal synechiae have formed below the ring which may be treated with dilators. Early implementation of mechanical and topical therapy can prevent the need for surgery. Dense fibrotic vaginal scarring or extensive labial fusion may require surgery [10–13, 21]. After surgery, use of topical immunosuppressive therapy with dilators may prevent the development of new scars [5]. For maintenance of vaginal patency, manually inserted dilators or frequent sexual intercourse is recommended [20].

Successful management of genital GVHD is dependent upon early recognition and implementation of topical immunosuppressive and estrogen therapy combined, if needed, with dilator use [2, 3, 6, 20]. Zantomio et al.'s study demonstrates that surgery for genital GVHD may be completely avoided by implementing a vulvovaginal GVHD surveillance program, including pretransplant education about genital cGVHD symptoms, regular genital self-examination, and scheduled pelvic examinations every 3 months posttransplant [2]. With early recognition of genital cGVHD and early implementation of topical therapy, dense vaginal scarring can be avoided [2]. Thus, systematic, regular examinations by a gynecologist appear pivotal in reducing morbidity and improving quality of life for these patients.

Human papillomavirus-related secondary cancer and disease

Incidence and risk factors

Human papillomavirus (HPV), the most common viral sexually transmitted infection worldwide, has a reported prevalence of 2–20% in healthy reproductive-aged women [22]. In healthy individuals, over 90% of these infections will regress within 2 years [23]. However, the infection can persist in a small proportion of women, leading to anogenital condylomata and dysplasia, and, if left untreated, may progress to cancers.

Reported HPV infection and dysplasia prevalence rates in the posttransplant population are increased compared with the general population, ranging from 27.9 to 34% [24]. In our population, approximately 40% of patients have abnormal cervical cytology, with 20% categorized as high-grade dysplasia [25]. In immunocompetent patients, the progression from cervical dysplasia to cervical cancer is protracted, with the mean time to invasive cancer 15 years from onset of dysplasia. In immunosuppressed patients, the timeline to cervical dysplasia and cancer is reported to be accelerated, and cervical cancer more rapidly progressive [26]. Cervical cancer is the fourth most common secondary malignancy (after skin, oral cavity, and thyroid) reported in long-term survivors of HSCT [27]. When compared with the general population, long-term survivors have a 13-fold higher risk of cervical cancer, increasing to 18-fold higher in survivors over the age of 34 [28].

The most consistently reported risk factor for abnormal cervical cytology, as with all squamous cell carcinomas (SCCs) [29], is cGVHD requiring prolonged systemic immunosuppressive therapy. Vulvovaginal cGVHD appears to incur additional risk [25–27]. In our population, we have noted increased prevalence of genital condylomata and cervical dysplasia in patients using topical immunosuppressants for the treatment of genital cGVHD. Additionally, allogeneic transplant recipients have been shown to have higher rates of cervical cytology abnormalities than their autologous counterparts [24, 26].

Pathogenesis

Both cell-mediated immunity (CMI) and neutralizing antibodies contribute to the defense against initial HPV infection and viral proliferation [30]. Cytotoxic T-lymphocyte responses are believed to participate in limiting the number of HPV-infected cells, as well as triggering an antiviral cytokine cascade (IFN-γ, IL-5, IL-10) [31]. Helper T-lymphocytes are recruited to activate B-lymphocyte responses, generating neutralizing antibodies and subsequently enhancing CMI [30].

New-onset HPV-related disease in long-term survivors is presumed to be the reactivation of previously existing HPV infection, rather than the acquisition of a new infection, as studies have demonstrated loss of HPV seroreactivity following transplant [32]. Hypothesized mechanisms for reactivation are centered on immunomodulation, including transplant-related loss of antibody titers, impaired T- and B-lymphocyte response, and the use of immunosuppressive therapies following transplant. Underlying disease and history of HPV disease of the genital tract are additional risk factors.

Clinical evaluation and current screening guidelines

Clinical manifestations of HPV infection include genital condyloma, vulvar, anal, vaginal, and cervical intraepithelial neoplasia, and anogenital SCC. For most patients, HPV infections are generally asymptomatic, with the exception of vulvar pruritis with vulvar HPV. Additionally, small vulvar condylomata, as well as cervical condylomata, may go unnoticed, thus necessitating regular cervical cytology screening and thorough inspection of the lower genital tract, with follow-up assessment as outlined in Table 23.2 [15].

The Center for International Blood & Marrow Transplant Research (CIBMTR) recommends speculum examination and cervical cytology testing with co-testing (or reflexive) HPV testing as a part of routine gynecological care prior to transplant. After transplant, annual screening is recommended by the European Bone Marrow Transplant registry, American Society for Blood and Marrow Transplantation, and Children's Oncology Group guidelines [20]. CIBMTR recommends screening every 1–3 years after transplant [33]. The American

Table 23.2 Care and screening recommendations for women post-HSCT

Contraception
- Encourage use of effective method with minimal side effects from time of transplant through assessment for engraftment, on multiple transplant medications, or at risk of disease recurrence
- Assess need for continuing contraception annually
- Assess contraindications to hormonal contraceptive therapy such as blood clots, liver function abnormalities, severe mucositis compromising absorption, hormone-dependent tumors
- Obtain pregnancy test in routine follow-up
- If amenorrhea occurs after menses have resumed
  - obtain pregnancy test
  - consider hypothalamic pituitary axis testing

Bone
- Dual-energy X-ray absorptiometry at beginning of follow-up period
- Continue calcium and vitamin D
- Treat osteoporosis with bisphosphonates or hormone therapy

Breast
- Annual clinical breast exam at puberty and mammogram annually starting at age 40
- Patients who underwent chest radiation begin annual mammography at age 25 or 8 years after treatment

HPV assessment
- Inspect vulva, vagina, and cervix for evidence of HPV disease
- Perform cervical cytology testing annually
- Perform HPV DNA testing for high-risk types at the time of cervical cytology testing or as reflex testing when cytology report is normal cytology or atypical cells of undetermined significance
- Refer for colposcopy for cytology reports of atypical cells suggestive of high-grade dysplasia or worse
- Consider HPV vaccination

Sexually transmitted disease
- Perform annual screening based on risk factors

Vulvovaginal symptoms
- Assess for vulvovaginal symptoms in the setting of other GVHD
- Refer for gynecologic evaluation if patient has vulvovaginal symptoms
- Assess for signs of genital GVHD at annual pelvic exam
- Consider gynecologic examination every 3 months for patients with severe GVHD or known genital GVHD
- Treat any genital GVHD with topical immunosuppression, dilators, and, if no contraindication, topical estrogens
- Treat labial fusion or complete vaginal stenosis with surgery followed by dilators, topical immunosuppression, and topical estrogens
- Assess for HPV disease if topical immunosuppression is used

Hypothalamic–pituitary–ovarian axis
- Assess pubertal status with Tanner stage at time of transplant
- Consider ovarian function at annual history and physical
- Check FSH, LH, estradiol
- Consider performing transvaginal ultrasound
- Check TSH when indicated

Hormone therapy in the setting of ovarian failure
- Assess contraindications to hormone therapy such as blood clots, liver function abnormalities, severe mucositis compromising absorption, hormone-dependent tumors
- Consider hormone therapy in women with ovarian failure less than age 35
  - may improve bone mass
  - likely improve sexual function
  - may improve overall morbidity and mortality [34]

Sexual function
- Assess for dyspareunia, hypoactive sexual desire, and dysfunction with arousal or orgasm
- Treat any underlying endocrine or medical conditions including genital GVHD
- Consider vaginal estrogen or lubricants for dyspareunia from atrophic vaginitis
- Refer to psychologist for individual or couples therapy

Adapted from [15]: Shanis D, Merideth M, Klepac Pulanic T, et al. Female long term survivors after allo-HSCT: evaluation and management. *Semin Hematol.* 2012;49(1):83–93.
Abbreviations: GnRH, gonadotropin-releasing hormone; FSH, follicle-stimulating hormone; LH, luteinizing hormone; TSH, thyroid-stimulating hormone.

College of Obstetricians and Gynecologists recommends more frequent screening for immunocompromised populations than their age-appropriate peers, agreeing that annual cytology screening and HPV testing at >21 years is reasonable [23]. Results of screening tests should be evaluated based on the general guidelines (Table 23.2) [15]. Additionally, inspection of the external genitalia should include the anal area. Abnormalities on inspection of the external genitalia, vagina, and cervix are further evaluated using colposcopy after topical application of 5% acetic acid, with biopsies of abnormal-appearing areas.

Prevention

Recombinant vaccines containing virus-like capsid particles are available for HPV infection prophylaxis: a bivalent vaccine containing HPV types 16 and 18 and a quadrivalent one containing types 6, 11, 16, and 18. HPV types 6 and 11 are responsible for 90% of anogenital condylomata, while types 16 and 18 have been isolated in 70% of cervical cancer and high-grade cervical intraepithelial neoplasia [35]. HPV type 16 appears to be more oncogenic and is responsible for 50% of all cervical cancers worldwide [36]. Currently, vaccination is recommended for use in healthy women, ages 9–26 years, where it has reduced the incidence of vulvar intraepithelial neoplasia, cervical cancer, and anogenital condylomata [35], even for oncogenic HPV types not included in the vaccine [37].

Although this vaccine has not been approved for use in populations older than age 26, vaccinating long-term survivors over this age has been proposed, and may decrease the morbidity and mortality caused by HPV-related cancers. Published guidelines propose vaccination schedules for patients following stem cell transplant, weighing the potential risks versus presumed benefits with the timing of these vaccinations [38]. In general, although evidence of seroreactivity to vaccines given as early as 6–9 months may be seen, immunoresponse is greater, and more predictable, when administered at least 12 months after HSCT. An additional, albeit theoretical, consideration is the potential for proinflammatory cascade initiated by vaccine administration triggering cGVHD flares, although this has not been documented [39]. Patients receiving intravenous immunoglobulin (IVIG) therapy as a component of their posttransplant regimen may be vaccinated. While IVIG is known to blunt the immune response and efficacy of vaccination with live vaccines, this is not known to happen with inactivated vaccines such as this one [40–42].

Quadrivalent HPV vaccination in HSCT patients is an area of active research, as it could potentially prevent reactivation of HPV (and thus the sequelae of anogenital condylomata, dysplasia and SCC) by triggering an immune response to HPV. A study examining whether quadrivalent HPV vaccination can induce seroreactivity in HSCT patients is currently underway at the National Institutes of Health (ClinicalTrials.gov Identifier: NCT01092195).

Ovarian failure, infertility, and sexual health

Greater than 90% of women in their reproductive years who undergo allo-HSCT will experience ovarian failure after radiation and myeloablative conditioning chemotherapy for HSCT [43]. The factors affecting the chance of permanent ovarian failure and posttransplantation infertility are the patient's age, pubertal status, radiation dose/location, and conditioning chemotherapy regimen [44–46]. Nearly all postpubertal females who undergo myeloablative regimens using high-dose total body irradiation (TBI) with the equivalent of direct ovarian radiation 10 Gy develop ovarian failure [47, 48]. Use of alkylating cytoreductive agents, particularly high-dose busulfan and cyclophosphamide, increases the risk of ovarian failure, as does increasing age [44, 45, 49]. In one study of women treated with cyclophosphamide and TBI preconditioning for marrow transplantation, all 68 women over the age of 25 years developed premature ovarian failure, defined as ovarian failure in a woman who is less than 40 years of age [43]. Radiation doses of 6 Gy cause irreversible ovarian injury in the majority of patients treated after age 40 years, while a much larger dose (two to three times) is required to cause ovarian failure in children [50, 51]. In addition to impairment of ovarian function, radiation-induced pelvic damage can also include impaired uterine function, particularly in the exposed prepubertal uterus [50, 51].

Myeloablative conditioning prior to transplant is known to impair fertility. The largest published series that has reported pregnancies in HSCT patients (17 950 autologous and 19 412 allogeneic transplants) reports

312 pregnancies in 232 (0.6%) of patients/partners of patients. Though sporadic pregnancies are reported after transplant [47], reduced-intensity HSCT is reported as more effective in preserving fertility than myeloablative transplantation [52]. Double transplant procedures are associated with lower fertility rates than single transplant procedures [53]. Gonadotropin-releasing hormone (GnRH) agonist-induced ovarian suppression is frequently used to protect ovarian function of women during chemotherapy with alkylating agents [54] and reduces the occurrence of chemotherapy-induced ovarian failure in premenopausal women with breast cancer [55]. Though the mechanism by which GnRH agonists help preserve ovarian function is not completely understood, proposed mechanisms for attenuating chemotherapy effects include suppression of the hypothalamic–pituitary–ovarian axis, activation of GnRH receptors, decreasing utero-ovarian perfusion, or protection of undifferentiated germ-line stem cells for upregulated intragonadal anti-apoptotic molecules like sphingosine-1-phosphate [55]. It is not yet known whether this strategy will be effective in HSCT. Options for preserving fertility are often discussed and must be implemented prior to transplantation, and include hormone stimulation and oocyte harvesting for fertilization/cryopreservation, as well as GnRH agonist treatment. Fertility issues are further addressed in Chapter 19.

Transient ovarian dysfunction resulting in amenorrhea or oligomenorrhea is common within the first year after treatment [56], arising as a result of chemotherapy and chronic disease, in addition to the use of immunosuppressive medications, especially steroids, to prevent GVHD. Women who resume menses after treatment may still develop early menopause (prior to age 40 years), with similar risk factors as those for acute ovarian failure [57, 58]. Women who are affected by early menopause experience not only menopausal symptoms (hot flashes, vaginal dryness, dyspareunia, sleep and mood disturbances) but also are at an increased risk of osteoporosis, cardiovascular disease, dementia, and sexual dysfunction [59–61]. Not surprisingly, the youngest transplant patients with ovarian failure are the ones most likely to report lower quality-of-life scores and an impaired sense of well-being [62].

Long-term survivors with ovarian dysfunction or failure may benefit from the use of hormone replacement therapy (HRT), which is known to improve vasomotor and urogenital menopausal symptoms, measures of psychological well-being, and may improve overall morbidity and mortality but has minimal effect on sexual desire and satisfaction [34, 63–65]. The use of testosterone has not improved libido in cancer survivors who were not taking estrogen [65]. The risks and benefits of using HRT in women after allo-HSCT must be individualized based on the patient's underlying disease status, the severity of her menopausal symptoms, and contraindications to hormone use (such as liver disease or history of deep venous thrombosis) [62]. Though the lowest dose that relieves symptoms is recommended, young women who have undergone premature ovarian failure may require higher doses of estrogen and progesterone to achieve physiologic levels compared with women who naturally go through menopause. Since these young women may be on HRT for an extended period of time, it may be reasonable to discontinue therapy every few years in order to assess the hypothalamic–pituitary–ovarian axis [66]. Menopausal patients who have contraindications to HRT use may benefit from the use of selective serotonin reuptake inhibitors or serotonin–norepinephrine reuptake inhibitors, which have been shown in placebo-controlled trials to decrease hot flashes by more than 50%, leading to increased energy, decreased sleep disturbances, and reduced psychological complaints [67].

Though most patients who have lost ovarian function as a result of myeloablative transplantation are unlikely to regain function, some may partially or completely regain ovarian function years after treatment [43, 68, 69]. Pregnancy outcome in long-term survivors is addressed in Chapter 19. Assessing for pregnancy in posttransplant patients who are not taking hormones and experience amenorrhea after the return of menses is important. Additionally, because it is difficult to predict who will have return of ovarian function and when it will occur, contraceptive use is recommended for all patients for whom pregnancy would be problematic for either health (e.g., those experiencing relapse, severe cGVHD, or are soon after transplant) or personal reasons.

Sexuality is a central aspect of an individual's self-esteem and identity and is discussed in Chapter 18. While intimacy and sexuality can decrease emotional distress and improve psychological response to a life-threatening disease and complications after treatment [55, 56], the sexual response cycle may be negatively altered by psychosocial factors such as anxiety, depression, body image changes, concurrent life stress, decreased self-confidence, fear of disease recurrence, and concerns related to infertility [52, 54, 68]. The impact of a serious illness on sexuality is often not a concern expressed by patients undergoing HSCT; additionally, sexual health, while important, may be overlooked by the healthcare team during recovery [43]. Discussion of sexual functioning has often been a taboo subject in the healthcare setting, leading to decreased awareness and undertreatment of this critical component of these patients' health.

The potential long-term sexual complications after transplant include decreased libido, vaginal alterations like scarring or genital tract atrophy, premature ovarian insufficiency, dysfunction in sexual hormones, dyspareunia, and infertility [43, 44, 47, 70]. In particular, sexual dysfunction in long-term female survivors of allo-HSCT may be related to ovarian failure, cGVHD, medication use, or psychosocial factors like depression and self-consciousness. Having either acute or chronic GVHD is associated with sexual dysfunction in allo-HSCT patients [47, 49]. In general, systemic cGVHD and treatment with high-dose corticosteroids may result in extensive changes in physical appearance such that sexuality and body image are seriously affected.

Sexual dysfunction can affect patients of all ages, and is reported to affect 80% of female survivors of allo-HSCT long term, with women reporting no significant improvement in sexual function 5 years after transplant [71]. Sexual function has been shown to be dependent upon the patient's psychological status and quality of the relationship with her partner [72]. Behavioral therapies can have a significant role in helping to improve sexual function, particularly those that address relationship conflicts and encourage communication about the patient's fears of feeling unattractive or rejected.

Little is known about sexual changes and their consequences experienced by patients following allo-HSCT. It is important to draw attention to the impact that HSCT has on the sexuality and sexual functioning in patients after HSCT. Sexual functioning is an important aspect of quality of life and needs further research (see Chapter 18).

As the number of women who undergo and survive allo-HSCT increases, it becomes increasingly important that gynecologic issues are identified and treated in this patient population. Identification and treatment of gynecologic issues such as chronic GVHD, HPV reactivation, ovarian failure and sexual dysfunction can lead to improved quality of life for these survivors. Table 23.2 provides both evaluation and management recommendations for the numerous gynecologic issues faced by long-term survivors. Given the complexity of medical issues in long-term survivors, it is important for the obstetrician–gynecologist, hematologist–oncologist, and other primary care providers to work together in providing optimal care for this patient population.

Acknowledgments

This work was funded, in part, by the Intramural Program of the NIH, Clinical Center, the Eunice Kennedy Shriver National Institute of Child Health and Human Development, and the National Human Genome Research Institute.

References

1. Spinelli S, Chiodi S, Costantini S, et al. Female genital tract graft-versus-host disease following allogeneic bone marrow transplantation. Haematologica. 2003;88(10):1163–1168.
2. Zantomio D, Grigg AP, Macgregor L, et al. Female genital tract graft-versus-host disease: incidence, risk factors and recommendations for management. Bone Marrow Transplant. 2006;38(8):567–572.
3. Stratton P, Turner ML, Childs R, et al. Vulvovaginal chronic graft-versus-host disease with allogeneic hematopoietic stem cell transplantation. Obstet Gynecol. 2007;110(5): 1041–1049.
4. Flowers ME, Parker PM, Johnston LJ, et al. Comparison of chronic graft-versus-host disease after transplantation of peripheral blood stem cells versus bone marrow in allogeneic recipients: long-term follow-up of a randomized trial. Blood. 2002;100(2):415–419.
5. Spiryda LB, Laufer MR, Soiffer RJ, et al. Graft-versus-host disease of the vulva and/or vagina: diagnosis and treatment. Biol Blood Marrow Transplant. 2003;9(12):760–765.
6. Turner ML, Stratton P. Gynecological disease. In: Vogelsang GB, Pavletic SZ (eds). Chronic Graft Versus Host Disease Interdisciplinary Management. Cambridge: Cambridge University Press, 2009; pp. 207–215.
7. Corson SL, Sullivan K, Batzer F, et al. Gynecologic manifestations of chronic graft-versus-host disease. Obstet Gynecol. 1982;60(4):488–492.
8. DeLord C, Treleaven J, Shepherd J, et al. Vaginal stenosis following allogeneic bone marrow transplantation for acute

myeloid leukaemia. Bone Marrow Transplant. 1999;23(5): 523–525.

9. Klepac Pulanic T, Turner M, Gemmill JA, et al. Female genital chronic graft versus host disease. 57th Annual Meeting of the Society for Gynecologic Investigation; March 17–21, 2010; Orlando, FL.
10. Hayes EC, Rock JA. Treatment of vaginal agglutination associated with chronic graft-versus-host disease. Fertil Steril. 2002;78(5):1125–1126.
11. Anguenot JL, Ibecheole V, Helg C, et al. Vaginal stenosis with hematocolpometra, complicating chronic graft versus host disease. Eur J Obstet Gynecol Reprod Biol. 2002;103(2): 185–187.
12. Jain SP, Henry RJ. Haematocolpos following allogenic bone marrow transplantation for chronic myeloid leukaemia. Br J Obstet Gynaecol. 2001;108(12):1309–1310.
13. Costantini S, Chiodi S, Spinelli S, et al. Complete vaginal obstruction caused by chronic graft-versus-host disease after haematopoietic stem cell transplantation: diagnosis and treatment. J Obstet Gynaecol. 2004;24(5):591–595.
14. Hirsch P, Leclerc M, Rybojad M, et al. Female genital chronic graft-versus-host disease: importance of early diagnosis to avoid severe complications. Transplantation. 2012;93: 1265–1269.
15. Shanis D, Merideth M, Pulanic TK, et al. Female long-term survivors after allogeneic hematopoietic stem cell transplantation: evaluation and management. Semin Hematol. 2012;49(1):83–93.
16. Prussick R. Adverse cutaneous reactions to chemotherapeutic agents and cytokine therapy. Semin Cutan Med Surg. 1996;15(4):267–276.
17. Cooper SM, Wojnarowska F. Influence of treatment of erosive lichen planus of the vulva on its prognosis. Arch Dermatol. 2006;142(3):289–294.
18. Anderson M, Kutzner S, Kaufman RH. Treatment of vulvovaginal lichen planus with vaginal hydrocortisone suppositories. Obstet Gynecol. 2002;100(2):359–362.
19. Couriel D, Carpenter PA, Cutler C, et al. Ancillary therapy and supportive care of chronic graft-versus-host disease: National Institutes of Health consensus development project on criteria for clinical trials in chronic graft-versus-host disease: V. Ancillary Therapy and Supportive Care Working Group Report. Biol Blood Marrow Transplant. 2006; 12(4):375–396.
20. Milroy CL, Jones KP. Gynecologic care in hematopoietic stem cell transplant patients: a review. Obstet Gynecol Surv. 2010;65(10):668–679.
21. Norian JM, Stratton P. Labial fusion: a rare complication of chronic graft-versus-host disease. Obstet Gynecol. 2008; 112(2 Pt 2):437–439.
22. Bosch FX, de Sanjosé S. Chapter 1: human papillomavirus and cervical cancer – burden and assessment of causality. J Natl Cancer Inst Monogr. 2003;(31):3–13.
23. Committee on Practice Bulletins – Gynecology. ACOG Practice Bulletin Number 131: screening for cervical cancer. Obstet Gynecol. 2012;120(5):1222–1238.
24. Sasadeusz J, Kelly H, Szer J, et al. Abnormal cervical cytology in bone marrow transplant recipients. Bone Marrow Transplant. 2001;28(4):393–397.
25. Savani BN, Stratton P, Shenoy A, et al. Increased risk of cervical dysplasia in long-term survivors of allogeneic stem cell transplantation – implications for screening and HPV vaccination. Biol Blood Marrow Transplant. 2008;14(9): 1072–1075.
26. Wang Y, Brinch L, Jebsen P, et al. A clinical study of cervical dysplasia in long-term survivors of allogeneic stem cell transplantation. Biol Blood Marrow Transplant. 2012; 18(5):747–753.
27. Kolb HJ, Socie G, Duell T, et al. Malignant neoplasms in long-term survivors of bone marrow transplantation. Late Effects Working Party of the European Cooperative Group for Blood and Marrow Transplantation and the European Late Effect Project Group. Ann Intern Med. 1999; 131(10):738–744.
28. Bhatia S, Louie AD, Bhatia R, et al. Solid cancers after bone marrow transplantation. J Clin Oncol. 2001;19(2):464–471.
29. Curtis RE, Metayer C, Rizzo JD, et al. Impact of chronic GVHD therapy on the development of squamous-cell cancers after hematopoietic stem-cell transplantation: an international case-control study. Blood. 2005;105(10): 3802–3811.
30. Zhang LF, Zhou J, Chen S, et al. HPV6b virus like particles are potent immunogens without adjuvant in man. Vaccine. 2000;18(11–12):1051–1058.
31. Pinto LA, Edwards J, Castle PE, et al. Cellular immune responses to human papillomavirus (HPV)-16 L1 in healthy volunteers immunized with recombinant HPV-16 L1 virus-like particles. J Infect Dis. 2003;188(2):327–338.
32. Lewensohn-Fuchs I, Ljungman P, Kjerrstrom A, et al. Loss of seroreactivity against human papillomavirus (HPV) in bone marrow transplant recipients. Bone Marrow Transplant. 1996;18(2):333–337.
33. Majhail NS, Rizzo JD, Lee SJ, et al. Recommended screening and preventive practices for long-term survivors after hematopoietic cell transplantation. Biol Blood Marrow Transplant. 2012;18(3):348–371.
34. Parker WH, Feskanich D, Broder MS, et al. Long-term mortality associated with oophorectomy compared with ovarian conservation in the nurses' health study. Obstet Gynecol. 2013;121(4):709–716. doi: 10.1097/AOG. 0b013e3182864350.

35. Garland SM, Hernandez-Avila M, Wheeler CM, et al. Quadrivalent vaccine against human papillomavirus to prevent anogenital diseases. N Engl J Med. 2007;356(19):1928–1943.
36. Bosch FX, Manos MM, Munoz N, et al. Prevalence of human papillomavirus in cervical cancer: a worldwide perspective. International biological study on cervical cancer (IBSCC) Study Group. J Natl Cancer Inst. 1995;87(11):796–802.
37. Brown DR, Kjaer SK, Sigurdsson K, et al. The impact of quadrivalent human papillomavirus (HPV; types 6, 11, 16, and 18) L1 virus-like particle vaccine on infection and disease due to oncogenic nonvaccine HPV types in generally HPV-naive women aged 16–26 years. J Infect Dis. 2009;199(7):926–935.
38. Savani BN, Griffith ML, Jagasia S, et al. How I treat late effects in adults after allogeneic stem cell transplantation. Blood. 2011;117(11):3002–3009.
39. Wilck MB, Baden LR. Vaccination after stem cell transplant: a review of recent developments and implications for current practice. Curr Opin Infect Dis. 2008;21(4):399–408.
40. Kroger AT, Sumaya CV, Pickering LK, Atkinson WL. General recommendations on immunization – recommendations of the Advisory Committee on Immunization Practices (ACIP). MMWR Recomm Rep. 2011;60(2):1–64.
41. Siber GR, Werner BG, Halsey NA, et al. Interference of immune globulin with measles and rubella immunization. J Pediatr. 1993;122(2):204–211.
42. Committee on Infectious Diseases. Recommended timing of routine measles immunization for children who have recently received immune globulin preparations. American Academy of Pediatrics Committee on Infectious Diseases. Pediatrics. 1994;93(4):682–685.
43. Sanders JE, Buckner CD, Amos D, et al. Ovarian function following marrow transplantation for aplastic anemia or leukemia. J Clin Oncol. 1988;6(5):813–818.
44. Warne GL, Fairley KF, Hobbs JB, et al. Cyclophosphamide-induced ovarian failure. N Engl J Med. 1973;289(22):1159–1162.
45. Jadoul P, Anckaert E, Dewandeleer A, et al. Clinical and biologic evaluation of ovarian function in women treated by bone marrow transplantation for various indications during childhood or adolescence. Fertil Steril. 2011;96(1):126–133.e3.
46. Schimmer AD, Quatermain M, Imrie K, et al. Ovarian function after autologous bone marrow transplantation. J Clin Oncol. 1998;16(7):2359–2363.
47. Salooja N, Szydlo RM, Socie G, et al. Pregnancy outcomes after peripheral blood or bone marrow transplantation: a retrospective survey. Lancet. 2001;358(9278):271–276.
48. Chatterjee R, Mills W, Katz M, et al. Prospective study of pituitary-gonadal function to evaluate short-term effects of ablative chemotherapy or total body irradiation with autologous or allogenic marrow transplantation in post-menarcheal female patients. Bone Marrow Transplant. 1994;13(5):511–517.
49. Teinturier C, Hartmann O, Valteau-Couanet D, et al. Ovarian function after autologous bone marrow transplantation in childhood: high-dose busulfan is a major cause of ovarian failure. Bone Marrow Transplant. 1998;22(10):989–994.
50. Thibaud E, Ramirez M, Brauner R, et al. Preservation of ovarian function by ovarian transposition performed before pelvic irradiation during childhood. J Pediatr. 1992;121(6):880–884.
51. Sarafoglou K, Boulad F, Gillio A, et al. Gonadal function after bone marrow transplantation for acute leukemia during childhood. J Pediatr. 1997;130(2):210–216.
52. Jackson GH, Wood A, Taylor PR, et al. Early high dose chemotherapy intensification with autologous bone marrow transplantation in lymphoma associated with retention of fertility and normal pregnancies in females. Scotland and Newcastle Lymphoma Group, UK. Leuk Lymphoma. 1997;28(1–2):127–132.
53. Salooja N, Chatterjee R, McMillan AK, et al. Successful pregnancies in women following single autotransplant for acute myeloid leukemia with a chemotherapy ablation protocol. Bone Marrow Transplant. 1994;13(4):431–435.
54. Somers EC, Marder W, Christman GM, et al. Use of a gonadotropin-releasing hormone analog for protection against premature ovarian failure during cyclophosphamide therapy in women with severe lupus. Arthritis Rheum. 2005;52(9):2761–2767.
55. Del Mastro L, Boni L, Michelotti A, et al. Effect of the gonadotropin-releasing hormone analogue triptorelin on the occurrence of chemotherapy-induced early menopause in premenopausal women with breast cancer: a randomized trial. JAMA. 2011;306(3):269–276.
56. Tauchmanova L, Selleri C, De Rosa G, et al. Endocrine disorders during the first year after autologous stem-cell transplant. Am J Med. 2005;118(6):664–670.
57. Sklar CA, Mertens AC, Mitby P, et al. Premature menopause in survivors of childhood cancer: a report from the childhood cancer survivor study. J Natl Cancer Inst. 2006;98(13):890–896.
58. Rutter MM, Rose SR. Long-term endocrine sequelae of childhood cancer. Curr Opin Pediatr. 2007;19(4):480–487.
59. Chiodi S, Spinelli S, Ravera G, et al. Quality of life in 244 recipients of allogeneic bone marrow transplantation. Br J Haematol. 2000;110(3):614–619.

60. Claessens JJ, Beerendonk CC, Schattenberg AV. Quality of life, reproduction and sexuality after stem cell transplantation with partially T-cell-depleted grafts and after conditioning with a regimen including total body irradiation. Bone Marrow Transplant. 2006;37(9):831–836.
61. Somali M, Mpatakoias V, Avramides A, et al. Function of the hypothalamic-pituitary-gonadal axis in long-term survivors of hematopoietic stem cell transplantation for hematological diseases. Gynecol Endocrinol. 2005;21(1): 18–26.
62. Fish JD. Part 1: hormone replacement for survivors of childhood cancer with ovarian failure – when is it worth the risk? J Pediatr Adolesc Gynecol. 2011;24(2):98–101.
63. Balleari E, Garre S, Van Lint MT, et al. Hormone replacement therapy and chronic graft-versus-host disease activity in women treated with bone marrow transplantation for hematologic malignancies. Ann N Y Acad Sci. 2002;966: 187–192.
64. Tauchmanova L, Selleri C, De Rosa G, et al. Estrogen-progestin therapy in women after stem cell transplant: our experience and literature review. Menopause. 2007;14(2): 320–330.
65. Heinonen H, Volin L, Uutela A, et al. Gender-associated differences in the quality of life after allogeneic BMT. Bone Marrow Transplant. 2001;28(5):503–509.
66. Cohen A, Bekassy AN, Gaiero A, et al. Endocrinological late complications after hematopoietic SCT in children. Bone Marrow Transplant. 2008;41(S2):S43–S48.
67. Stearns V. Serotonergic agents as an alternative to hormonal therapy for the treatment of menopausal vasomotor symptoms. Treat Endocrinol. 2006;5(2):83–87.
68. Liu J, Malhotra R, Voltarelli J, et al. Ovarian recovery after stem cell transplantation. Bone Marrow Transplant. 2008; 41(3):275–278.
69. Spinelli S, Chiodi S, Bacigalupo A, et al. Ovarian recovery after total body irradiation and allogeneic bone marrow transplantation: long-term follow up of 79 females. Bone Marrow Transplant. 1994;14(3):373–380.
70. Critchley HO, Wallace WH. Impact of cancer treatment on uterine function. J Natl Cancer Inst Monogr. 2005;(34): 64–68.
71. Syrjala KL, Kurland BF, Abrams JR, et al. Sexual function changes during the 5 years after high-dose treatment and hematopoietic cell transplantation for malignancy, with case-matched controls at 5 years. Blood. 2008;111(3):989–996.
72. Watson M, Wheatley K, Harrison GA, et al. Severe adverse impact on sexual functioning and fertility of bone marrow transplantation, either allogeneic or autologous, compared with consolidation chemotherapy alone: analysis of the MRC AML 10 trial. Cancer. 1999;86(7):1231–1239.

24

CHAPTER 24

Cardiac and vascular complications in long-term survivors after hematopoietic stem cell transplantation

Alicia Rovó and André Tichelli

Hematology Department, University Hospital of Basel, Basel, Switzerland

Late cardiac complications

Late cardiotoxicity in long-term survivors after hematopoietic stem cell transplantation (HSCT) includes cardiomyopathy, overt congestive heart failure (CHF), valvular dysfunction, arrhythmia, and pericarditis. After autologous HSCT, 43% of the late deaths were attributed to treatment-related causes, and 2.4% of them were due to cardiac events [1]. After allogeneic HSCT, mortality was attributed to transplant-related causes in 25%, and cardiac toxicity was the cause of death in 3% [2]. Compared with relapse of the primary disease and other nonrelapse-related complications, cardiac late effects are, though, considered to be a rare complication and have so far not been a major concern in long-term HSCT survivors. Publications on long-term cardiac complications after HSCT are consequently scarce. Based on the experiences of cancer survivors, follow-up time after HSCT might still be too short to assess the full magnitude of risk. For example, long-term survivors of Hodgkin lymphoma with considerably longer follow-up are at increased risk of nonrelapse mortality, with cardiovascular complications being the most common nonmalignant cause of death [3].

Late cardiac complications in long-term cancer survivors

Anthracyclines and their derivatives are the main cause of cardiomyopathy. A number of risk factors for the development of chronic anthracycline cardiotoxicity have been identified. The strongest predictor is its cumulative dose. However, age at the time of drug exposure, concomitant administration of other cardiotoxic chemotherapeutic agents, concurrent or prior chest irradiation, and preexisting cardiovascular disease (CVD) are also well-recognized risk factors [4, 5].

Anthracycline-induced cardiotoxicity incidence approaches 26% in non-HSCT survivors treated with doses exceeding 550 mg/m^2 [6]. However, there is no safe cumulative dose of anthracycline. Elderly patients are at higher risk for anthracycline-induced cardiotoxicity; hence, in a large cohort of 3164 patients aged ≥65 years with *diffuse large B-cell lymphoma*, any doxorubicin use was associated with a 29% increase in risk of CHF (95% confidence interval (CI), 1.02–1.62). Patients treated with doxorubicin were at higher risk to develop CHF than those treated without. In this population, various factors increased CHF risk, but only hypertension was synergistic with doxorubicin [7]. Longer interval since exposure

Blood and Marrow Transplantation Long-Term Management: Prevention and Complications, First Edition. Edited by Bipin N Savani.

is also at risk for cardiac toxicity. In pediatric patients, a continuous deterioration of cardiac function was observed for up to 30 years after treatment [8].

Mediastinal radiotherapy can produce inflammation and fibrosis of any structure of the heart, causing a restrictive cardiomyopathy. Fibrosis may also affect electrical conduction pathways, causing intra-cardiac conduction delay, arrhythmias, and autonomic dysfunction, and develop valvular defects. Cardiac damage induced by radiation is dose dependent through several different mechanisms. In animal models, radiation can incite a pro-inflammatory response that facilitates the development or destabilization of coronary artery plaques [9]. In addition, intimal thickening in large vessels and microvascular damage with impairment of myocardial perfusion can be seen after radiation exposure [10]. Among survivors treated with mantle radiation therapy at doses of 35–45 Gy, the standardized incidence ratio of significant cardiac morbidity is elevated by two- to four-fold, and the cumulative risks of significant heart disease among survivors of adult Hodgkin disease are 5–10% at 15 years [4], 16% at 20 years [8], and 34% at 30 years [11]. Mediastinal radiation additionally increases the risk of myocardial infarction, angina pectoris, and CHF two- to seven-fold.

Late cardiac complications after HSCT

In adult patients treated with HSCT, the follow-up is still substantially shorter than in survivors of Hodgkin lymphoma. Compared with the general population, the risk of late death due to cardiac complications is fourfold higher after autologous HSCT in females only [1] and 2.3-fold higher after allogeneic HSCT in males and females [2]. In a cohort of aggressive lymphoma treated with autologous HSCT, nonmalignant late complications observed within the first 3 years were most often related to infections (19%), or were neurological (18%) and gastrointestinal (15%) late events. Cardiovascular late effects were reported in 6% of the patients, with a 3-year cumulative incidence of 9% [12]. All these patients presented with left ventricular ejection fraction (LVEF) dysfunction, but only one-third of them had clinical symptoms requiring treatment. More late cardiac complications were noted when mitoxantrone was used as part of the conditioning regimen. In a large study of 425 lymphoma survivors after autologous HSCT, a high prevalence of CHF with exercise-induced shortness of breath was reported. Females had a greater likelihood of developing CHF (odds ratio (OR): 4.3; 95% CI: 1.1–17.2) [13]. In pediatric patients, late cardiac complications after HSCT are less frequent [14]. With a median follow-up of 10 years, 87% of 155 long-term survivors after allogeneic HSCT had at least one late effect. Pulmonary dysfunction was observed in 63.2%, but cardiovascular events in only 15% of the patients. In a prospective multicenter European Group for Blood and Marrow Transplantation (EBMT) study, cardiac shortening fraction measured by echocardiogram before and yearly up to 5 years of follow-up was evaluated in 119 children treated with allogeneic HSCT [15]. The 5-year cumulative incidence of cardiac impairment was 26%. Total body irradiation (TBI) alone and TBI together with pretransplant anthracycline administration were significant risk factors for reduced cardiac function. Of the patients who received TBI and anthracyclines, 26% had abnormal cardiac shortening fraction, as compared with only 2% of patients without TBI and anthracyclines. At last follow-up 5 years after HSCT, only 13% of the patients had cardiac dysfunction, and all of them were asymptomatic. In another study on children surviving 1 year after allogeneic HSCT for a hematological malignancy, the probability of developing cardiac and cardiovascular complications at 10 years increased up to 11% [16]. Eleven out of 48 children had abnormal echocardiography, eight patients had high blood pressure, and two patients had cerebrovascular injuries. All 11 patients had received TBI. Most studies on long-term survivors are based on functional cardiac tests at rest. In a pediatric population, longitudinal assessment of cardiovascular performance with exercise testing was significantly impaired after HSCT [17].

The relative contributions of fludarabine or cyclophosphamide-based conditioning, as well as iron overload in the development of late cardiac toxicity, are not well known. Some studies describe early cyclophosphamide cardiotoxicity with left ventricular diastolic rather than systolic dysfunction [18–20]. The late cardiotoxicity of cyclophosphamide remains obscure and is more considered as an adjuvant player when administrated in combination with TBI or given to patients with previous exposure to anthracycline. Fludarabine used as conditioning with melphalan has been associated with severe cardiac toxicity in at least seven cases [21]. A longer follow-up is needed to clearly define the cardiac harm extent of these compounds in transplanted patients.

Iron-induced cardiac disease is the primary cause of death in transfused patients with thalassemia major. The beneficial effects of deferoxamine on clinical cardiac disease have been well described, but the impact of iron chelation on subclinical cardiac dysfunction is unknown. Transplanted thalassemia patients with early cardiac involvement can show complete regression of these subclinical cardiac abnormalities after phlebotomy [22]. Pretransplantation transfusion history and serum ferritin have significant prognostic value in patients with myelodysplastic syndrome undergoing myeloablative allogeneic stem cell transplantation, inducing a significant increase of nonrelapse mortality [23–25]. However, so far there is no proof that iron-induced cardiotoxicity is responsible for the increased death rates.

In long-term HSCT survivors, transplantation-related risk factors include conditioning with high-dose chemotherapy, TBI and chronic graft-versus-host disease (GVHD). In a case–control [26], 63 survivors with clinical CHF were compared with 186 matched controls (HSCT survivors without CHF) to identify predictors for late cardiovascular complications after HSCT. The mean ejection fraction of the patients with CHF was 36.7% (range: 13–53%). Multivariate analysis revealed the following factors independently associated with risk of CHF: female gender (OR: 2.1; $p < 0.01$), high-dose ($\geq$250 mg/m^2) anthracycline alone (OR: 3.9; $p < 0.01$) or with chest radiation (OR: 6.7; $p < 0.01$), and the presence of multiple post-HSCT comorbidities (OR: 3.0; $p < 0.01$). Overall survival following CHF was 46.1% at 5 years. High-dose chemotherapy or TBI used for conditioning did not contribute significantly to the risk of CHF. The same group evaluated the incidence and predictors of CHF in 1244 patients undergoing autologous HSCT for a hematologic malignancy between 1988 and 2002. The cumulative incidence of CHF was 4.8% at 5 years and 9.1% at 15 years after transplantation. Compared with a matched general population, the standardized incidence ratio was 4.5-fold increased. The risk of CHF increased substantially for patients receiving >250 mg/m^2 of cumulative anthracycline exposure (OR: 9.9, $p < 0.01$). This means that, compared with cancer patients, the threshold for anthracycline-related cardiotoxicity is lower in HSCT patients (Figure 24.1). Among recipients with a cumulative anthracycline dose of >250 mg/m^2, the presence of hypertension (OR: 35.3, $p < 0.01$) or diabetes (OR: 26.8; $p < 0.01$) resulted in a significant increased relative risk of CHF, providing evidence that hypertension and

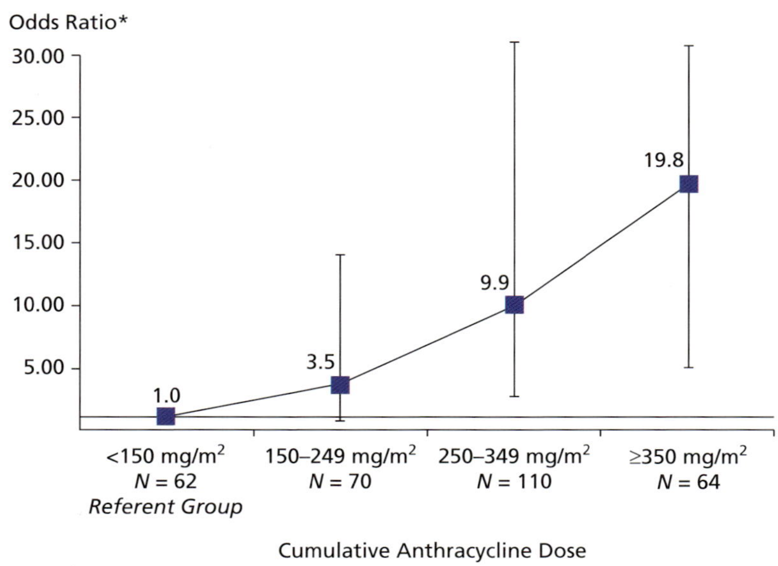

Figure 24.1 Magnitude of risk of CHF of patients treated with HSCT by increments of anthracycline dose. Compared with the reference group of patients who received a cumulative dose of anthracycline <150 mg/m^2, the relative risk for CHF is significantly increased for patients with anthracycline $\geq$250 mg/m^2. Adapted from Armenian S et al. *Blood*. 2011;118(23):6023–6029.

diabetes may be critical modifiers of anthracycline-related myocardial injury after HSCT [27].

Monitoring and management of cardiac late effects

Routine clinical assessment is indicated for all HSCT recipients [28]. Closer monitoring of cardiac function before, during, and after HSCT is highly recommended for patients at risk for cardiac complications to detect subclinical cardiac impairment. The most frequent approach used to monitor cardiac function is the evaluation of LVEF. Echocardiography and radionuclide angiography are the standard approaches for noninvasive monitoring of LVEF. All the conventional echocardiographic parameters of M-mode, 2-D, and Doppler techniques can be used. When echocardiography is suboptimal or suggestive of cardiac dysfunction, radionuclide ventriculography [29] or cardiac magnetic resonance imaging can be helpful to quantify the ejection fraction [30].

The leading risk factors for late cardiac toxicity after HSCT are previous exposure to anthracyclines, having TBI as part of the conditioning regimen, and cardiac comorbidity. Other factors, like standard cardiovascular risks (CVRs), gender, advanced age at transplantation, and presence of noncardiac comorbidities emerge as potential contributors in the development of late cardiac effects. All patients with increased risk profile should therefore undergo a surveillance program where the main goal is to detect early changes in cardiac function. A multidisciplinary approach involving the expertise of internist, cardiologist and diagnostic imaging services, together with the transplantation team, is paramount in following these patients.

Vascular complications

Vascular complications have been recently recognized as late effects after HSCT [31, 32]. The high prevalence of CVDs in the general population and the very late presentation of CVDs after HSCT were the main reasons for underestimating the relationship between the CVD and HSCT. CVDs belong to the nonmalignant late events that affect the arterial blood vessels, and refer usually to diseases related to atherosclerosis. They can present as cerebrovascular accidents, coronary heart diseases, or peripheral vascular diseases.

Cardiovascular diseases after HSCT

Therapy-related CVDs have been recently acknowledged as one of the more serious complications in long-term survivors after HSCT [33, 34]. A retrospective single-center study first showed that vascular events are increased after allogeneic HSCT [31]. Eighteen out of 265 (6.8%) patients were diagnosed with an arterial event. The patients at first vascular event were unexpectedly young (median age 49 years), with a long time interval from transplantation to the first event (median 9 years; range 2–12 years). The cumulative incidence of a late CVD was 22% at 25 years. Adjusted for age of the patients, recipients of allogeneic HSCT presented significantly more arterial events than patients did treated with autologous HSCT (Figure 24.1), with a cumulative incidence of an arterial event at 15 years posttransplant of 2.3% for autologous HSCT and 7.5% for allogeneic HSCT. From these data, it appears that, in patients treated with allogeneic HSCT, arterial events occur prematurely.

These data were confirmed in a retrospective multicenter study of the Late Effects Working Party of the EBMT [35]. Twenty of 548 long-term survivors treated with allogeneic HSCT between 1990 and 1995 were reported with an arterial event, with a cumulative incidence at 15 years of 6%. The lower incidence of CVD in this study could be explained by a shorter follow-up time and a higher rate of underreporting of vascular events owing to the multicenter design of the study. The incidence rate of new CVDs was increased to 4.1 new events per 1000 person-years over what is expected (<1.0 new event per 1000 person-years).

Recently, cardiovascular-related hospitalization and death were evaluated among persons still alive at least 2 years after HSCT. Transplant recipients experienced increased cardiovascular deaths (adjusted incidence rate difference: 3.6 per 1000 person-years; 95% CI: 1.7–5.5) and showed an increased cumulative incidence of ischemic heart disease, cardiomyopathy or heart failure, stroke, vascular diseases, and rhythm disorders, when compared with a matched control population [36]

Among long-term survivors, CVDs present more frequently as coronary heart disease and/or cerebrovascular accidents. Isolated peripheral artery disease has been rarely reported. In a case–control study of 63 patients with late CVDs, 44 presented with coronary artery disease and 19 with cerebrovascular disease. The median time from HSCT to CVD was 4 years, though with a broad range (1.1–19.4 years). Thirty-four of these 63 patients with a CVD died, 31% of them from a cardiovascular event [37]. CVD directly affects the health condition in long-term survivors. In a study on 1022 HSCT survivors, the cumulative incidence of a chronic health condition was 59% at 10 years after HSCT. Long-term survivors were more likely to have gastrointestinal, musculoskeletal, and cardiovascular problems, compared with siblings after adjustment for age, sex, and race/ethnicity, both after allogeneic and autologous HSCT [38].

The risk of developing CVDs is thus increased after HSCT, and cardiovascular complications appear prematurely compared with the expectation in the general population.

Cardiovascular risk factors

Atherosclerosis is a slow, chronic inflammatory process that typically starts in childhood and leads to cardiovascular manifestations in adults past the age of 60 years. Established risk factors for CVD include family history, dyslipidemia, hypertension, diabetes mellitus, obesity, chronic kidney disease, and lifestyle factors. A number of pretransplant and posttransplant factors may accelerate atherosclerosis, and therefore contribute to the development of premature CVDs after HSCT.

In a large cohort of 1089 HSCT recipients who survived at least 2 years and who were not currently taking immunosuppressant agents, the prevalence of diabetes and hypertension was increased. Diabetes was at least three times more likely to occur in allogeneic transplant patients than in siblings [32]. This risk was even higher for patients conditioned with TBI. In contrast, recipients of autologous HSCT did not have a higher risk than siblings to develop diabetes or hypertension.

A clear relationship between posttransplant CVRs and late CVDs in long-term survivors has been demonstrated in the two aforementioned studies [31, 35]. CVRs, such as hypertension, diabetes, and dyslipidemia appearing after HSCT, as well as physical inactivity and ongoing tobacco smoking, were related to increased risk of late CVDs. In a case–control study, the presence of two or more post-HSCT CVRs resulted in a greater than fivefold increased risk of CVDs, and a high cardiovascular risk score was associated with a 20-fold increased risk for cerebrovascular complications after HSCT [37].

In a cross-sectional study, patients treated with allogeneic HSCT showed a 2.2-fold increase of risk of a metabolic syndrome [39], a clustering of CVRs characterized by abdominal obesity, dyslipidemia, hypertension, and elevated fasting glucose, compared with age- and gender-matched controls [40]. In a case-matched comparison performed in 44 recipients and their respective donors with a very long term follow-up after allogeneic HSCT (median: 17.5 years; range: 11–26 years), recipients had more frequent hypertension ($p = 0.015$), dyslipidemia ($p = 0.002$), thyroid dysfunction ($p = 0.002$), and showed systematically lower glomerular filtration rates ($p < 0.0001$) [41]. Dyslipidemia appearing after HSCT seems to play a central role in therapy-related CVDs [42]. Estimates of dyslipidemia in long-term survivors after allogeneic HSCT range from 8.9% to 56%, and are even higher in patients still on immunosuppressive treatment. In a small study on 23 children treated with allogeneic HSCT, hypertriglyceridemia was observed in 39%, which was significantly higher than in patients treated with chemotherapy alone (8%) for acute lymphoblastic leukemia [43]. Risk factors emerging after HSCT are probably responsible for the premature onset of CVDs rather than those present at time of transplantation. Cardiovascular risk factors are increased after allogeneic HSCT compared with autologous HSCT, with relative risks of new-onset dyslipidemia and hypertension of 2.31 and 2.5, respectively [31]. In a recent publication, these posttransplant CVRs were shown to be increased after allogeneic HSCT compared with autologous HSCT, with a relative risk of new onset for hypertension, diabetes, and dyslipidemia of 5.2, 2.6, and 2.2, respectively. Multivariate regression analysis revealed that survivors with a history of grade II–IV acute GVHD were at a ninefold risk of hypertension, sixfold risk of diabetes, and threefold risk of dyslipidemia when compared with autologous HSCT survivors. TBI has a significant risk for post-HSCT diabetes and dyslipidemia [44].

Role of endothelial injury in the pathogenesis of cardiovascular disease

There is evidence now that CVRs are associated with the development of CVDs after allogeneic HSCT. But why do long-term survivors develop CVRs more frequently after

HSCT even once they are off immunosuppressive treatment? Endocrine dysfunctions, growth hormone insufficiency, hypothyroidism, and particularly gonadal dysfunction may all be involved in this process.

Insulin sensitivity is impaired in adults with growth hormone deficiency, inducing hypertriglyceridemia, low high-density lipoprotein (HDL) cholesterol, and hypertension [45]. In children treated with allogeneic HSCT, insufficient growth hormone secretion is associated with a higher risk of metabolic syndrome. Indeed, in a study of 34 transplanted children, the majority of those with metabolic syndrome had growth hormone deficiency [46].

Hypothyroidism has an adverse effect on serum lipids. Hypercholesterolemia is present in 95% and high serum cholesterol and hypertriglyceridemia in 40–70% of the patients with thyroid dysfunction. While patients with overt hypothyroidism have an increased risk for CVDs, which is most likely due to this unfavorable lipid profile, the situation is less clear for patients with subclinical hypothyroidism. Hypothyroidism is a common late effect in patients treated with HSCT, particularly when conditioned with TBI. After HSCT, overt hypothyroidism, and probably also subclinical dysfunction of the thyroid, induces changes resembling a metabolic syndrome, and is probably in part responsible for the increased CVRs [47].

Gonadal dysfunction is one of the most frequent complications after HSCT, particularly when conditioned with TBI. There is a strong association between hypogonadism and metabolic syndrome in these patients, with severe insulin resistance and dyslipidemia [48]. Metabolic syndrome is common in males with low androgen levels [49], and patients with testosterone deficiency may improve insulin sensitivity on receiving testosterone replacement therapy. In females, estrogens are known to influence the body composition, lipid metabolism, blood pressure, and vascular tone [47, 50].

Physiologically, leptin acts as a regulator of food intake and energy metabolism. Obesity is associated with hyperleptinemia, reflecting either leptin tolerance or leptin resistance. Hyperleptinemia could be pathophysiologically involved in the development of metabolic syndrome after HSCT. A potential interaction among circulating leptin, components of metabolic syndrome, and immune function might explain the role of this adipokine in mediating cardiovascular risk after HSCT [51, 52].

Nonendocrinal factors could also be involved in the development of hypertension and metabolic syndrome after HSCT. Plasma magnesium levels may modify insulin sensitivity. Chronic magnesium deficiency has been associated with the development of insulin resistance, diabetes, and metabolic syndrome [53, 54]. Hypomagnesemia is a common finding in patients after HSCT. Magnesium depletion may be due to reduced dietary intake, intestinal loss during chronic gastrointestinal GVHD, and the use of calcineurin inhibitors suppressing magnesium reabsorption from renal tubules [55]. The role of magnesium levels on metabolic syndrome after HSCT is still unknown. However, magnesium deficiency could contribute to the risk of atherosclerosis and CVDs, and therefore deserves wider attention.

Endothelial injury occurring during HSCT might be the primary event leading to premature atherosclerosis and subsequent development of CVD in long-term survivors after HSCT. The vascular endothelium can be the target of TBI. Radiation exposure induces direct endothelial damage of the microvasculature system and vascular stiffening, both findings of CVD. In an animal model, radiation exposure significantly reduces endothelial cell outgrowth in a dose-dependent manner. This effect may inhibit re-endothelialization or angiogenesis after vascular injury and, therefore, contribute to radiation-induced endothelial dysfunction and leave the vascular system vulnerable to future vascular injury [56]. In a rat model, 10 Gy TBI decreases the density of the smaller caliber coronary vessels in the heart, resulting in coronary microvasculature injury [57].

The vascular endothelium can also be damaged by a graft-versus-host reaction. At engraftment, the host vascular endothelium is the first cell type that comes into contact with the emerging donor T lymphocytes. The accelerated atherosclerosis occurring after allogeneic HCT could therefore result from an inflammatory process initiated by transplant-related endothelial damage. Cutaneous chronic GVHD is characterized by progressive loss of dermal microvessels [44, 58, 59]. Furthermore, indicators of inflammation are more frequent in long-term survivors after HSCT with ongoing chronic GVHD as measured by higher c-reactive protein ($p = 0.001$) and higher von Willebrand factor ($p = 0.002$) [41]. A diagram of the hypothetical atherosclerotic process occurring in long-term survivors after HSCT and leading eventually to a therapy-related CVDs is outline in Figure 24.2.

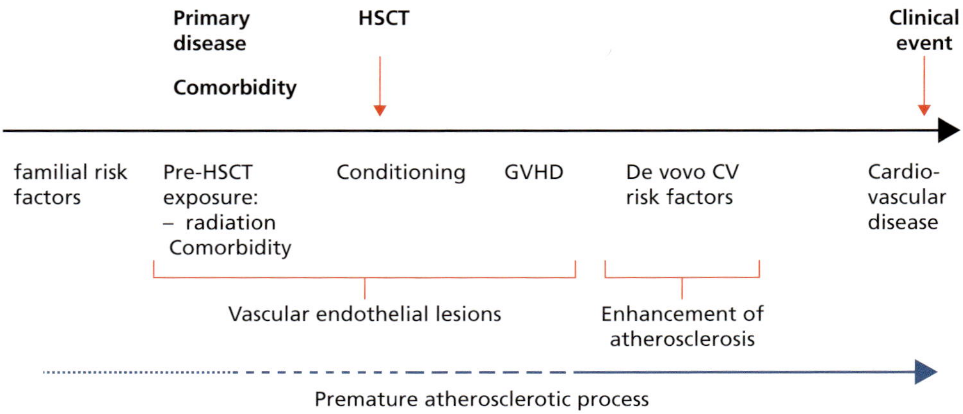

Figure 24.2 Diagram of the hypothetical atherosclerotic process occurring in long-term survivors after HSCT and leading eventually to a therapy-related CVD. In patients treated with HSCT, early endothelial injury, various hormonal deficiencies, and hypomagnesemia secondary to the conditioning regimen and/or GVHD might represent the basis of the accelerated process of atherosclerosis. As a consequence, metabolic alterations such as hypertension, insulin resistance, dyslipidemia, and glucose abnormalities will occur in patients treated with HSCT. Such changes will continuously harm the already more vulnerable vascular endothelium. The clinical manifestations of a CVD, which are the final consequences of this atherosclerotic process, appear much later in the course of HSCT. Individually, genetic factors, heart-healthy lifestyle, and pretransplant injuries such as local radiation therapy may reinforce the process of atherosclerosis. The correction of endocrine dysfunctions and the early management of the metabolic alterations are the modifiable factors which might prevent or postpone the further development of therapy-related atherosclerosis and consecutive CVD [78].

Monitoring and management of long-term survivors at risk for cardiovascular disease

The management of a patient with symptomatic CVD after HSCT is no different than it is for a nontransplant population. However, since patients may develop a CVD at premature age, the question is how to prevent or postpone such an event. For accurate management of the long-term survivors, patients at risk have to be defined (I), the type and timing for optimal screening need to be decided (II), and preventive and therapeutic practices should be implemented promptly (III). This way of proceeding makes sense, assuming that prevention and intervention measures have a similar benefit in transplanted patients as they have in the general population, even though this has not yet been proven.

(I) Identification of patients at risk for cardiovascular disease

Patients treated with mediastinal, neck, or head radiation before HSCT [60, 61] as well as those conditioned with TBI [31, 35] are at particularly high risk for CVD. Furthermore, the development of endocrine dysfunctions after HSCT is associated with an increased probability of a metabolic syndrome, which in turn represents the main risk factor for CVD [43, 46, 48]. Finally, long-lasting immunosuppressive therapy and ongoing chronic GVHD have been associated with increased risk for CVD.

(II) When and how to start screening

The ultimate aim is to prevent CVD after HSCT and, therefore, to manage risk factors. Age, sex, and hereditary factors are nonmodifiable CVRs. Additionally, we assume that pretransplant factors, as well as conditioning regimen and the type of transplantation, are determined by other considerations. The obvious modifiable CVRs are obesity, diabetes, dyslipidemia, hypertension, and lifestyle factors such as cigarette smoking, physical inactivity, and food habits (Table 24.1).

Preventive practices should not be deferred until immunosuppressive drugs are withdrawn , since even patients off immunosuppression for a long time may be at increased risk for metabolic-syndrome-like changes. Furthermore, long-term survivors will return to their local hematologist/oncologist or primary care physician, who may not be familiar with specific management of

Table 24.1 Approach of CRFs in long-term survivors after HSCT [78]

Risk factors	Common causes	HSCT-related causes	Monitoring	Intervention
Dyslipidemia	• Obesity • Atherogenic diet • Familial dyslipidemia • Alcohol • Uncontrolled diabetes mellitus	• Gonadal dysfunction • Growth hormone • deficiency • Hypothyroidism • Chronic GVHD (cholestatic liver) • Immunosuppression	• Regular control of fasting lipid profile even after immunosuppression has been stopped • Monitoring HSCT-related causes: evaluate hormonal levels	• Weight control • Counseling healthy heart life style • Intervention of HSCT-related causes; i.e. ,evaluate need of hormonal replacement • By persistence of high values: – statin therapy – high-risk patients – consider early onset
Arterial hypertension	• Obesity • Sodium sensitivity • Role of renin • Insulin resistance • Diabetes • Sleep apnea • Kidney disease • Nonsteroidal anti-inflammatory drugs • Aging	• Corticosteroids • Calcineurin inhibitors • Insulin resistance • Endocrine dysfunction • Kidney disease	• Blood pressure check performed at least every 2 years • Unclear cases: ambulatory blood pressure monitoring • Cases with arterial hypertension: – periodic evaluation of target organ damage (heart, kidney, lung, brain, arterial vessels)	• Intervention is indicated for readings >140/90 mmHg in adults on two separate visits at least 1 week apart *or* >130/80 mmHg in diabetes or renal disease: – weight reduction – dietary sodium reduction – moderate alcohol consumption – regular physical activity – choice of antihypertensive drugs based on general recommendations – angiotensin receptor blockers and angiotensin-converting enzyme inhibitors preferred in patients with chronic kidney disease or diabetes
Diabetes	• Obesity • Aging • Physical inactivity	• Corticosteroids • Endocrine dysfunction	• HbA1C • Fasting glucose • 2-h postchallenge glucose	Stepwise approach, consider: 1. Counseling for appropriate diet and physical activity 2. By corticosteroids therapy, evaluate reduction or replacement by another immune-suppressive drug 3. Oral hypoglycemic 4. Insulin
Kidney disease	• Atherosclerosis • Diabetes • Arterial hypertension • Nonsteroidal anti-inflammatory drugs • Glomerulonephritis	• TBI • Chemotherapy (carboplatin) • Nephrotoxic drugs • Calcineurin inhibitors • GVHD	• Yearly control of renal function, • Glomerular filtration rate • Urine protein analysis • Unclear chronic kidney disease: consider renal biopsy	• Control of hypertension • Treatment of GVHD • Dialysis • Consider renal transplantation

long-term survivors. Therefore, transplantation centers should play a central role in counseling health providers on screening and prevention of long-time survivors [62].

The screening of the modifiable CVRs after HSCT includes regular control of blood pressure, body weight, inclusive of waist circumference, and the laboratory tests to detect dyslipidemia and abnormal glucose profile. According to the recommendations on screening and preventive practices for long-term survivors after HSCT, a blood pressure check should be performed at least every 2 years in long-term survivors [62]. There is a debate about the ideal screening test for early detection of type 2 diabetes. Measurement of glycated hemoglobin (HbA1C), fasting glucose, or 2-h postchallenge glucose can be used [39, 63]. Despite these parameters not having been validated in transplanted patients, a number of publications have proven to be useful [40, 43, 47].

Lipid and glucose profiles for all patients 1 year after HSCT should be performed. Thereafter, it depends on the risk profile of the patients. Patients with a high probability to develop CVRs should be controlled yearly. When a treatment for dyslipidemia is started, the effect on lipid serum values has to be controlled after 4–6 weeks until normalization of the values. In low-risk patients with a normal profile at 1 year, the posttransplant evaluation should be done according to the recommendations as for the general population.

(III) Prevention and treatment of cardiovascular risks

The main effort has to be brought to the management of the modifiable CVRs. Two main complementary approaches can be considered: treatment of the endocrine dysfunctions that may be responsible for the development of the CVRs, and treatment of these CVRs themselves, which are hypertension, diabetes, obesity, and dyslipidemia. The counseling of a healthy heart lifestyle is an integral part of the preventive practices.

There are conflicting data on improvement of CVRs by treatment of endocrine dysfunctions. All data come from interventions tested in nontransplant cohorts with endocrine dysfunction. Patients with overt hypothyroidism are usually treated with hormonal substitution, while treatment of asymptomatic patients remains controversial. The effect of the treatment of hypothyroidism on metabolic syndrome after HSCT is largely unknown. In a nontransplant setting, modest reductions in serum cholesterol and triglyceride levels have been demonstrated after hormonal substitution. However, replacement therapy seems not to have a marked effect on weight or blood pressure [64–66].

The effect of gonadal substitution on metabolic changes in females is not clear. In postmenopausal women with documented coronary heart disease, a decrease in low-density lipoprotein (LDL) cholesterol and an increase in HDL cholesterol levels have been observed in the group of patients with hormonal substitution, but not in patients of the placebo group. However, no difference was observed between both groups in respect of the incidence of CVD [67]. In an interventional study of cancer treatment, males with hypogonadal function and growth hormone deficiency have shown benefits of hormonal substitution on lipid profile, body mass index, and glucose metabolism [68, 69]. Testosterone therapy has also significantly improved lipid profiles, reduced body fat, increased lean muscle mass, and lowered blood pressure in men with hypogonadism [70]. In another situation with only relative testosterone deficiency as observed in elderly patients, testosterone substitution could not improve and correct metabolic changes [71]. It could be a similar situation for post-transplant male recipients who actually have normal or only slightly decreased testosterone levels and are usually asymptomatic.

There are no data on the effects of growth hormone substitution on metabolic syndrome in patients treated with HSCT. In nontransplant patients, replacement therapy can reduce CVRs, and a treatment with growth hormone seems to increase the lean body mass and decrease the fat mass. Growth hormone substitution has a lowering effect on total and LDL cholesterol, particularly in patients with higher pretreatment cholesterol levels. Furthermore, growth hormone replacement is shown to exert additional beneficial effects on lipoprotein profiles in patients on maintenance statin therapy [72–74].

Post-HSCT recipients with endocrine deficiency treated with hormonal substitution may have a beneficial and additive effect to the standard treatment on lipid profile, glucose tolerance, and body fat. So far, the indication for the treatment of an endocrine dysfunction with hormonal supplementation should be based on classical recommendations. The initiation of hormonal substitution should not be an argument to postpone the specific treatment of dyslipidemia, diabetes, or hypertension.

The key to CVD prevention is mainly based on the treatment of the modifiable CVRs, but no formal recommendations exist for the management of the patients treated with HSCT. Treatment of hypertension, diabetes, and dyslipidemia does not principally differ to the treatment in the general population; therefore, the general recommendations should be applied. However, some specific differences have to be observed mainly because of drug interactions and toxicity [75].

The treatment of diabetes mellitus after HSCT necessitates special consideration; essentially, the treatment goal is similar to nontransplanted patients with diabetes. Counseling for appropriate diet and physical activity is the first step to improving glucose metabolism. However, post-HSCT recipients may present with reduced health status imposing a limitation for regular exercise. Post-transplant medications, particularly corticosteroids used to control GVHD, play a key role triggering or worsening diabetes. Reduction of corticosteroids and even replacement by another immunosuppressive drug should be considered. If these initial measures cannot control the diabetes, drug therapy to improve glucose metabolism is indicated. There are only limited data on oral hypoglycemic agents for posttransplant patients. In clinically unstable patients receiving high-dose corticosteroids, or patients with gastrointestinal problems, insulin therapy is usually preferred until further stabilization [42].

There are currently no established guidelines for management of dyslipidemia after HSCT. The use of the guidelines from the National Cholesterol Education Program ATP III represent the basis for management [39]. A review with a suggested approach on the management of dyslipidemia after HSCT has recently been published [42]. The focus was on aspects that may interfere with the therapy for dyslipidemia post-HSCT. The main target of the treatment is to normalize LDL cholesterol. According to the ATP III recommendations, in the case of excess of LDL cholesterol, a stepwise procedure is indicated. The first step is counseling lifestyle changes. The patients should decrease the intake of saturated fat and dietary cholesterol, minimize trans-fatty acid ingestion, and increase regular physical activity. For patients who are still under immunosuppressive treatment, thoughts about dose reduction or drug replacement by an immunosuppressive medicament with less effect on lipid profile should be considered. In the last step, when therapeutic lifestyle changes and medicament adjustment have not corrected the lipid profile adequately, drug therapy has to be discussed. In this case, special attention should be given to drug interactions and toxicity. The statins are the most commonly used drugs in the treatment of hypercholesterolemia for lowering LDL cholesterol. The effects of statin therapy are additive to those of therapeutic lifestyle changes.

Hypertension in long-term survivors should be treated according to the Joint National Committee (JNC7) guidelines [76, 77]. In a first step, lifestyle modification alone can be tried to correct mild hypertension. This includes weight reduction if indicated, adoption of a DASH eating plan (Dietary Approaches to Stop Hypertension), dietary sodium reduction, moderate alcohol consumption, and regular physical activity. In more refractory forms of hypertension or in hypertension associated with chronic kidney disease, a treatment with an antihypertensive agent is usually necessary. The choice of antihypertensive drugs is based on the general recommendations mentioned before. Angiotensin receptor blockers and angiotensin-converting enzyme inhibitors are generally preferred in patients with chronic kidney disease or diabetes because of their renal protective effect [75].

Conclusions

After HSCT, patients are at risk for therapy-related CVD. The "standard" CVRs play a major role in the appearance of premature cardiovascular events after HSCT. The role of endothelium injury in the pathogenesis of CVD seems to be crucial. Previous exposure to radiotherapy, TBI used as part of the conditioning regimen, and GVHD are the main players involved in triggering the atherosclerotic process leading to premature endothelial aging and enhanced late cardiovascular complications. The reasons for the higher incidence of CVRs responsible for late CVDs are probably multifactorial and due to multiple endocrine dysfunctions, magnesium dysbalance, treatment with immunosuppressive drugs, and changes in healthy lifestyle. So far, the best way to reduce the risk of premature CVDs is to manage the modifiable CVRs. Regular screening allows early detection of CVRs. Adequate preventive and therapeutic interventions when necessary may be introduced. In all cases, counseling of healthy heart lifestyle should be an integral part of the management. A steady growth in late CVD after allogeneic HSCT can be expected in the forthcoming decades. Hence, late CVDs emerge as one of the most harmful nonmalignant late effects after HSCT; this trend could possibly be delayed by applying early screening and systematic management of the modifiable risk factors.

Disclosures

Conflict-of-interest disclosure: AR and AT declare no competing financial interests.

References

1. Bhatia S, Robison LL, Francisco L, et al. Late mortality in survivors of autologous hematopoietic-cell transplantation: report from the Bone Marrow Transplant Survivor Study. Blood. 2005;105:4215–4222.
2. Bhatia S, Francisco L, Carter A, et al. Late mortality after allogeneic hematopoietic cell transplantation and functional status of long-term survivors: report from the Bone Marrow Transplant Survivor Study. Blood. 2007;110:3784–3792.
3. Ng AK. Review of the cardiac long-term effects of therapy for Hodgkin lymphoma. Br J Haematol. 2011;154:23–31.
4. Myrehaug S, Pintilie M, Tsang R, et al. Cardiac morbidity following modern treatment for Hodgkin lymphoma: supra-additive cardiotoxicity of doxorubicin and radiation therapy. Leuk Lymphoma. 2008;49:1486–1493.
5. Hooning MJ, Botma A, Aleman BM, et al. Long-term risk of cardiovascular disease in 10-year survivors of breast cancer. J Natl Cancer Inst. 2007;99:365–375.
6. Yahalom J, Portlock CS. Long-term cardiac and pulmonary complications of cancer therapy. Heart Fail Clin 2011;7: 403–411.
7. Hershman DL, McBride RB, Eisenberger A, et al. Doxorubicin, cardiac risk factors, and cardiac toxicity in elderly patients with diffuse B-cell non-Hodgkin's lymphoma. J Clin Oncol. 2008;26:3159–3165.
8. Galper SL, Yu JB, Mauch PM, et al. Clinically significant cardiac disease in patients with Hodgkin lymphoma treated with mediastinal irradiation. Blood. 2011;117:412–418.
9. Hendry JH, Akahoshi M, Wang LS, et al. Radiation-induced cardiovascular injury. Radiat Environ Biophys. 2008;47: 189–193.
10. Darby SC, Cutter DJ, Boerma M, et al. Radiation-related heart disease: current knowledge and future prospects. Int J Radiat Oncol Biol Phys. 2010;76:656–665.
11. Aleman BMP, van den Belt-Dusebout A, De Bruin ML, et al. Late cardiotoxicity after treatment for Hodgkin lymphoma. Blood. 2007;109:1878–1886.
12. Ruiz-Soto R, Sergent G, Gisselbrecht C, et al. Estimating late adverse events using competing risks after autologous stem-cell transplantation in aggressive non-Hodgkin lymphoma patients. Cancer. 2005;104:2735–2742.
13. Majhail NS, Ness KK, Burns LJ, et al. Late effects in survivors of Hodgkin and non-Hodgkin lymphoma treated with autologous hematopoietic cell transplantation: a report from the Bone Marrow Transplant Survivor Study. Biol Blood Marrow Transplant. 2007;13:1153–1159.
14. Leung W, Ahn H, Rose SR, et al. A prospective cohort study of late sequelae of pediatric allogeneic hematopoietic stem cell transplantation. Medicine (Baltimore). 2007;86:215–224.
15. Uderzo C, Pillon M, Corti P, et al. Impact of cumulative anthracycline dose, preparative regimen and chronic graft-versus-host disease on pulmonary and cardiac function in children 5 years after allogeneic hematopoietic stem cell transplantation: a prospective evaluation on behalf of the EBMT Pediatric Diseases and Late Effects Working Parties. Bone Marrow Transplant. 2007;39:667–675.
16. Ferry C, Gemayel G, Rocha V, et al. Long-term outcomes after allogeneic stem cell transplantation for children with hematological malignancies. Bone Marrow Transplant. 2007;40:219–224.
17. Hogarty AN, Leahey A, Zhao H, et al. Longitudinal evaluation of cardiopulmonary performance during exercise after bone marrow transplantation in children. J Pediatr. 2000; 136:311–317.
18. Katayama M, Imai Y, Hashimoto H, et al. Fulminant fatal cardiotoxicity following cyclophosphamide therapy. J Cardiol. 2009;54:330–334.
19. Mori T, Yanagi N, Maruyama T, et al. Left ventricular diastolic dysfunction induced by cyclophosphamide in blood stem cell transplantation. Jpn Heart J. 2002;43:249–261.
20. Zver S, Zadnik V, Cernelc P, Kozelj M. Cardiac toxicity of high-dose cyclophosphamide and melphalan in patients with multiple myeloma treated with tandem autologous hematopoietic stem cell transplantation. Int J Hematol. 2008;88:227–236.
21. Van BK, Devine S, Wickrema A, et al. Regimen-related toxicity after fludarabine-melphalan conditioning: a prospective study of 31 patients with hematologic malignancies. Bone Marrow Transplant. 2003;32:471–476.
22. Mariotti E, Angelucci E, Agostini A, et al. Evaluation of cardiac status in iron-loaded thalassaemia patients following bone marrow transplantation: improvement in cardiac function during reduction in body iron burden. Br J Haematol. 1998;103:916–921.

23. Alessandrino EP, Della Porta MG, Bacigalupo A, et al. Prognostic impact of pre-transplantation transfusion history and secondary iron overload in patients with myelodysplastic syndrome undergoing allogeneic stem cell transplantation: a GITMO study. Haematologica. 2010;95:476–484.
24. Deeg HJ, Spaulding E, Shulman HM. Iron overload, hematopoietic cell transplantation, and graft-versus-host disease. Leuk Lymphoma. 2009;50:1566–1572.
25. Kataoka K, Nannya Y, Hangaishi A, et al. Influence of pre-transplantation serum ferritin on nonrelapse mortality after myeloablative and nonmyeloablative allogeneic hematopoietic stem cell transplantation. Biol Blood Marrow Transplant. 2009;15:195–204.
26. Armenian SH, Sun CL, Francisco L, et al. Late congestive heart failure after hematopoietic cell transplantation. J Clin Oncol. 2008;26:5537–5543.
27. Armenian SH, Sun CL, Shannon T, et al. Incidence and predictors of congestive heart failure after autologous hematopoietic cell transplantation. Blood. 2011;118:6023–6029.
28. Majhail NS, Rizzo JD, Lee SJ, et al. Recommended screening and preventive practices for long-term survivors after hematopoietic cell transplantation. Hematol Oncol Stem Cell Ther. 2012;5:1–30.
29. Kremer LC, Caron HN. Anthracycline cardiotoxicity in children. N Engl J Med. 2004;351:120–121.
30. Oberholzer K, Kunz RP, Dittrich M, Thelen M. Anthracycline-induced cardiotoxicity: cardiac MRI after treatment for childhood cancer. Rofo. 2004;176:1245–1250 (in German).
31. Tichelli A, Bucher C, Rovó A, et al. Premature cardiovascular disease after allogeneic hematopoietic stem-cell transplantation. Blood. 2007;110:3463–3471.
32. Baker KS, Ness KK, Steinberger J, et al. Diabetes, hypertension, and cardiovascular events in survivors of hematopoietic cell transplantation: a report from the bone marrow transplantation survivor study. Blood. 2007;109:1765–1772.
33. Armenian SH, Bhatia S. Cardiovascular disease after hematopoietic cell transplantation – lessons learned. Haematologica. 2008;93:1132–1136.
34. Tichelli A, Bhatia S, Socie G. Cardiac and cardiovascular consequences after haematopoietic stem cell transplantation. Br J Haematol. 2008;142:11–26.
35. Tichelli A, Passweg J, Wojcik D, et al. Late cardiovascular events after allogeneic hematopoietic stem cell transplantation: a retrospective multicenter study of the Late Effects Working Party of the European Group for Blood and Marrow Transplantation. Haematologica. 2008;93:1203–1210.
36. Chow EJ, Mueller BA, Baker KS, et al. Cardiovascular hospitalizations and mortality among recipients of hematopoietic stem cell transplantation. Ann Intern Med. 2011;155:21–32.
37. Armenian SH, Sun CL, Mills G, et al. Predictors of late cardiovascular complications in survivors of hematopoietic cell transplantation. Biol Blood Marrow Transplant. 2010;16:1138–1144.
38. Sun CL, Francisco L, Kawashima T, et al. Prevalence and predictors of chronic health conditions after hematopoietic cell transplantation: a report from the Bone Marrow Transplant Survivor Study. Blood. 2010;116:3129–3139.
39. Kuhar MB. Update on managing hypercholesterolemia. The new NCEP guidelines. AAOHN J. 2002;50:360–364.
40. Majhail NS, Flowers ME, Ness KK, et al. High prevalence of metabolic syndrome after allogeneic hematopoietic cell transplantation. Bone Marrow Transplant. 2009;43:49–54.
41. Rovó A, Daikeler T, Halter J, et al. Late altered organ function in very long-term survivors after allogeneic hematopoietic stem cell transplantation: a paired comparison with their HLA-identical sibling donor. Haematologica. 2011;96:150–155.
42. Griffith ML, Savani BN, Boord JB. Dyslipidemia after allogeneic hematopoietic stem cell transplantation: evaluation and management. Blood. 2010;116:1197–1204.
43. Taskinen M, Saarinen-Pihkala UM, Hovi L, Lipsanen-Nyman M. Impaired glucose tolerance and dyslipidaemia as late effects after bone-marrow transplantation in childhood. Lancet. 2000;356:993–997.
44. Armenian SH, Sun CL, Vase T, et al. Cardiovascular risk factors in hematopoietic cell transplantation (HCT) survivors: role in development of subsequent cardiovascular disease. Blood. 2012;120:4502–4512.
45. Murray RD, Shalet SM. Insulin sensitivity is impaired in adults with varying degrees of GH deficiency. Clin Endocrinol (Oxf). 2005;62:182–188.
46. Taskinen M, Lipsanen-Nyman M, Tiitinen A, et al. Insufficient growth hormone secretion is associated with metabolic syndrome after allogeneic stem cell transplantation in childhood. J Pediatr Hematol Oncol. 2007;29:529–534.
47. Nuver J, Smit AJ, Postma A, et al. The metabolic syndrome in long-term cancer survivors, an important target for secondary preventive measures. Cancer Treat Rev. 2002;28:195–214.
48. Steffens M, Beauloye V, Brichard B, et al. Endocrine and metabolic disorders in young adult survivors of childhood acute lymphoblastic leukaemia (ALL) or non-Hodgkin lymphoma (NHL). Clin Endocrinol (Oxf). 2008;69:819–827.
49. Singh SK, Goyal R, Pratyush DD. Is hypoandrogenemia a component of metabolic syndrome in males? Exp Clin Endocrinol Diabetes. 2011;119:30–35.

50. Rutter MM, Rose SR. Long-term endocrine sequelae of childhood cancer. Curr Opin Pediatr. 2007;19:480–487.
51. Airaghi L, Usardi P, Forti S, et al. A comparison between metabolic syndrome post-hematopoietic stem cell transplantation and spontaneously occurring metabolic syndrome. J Endocrinol Invest. 2011;34:e6–e11.
52. Annaloro C, Usardi P, Airaghi L, et al. Prevalence of metabolic syndrome in long-term survivors of hematopoietic stem cell transplantation. Bone Marrow Transplant. 2008; 41:797–804.
53. Champagne CM. Magnesium in hypertension, cardiovascular disease, metabolic syndrome, and other conditions: a review. Nutr Clin Pract. 2008;23:142–151.
54. Chaudhary DP, Sharma R, Bansal DD. Implications of magnesium deficiency in type 2 diabetes: a review. Biol Trace Elem Res. 2010;134:119–129.
55. Aisa Y, Mori T, Nakazato T, et al. Effects of immunosuppressive agents on magnesium metabolism early after allogeneic hematopoietic stem cell transplantation. Transplantation. 2005;80:1046–1050.
56. Soucy KG, Attarzadeh DO, Ramachandran R, et al. Single exposure to radiation produces early anti-angiogenic effects in mouse aorta. Radiat Environ Biophys. 2010;49: 397–404.
57. Baker JE, Fish BL, Su J, et al. 10 Gy total body irradiation increases risk of coronary sclerosis, degeneration of heart structure and function in a rat model. Int J Radiat Biol. 2009;85:1089–1100.
58. Biedermann BC, Sahner S, Gregor M, et al. Endothelial injury mediated by cytotoxic T lymphocytes and loss of microvessels in chronic graft versus host disease. Lancet. 2002;359:2078–2083.
59. Hausermann P, Walter RB, Halter J, et al. Cutaneous graft-versus-host disease: a guide for the dermatologist. Dermatology. 2008;216:287–304.
60. Dorresteijn LD, Kappelle AC, Boogerd W, et al. Increased risk of ischemic stroke after radiotherapy on the neck in patients younger than 60 years. J Clin Oncol. 2002;20: 282–288.
61. Smith GL, Smith BD, Buchholz TA, et al. Cerebrovascular disease risk in older head and neck cancer patients after radiotherapy. J Clin Oncol. 2008;26:5119–5125.
62. Rizzo JD, Wingard JR, Tichelli A, et al. Recommended screening and preventive practices for long-term survivors after hematopoietic cell transplantation: joint recommendations of the European Group for Blood and Marrow Transplantation, Center for International Blood and Marrow Transplant Research, and the American Society for Blood and Marrow Transplantation (EBMT/CIBMTR/ASBMT). Bone Marrow Transplant. 2006;37:249–261.
63. Carter BL. Implementing the new guidelines for hypertension: JNC 7, ADA, WHO-ISH. J Manag Care Pharm. 2004; 10:S18–S25.
64. Cooper DS, Halpern R, Wood LC, et al. L-Thyroxine therapy in subclinical hypothyroidism. A double-blind, placebo-controlled trial. Ann Intern Med. 1984;101: 18–24.
65. Iqbal A, Jorde R, Figenschau Y. Serum lipid levels in relation to serum thyroid-stimulating hormone and the effect of thyroxine treatment on serum lipid levels in subjects with subclinical hypothyroidism: the Tromsø Study. J Intern Med. 2006;260:53–61.
66. Meier C, Staub JJ, Roth CB, et al. TSH-controlled L-thyroxine therapy reduces cholesterol levels and clinical symptoms in subclinical hypothyroidism: a double blind, placebo-controlled trial (Basel Thyroid Study). J Clin Endocrinol Metab. 2001;86:4860–4866.
67. Heckbert SR, Kaplan RC, Weiss NS, et al. Risk of recurrent coronary events in relation to use and recent initiation of postmenopausal hormone therapy. Arch Intern Med. 2001;161:1709–1713.
68. Meriggiola MC, Marcovina S, Paulsen CA, Bremner WJ. Testosterone enanthate at a dose of 200 mg/week decreases HDL-cholesterol levels in healthy men. Int J Androl. 1995; 18:237–242.
69. Ginzburg E, Klimas N, Parvus C, et al. Long-term safety of testosterone and growth hormone supplementation: a retrospective study of metabolic, cardiovascular, and oncologic outcomes. J Clin Med Res. 2010;2:159–166.
70. Traish AM, Guay A, Feeley R, Saad F. The dark side of testosterone deficiency: I. Metabolic syndrome and erectile dysfunction. J Androl. 2009;30:10–22.
71. Basu R, Dalla MC, Campioni M, et al. Effect of 2 years of testosterone replacement on insulin secretion, insulin action, glucose effectiveness, hepatic insulin clearance, and postprandial glucose turnover in elderly men. Diabetes Care. 2007;30:1972–1978.
72. Chrisoulidou A, Beshyah SA, Rutherford O, et al. Effects of 7 years of growth hormone replacement therapy in hypopituitary adults. J Clin Endocrinol Metab. 2000;85:3762–3769.
73. Florakis D, Hung V, Kaltsas G, et al. Sustained reduction in circulating cholesterol in adult hypopituitary patients given low dose titrated growth hormone replacement therapy: a two year study. Clin Endocrinol (Oxf). 2000; 53:453–459.
74. Monson JP, Jonsson P, Koltowska-Haggstrom M, Kourides I. Growth hormone (GH) replacement decreases serum total and LDL-cholesterol in hypopituitary patients on maintenance HMG CoA reductase inhibitor (statin) therapy. Clin Endocrinol (Oxf). 2007;67:623–628.

75. Savani BN, Griffith ML, Jagasia S, Lee SJ. How I treat late effects in adults after allogeneic stem cell transplantation. Blood. 2011;117:3002–3009.

76. Chobanian AV, Bakris GL, Black HR, et al. The Seventh Report of the Joint National Committee on Prevention, Detection, Evaluation, and Treatment of High Blood Pressure: the JNC 7 report. JAMA. 2003;289:2560–2572.

77. Chobanian AV, Bakris GL, Black HR, et al. Seventh report of the Joint National Committee on Prevention, Detection, Evaluation, and Treatment of High Blood Pressure. Hypertension. 2003;42:1206–1252.

78. Rovó A, Tichelli A. Cardiovascular complications in long-term survivors after allogeneic hematopoietic stem cell transplantation. Semin Hematol. 2012;49:25–34.

25

CHAPTER 25

Hyperlipidemia: prevalence, monitoring, management, interactions with immunosuppressive agents, and follow-up

Dara L Eckerle Mize[1], *Shubhada Jagasia*[1], *and Jeffrey B Boord*[2]

[1]Division of Diabetes, Endocrinology & Metabolism, Vanderbilt University Medical Center, Nashville, TN, USA

[2]Division of Cardiovascular Medicine, Vanderbilt Heart and Vascular Institute, Nashville, TN, USA

Prevalence and incidence

Long-term follow-up studies have shown that allogeneic hematopoietic stem cell transplantation (HSCT) recipients are at increased risk of cardiovascular disease (CVD) compared with both autologous HSCT recipients and age-matched population counterparts [1]. Some of this increased risk may be due to the direct effects of radiation, chemotherapeutic agents, and immunosuppressive therapy (IST). However, HSCT recipients also experience an independent increase in several cardiovascular risk factors, including dyslipidemia, hypertension, and diabetes mellitus. The reports on prevalence and incidence of hyperlipidemia following HSCT are highly variable, ranging from a prevalence of 8.9% in one Canadian study examining long-term (>2 years) complications in 369 patients after HSCT [2] to an incidence of hypercholesterolemia (total cholesterol ≥200 mg/dL) as high as 73% in the largest study to date of 761 allogeneic HSCT patients evaluated within the first 2 years following transplant [3]. In the latter study, the baseline prevalence of hypercholesterolemia (total cholesterol ≥200 mg/dL) was 32% pretransplantation, and hypertriglyceridemia (triglyceride ≥200 mg/dL) was 39.3%. Among the patients with a pretransplant total cholesterol <200 mg/dL, 65% became newly hypercholesterolemic after transplantation, and in those with pretransplant triglyceride <200 mg/dL, 64% developed hypertriglyceridemia after transplantation. Multivariable regression analysis showed that development of grade II–IV graft-versus-host disease (GVHD) and being overweight at time of transplant (body mass index ≥25 kg/m^2) were independent risk factors for posttransplant total cholesterol ≥200 mg/dL or triglyceride ≥200 mg/dL [3]. Lee et al. found a fasting hyperlipidemia prevalence of 56% in 118 patients 1 year after transplant, but their pretransplant lipid status was not reported [4]. In that study, medication use at 1 year after allogeneic HSCT included antihypertensive therapy in 32%, diabetes therapy in 15%, and lipid-lowering therapy in 9%. A small study of 23 long-term survivors of HSCT in childhood found higher rates of hypertriglyceridemia and low high-density lipoprotein (HDL), 39% and 26%, respectively, when compared with prevalence of 4% for each in age-matched controls [5]. A more

Blood and Marrow Transplantation Long-Term Management: Prevention and Complications, First Edition. Edited by Bipin N Savani.

recent Japanese study of 194 patients (5.7% with hypercholesterolemia and 18.1% hypertriglyceridemia pretransplant) showed that 83 patients (42.8%) developed hypercholesterolemia (≥240 mg/dL) and 99 (50.8%) developed hypertriglyceridemia (≥200 mg/dL) more than 100 days after HSCT. The cumulative incidence at 3 years after HSCT was 38.5% for hypercholesterolemia (≥240 mg/dL) and 47.7% for hypertriglyceridemia (≥200 mg/dL) [6]. Multivariate analysis of risk factors for posttransplant hypercholesterolemia included family history of hyperlipidemia, chronic GVHD, posttransplant elevation of liver function tests >3 months, and steroid use. Thus, hyperlipidemia is a very common problem among allogeneic HSCT patients, and requires a reasoned approach to evaluation and management.

Mechanisms of dyslipidemia in transplant patients

Many factors contribute to increased risk of hyperlipidemia, including traditional considerations such as obesity, genetic lipid disorders, diet, and uncontrolled diabetes mellitus. However, the underlying diseases, complications of disease treatment, and post-HSCT immunosuppressive agents also increase the risk of dyslipidemia [1]. Long-term childhood survivors of hematologic malignancies will frequently experience gonadal failure or growth hormone deficiency from chemotherapy agents or from conditioning total body irradiation (TBI) prior to HSCT. This places them at increased risk for insulin resistance and dyslipidemia [7]. Hypothyroidism is also a common adverse effect of TBI and promotes dyslipidemia [7], and nephrotic syndrome can lead to or worsen underlying dyslipidemia [1].

Chronic GVHD of the liver is another rare but important cause of hyperlipidemia in both the adult and pediatric allogeneic HSCT populations and can cause severe hypercholesterolemia (>500 mg/dL). This syndrome presents with a cholestatic pattern of liver injury which leads to the reflux of bile lipoproteins into the bloodstream [8]. The formation of one of these abnormal lipoproteins, lipoprotein X, appears to be responsible for most of the serum cholesterol elevation in this setting, which differentiates it from other transplant-related causes of hyperlipidemia [8]. The severity of acute GVHD also appears to correlate with the risk of development of post-HSCT dyslipidemia, with rates of 71% of patients with grade 0 to I GVHD and up to 81% of those with grade II to IV GVHD [3].

Immunosuppressant medications are the most common cause of secondary hyperlipidemia following HSCT. Several of the agents used in this setting have been shown to have adverse effects on the lipid profile, typically increased low-density lipoprotein (LDL) cholesterol and triglycerides and reduced HDL. The magnitude of this effect usually leads to total cholesterol in the range of 200–300 mg/dL and triglycerides between 200 and 350 mg/dL [9]. The incidence of dyslipidemia in solid organ transplant patients on IST has ranged from 45% to 80% in different studies and is influenced by the organ transplanted, age, proteinuria, obesity, antihypertensive medication, glucocorticoid dose, preexisting hyperlipidemia, treatment with cyclosporine or sirolimus, male gender, renal dysfunction, and diabetes [9].

Glucocorticoids may cause dyslipidemia both through their direct effects on lipid metabolism by enhancing activity of 3-hydroxy-3-methylglutaryl coenzyme A (HMG-CoA) reductase and by inhibiting lipoprotein lipase [9]. But they can also cause dyslipidemia indirectly as a result of weight gain, hyperglycemia, and insulin resistance, and it is the cumulative dose of glucocorticoids that appears to show the greatest correlation with increased risk [9]. Several studies have examined differing glucocorticoid dosing regimens, such as low-dose therapy, alternate-day therapy, and early withdrawal and while some of these have suggested improvement in dyslipidemia outcomes, their effects on transplant rejection, morbidity, and mortality are not well established [9, 10].

Cyclosporine has also been shown to have adverse effects on total cholesterol, LDL, and triglycerides in patients following transplant [9], but also in amyotrophic lateral sclerosis (ALS) patients who were not receiving co-administration of glucocorticoids [11]. Proposed mechanisms for this effect include the inhibition of bile acid synthesis limiting the breakdown of cholesterol and the binding and inhibition of the LDL receptor. Cyclosporine also decreases the activity of lipoprotein lipase and enhances activity of hepatic lipase, resulting in decreased clearance of very low density lipoprotein (VLDL) and LDL [9, 10]. In transplant patients treated with both cyclosporine and glucocorticoids, cyclosporine can attenuate the metabolism of glucocorticoids, worsening steroid-induced dyslipidemia [1].

Secondary hyperlipidemia generally improves with discontinuation of therapy.

Tacrolimus (FK506), another calcineurin inhibitor, has been known to worsen hyperlipidemia when given in combination with a glucocorticoid, but to a lesser degree than cyclosporine [1, 9, 10]. Changing a treatment regimen from cyclosporine to tacrolimus may yield significant improvements in the lipid profile [9, 10, 12, 13]. This benefit was previously attributed to the lower dose of glucocorticoids patients may receive when on a tacrolimus- rather than cyclosporine-based regimen; however, some studies have shown significant improvement in the lipid profile with this change in regimen even when there was no significant difference in the dose of glucocorticoids being coadministered [12, 13]. In one study of approximately 1600 renal transplant recipients, patients in the tacrolimus arm had significantly lower LDL and triglyceride levels at 1 year when compared with the sirolimus group and were less likely to be on lipid-lowering therapy at any time during the study period [14].

Sirolimus, a mammalian target of rapamycin inhibitor, has been known to cause dyslipidemia in 40–50% of solid-organ transplant recipients [10]. Elevations in total cholesterol and triglyceride levels may be seen as early as 2 weeks after the initiation of therapy in a dose-related fashion and may not return to pretreatment levels until 4 weeks following discontinuation of the drug [9]. Mycophenolate mofetil and azathioprine have not been independently associated with the development of dyslipidemia [1].

Screening and evaluation

Joint recommendations for lipid monitoring by the Center for International Blood and Marrow Transplant Research, the European Group for Blood and Marrow Transplantation, and the American Society for Blood and Marrow Transplantation (published in 2006 and revised in 2011) suggest that cardiovascular risk-factor assessment should begin 1 year post-HSCT and continue annually for all transplant recipients. Their recommendations advise that screening begin earlier, at 6 months post-HSCT, in patients with previously abnormal testing [15]. The guidelines recommend that total cholesterol and HDL levels be checked every 5 years starting at age 35 in men and 45 in women, but recommend screening start at age 20 in patients who smoke, have diabetes, hypertension, obesity (BMI >30 kg/m^2) or a family history of premature coronary artery disease [15]. A full fasting lipid profile should be obtained if total cholesterol levels are found to be >200 mg/dL or HDL levels <40 mg/dL [15].

However, others suggest a more intensive screening approach given the emerging data regarding the significant late cardiovascular risks seen in post-allogeneic HSCT patients, particularly those receiving chronic IST [1, 3]. Our suggested approach is outlined in Table 25.1.

Prior to transplantation, all patients, but particularly those with a history of dyslipidemia or CVD, should have an evaluation of their lipid profile after 9–12 h of fasting. LDL cannot be calculated accurately using the Friedwald formula if the triglycerides are >400 mg/dL but can now be measured directly at most laboratories [1]. Non-HDL cholesterol, which is the total cholesterol minus the HDL, may be used to determine treatment goals if triglycerides are >400 mg/dL and a direct measurement of LDL is not available. Non-HDL cholesterol represents the measurement of VLDL and LDL, the atherogenic lipid particles containing apoprotein B lipoproteins [1]. The goal for non-HDL cholesterol is the patient's LDL goal plus 30 mg/dL. It is generally not necessary to perform advanced lipoprotein analysis (e.g., LDL particle number, lipoprotein subfractions) in post-HSCT patients [1]. Other cardiovascular biomarkers such as high-sensitivity C-reactive protein and lipoprotein(a) have been studied in general populations and can provide additional information for cardiovascular risk assessment. However, none of these measures has been validated in the post-HSCT population and cannot be recommended at this point.

Management

Many factors must be considered when determining the appropriate management of dyslipidemia in post-HSCT patients. These include an estimation of the patient's CVD risk, pattern and degree of dyslipidemia, risk of drug interactions, the patient's age at time of HSCT, and use of IST (Table 25.1) [1]. It is also important to remember that the two goals of treatment of dyslipidemia are to decrease the risk of cardiovascular events in the future

Table 25.1 Suggested approach to lipid management in HSCT patients [1]

Evaluation

Obtain fasting lipid profile before transplantation

Evaluate coronary heart disease (CHD) risk

1. If patient has CHD or CHD risk equivalent, then manage as high risk with appropriate therapy to reach LDL goal.
   (i) Option to consider allogeneic HSCT patients 40 years of age or older as high risk.
2. Otherwise, calculate 10-year risk with online risk assessment tool (hp2010.nhlbihin.net/atpiii/calculator.asp?usertype=prof) and manage LDL per ATP-III guidelines.

Monitor lipid profiles after HSCT

1. Check lipid profile within 4 weeks after HSCT and then at least every 3 months for patients on IST.
2. For patients at treatment goal on stable therapy every 6–12 months as indicated, or after significant change in IST regimen in patients with dyslipidemia.
3. If patients develop significant dyslipidemia after HSCT compared with baseline, consider secondary causes of dyslipidemia (IST diabetes, hypothyroidism).
4. Even patients without dyslipidemia should have lipids monitored every 1–2 years after allogeneic HSCT given increased cardiovascular risk.

Management

If patient has high CHD risk (>20% 10-year risk), treat dyslipidemia with appropriate agent(s) to meet LDL goal, but monitor clinically if on IST or renal dysfunction.

In patients with low (<10%) or moderate CHD risk (10–20%), consider drug treatment based upon severity of dyslipidemia, estimated prognosis after HSCT, and risks of lipid drug therapy (if on long-term IST for GVHD).

1. In patients with low CHD risk that develop moderate secondary dyslipidemia on IST, this can be managed conservatively if IST will be tapered off.
2. Patients with low to moderate CHD risk that develop severe hypertriglyceridemia (>500 mg/dL) should be treated to prevent pancreatitis.

Consider referral to a lipid specialist for the following:

1. severe dyslipidemia (total cholesterol >300 or LDL >180, triglycerides >500–1000 mg/dL);
2. patients with dyslipidemia refractory to treatment and not meeting goals;
3. patients with intolerance or contraindications to lipid-lowering therapy;
4. patients requiring combination lipid therapy, particularly in the setting of IST;
5. patients needing individualized cardiovascular risk assessment because of strong family history of premature CHD or other factors.

This research was originally published in *Blood*. Griffith ML, Savani BN, Boord JB. Dyslipidemia after allogeneic hematopoietic stem cell transplantation: evaluation and management. *Blood*. 2010;116:1197–1204.

and to prevent risk of pancreatitis. Therefore, malignancy-specific considerations, such as prognosis, risk of recurrent disease, and life-expectancy, may alter the decision to treat or treatment goals. For example, if there is a high likelihood of recurrent malignancy or decreased life expectancy, aggressive lipid-lowering therapy to target LDL goals may not be warranted. However, if the likelihood of malignancy recurrence is low and the patient's life expectancy is at least 5–10 years more, then treatment of dyslipidemia to reduce risk of future cardiovascular events is recommended [1]. Treatment of severe hypertriglyceridemia (triglycerides >500 mg/dL) is generally recommended to prevent pancreatitis.

The National Cholesterol Education Program (NCEP) Expert Panel on Detection, Evaluation, and Treatment of High Blood Cholesterol in Adults (Adult Treatment Panel III) makes recommendations, regarding when to initiate lifestyle modifications and drug therapy based on cardiovascular risk category for adults in the general population [16]. While the current guidelines have no specific recommendations for post-HSCT patients and have not directly been studied in this population, they provide a well-known and widely used framework for evaluating individual risk and guiding management [15]. High-sensitivity C-reactive protein is another marker which has been useful in the evaluation of CVD risk in the

Table 25.2 Summary of ATP-III LDL cholesterol and triglyceride goals by risk category [32]

Risk category	Threshold to initiate TLC[a]	Threshold to consider drug therapy
High risk: LDL goal <100 mg/dL (optional <70)		
CHD or equivalents[b] (10-year risk >20%)	LDL ≥100 mg/dL	LDL ≥100 mg/dL (<100 mg/dL consider drug)
Moderately high risk: LDL goal <130 mg/dL (optional <100)		
Two or more risk factors (10-year risk 10–20%)	LDL ≥130 mg/dL	LDL ≥130 mg/dL (100–129 mg/dL consider drug)
Moderate risk: LDL goal <130 mg/dL		
Two or more risk factors (10-year risk <10%)	LDL ≥130 mg/dL	LDL ≥160 mg/dL
Lower risk: LDL goal <160 mg/dL		
Zero or one risk factor	LDL ≥160 mg/dL	LDL ≥190 mg/dL (160–189 mg/dL drug optional)
Severe hypertriglyceridemia (>500 mg/dL): triglyceride goal <500 mg/dL	>500 mg/dL	>500 mg/dL
Moderate hypertriglyceridemia (200-250 mg/dL): triglyceride goal <200 mg/dL	>200 mg/dL	Consider modifying therapy to reach secondary non-HDL cholesterol goal (after LDL goal reached)

[a]TLC: therapeutic lifestyle change.
[b]CHD equivalents are diabetes mellitus, abdominal aortic aneurysm, carotid stenosis, and peripheral vascular disease.

general population. However, this test is likely to be susceptible to effects of multiple confounding variants in the HSCT patient population and is not recommended for use in that setting [1]. The ATP-IV guidelines are due to be published in 2013 but have not been released at the time of writing.

According to the most recent NCEP ATP III guidelines, as outlined in Table 25.2, individuals in higher risk categories should have lower LDL goals and thresholds for lifestyle modification and drug therapy. While LDL should be the primary target of therapy, if a calculated LDL is inaccurate due to triglycerides >400 mg/dL and a direct LDL cannot be measured, then non-HDL (total cholesterol minus HDL) can be used to target therapy and the non-HDL goal is determined by adding 30 points to the LDL goal [16]. A patient's 10-year risk of CHD events can be calculated using The National Heart, Lung and Blood Institute website (www.nhlbi.nih.gov) 10-year CVD risk calculator. This helps stratify patients into low (10-year risk <10%), moderate (10-year risk 10–20%), and high (10-year risk >20%) risk based on major risk factors which modify the LDL goal. These risk factors include current cigarette smoking, hypertension (BP ≥140/90 mmHg or currently taking antihypertensive medication), low HDL cholesterol (<40 mg/dL), family history of premature CVD (in male first-degree relative <55 years; in female first-degree relative <65 years) and age (men ≥45 years; women ≥55 years). HDL ≥60 mg/dL is a negative risk factor and subtracts one risk factor from the total. Diabetes is considered a CVD equivalent. Other CVD equivalents are abdominal aortic aneurysm, carotid stenosis, and peripheral vascular disease [16]. Similarly, patients older than 40 years who have received an allogeneic HSCT have a 10-year CVD event risk of >20% and so we believe that they should be considered high risk with respect to cholesterol treatment and risk reduction until further data prove otherwise. Though the risk calculator can be used to establish baseline CHD event risk prior to transplantation, the risk calculator should not be used as the sole determinant of cardiovascular risk assessment in patients after allogeneic HSCT. The risk calculator cannot factor in late CVD effects of transplantation and would be confounded by posttransplant issues such as secondary dyslipidemia and hypertension related to IST.

The American Heart Association recommends a specific approach to TLC for patients with dyslipidemia and/or CVD. In addition to recommendations made to the general population regarding limiting intake of trans-fatty acids and increasing physical activity level so as to balance caloric intake with energy expenditure, patients with elevated LDL or CVD should consume <7% of their daily calories from saturated fat and <200 mg of cholesterol per day [17]. In all patients, TLC should be initiated once it is recognized that their LDL exceeds goal for their CVD risk category. TLC alone may be adequate for management of mild to moderate dyslipidemia in patients with low to moderate CVD risk. In clinical practice, TLC may be difficult to implement in some patients owing to gut GVHD and concerns regarding malnutrition, as well as poor exercise capacity related to deconditioning or other comorbid conditions. TLC, therefore, should be tailored to individual patient circumstances.

IST is a common cause of dyslipidemia in post-HSCT patients, particularly in the early posttransplant period. Secondary dyslipidemia from IST may improve with adjustments to medication dose or immunosuppressant regimen [9, 10, 12, 13]. In the appropriate clinical setting, an evaluation for other secondary causes in post-HSCT patients, including uncontrolled diabetes mellitus, obesity, alcohol use, hypogonadism, hypothyroidism, or nephrotic syndrome, may need to be performed. As previously mentioned, reducing the dose, frequency, or duration of treatment with glucocorticoids when clinically feasible can improve dyslipidemia. Another option is to change from cyclosporine to tacrolimus, which is known to have less deleterious effects on the lipid profile.

If TLCs and IST modifications do not lead to sufficient improvement in dyslipidemia, conventional drug therapy may be needed to reach treatment goals. Commonly used agents are summarized in Table 25.3. If a patient is no longer on IST and does not have GVHD, treatment of their dyslipidemia would follow the recommendations outlined for the general population and the mainstay of therapy would be an HMG-CoA reductase inhibitor (statin). Statins have excellent LDL-lowering and modest triglyceride-lowering effects, making them useful in patients with a mixed dyslipidemia if the hypertriglyceridemia is mild (<300–400 mg/dL) [1]. Historically, use of statins in the post-HSCT patient population was limited due to concerns for liver toxicity, myopathy related to interactions with IST, and confounding effects of liver GVHD on liver function test monitoring. However, their use in this population is becoming more common. Blaser et al. conducted a retrospective analysis of 220 patients who received a statin within 2 years of allogeneic HSCT and were able to document a significant improvement in total cholesterol, LDL cholesterol, and triglycerides without any significant adverse effects [3]. Data from use in patients with solid organ transplants [18–21] and HSCT [3] suggests that, with careful selection of statin dose and preparation and monitoring, adverse side effects are uncommon. Statins have also been safely administered to patients with stable chronic liver disease, and mild baseline elevation of transaminases does not appear to predispose to increased risk of statin toxicity [22, 23]. However, these effects have not been studied in HSCT patients with liver GVHD. Statins should not be administered to patients with severe baseline elevations in transaminases, or in the setting of decompensated or acute liver failure. While the effect of treatment in post-HSCT patients has not been established, there are data that statins reduce risk of cardiovascular events in patients following renal and cardiac transplantation [18–21].

The data regarding interaction of ezetimibe with IST is mixed, but several small studies in solid organ transplant patients have shown good safety, tolerability, and cholesterol reduction with ezetimibe used alone or in combination with a statin [24]. Ezetimibe has a more modest LDL-lowering effect than statins have and has not yet been proven independently to reduce risk of cardiovascular events. Therefore, it should not be considered first-line therapy for LDL reduction [1].

The bile acid sequestrants have moderate LDL-lowering effects but have not been studied in posttransplant patients. The two oldest bile acid resins, colestipol and cholestyramine, can potentially interfere with gastrointestinal absorption of IST and other medications if not administered at least 1 h before or 4 h after the resin dose. Use of colestipol and cholestyramine should be avoided in all patients on IST and in patients with complex medication regimens. Compared with the older medications in this class, colesevelam has more specificity for binding bile acids and can be safely co-administered with other narrow therapeutic index medications such as warfarin and digoxin. Thus, colesevelam is more suitable for use with IST in post-HSCT patients based on its pharmacology [25]. However, this agent has not been used in

Table 25.3 Pharmacologic therapy used in the treatment of dyslipidemia[a] [1]

Predominant dyslipidemia/ drug class	Agent/daily dose range[b]	Expected effect	Major side effects	Important interactions
Elevated LDL-C predominant				
HMG-CoA reductase inhibitors	Pravastatin, lovastatin or atorvastatin /10–80 mg; fluvastatin 20–80 mg; simvastatin 5–80 mg; rosuvastatin 5–40 mg; pitavastatin 1–4 mg	↓ LDL-C 30–45%; ↓ triglycerides 7–30%; ↑HDL-C up to 10% (variable by agent)	Myopathy; elevated liver tests	Increased myopathy risk with renal dysfunction and cyclosporine; fibrates; CYP3A4 inhibitors
Cholesterol absorption inhibitor	Ezetimibe 10 mg	↓ LDL-C 17%	Gastrointestinal upset, elevated liver tests, myalgias (rare)	No major drug interactions
Bile acid sequestrants	Colesevelam 2400–3750 mg	↓ LDL 15–30%; can raise triglycerides	Constipation, dyspepsia	Monitor drug levels in IST
Hypertriglyceridemia predominant				
Omega-3 fatty acids	Omega-3-acid ethyl esters 2–4 g daily divided BID	↓ Triglycerides 35–45%; ↑ HDL-C 3%, ↑ LDL-C 5%	Gastrointestinal upset, diarrhoea	No major drug interactions
Fibric acid derivatives	Fenofibrate, fenofibric acid 45–200 mg daily; gemfibrozil 600–1200 mg daily divided BID	↓ Triglycerides 20–50%; ↑ HDL-C 10–20%	Myopathy, elevated liver tests, gallstones, rash; renal dysfunction (fenofibrate)	Use with caution in combination with statins and cyclosporine
Mixed hyperlipidemia				
Niacin	Niacin 500–2000 mg	↓ LDL-C 20–30%; ↓ triglycerides 35–55%; ↑ HDL-C 20–35%	Dyspepsia, flushing, elevated liver tests, ↑ glucose, ↑ uric acid	No major drug interactions

This research was originally published in *Blood*. Griffith ML, Savani BN, Boord JB. Dyslipidemia after allogeneic hematopoietic stem cell transplantation: evaluation and management. *Blood*. 2010;116:1197–1204.

[a] LDL-C: low-density lipoprotein-cholesterol; HDL-C: high-density lipoprotein-cholesterol; BID: twice daily.

[b] We recommend submaximal statin dosing in patients on IST agents that may alter metabolism of the statin agents. In general, patients gain only 6% additional LDL-C lowering with each doubling of statin dose.

controlled studies in posttransplant patients on IST and should only be used as a second-line agent, with regular IST drug level monitoring [1]. Since bile acid resins can increase VLDL production, they should be avoided in patients with significant hypertriglyceridemia (>200–300 mg/dL).

In patients with moderate to severe hypertriglyceridemia (>400 mg/dL), statins may not provide enough triglyceride-lowering effect to be used as monotherapy and additional medications may be needed to reduce the risk of pancreatitis. Niacin and omega-3 fatty acids provide a greater degree of triglyceride-lowering effects and should be used in cases of moderate or severe hypertriglyceridemia. Niacin can lower LDL and raise HDL in addition to its effects on triglycerides and is, therefore, useful in patients with a both hypercholesterolemia and hypertriglyceridemia. It is not known to have any significant interactions with IST, but it can worsen hyperuricemia and hyperglycemia in some cases. Older rapid-acting preparations of niacin were often not well tolerated owing to gastrointestinal side effects and flushing, but the newer extended release form has an improved side-effect profile and should be used preferentially. Omega-3 fatty acids (supplied in fish oil) lower triglycerides but not total cholesterol. They demonstrate a good safety profile and, despite their ability to decrease platelet aggregation, have not been shown to cause a significant increase in bleeding, even in patients receiving aspirin and clopidogrel for dual antiplatelet therapy [1]. They have few adverse reactions, no significant drug interactions, and have safely treated hypertriglyceridemia caused by sirolimus [1]. The effective dose of omega-3 fatty acids for treatment of hypertriglyceridemia is 2–4 g per day, given in divided doses. It is important to recognize that over-the-counter preparations vary widely in the content of omega-3 fatty acids per capsule, and that the label must be evaluated to calculate the appropriate total daily dose. For example, a fish oil preparation where each 1000 mg capsule contains 300 mg of omega-3 fatty acids would need to be given at a dose of three capsules three times a day to provide an effective dose of 2700 mg of omega-3 fatty acids per day.

Fibric acid derivatives such as fenofibrate and gemfibrozil can also significantly lower triglycerides, but owing to their side-effect profile and increased risk of such reactions in patients receiving IST they should be used with caution in the post-HSCT patient population and only for severe hypertriglyceridemia (>500 mg/dL) not responsive to other therapy. Adverse reactions associated with their use include gastrointestinal upset, myopathy, and cholelithiasis. The incidence of myopathy is higher in patients receiving concomitant statin therapy, especially when administered with cyclosporine or in individuals with decreased renal function. Fenofibrate appears to increase statin levels to a lesser degree when compared with gemfibrozil and so is the preferable fibrate if used in combination with a statin [1]. Fenofibrate can also cause a modest increase in the serum creatinine level in some patients, particularly those with preexisting renal dysfunction [26]. The mechanism of this effect is not fully understood, but it is generally reversible with dose reduction or discontinuation and has not been associated with serious adverse renal outcomes in large clinical trials. However, given the high incidence of renal dysfunction in the setting of calcineurin inhibitor use in posttransplant patients, this issue should be carefully considered, and fenofibrate should be avoided in patients with moderate to severe renal dysfunction. It is important to remember that, in patients with uncontrolled diabetes and hypertriglyceridemia, achieving better glucose control will improve triglycerides and may help minimize the need for other lipid therapy.

Patients with complex dyslipidemia should be considered for referral to a lipid specialist. This would include patients who are not reaching treatment goals on current therapy, those who are experiencing adverse side effects from current treatment regimen, the need for multidrug therapy in the setting of IST, or any patient who needs a more personalized risk assessment.

Interactions with immunosuppressant agents

Table 25.3 summarizes several pharmacologic options used in the treatment of dyslipidemia, but statins are the class of medication most commonly prescribed. Rare but serious potential adverse effects associated with statins are myopathy, hepatotoxicity, and rhabdomyolysis. Several of the drugs in this class, specifically lovastatin, simvastatin, and atorvastatin, are metabolized by the microsomal enzyme cytochrome P450 3A4, a pathway which is inhibited by cyclosporine, tacrolimus, and sirolimus. This can result in increased serum statin levels and potentiate the risk for adverse side effects [1, 9, 27, 28]. Of these three immunosuppressive agents, cyclosporine appears to be the strongest inhibitor of this pathway [27, 28], but it also increases statin serum levels by inhibiting the effect of a hepatic cell membrane transporter [29], which may increase the risk of adverse side effects associated with any statin. Cyclosporine's effect through both mechanisms may explain why there appears to be higher risk for statin-related toxicity with its use compared with some other immunosuppressive medications [29]. Simvastatin [30] and pitavastatin [31] are specifically contraindicated for use with cyclosporine, while other statins should be used with caution, and use of the lowest effective dose is prudent. Several other drugs which are known to inhibit cytochrome P450 3A4 are commonly used in patients following HSCT and may also increase the risk of statin-associated toxicity. Common cytochrome P450 3A4 inhibitors include amiodarone, azole antifungals, cyclosporine, gemfibrozil, grapefruit, macrolide antibiotics, non-dihydropyridine calcium channel blockers, and sirolimus. To reduce the risk of statin-related toxicity in patients receiving medications which are known to inhibit cytochrome P450

3A4, it is recommended to use one of the statins not metabolized through this pathway, which include pravastatin, rosuvastatin, and fluvastatin.

As previously discussed, the older bile acid sequestrants, such as colestipol and cholestyramine, should not be prescribed to patients receiving IST as they bind these drugs and may significantly reduce absorption. A newer medication in this class, colesevelam, is safer to use in post-HSCT patients receiving IST owing to its increased specificity for binding bile acids. However, IST drug levels should be monitored more closely in patients receiving colesevelam [1]. Niacin and omega-3 fatty acids are not known to interact with IST. Because of an increased risk of myopathy in patients on IST who receive fibrates, it is recommended to limit fibrate use to patients with severe hypertriglyceridemia (>500 mg/dL) not responsive to other therapy [1].

Follow-up

In all patients, fasting lipid profile should ideally be measured prior to transplantation, 4 weeks after HSCT, and then every 3 months while on IST. Prior to initiating statin therapy, baseline transaminase levels should be evaluated. In the general population, transaminases should be measured approximately 12 weeks after starting statin therapy and then, if normal, yearly unless indicated earlier, such as for an increase in dose. There are no studies which establish evidence-based recommendations for transaminase monitoring in patients receiving a statin post-HSCT. However, in patients with potential for active GVHD or who are receiving IST, there is increased risk for hepatotoxicity, and so transaminases should be checked earlier than in the general population, approximately 2–4 weeks after the initiation of therapy [1]. Mild elevations in transaminases (greater than three times the upper limit of normal) following statin administration are uncommon and are not typically associated with any significant histopathological changes. This mild elevation is usually asymptomatic and transient; therefore, continued treatment with close monitoring of transaminases and clinical status is appropriate [1, 23]. If transaminases rise to a level greater than three times the upper limit of normal, statin therapy should be discontinued and transaminases monitored for return to normal. If they return to normal, it is reasonable to restart therapy with the same drug at a lower dose or a different statin medication. If they remain persistently elevated, screening should be conducted for other potential causes of elevated liver enzymes [1, 23]. Patients receiving colesevalam while on IST should have closer monitoring of drug levels owing to the potential for decreased drug absorption. All patients initiated on statin therapy should be advised of risk for myopathy and educated on signs and symptoms of this disorder.

Conclusions

Dyslipidemia after allogeneic HSCT is a common problem and requires consideration of multiple factors to determine the best course of treatment. Data from long-term follow-up studies suggest that allogeneic HSCT patients have high long-term cardiovascular risk, especially those undergoing transplantation after the age of 40. There are currently no established guidelines for the management of dyslipidemia in HSCT patients, but studies in solid organ transplant recipients indicate that lipid-lowering therapy can be safe and effective in patients receiving long-term IST. Selection of lipid therapy and treatment goals should be based on individualized assessment of the patient's cardiovascular risk, type and severity of dyslipidemia, and risk of adverse reactions from lipid treatment.

References

1. Griffith ML, Savani BN, Boord JB. Dyslipidemia after allogeneic hematopoietic stem cell transplantation: evaluation and management. Blood. 2010;116(8):1197–1204.
2. Abou-Mourad YR, Lau BC, Barnett MJ, et al. Long-term outcome after allo-SCT: close follow-up on a large cohort treated with myeloablative regimens. Bone Marrow Transplant. 2010;45(2):295–302.
3. Blaser BW, Kim HT, Alyea EP III, et al. Hyperlipidemia and statin use after allogeneic hematopoietic stem cell transplantation. Biol Blood Marrow Transplant. 2012;18(4): 575–583.
4. Lee SJ, Seaborn T, Mao FJ, et al. Frequency of abnormal findings detected by comprehensive clinical evaluation at 1

year after allogeneic hematopoietic cell transplantation. Biol Blood Marrow Transplant. 2009;15(4):416–420.
5. Taskinen M, Saarinen-Pihkala UM, Hovi L, Lipsanen-Nyman M. Impaired glucose tolerance and dyslipidaemia as late effects after bone-marrow transplantation in childhood. Lancet. 2000;356(9234):993–997.
6. Kagoya Y, Seo S, Nannya Y, Kurokawa M. Hyperlipidemia after allogeneic stem cell transplantation: prevalence, risk factors, and impact on prognosis. Clin Transplant. 2012; 26(2):E168–E175.
7. Siviero-Miachon AA, Spinola-Castro AM, Guerra-Junior G. Detection of metabolic syndrome features among childhood cancer survivors: a target to prevent disease. Vasc Health Risk Manag. 2008;4(4):825–836.
8. Turchin A, Wiebe DA, Seely EW, et al. Severe hypercholesterolemia mediated by lipoprotein X in patients with chronic graft-versus-host disease of the liver. Bone Marrow Transplant. 2005;35(1):85–89.
9. Miller LW. Cardiovascular toxicities of immunosuppressive agents. Am J Transplant. 2002;2(9):807–818.
10. Subramanian S, Trence DL. Immunosuppressive agents: effects on glucose and lipid metabolism. Endocrinol Metab Clin North Am. 2007;36(4):891–905, vii.
11. Ballantyne CM, Podet EJ, Patsch WP, et al. Effects of cyclosporine therapy on plasma lipoprotein levels. JAMA. 1989;262(1):53–56.
12. Aguirrezabalaga J, Fernandez-Selles C, Fraguela J, et al. Lipid profiles after liver transplantation in patients receiving tacrolimus or cyclosporin. Transplant Proc. 2002;34(5): 1551–1552.
13. McCune TR, Thacker LR II, Peters TG, et al. Effects of tacrolimus on hyperlipidemia after successful renal transplantation: a Southeastern Organ Procurement Foundation multicenter clinical study. Transplantation. 1998;65(1): 87–92.
14. Claes K, Meier-Kriesche HU, Schold JD, et al. Effect of different immunosuppressive regimens on the evolution of distinct metabolic parameters: evidence from the Symphony study. Nephrol Dial Transplant. 2012;27(2): 850–857.
15. Majhail NS, Rizzo JD, Lee SJ, et al. Recommended screening and preventive practices for long-term survivors after hematopoietic cell transplantation. Bone Marrow Transplant. 2012;47(3):337–341.
16. National Cholesterol Education Program, National Heart, Lung, and Blood Institute, and National Institutes of Health. Third Report of the National Cholesterol Education Program (NCEP) Expert Panel on Detection, Evaluation, and Treatment of High Blood Cholesterol in Adults (Adult Treatment Panel III) final report. Circulation. 2002;106(25): 3143–3421.
17. Krauss RM, Eckel RH, Howard B, et al. AHA Dietary Guidelines: revision 2000: a statement for healthcare professionals from the Nutrition Committee of the American Heart Association. Circulation. 2000;102(18): 2284–2299.
18. Wenke K, Meiser B, Thiery J, Reichart B. Impact of simvastatin therapy after heart transplantation an 11-year prospective evaluation. Herz. 2005;30(5):431–432.
19. Holdaas H, Fellstrom B, Cole E, et al. Long-term cardiac outcomes in renal transplant recipients receiving fluvastatin: the ALERT extension study. Am J Transplant. 2005;5(12): 2929–2936.
20. Soveri I, Abedini S, Holdaas H, et al. Metabolic syndrome and cardiovascular risk in renal transplant recipients: effects of statin treatment. Clin Transplant. 2009;23(6): 914–920.
21. Navaneethan SD, Perkovic V, Johnson DW, et al. HMG CoA reductase inhibitors (statins) for kidney transplant recipients. Cochrane Database Syst Rev. 2009;(2):CD005019.
22. Russo MW, Scobey M, Bonkovsky HL. Drug-induced liver injury associated with statins. Semin Liver Dis. 2009; 29(4):412–422.
23. Calderon RM, Cubeddu LX, Goldberg RB, Schiff ER. Statins in the treatment of dyslipidemia in the presence of elevated liver aminotransferase levels: a therapeutic dilemma. Mayo Clin Proc. 2010;85(4):349–356.
24. Savvidaki E, Koukoulaki M, Benou A, et al. Ezetimibe is effective in the treatment of persistent hyperlipidemia of renal allograft recipients. Clin Nephrol. 2011;75(2): 107–112.
25. Steinmetz KL, Schonder KS. Colesevelam: potential uses for the newest bile resin. Cardiovasc Drug Rev. 2005;23(1): 15–30.
26. Zhao YY, Weir MA, Manno M, et al. New fibrate use and acute renal outcomes in elderly adults: a population-based study. Ann Intern Med. 2012;156(8):560–569.
27. Riella LV, Gabardi S, Chandraker A. Dyslipidemia and its therapeutic challenges in renal transplantation. Am J Transplant. 2012;12(8):1975–1982.
28. Jardine AG, Gaston RS, Fellstrom BC, Holdaas H. Prevention of cardiovascular disease in adult recipients of kidney transplants. Lancet. 2011;378(9800):1419–1427.
29. Kasiske B, Cosio FG, Beto J, et al. Clinical practice guidelines for managing dyslipidemias in kidney transplant patients: a report from the Managing Dyslipidemias in Chronic Kidney Disease Work Group of the National Kidney Foundation Kidney Disease Outcomes Quality Initiative. Am J Transplant. 2004;4(Suppl 7):13–53.
30. FDA Website: Food and Drug Administration. Safety Labeling Changes Approved By FDA Center for Drug Evaluation and Research (CDER). 2012. Available from: http://

www.fda.gov/Safety/MedWatch/SafetyInformation/ucm208610.htm (accessed 20 May 2013).

31. Kowa Pharmaceuticals America, Inc. Livalo Website and Package Insert. 2012. Available from: http://www.livalorx.com/Pages/index.aspx#ISI (accessed 20 May 2013).

32. Grundy SM, Cleeman JI, Merz CN, et al. Implications of recent clinical trials for the National Cholesterol Education Program Adult Treatment Panel III guidelines. Circulation. 2004;110(2):227–239.

26

CHAPTER 26

Hypertension management in long-term survivors

Imad Abboud

Nephrology Department, Saint Louis Hospital (Assistance Publique – Hôpitaux de Paris), Paris, France

Background

Hematopoietic stem cell transplantation (HSCT) is an established and increasingly used treatment for a wide range of hematological malignancies, as well as autoimmune and metabolic diseases. With the recent improvement in overall survival [1] there is an increased awareness of the long-term burden of organ damage [2], specifically chronic kidney disease (CKD) and hypertension (HTN). HTN is a well-established risk factor for cardiovascular events and end-stage renal disease. It represents a significant health risk for pediatric HSCT survivors.

Definition of hypertension

There is a continuous, consistent, and independent relationship between elevated blood pressure (BP) and risk of cardiovascular events [3]. Normal or optimal BP is defined as the level above which vascular damage occurs. The seventh report of the Joint National Committee on Prevention, Detection, Evaluation, and Treatment of High BP (JNC 7) defines normal BP as a systolic BP less than 120 mmHg and diastolic BP less than 80 mmHg [4].

Most guidelines for the general population define HTN as persistent systolic BP on at least 2 days ≥140 mmHg and/or diastolic BP ≥90 mmHg if age ≥18 years, and ≥95th percentile for gender, age, and height if age <18 years [5]. These same guidelines establish treatment goals for high-risk subpopulations (e.g. diabetes and CKD) that are generally systolic <130 mmHg and/or diastolic <80 mmHg for adults, and <90th percentile for gender, age, and height for adolescents and children.

Incidence and prevalence of HTN after HSCT

It is estimated that 29% of the adult US population has HTN or are taking anti-hypertensive medication [6]. The prevalence of HTN increases progressively with age [7].

HTN following pediatric HSCT has been reported to occur in up to 12% of patients in many studies [8–14]. Recently, the Fred Hutchinson Cancer Research Center team (Seattle, WA) conducted a retrospective study [13] to determine risk factors for the development of HTN and to describe the prevalence among long-term survivors of pediatric HSCT. Among 689 pediatric patients who survived at least 5 years after HSCT from 1969 to 2004, 120 (17%) developed HTN during a median follow-up period of 16 years (range: 5–36 years). The prevalence of HTN increased with time after transplantation from 7% at 5–9 years post-HSCT, 12% at 10–19 years, 17% at 20–29 years, and 36% (cumulative incidence) at ≥30 years. The prevalence of HTN was higher in obese (33%) versus nonobese (5%) children and higher in obese (26%) versus nonobese (15%) adults HTN was also more prevalent in patients with diabetes

Blood and Marrow Transplantation Long-Term Management: Prevention and Complications, First Edition. Edited by Bipin N Savani.

than without (52% versus 11%). Isolated diastolic HTN was found in 30% of adults and only 13% of children, whereas isolated systolic HTN was more common in children (41%) than in adults (25%). Among HSCT survivors 11–17 years old and 18–39 years old [13], the prevalence of HTN was triple (10% versus 3.2%) [15] and double (14% versus 7.3%) [6] that of the general US population, respectively. Also, the patients developed HTN at an average age of 25 years old; this is much earlier than the general population, which typically develops HTN after 40 years of age [6].

Risk factors of hypertension after HSCT

In the general population, HTN is primary (or idiopathic) 95% of the time, when there is no identifiable risk factor, and is of secondary etiologies like renovascular disease, primary aldosteronism, and others in 5% of patients. A number of factors are associated with increased BP, including older age, obesity, insulin resistance, physical inactivity, excess alcohol consumption, stress, and dietary factors [16]. Other factors include kidney disease, sleep apnea, nicotine, and endocrine disorders [17].

The early onset of HTN after HSCT appears to be multifactorial, resulting from both multiple risk factors at the time of transplantation and the development of diabetes and obesity after transplantation. Risk factors associated with HTN in different studies were mainly:

- acute kidney injury (doubling of baseline creatinine by day 100 after HSCT) [13], suggesting that renal damage plays a role in the pathophysiology of HTN;
- total body irradiation (TBI) in some studies [13], but not all [12];
- donor type, which was variably reported as an HTN risk factor in different studies [10, 12, 13];
- obesity and diabetes, which are well-established risk factors for HTN [12, 13], as in the general population;
- CKD [18].

Interestingly, although one could hypothesize that calcineurin inhibitors (CNIs) use, corticosteroids, and systemic inflammatory state could facilitate HTN, no association was found between graft-versus-host disease and posttransplantation HTN [12, 13].

Screening for hypertension after HSCT

Screening recommendations for patients beyond 6 months following transplantation were developed by a consensus panel formed by members of the Center for International Blood and Marrow Transplant Research, the European Group for Blood and Marrow Transplantation, and the American Society for Bone Marrow Transplantation [19]: BP should be checked at every clinic visit and at least every year, and HTN should be investigated and managed aggressively.

In fact, there are few data to suggest how often patients should be screened for HTN after HSCT. However, the high incidence of HTN, the high cardiovascular disease (CVD) risk after HSCT, and the ease of obtaining BP measurements are compelling arguments for measuring BP at every clinic visit. Medical providers should screen patients and refer cases to a nephrologist for specialized care.

Office blood pressure measurement

Because BP inaccuracies are common in clinical practice, the following guidelines should be followed when measuring a patient's BP. The patient should be seated comfortably for at least 5 min with the back supported, the feet on the floor, and the upper arm bared without constrictive clothing. The legs should not be crossed. The arm should be supported at heart level. An appropriately sized cuff with bladder encircling at least 80% of the arm should be used. At least two measurements should be made. Systolic BP is the point at which the first of two or more sounds is heard (phase 1), and diastolic BP is the point before the disappearance of sounds (phase 5) [4]. Neither the patient nor the observer should talk during the measurement.

Ambulatory blood pressure monitoring

In addition to office BP measurements, 24-h ambulatory BP monitoring is indicated to rule out white-coat HTN, to uncover apparent drug resistance (office resistance), to better define resistant HTN, to identify hypotensive symptoms while the patient is being treated with antihypertensives, to monitor episodic HTN, and to identify autonomic dysfunction states [4]. Ambulatory BP readings are lower than office BP readings, with

Table 26.1 Adult BP thresholds for defining HTN [5]

Method of measurement	Threshold (mmHg)
Office or clinic	140/90
24-h average	125–130/80
Daytime	130–135/85
Night-time	120/70
Home (daytime)	130–135/85

daytime values being higher than values during sleep (Table 26.1) [5].

Home blood pressure monitoring

Self-measured BP is also useful in assessing treatment of HTN and improving adherence to treatment [4].

Several prospective trials have demonstrated that home BP is a better predictor of cardiovascular morbidity and mortality than office BP measurements are. Based on these data, the first home BP monitoring guidelines endorsed by national societies, including the American Heart Association and the American Society of Hypertension, among others, have been published [20]. BP measurements using validated devices should be taken before an office visit, with at least two morning and two evening readings every day for 1 week (but discarding the readings of the first day), which gives a total of 12 BP readings with which clinical decisions can be made. Home measurement devices should be checked regularly for accuracy.

Workup of hypertension after HSCT

Baseline laboratory tests are recommended by JNC 7 to identify patients at risk for future events [4]:

- urinalysis;
- measurement of urinary albumin excretion or albumin/creatinine ratio;
- serum creatinine, or the corresponding estimated glomerular filtration rate;
- serum potassium;
- serum calcium;
- hematocrit;
- blood glucose;

Table 26.2 Tests and their clues to the etiology in patients with resistant or secondary HTN

Laboratory test	Possible clinical implication	Change in management
Abnormal urinalysis	Renal disease	Lower BP goal
		Consider specialist referral
Serum creatinine concentration	Renal disease and renovascular disease	Further evaluation and more aggressive therapy
Low serum potassium	Primary aldosteronism–Cushing's syndrome	Further evaluation for secondary HTN
Hematocrit	Polycythemia	Further evaluation
Electrocardiogram	Left ventricular hypertrophy	More aggressive therapy
Fasting lipid profile	Elevated risk for cardiovascular events	Aggressive lifestyle modifications

- lipid profile, after 9–12-h fast, that includes high-density and low-density lipoprotein cholesterol, and triglycerides;
- electrocardiogram.

In addition, these tests can provide clues to the etiology in those with resistant or secondary HTN (Table 26.2) [4]. More extensive testing for identifiable causes is not generally indicated unless BP control is not achieved.

Long-term implications of hypertension

HTN is an important risk factor in the general population for a variety of serious diseases and conditions, including heart disease (ischemic heart disease and heart failure), stroke, CKD, peripheral artery disease, retinopathy, and dementia [4, 21]. In addition, evidence from randomized clinical trials in the general population has conclusively shown that reducing BP reduces the risk of CVD and progression of CKD. In the study of Hoffmeister et al. [13], 72% of treated patients achieved adequate BP control, but 27 hypertensive patients were untreated. Unfortunately, three patients developed end-stage renal disease, four developed congestive heart failure, four had strokes, and one patient died of HTN-related complications.

Life expectancy is lower in HSCT survivors than in the general population [1], and it is possible that the benefits and harm of HTN treatment in HSCTs are different than in the general population. Also, unsurprisingly, no randomized controlled studies have demonstrated improved long-term outcomes by decreasing BP after HSCT transplantation. However, there is little reason to believe that the prevention and treatment of HTN would not also prevent CVD in this patient population. As part of best medical practice, it is therefore appropriate to treat post-transplantation HTN whenever possible [19]. In the absence of specific guidelines for HTN after HSCT, physicians should follow recommendations for BP target values in the general population [4]. Based on JNC 7, patients with sustained HTN are divided into stage 1 HTN (systolic BP 140–159 mmHg or diastolic BP 90–99 mmHg), stage 2 HTN (systolic BP ≥160 mmHg or diastolic BP ≥100 mmHg), and those with compelling indications that include diabetes, CVD, and renal disease [4] (Table 26.3).

Treatment strategy

Management of HTN should include:
• adjusting modifiable causes (reduction or withdrawal of steroid or CNI, etc.);
• encouraging nonpharmacologic treatments;
• administering antihypertensive medications; and
• managing other CVD risk factors.

Treatment is indicated for BP readings of greater than 140/90 mmHg in adults (greater than the 95th percentile for age, sex, and height in children) on two separate visits at least 1 week apart, unless HTN is mild and/or can be attributed to a temporary acute condition or medication (e.g., cyclosporine) [4]. Nonpharmacologic treatments may also be tried for mild HTN and include moderate dietary sodium restriction, weight reduction in the obese, avoidance of excess alcohol intake, and regular aerobic exercise [19].

Guidelines from the general population recommend targeting <140/90 mmHg for all patients, even low-risk patients. However, these same guidelines recommend targeting <130/80 mmHg for high-risk patients, such as patients with diabetes and CKD [4, 22].

Table 26.3 BP classification for adults

SPB: <120	and	DBP: <80	→	Normal
SBP: 120–139	and/or	DBP: 80–89	→	Prehypertension
SBP: 140–159	and/or	DBP: 90–99	→	Stage 1 HTN
SBP: >160	and/or	DBP: >100	→	Stage 2 HTN

Data from [4]. Available at http://www.nhlbi.nih.gov/guidelines/hypertension/index.htm (accessed November 30, 2012).
SBP, systolic BP; DBP, diastolic BP.

Lifestyle modifications

Lifestyle modifications not only reduce BP but also enhance the efficacy of antihypertensive drugs and decrease cardiovascular risk; they include [4]:
• Weight reduction in the obese – maintain normal body weight (body mass index, 18.4–24.9 kg/m^2).
• A DASH (Dietary Approaches to Stop Hypertension) eating plan [23] – the DASH trial has provided substantial data that a diet rich in fruits, vegetables, low-fat dairy products, with reduced content of saturated and total fats lowered BP even without weight reduction.
• A dietary sodium reduction – reducing sodium intake to no more than 100 mmol/day (i.e., 2.4 g sodium or 6 g sodium chloride).
• Increasing physical activity – engage in regular aerobic physical activity (e.g., brisk walking) at least 30 min/day, most days of the week.
• Limiting alcohol intake.
• Cigarette smoking is a recognized accelerator of CVD. Smoking cessation should therefore be strongly encouraged for all patients, and education, counseling, and medication should be provided as needed.

Drug choice

Most classes of antihypertensive medications can be used in HSCT, and there is insufficient evidence to recommend any class as a preferred long-term therapy for reducing CVD or improving a patient's survival.

Based on the Antihypertensive and Lipid Lowering to Reduce Heart Attack Trial data, JNC 7 recommends diuretics as first-line therapy for the management of stage 1 HTN and a combination of two drugs as an initial therapy in those with stage 2 HTN, one of which should preferably be a diuretic [24]. In addition to thiazide

Table 26.4 Recommended antihypertensive drugs for compelling indications

	CKD	Diabetes	Heart failure	Post-myocardial infarction	High coronary disease risk	Recurrent stroke prevention
ACEI	✓	✓	✓	✓	✓	✓
ARB	✓	✓	✓			
Diuretic		✓	✓		✓	✓
Calcium channel blocker		✓			✓	
Aldosterone antagonist			✓	✓		
β-blocker		✓	✓	✓	✓	

Data from [4]. Available at http://www.nhlbi.nih.gov/guidelines/hypertension/index.htm (accessed November 30, 2012).

diuretics, JNC 7 guidelines also recommend angiotensin-converting enzyme inhibitors (ACEIs), angiotensin receptor blockers (ARBs), beta blockers, and calcium channel blockers as first-line therapy for HTN. Since publication of the JNC 7 guidelines, studies have shown that beta-blocker therapy might not be effective and in fact might increase the risk of stroke [25, 26]. In the newer guidelines published by various national societies, beta blockers have been removed as first-line therapy and are recommended only with a compelling indication in those with cardiac disease [5]. Based on evidence of improved outcomes, JNC 7 has recommended several medications for compelling indications (Table 26.4 and Table 26.5). These include beta blockers and aldosterone antagonists in those with cardiac disease, ACEIs and ARBs in those with CKD, and diuretics and calcium channel blockers in those with isolated systolic HTN. A combination of ACEIs and diuretics is recommended for preventing recurrence of stroke. Many patients will require combination therapy to control BP. Most combinations should include a thiazide diuretic, unless it is contraindicated.

ACEIs and ARBs have been used in rodent models of HSCT-related renal injury, specifically of radiation-induced haemolytic–uremic syndrome. The use of captopril or enalapril at the time of TBI in these animals resulted in less azotemia, lower BPs, decreased proteinuria, and long-term preservation of renal function [27]. In a randomized controlled trial, captopril demonstrated a trend toward improvement in 1-year glomerular filtration rate and serum creatinine [28]. ACEIs and ARBs also help reduce inflammation and inflammatory markers and reduce circulating levels of TGF-β1 in patients after

Table 26.5 Management of BP in adults

Prehypertension	• If diabetes or CKD: treat to a BP goal <130/80 mmHg (using drugs for the compelling indications) • Otherwise, no antihypertensive drug is indicated
Stage 1 HTN	• If compelling indication(s), use corresponding drug(s) • Otherwise, may use a thiazide-type diuretic for most
Stage 2 HTN	• If compelling indication(s), use corresponding drug(s) • Otherwise, begin with a two-drug combination for most

Data from [4]. Available at http://www.nhlbi.nih.gov/guidelines/hypertension/index.htm (accessed November 30, 2012).

transplant [29]. Because renin–angiotensin system antagonists have also been shown to slow CKD progression and decrease proteinuria in patients with renal disease from various causes, they could be proposed as first-line agents to manage HTN in patients after HSCT. A close follow-up (1 week after starting treatment and 1 month later) of BP, serum creatinine, and electrolytes is recommended, and caution is advised in individuals with pre-existing hyperkalemia and/or anemia.

Conclusion

In addition to transplant-specific diseases and complications, HSCT survivors remain at risk of common diseases found in the general population, particularly HTN, a frequent and modifiable cardiovascular and renal risk factor. Although a majority of patients with HTN remain asymptomatic, a careful early evaluation identifies those with or at risk for target organ damage. Early identification of these patients and achieving BP goals could potentially reverse early end-organ damage and improve outcomes in these patients.

References

1. Socié G, Stone JV, Wingard JR, et al. Long-term survival and late deaths after allogeneic bone marrow transplantation. Late Effects Working Committee of the International Bone Marrow Transplant Registry. N Engl J Med. 1999; 341(1):14–21.
2. Socié G, Salooja N, Cohen A, et al. Nonmalignant late effects after allogeneic stem cell transplantation. Blood. 2003; 101(9):3373–3385.
3. Lewington S, Whitlock G, Clarke R, et al. Blood cholesterol and vascular mortality by age, sex, and blood pressure: a meta-analysis of individual data from 61 prospective studies with 55,000 vascular deaths. Lancet. 2007;370(9602): 1829–1839.
4. Chobanian AV, Bakris GL, Black HR, et al. The Seventh Report of the Joint National Committee on Prevention, Detection, Evaluation, and Treatment of High Blood Pressure: the JNC 7 report. JAMA. 2003;289(19):2560–2572.
5. Mancia G, De Backer G, Dominiczak A, et al. 2007 Guidelines for the management of arterial hypertension: the task force for the management of arterial hypertension of the European Society of Hypertension (ESH) and of the European Society of Cardiology (ESC). J Hypertens. 2007; 25(6):1105–1187.
6. Ong KL, Cheung BM, Man YB, et al. Prevalence, awareness, treatment, and control of hypertension among United States adults 1999–2004. Hypertension. 2007;49(1):69–75.
7. Vasan RS, Beiser A, Seshadri S, et al. Residual lifetime risk for developing hypertension in middle-aged women and men: the Framingham Heart Study. JAMA. 2002;287(8): 1003–1010.
8. Kumar M, Kedar A, Neiberger RE. Kidney function in long-term pediatric survivors of acute lymphoblastic leukemia following allogeneic bone marrow transplantation. Pediatr Hematol Oncol. 1996;13(4):375–379.
9. Leahey AM, Teunissen H, Friedman DL, et al. Late effects of chemotherapy compared to bone marrow transplantation in the treatment of pediatric acute myeloid leukemia and myelodysplasia. Med Pediatr Oncol. 1999;32(3):163–169.
10. Frisk P, Bratteby LE, Carlson K, Lonnerholm G. Renal function after autologous bone marrow transplantation in children: a long-term prospective study. Bone Marrow Transplant. 2002;29(2):129–136.
11. Kist-van Holthe JE, Bresters D, Ahmed-Ousenkova YM, et al. Long-term renal function after hemopoietic stem cell transplantation in children. Bone Marrow Transplant. 2005; 36(7):605–610.
12. Baker KS, Ness KK, Steinberger J, et al. Diabetes, hypertension, and cardiovascular events in survivors of hematopoietic cell transplantation: a report from the bone marrow transplantation survivor study. Blood. 2007;109(4):1765–1772.
13. Hoffmeister PA, Hingorani SR, Storer BE, et al. Hypertension in long-term survivors of pediatric hematopoietic cell transplantation. Biol Blood Marrow Transplant. 2010; 16(4):515–524.
14. Majhail NS, Challa TR, Mulrooney DA, et al. Hypertension and diabetes mellitus in adult and pediatric survivors of allogeneic hematopoietic cell transplantation. Biol Blood Marrow Transplant. 2009;15(9):1100–1107.
15. McNiece KL, Poffenbarger TS, Turner JL, et al. Prevalence of hypertension and pre-hypertension among adolescents. J Pediatr. 2007;150(6):640–644, 4 e1.
16. Carretero OA, Oparil S. Essential hypertension. Part I: definition and etiology. Circulation. 2000;101(3):329–335.
17. Onusko E. Diagnosing secondary hypertension. Am Fam Physician. 2003;67(1):67–74.
18. Kersting S, Verdonck LF. Chronic kidney disease after nonmyeloablative stem cell transplantation in adults. Biol Blood Marrow Transplant. 2008;14(4):403–408.
19. Rizzo JD, Wingard JR, Tichelli A, et al. Recommended screening and preventive practices for long-term survivors after hematopoietic cell transplantation: joint recommendations of the European Group for Blood and Marrow Transplantation, the Center for International Blood and Marrow Transplant Research, and the American Society of Blood and Marrow Transplantation. Biol Blood Marrow Transplant. 2006;12(2):138–151.
20. Pickering TG, Miller NH, Ogedegbe G, et al. Call to action on use and reimbursement for home blood pressure monitoring: a joint scientific statement from the American Heart Association, American Society Of Hypertension, and Preventive Cardiovascular Nurses Association. Hypertension. 2008;52(1):10–29.
21. National High Blood Pressure Education Program Working Group on High Blood Pressure in Children and Adolescents. The fourth report on the diagnosis, evaluation, and treatment of high blood pressure in children and adolescents. Pediatrics. 2004 ;114(2 Suppl 4th Report):555–576.

22. Kidney Disease Outcomes Quality Initiative (K/DOQI). K/DOQI clinical practice guidelines on hypertension and antihypertensive agents in chronic kidney disease. Am J Kidney Dis. 2004 May;43(5 Suppl 1):S1–S290.
23. Appel LJ, Moore TJ, Obarzanek E, et al. A clinical trial of the effects of dietary patterns on blood pressure. DASH Collaborative Research Group. N Engl J Med. 1997;336(16):1117–1124.
24. The ALLHAT Officers and Coordinators for the ALLHAT Collaborative Research Group. Major outcomes in high-risk hypertensive patients randomized to angiotensin-converting enzyme inhibitor or calcium channel blocker vs diuretic: the Antihypertensive and Lipid-Lowering Treatment to Prevent Heart Attack Trial (ALLHAT). JAMA. 2002;288(23):2981–2997.
25. Sever PS, Poulter NR, Dahlof B, Wedel H. Different time course for prevention of coronary and stroke events by atorvastatin in the Anglo-Scandinavian Cardiac Outcomes Trial-Lipid-Lowering Arm (ASCOT-LLA). Am J Cardiol. 2005;96(5A):39F–44F.
26. Carlberg B, Samuelsson O, Lindholm LH. Atenolol in hypertension: is it a wise choice? Lancet. 2004;364(9446):1684–1689.
27. Cohen EP. Radiation nephropathy after bone marrow transplantation. Kidney Int. 2000;58(2):903–918.
28. Cohen E, Irving A, Drobyski W, et al. Captopril to mitigate chronic renal failure after hematopoietic stem cell transplantation: a randomized controlled trial. Int J Radiat Oncol Biol Phys. 2008;70(5):1546–1551.
29. Dagenais NJ, Jamali F. Protective effects of angiotensin II interruption: evidence for antiinflammatory actions. Pharmacotherapy. 2005;25(9):1213–1229.

27

CHAPTER 27
Gastrointestinal complications of hematopoietic cell transplantation

Preet Bagi[1], *Niharika Samala*[2], *Steven Pavletic*[3], *and Theo Heller*[2]

[1]The National Institute of Diabetes and Digestive and Kidney Diseases (NIDDK), National Institutes of Health, Bethesda, MD, USA
[2]Liver Disease Branch, The National Institute of Diabetes and Digestive and Kidney Diseases (NIDDK), National Institutes of Health, Bethesda, MD, USA
[3]Graft-versus-Host and Autoimmunity Unit, Center for Cancer Research, National Cancer Institute, Bethesda, MD, USA

Introduction

Over recent years, there has been a rise in the number of indications for hematopoietic cell transplantation (HCT) resulting in increasing numbers of patients who are long-term survivors. Progress has been made in the realm of both allogeneic and autologous hematopoietic cells which can be harvested from bone marrow, umbilical cord blood, or peripheral blood stem cells. Patients are living longer after HCT, and some even undergo more than one transplant [1]. HCT indications have broadened to include immunologic and nonmalignant hematologic diseases [2]. Associated with this has been an increase in the nonmalignant complications of HCT, including gastrointestinal (GI) complications. Therefore, recognition of the GI complications surrounding HCT is imperative [3]. GI complications can occur due to transplant conditioning, immunosuppressive medication effects, opportunistic infections, and acute or chronic graft-versus-host disease (GVHD). GI toxicity is a major cause of transplant-associated morbidity and mortality, which highlights the need for quick recognition followed by corrective strategies. This chapter will provide an up-to-date overview of the diagnosis and management of GI complications that occur before, during, and after HCT.

Preconditiong-related gastrointestinal complications

Preexisting gastrointestinal conditions

Preexisting GI conditions must be evaluated pretransplant, as several GI conditions have symptoms that overlap with HCT-related GI complications. These include, but are not limited to, gastroesophageal reflux disease (GERD), inflammatory bowel disease (IBD), irritable bowel syndrome, symptomatic cholelithiasis, and autoimmune or chronic pancreatitis. For example, a patient with Crohn's or ulcerative colitis should be well controlled and in remission prior to undergoing HCT, as afterward the symptoms such as abdominal pain and diarrhea may be confused with active GVHD. Of note, protocols have examined high-dose immunosuppression followed by autologous hematopoietic stem cell transplant with variable success in refractory Crohn's; however, this is not currently part of standard IBD therapy [4–7]. Additionally, some posttransplant immunosuppressive

Blood and Marrow Transplantation Long-Term Management: Prevention and Complications, First Edition. Edited by Bipin N Savani.

therapies, such as cyclosporine and tacrolimus, are considered second-line treatments for IBD and can be effective in maintaining IBD remission [8].

Transplant-conditioning gastrointestinal effects

Transplant conditioning itself can cause significant GI side effects. Conditioning regimens involve radiotherapy with or without chemotherapy. Typical myeloablative preparative regimens include: high-dose radiation with or without an alkylating agent such as busulfan, cyclophosphamide, or, less commonly, melphan, thiotepa, etoposide, or dimethylbusulfan [9]. Nonmyelcablative regimens will cause minimal cytopenia or other side effects and typically include fludarabine, cyclophosphamide, cytarabine, antithymocyte globulin, or total body irradiation [9]. Reduced-intensity conditioning is an intermediate category that uses various combinations of the above-mentioned regimens. GI side effects are typically noted very early prior to engraftment, which is within 15 days posttransplant [1]. Total body irradiation acutely can cause nausea and vomiting [10]. Although there are several possible early GI effects of conditioning chemotherapy, the most common effects are mucositis, nausea, vomiting, and diarrhea (Table 27.1).

Table 27.1 GI effects of conditioning agents [1, 16]

Agent	GI effect
Antithymocyte globulin	Nausea, abdomina pain, gastritis, diarrhea, GI candiciasis
Busulfan	Mucositis, nausea, emesis, dyspepsia, anorexia, diarrhea, abdominal pain, abdominal fullness, constipation
Cyclophosphamide	Mucositis, nausea, emesis anorexia, abdominal pain, GI bleed, mesenteric ischemia
Cytarabine	Mucositis, nausea, vomiting, anorexia, abdominal pain, diarrhea, anal inflammation/ulceration, bowel necrosis, esophageal ulceration/ esophagitis, pancreatitis
Etoposide	Nausea, emesis, anorexia abdominal pain, diarrhea
Fludarabine	Mucositis, nausea, emesis, dysphagia, esophagitis, anorexia, diarrhea, GI bleeding, constipation
Melphalan	Musositis, nausea, emesis, diarrhea, ileus
Thiotepa	Nausea, emesis, anorexia, abdominal pain
Total body irradiation	Mucositis, sicca syndrome, nausea, vomiting

Acute and subacute gastrointestinal HCT complications

Oral pain

Conditioning-induced mucositis

Oral mucositis occurs in up to 40% of patients during chemotherapy and appears 5–10 days after conditioning starts [1, 11]. The incidence of grade 3–4 oral mucositis is 30–50% during HCT, and if also undergoing total body irradiation it rises to greater than 60% [11]. There are several grading systems for the severity of mucositis, such as the commonly used National Cancer Institute Common Terminology for Adverse Events Criteria, which combines symptoms and clinical findings (Table 27.2). A separate scoring system exists for patients with mucositis after autologous or allogeneic stem cell transplant [12]. Outcomes of patients with grade 3–4 oral mucositis are worse, as 80% require narcotic analgesics, 70% require feeding tubes to maintain nutrition, which should be considered after inability to tolerate oral intake

Table 27.2 National Cancer Institute common terminology criteria for adverse events [55]

Grade	Description
1	Asymptomatic or mild symptoms; intervention not indicated
2	Moderate pain, not interfering with oral intake; modified diet indicated
3	Severe pain, interfering with oral intake
4	Life-threatening consequences; urgent intervention indicated
5	Death

over 7 days, 62% require hospitalization, and 60% develop fever [11]. Prophylaxis against conditioning-induced oral mucositis after HCT includes the use of saline plus bicarbonate mouth washes and the keratinocyte growth factor-1, palifermin, at 60 μg/kg intravenously for three consecutive days before and three consecutive days after conditioning therapy [1, 13]. Guidelines advocate against the use of sucralafate, antimicrobial lozenges, and granulocyte–macrophage colony-stimulating factor mouthwashes for radiation-induced oral mucositis [14].

Oral infections

Infectious mucositis can exist as a distinct entity, but it occurs commonly superimposed upon an already damaged oral mucosal barrier after conditioning. Neutropenia further increases the chance of oral infections, and the most common are oral candidiasis and herpes simplex virus (HSV) and less commonly cytomegalovirus (CMV), varicella zoster virus (VZV), and bacteria [1]. These all occur with decreased frequency as a result of prophylaxis with antifungal and antiviral medications.

Dysphagia and odynophagia

During the acute phase, new-onset and persistent dysphagia/odynophagia warrants an infectious work-up. During conditioning, prophylactic daily proton pump inhibitors are often used, and if symptoms persist then upper endoscopy is required. Endoscopy can evaluate for viral esophagitis due to CMV, HSV, and VZV, whose lesions appear as ulcers, exudates, plaques, or erosive esophagitis [15]. Immunohistochemical stains must be specifically performed to identify the virus in pathology specimens, and viral culture in saline can identify resistant viral strains that will not respond to acyclovir. Additionally, one must exclude fungal esophagitis, such as esophageal candidiasis, which can occur independent of oral candidiasis.

Nausea, vomiting, and diarrhea

Chemotherapy effects

Nausea and vomiting within the first 15 days after transplantation are almost always due to the chemotherapy or total-body radiotherapy used for conditioning. The pathogenesis of nausea and vomiting after chemotherapy include: (1) direct activation of the vomiting center in the brainstem by chemotherapy, which triggers target organs in the GI tract, and (2) direct damage to the GI mucosa, causing vagal stimulation and neuropeptide release causing positive feedback on the vomiting center [1]. Prophylaxis will aid in preventing or minimizing this phase of nausea and vomiting and can be accomplished with corticosteroids plus 5-hydroxytryptamine-3 receptor antagonists in the acute phase up to 24 h after chemotherapy infusion and with corticosteroids alone during the subacute phase up to 5 days after [1]. If symptoms persist, then alternative therapies include metoclopramide, lorazepam, pheothiazines, haloperidol, dronabinol, scopolamine, and corticosteroids [16].

Acute GVHD

Background

The greater is the intensity of the pretransplant radiotherapy and/or chemotherapy, the higher are the risk and severity of acute GVHD. This is from conditioning-related release of cytokines such as tumor necrosis factor-α, interleukin-1, and interleukin-6 [17]. Proposed mechanisms by which this occurs include increased antigen presentation from the host to donor T-cells and cytokine activation of donor T-cells [18]. This is further supported by the decreased incidence of and decreased severity of acute GVHD in severe combined immunodeficiency patients who undergo allogeneic HCT without conditioning [19]. Additionally, the GI tract is thought to play a key role in the development of GVHD, as acute GI mucosal damage leads to a release of endotoxins which fuels the cytokine release that leads to acute GVHD [20].

Symptoms

Acute GI GVHD develops typically within 3 months of HCT or donor leukocyte infusion [21]. Of note, there is an overlap syndrome that has been defined as occurring with features of both the acute and chronic phases [1]. This overlap syndrome is more commonly seen with reduced-intensity conditioning regimens. The development of acute GI GVHD is relevant as it predicts prognosis, and the overall mortality rate is 30–60% [22]. Symptoms of acute GI GVHD may include nausea, vomiting, loss of appetite, abdominal pain, and/or diarrhea. The diarrhea can be quite severe and voluminous, making maintenance of adequate fluid balance essential (Table 27.3). Initially the diarrhea is watery, which is due to small and large intestinal malabsorption. As the disease progresses, bloody diarrhea and paralytic ileus may

Table 27.3 Staging of acute GVHD [56]

Stage	Skin	Liver	GI tract
1	Maculopapular rash <25% of body surface	Bilirubin 34–50 μmol/L	Diarrhea >30 ml/kg or >500 ml/day
2	Maculopapular rash <25% of body surface	Bilirubin 51–102 μmol/L	Diarrhea >60 ml/kg or >1000 ml/day
3	Generalized erythoderma	Bilirubin 103–225 μmol/L	Diarrhea >90 ml/kg or >1500 ml/day
4	Generalized erythroderma with bullous formation and desquamation	Bilirubin >225 μmol/L	Diarrhea >100 ml/kg or >2000 ml/day or severe abdominal pain with or without ileus

Table 27.4 Grading of acute GVHD: Glucksberg criteria (modified) [56–58]

Grade	Skin	Liver	GI tract	Clinical performance	Frequency post-HCT (%)	Mortality
1	1–2	0	0	No decrease	12–36	~0%
2	1–3	1	[illegible]	Mild decrease	12–25	~60%
3	2–3	2–3	2–3	Marked decrease	10–24	~60%
4	2–4	2–4	2–4	Extreme decrease	5–16	>90%

develop. Upper GI symptoms may be subtle and may include dyspepsia, anorexia, food intolerance, nausea, and vomiting [23]. Grading acute GVHD is important, as survival directly correlates with GVHD severity as the risk of morbidity and mortality rises from complications such as hemorrhage, infection and sepsis (Table 27.4). It is rare for GI involvement to occur alone, and GI manifestations typically occur at the same time as skin GVHD or liver [24].

Table 27.5 Endoscopic scoring of acute GI GVHD [1]

Stage	Endoscopic appearance
I	Loss of vascular pattern and/or focal moderate erythema
II	Edema and/or diffuse erythema
III	Edema, erythema, erosions, possible bleeding
IV	Ulceration, exudates, possible bleeding

Endoscopy

Endoscopic findings may include erythema, edema, ulceration, and bleeding. Severe cases may result in loss of vascularity, mucosal sloughing, desquamation, and endoscope contact bleeding. An endoscopic scoring system has been proposed; the severity of endoscopic findings can be suggestive of the degree of histologic severity, but it does not always correlate with the degree of clinical severity [1, 25] (Table 27.5).

Histology

In order to diagnose acute GI GVHD, biopsies must be taken and pathologic criteria must be met. However, in many situations the results of these biopsies are inconclusive and the ultimate clinical diagnosis depends on the integration of all clinical information (e.g., presence of concurrent acute GVHD in other organs, ruling out other causes of GI symptoms, clinical circumstances). Although GI GVHD symptoms can develop as early as at 15 days posttransplant, which is the expected day of engraftment, biopsies initially permit recognition of GVHD by day 21 [26]. Furthermore, the pathologic changes due to conditioning may still be present up until day 20 [27]. Any and all parts of the GI tract can be affected, and there is no consensus on which region of the GI tract to biopsy in order to best diagnose acute GVHD. Typically, the location in which symptoms are occurring is where biopsies should be obtained, as gastric/duodenal biopsies are used for nausea, vomiting, or upper abdominal pain, and rectosigmoid biopsies are used for diarrhea [28]. Although postmortem studies have shown the highest yield to be from the small intestine, this region can be difficult to sample [22]. The rectosigmoid region has been shown to have a high sensitivity and specificity for diagnosing GVHD and is at least as good as duodenal biopsies; therefore, given this, the ideal location from which to make a diagnosis of GVHD is the rectosigmoid, as an unsedated flexible sigmoidoscopy procedure is lower risk than an upper endoscopy or colposcopy with ileoscopy [29, 30]. There has been some concern regarding the higher risk of bleeding while obtaining duodenal biopsies as it is a difficult region in which to achieve hemostasis after bleeding and patients are often thrombocytopenic [31, 32]. The type of presenting GI symptom and ultimate region of positive pathology do not appear to correlate [29].

The initial histology changes involve a focal increase in the number of lymphocytes in the lamina propria, edema, and granular necrosis/apoptotic cell death of individual epithelial cells within crypts [33]. Acutely, as patients often have leukopenia, there is little to no inflammatory infiltration [33]. These early lesions are quite nonspecific and nondiagnostic, yet one exception is that the stomach may be an area from which to diagnose early acute GVHD given a general lack of physiologic inflammation in this area [28, 34].

As the graft-versus-host reaction continues, the defining characteristics of acute GVHD become more established. Crypts develop a dilated lumen and contain significant cellular debris, and several apoptotic bodies and have been described as a characteristic finding and have been named "exploding crypts" [35]. These lesions further progress to become crypt abscesses and display increased numbers of intraepithelial lymphocytes [33, 35]. If uncontrolled, the evolution of the disease involves focal or diffuse mucosal ulceration, crypt dropout, and epithelial denudement [33]. Of note, there are no pathognomic findings for acute GVHD, but exploding crypts are considered a pathologic hallmark. Single apoptotic bodies that can be found within the first 20–30 days posttransplant as a result of radiation, therefore, are nondiagnostic, and biopsies after day 20–30 will be of higher yield for acute GVHD [28]. During this early time period, the concomitant presence of acute skin or liver GVHD would support the diagnosis.

Table 27.6 Lerner histologic GVHD grading [36]

Grade 1	Isolated apoptotic epithelial cell
Grade 2	Loss of isolated crypts, glandular abscesses, epithelial flattening, glandular/crypt dilation
Grade 3	Drop out of one or more crypts/glands
Grade 4	Extensive crypt loss, mucosal denudement

A method to stage the pathologic findings in acute GI GVHD exists [36] (Table 27.6). Biopsies should be taken even if the mucosa appears normal, as pathology can be positive without endoscopic abnormalities. There is inconclusive evidence as to whether a higher grade of histologic acute GVHD correlates with clinical severity [27, 29]. A higher severity of histologic findings does not appear to correlate with an increased severity of endoscopic findings [27].

Radiology

There is no established radiologic finding that is pathognomic for acute GI GVHD, but radiologic abnormalities are common in GVHD and worth mentioning. Imaging is not highly specific, but abdominal imaging is often done to exclude other etiologies of GI symptoms. Abdominal plain films are often abnormal and may show separated bowel loops, decreased luminal gas, and small intestinal dilation, whereas a computed axial tomography (CAT) scan most commonly reveals luminal narrowing, moderate (<8 mm) bowel wall thickening, and mucosal enhancement [37]. The most common location of imaging abnormality is within the small intestine [38]. Other possible findings include bowel dilation, mesenteric infiltration, ascites, engorgement of the vasa recta, or increased small bowel fluid [37].

Infection

Any posttransplant patient with vomiting and/or diarrhea may be infected with common causes of viral gastroenteritis, such as rotavirus, adenovirus, or norovirus, and may take longer to recover. Any vomiting or diarrhea that persists warrants further work-up. Stool studies must be done on persistent diarrhea mainly to exclude *Clostridium difficile*, bacterial colitis, and *Giardia* or *Cryptosporidia* opportunistic infections. If this work-up is negative and symptoms persist or progress, an endoscopy should be performed to exclude acute GVHD; and any lesions, such as erythema, erosions, or ulcers, require biospies for viral staining and to exclude CMV or HSV. Fungal staining may be done if applicable. These concomitant infections that require endoscopic diagnosis must be considered as they have been reported in up to 23% of acute GI GVHD cases [30].

Medications

Posttransplant prophylactic medications (cyclosporine, mycophenolate, or methotrexate) can cause GI upset in the form of nausea, vomiting, or diarrhea. The symptom severity is dependent upon the medication dose and typically will occur early after the medication has been begun but can cause symptoms later.

Systemic antibiotics, antifungals, and antivirals which may be given for chronic antimicrobial prophylaxis can also cause nausea, vomiting, or diarrhea during the posttransplant time period.

Abdominal pain

Typhilitis

Typhilitis will present within 30 days after transplant with abdominal pain with fever, diarrhea, and, as it progresses, decreased bowel movements [39]. Radiographically, bowel wall thickening may be limited to a single region such as the ileocecal area or ascending colon [37]. If unrecognized, bowel perforation may occur and air may be seen within the intestinal wall [37]. Treatment includes antibiotics and bowel rest.

Lymphoproliferative disease

If a donor is infected with Epstein–Barr virus, in the late posttransplant period beyond 100 days, B- or T-cell proliferation can lead to malignant lymphoma which can occur almost anywhere and also in the GI tract [40, 41].

Other

A few of the chemotherapy medications can cause abdominal pain and may be associated with ileus or bowel ischemia. Also, acute GVHD may histologically resemble other conditions that are not associated with transplant, such as IBD, intestinal vasculitis, or ischemic colitis; therefore, other clues must be used, such as location of the area affected (e.g., ischemic colitis occurs in watershed regions).

Rectal pain and bleeding

Radiation-induced GI damage can manifest as early as 3 weeks after transplant, which typically presents as painless rectal bleeding. A commonly affected area is the rectum, and radiation proctitis can be prevented with amifostine and treated with endoscopic cautery. Infectious proctitis is also on the differential. Anal fissures can become superinfected during the neutropenic phase after conditioning. Significant rectal bleeding can be from a proximal source such as acute GVHD ulcerations, friable mucosa, CMV/HSV ulcerations, or a brisk upper GI bleed.

Chronic gastrointestinal HCT complications

Chronic GI complications after transplant are most commonly related to chronic GVHD, infections, or medications. Chronic GVHD is common and occurs in 50% of survivors of human leukocyte antigen-identical sibling transplants [42]. Chronic GI GVHD significantly affects long-term survival, but also quality of life.

Oral pain and xerostomia

Chronic oral GVHD can cause painful ulcerations, lichenoid lesions, and poor dentition. Progression of these lesions suggests progressive chronic oral GVHD [43]. Salivary gland damage from GVHD and/or radiation can cause xerostomia. Most patients with extensive GVHD will have oral mucosa involvement [44].

Dysphagia, odynophagia, and gastroesophageal reflux disease

Dysmotility

Oropharyngeal dysphagia results as a combination of multiple problems: tongue/hypopharyngeal inflammation from chronic GVHD and a poorly coordinated tongue/hypopharyngeal pressure wave [45]. The result is difficulty initiating a swallow and possible food regurgitation through the nose. Although rare, myasthenia gravis can even result from severe hypopharyngeal dysmotility [46].

Chronic esophageal GVHD

Esophageal dysphagia must be distinguished from oropharyngeal dysphagia, as this may be overshadowed

	SCORE 0	SCORE 1	SCORE 2	SCORE 3
GI Tract	☐ No symptoms	☐ Symptoms such as dysphagia, anorexia, nausea, vomiting, abdominal pain or diarrhea without significant weight loss (<5%)	☐ Symptoms associated with mild to moderate weight loss (5-15%)	☐ Symptoms associated with significant weight loss >15%, requires nutritional supplement for most calorie needs OR esophageal dilation
Liver	☐ Normal LFT	☐ Elevated Bilirubin, AP*, AST or ALT <2 × ULN	☐ Bilirubin >3 mg/dl or Bilirubin, enzymes 2-5 × ULZ	☐ Bilirubin or enzymes > 5 × ULN

Figure 27.1 Scoring of chronic GI and liver GVHD [49].

by oral symptoms. Severe esophageal disease from chronic GVHD presents with dysphagia to solids, chest discomfort, and possible aspiration. This was prevalent at 13% in the past but has decreased owing to routine prophylaxis with cyclosporine [47]. A diagnosis is made using a barium esophagram or upper endoscopy. A barium study can identify esophageal abnormalities that may be a perforation risk [47]. Esophagram findings include mid/upper esophageal strictures (which can be long and tapered), webs, rings, bullae, and desquamation. Endoscopic findings are similar, and desquamation appears as erythematous, friable sloughed mucosa. Pathology shows basal-layer squamous cell necrosis, epithelial desquamation, and mucosal infiltration with neutrophils, lymphocytes, and eosinophils [45]. If unrecognized, then chronic esophageal GVHD can lead to insidious weight loss and malnutrition; and once severe, chronic strictures often need serial dilations with a Savary dilator over a guidewire, possibly under fluoroscopy, and enteral feeding tube placement may be required or esophagectomy may be needed [45].

Infectious esophagitis

Esophageal infections similar to the acute phase can occur due to immunosuppression but are much less common [48]. Additionally, this risk has decreased by the use of chronic antimicrobial prophylaxis.

Gastroesophageal reflux disease

There are several mechanisms by which GERD occurs, including decreased oral bicarbonate production due to damaged salivary glands, which leads to decreased neutralization of gastric acid or decreased esophageal/gastric motility. Often, patients require chronic proton pump inhibitor therapy and can develop lower esophageal peptic esophagtitis, strictures, and Barrett's esophagus.

Secondary malignancy

There have also been reports of an increased incidence of esophageal squamous cell carcinoma and adenocarcinoma in patients, and these patients typically also have oral GVHD [45, 49].

Nausea, vomiting, anorexia, diarrhea

Late acute gastrointestinal GVHD

The phenomenon of GVHD-related nausea, vomiting, diarrhea, and anorexia beyond 100 days after transplant is actually very similar to classic acute GI GVHD both endoscopically and pathologically. This phenomenon is termed "late" acute GI GVHD and it includes cases of persistent, recurrent, or late-onset acute GVHD [49]. If these manifestations occur in the presence of diagnostic signs of chronic GVHD this entity is called "chronic GVHD-overlap syndrome subtype". Such chronic GI GVHD manifestations can present with diarrhea, abdominal distention, malabsorption, and possibly vomiting (Figure 27.1). Chronic GVHD is defined by pathology that shows the chronic changes of submucosal and subserosal fibrosis. These chronicity pathology findings are now rare owing to prophylaxis. More commonly, pathology will show changes similar to the acute stage: apoptosis, mucosal crypt destruction, and lamina propria plasma cell/lymphocyte infiltrates [45]. Gastroparesis can develop owing to altered gastric motility from chronic fibrosis, which in turn leads to symptoms of nausea, vomiting, and early satiety. A gastric emptying study can be used to make this diagnosis, and reglan or erythromycin can be used as promotility agents.

Infectious

Similar to the acute phase, chronic infections can occur involving the stomach, small intestine, and/or colon and include *Helicobacter pylori* (gastric only), CMV, HSV, VZV, candidiasis, *Giardia*, and *Cryptosporidia*.

Medication induced

Other than antibiotics and immunosuppressives, chronic corticosteroid use can cause secondary adrenal insufficiency with symptoms of anorexia and vomiting.

Pancreatic disease

Pancreatic insufficiency and atrophy has been reported after transplant and is rare [50]. The etiology remains uncertain and treatment relies on pancreatic enzyme replacement. Acute pancreatitis can be detected by elevated amylase and lipase and fat malabsorption is determined by elevated fecal fat. Chronic pancreatitis will show low serum trypsinogen and high fecal elastase-1 and possible pancreatic atrophy on CAT or magnetic resonance imaging [48]. Some proposed causes of pancreatic disease include medications (prednisone, tacrolimus), stones, or sludge passing, which causes pancreatic duct obstruction or direct damage of the pancreatic tissue from GVHD [45].

Abdominal pain

Strictures

If not suppressed by adequate treatment, acute GI GVHD can lead to small or large intestinal strictures from chronic, severe segmental fibrotic changes [45]. These require serial endoscopic dilation or surgical resection.

Biliary disease

Biliary sludge and stones increase posttransplant and are thought to be due to conditioning medications [45].

Rectal pain and bleeding

Radiation proctitis

Depending upon the strength of the initial radiation dose, radiation proctitis can persist long term with bleeding and sometimes pain. Persistent bleeding requires serial cautery via sigmoidoscopy in conjunction with medical therapy and is best managed by an experienced team.

Future directions

GI GVHD remains a formidable diagnostic challenge and major cause of mortality and morbidity after HCT. Further progress is expected in the area of developing better biomarkers of the disease to improve ability to do early diagnosis, risk-stratify, and monitor therapy of such manifestations [51, 52]. Better understanding of GVHD biology should also lead to developing better methods for prevention therapy of GI GVHD. Progress is also expected to come from further advancement of diagnostic methods, including imaging such as confocal microscopy and positron emission tomography scanning [53, 54].

References

1. Tuncer HH, Rana N, Milani C, et al. Gastrointestinal and hepatic complications of hematopoietic stem cell transplantation. World J Gastroenterol. 2012;18:1851–1860.
2. Burt RK, Loh Y, Pearce W, et al. Clinical applications of blood-derived and marrow-derived stem cells for nonmalignant diseases. JAMA. 2008;299:925–936.
3. Gratwohl A, Baldomero H, Aljurf M, et al. Hematopoietic stem cell transplantation: a global perspective. JAMA. 2010;303:1617–1624.
4. Burt RK, Traynor A, Oyama Y, Craig R. High-dose immune suppression and autologous hematopoietic stem cell transplantation in refractory Crohn disease. Blood. 2003;101:2064–2066.
5. Burt RK, Craig RM, Milanetti F, et al. Autologous nonmyeloablative hematopoietic stem cell transplantation in patients with severe anti-TNF refractory Crohn disease: long-term follow-up. Blood. 2010;116:6123–6132.
6. Oyama Y, Craig RM, Traynor AE, et al. Autologous hematopoietic stem cell transplantation in patients with refractory Crohn's disease. Gastroenterology. 2005;128:552–563.
7. Hommes DW, Duijvestein M, Zelinkova Z, et al. Long-term follow-up of autologous hematopoietic stem cell transplantation for severe refractory Crohn's disease. J Crohns Colitis 2011;5:543–549.
8. Girardin M, Manz M, Manser C, et al. First-line therapies in inflammatory bowel disease. Digestion. 2012;86(Suppl 1):6–10.
9. Bacigalupo A, Ballen K, Rizzo D, et al. Defining the intensity of conditioning regimens: working definitions. Biol Blood Marrow Transplant. 2009;15:1628–1633.
10. Ozsahin M, Pene F, Cosset JM, Laugier A. Morbidity after total body irradiation. Semin Radiat Oncol. 1994;4:95–102.
11. Sonis ST, Elting LS, Keefe D, et al. Perspectives on cancer therapy-induced mucosal injury: pathogenesis, measurement, epidemiology, and consequences for patients. Cancer. 2004;100:1995–2025.

12. Rapoport AP, Miller Watelet LF, Linder T, et al. Analysis of factors that correlate with mucositis in recipients of autologous and allogeneic stem-cell transplants. J Clin Oncol. 1999;17:2446–2453.
13. Langner S, Staber P, Schub N, et al. Palifermin reduces incidence and severity of oral mucositis in allogeneic stem-cell transplant recipients. Bone Marrow Transplant. 2008;42: 275–279.
14. Keefe DM, Schubert MM, Elting LS, et al. Updated clinical practice guidelines for the prevention and treatment of mucositis. Cancer. 2007;109:820–831.
15. Wong RF, Davis TV, Peterson KA. Complications involving the mediastinum after injection of Enteryx for GERD. Gastrointest Endosc. 2005;61:753–756.
16. Basch E, Prestrud AA, Hesketh PJ, et al. Antiemetics: American Society of Clinical Oncology clinical practice guideline update. J Clin Oncol. 2011;29:4189–4198.
17. Deeg HJ, Klingemann H-G, Phillips GL, Van Zant G. A Guide to Blood and Marrow Transplantation. Berlin: Springer, 1999.
18. Hill GR, Krenger W, Ferrara JL. The role of cytokines in acute graft-versus-host disease. Cytokines Cell Mol Ther. 1997;3:257–266.
19. Fischer A, Landais P, Friedrich W, et al. Bone marrow transplantation (BMT) in Europe for primary immunodeficiencies other than severe combined immunodeficiency: a report from the European Group for BMT and the European Group for Immunodeficiency. Blood. 1994;83:1149–1154.
20. Hill GR, Ferrara JL. The primacy of the gastrointestinal tract as a target organ of acute graft-versus-host disease: rationale for the use of cytokine shields in allogeneic bone marrow transplantation. Blood. 2000;95:2754–2759.
21. Ferrara JL, Levine JE, Reddy P, Holler E. Graft-versus-host disease. Lancet. 2009;373:1550–1561.
22. Chirletti P, Caronna R, Arcese W, et al. Gastrointestinal emergencies in patients with acute intestinal graft-versus-host disease. Leuk Lymphoma. 1998;29:129–137.
23. Weisdorf DJ, Snover DC, Haake R, et al. Acute upper gastrointestinal graft-versus-host disease: clinical significance and response to immunosuppressive therapy. Blood. 1990;76:624–629.
24. Ferrara J, Deeg HJ, Burakoff SJ (eds). Graft-vs.-Host Disease. New York: Marcel Dekker, 1997.
25. Cruz-Correa M, Poonawala A, Abraham SC, et al. Endoscopic findings predict the histologic diagnosis in gastrointestinal graft-versus-host disease. Endoscopy. 2002; 34:808–813.
26. Wu D, Hockenberry DM, Brentnall TA, et al. Persistent nausea and anorexia after marrow transplantation: a prospective study of 78 patients. Transplantation. 1998;66: 1319–1324.
27. Velasco-Guardado A, Lopez-Corral L, Alvarez-Delgado A, et al. Endoscopic evaluation and histological findings in graft-versus-host disease. Rev Esp Enferm Dig. 2012;104: 310–314.
28. Snover DC. Graft-versus-host disease of the gastrointestinal tract. Am J Surg Pathol. 1990;14(Suppl 1):101–108.
29. Ross WA, Ghosh S, Dekovich AA, et al. Endoscopic biopsy diagnosis of acute gastrointestinal graft-versus-host disease: rectosigmoid biopsies are more sensitive than upper gastrointestinal biopsies. Am J Gastroenterol. 2008;103:982–989.
30. Terdiman JP, Linker CA, Ries CA, et al. The role of endoscopic evaluation in patients with suspected intestinal graft-versus-host disease after allogeneic bone-marrow transplantation. Endoscopy. 1996;28:680–685.
31. Lipson SA, Perr HA, Koerper MA, et al. Intramural duodenal hematoma after endoscopic biopsy in leukemic patients. Gastrointest Endosc. 1996;44:620–623.
32. Murakami CS, Louie W, Chan GS, et al. Biliary obstruction in hematopoietic cell transplant recipients: an uncommon diagnosis with specific causes. Bone Marrow Transplant. 1999;23:921–927.
33. Heymer B. Clinical and Diagnostic Pathology of Graft-versus-Host Disease. London: Springer, 2002.
34. Sale GE, Beauchamp M, Myerson D. Immunohistologic staining of cytotoxic T and NK cells in formalin-fixed paraffin-embedded tissue using microwave TIA-1 antigen retrieval. Transplantation. 1994;57:287–289.
35. Sale GE, Shulman HM, McDonald GB, Thomas ED. Gastrointestinal graft-versus-host disease in man. A clinicopathologic study of the rectal biopsy. Am J Surg Pathol. 1979;3:291–299.
36. Lerner KG, Kao GF, Storb R, et al. Histopathology of graft-vs.-host reaction (GvHR) in human recipients of marrow from HL-A-matched sibling donors. Transplant Proc. 1974;6:367–371.
37. Mahgerefteh SY, Sosna J, Bogot N, et al. Radiologic imaging and intervention for gastrointestinal and hepatic complications of hematopoietic stem cell transplantation. Radiology. 2011;258:660–671.
38. Brodoefel H, Bethge W, Vogel M, et al. Early and late-onset acute GvHD following hematopoietic cell transplantation: CT features of gastrointestinal involvement with clinical and pathological correlation. Eur J Radiol. 2010; 73:594–600.
39. Taylor AJ, Dodds WJ, Gonyo JE, Komorowski RA. Typhlitis in adults. Gastrointest Radiol. 1985;10:363–369.
40. Day DL, Shapiro RS, Yueh N, et al. B-cell lymphoproliferative disorders in children after bone marrow transplantation: radiologic manifestations. Radiology. 1987;162: 807–810.

41. Lones MA, Lopez-Terrada D, Shintaku IP, et al. Posttransplant lymphoproliferative disorder in pediatric bone marrow transplant recipients: disseminated disease of donor origin demonstrated by fluorescence in situ hybridization. Arch Pathol Lab Med. 1998;122:708–714.
42. Atkinson K, Horowitz MM, Gale RP, et al. Consensus among bone marrow transplanters for diagnosis, grading and treatment of chronic graft-versus-host disease. Committee of the International Bone Marrow Transplant Registry. Bone Marrow Transplant. 1989;4:247–254.
43. McDonald GB, Sullivan KM, Plumley TF. Radiographic features of esophageal involvement in chronic graft-vs.-host disease. AJR Am J Roentgenol. 1984;142:501–506.
44. Mays J, Fassil H, Edwards D, et al. Oral chronic graft-versus-host disease: current pathogenesis, therapy, and research. Oral Dis. 2013;19:327–346.
45. Kida A, McDonald GB. Gastrointestinal, hepatobiliary, pancreatic, and iron-related diseases in long-term survivors of allogeneic hematopoietic cell transplantation. Semin Hematol. 2012;49:43–58.
46. Mackey JR, Desai S, Larratt L, et al. Myasthenia gravis in association with allogeneic bone marrow transplantation: clinical observations, therapeutic implications and review of literature. Bone Marrow Transplant. 1997;19:939–942.
47. McDonald GB, Sullivan KM, Schuffler MD, et al. Esophageal abnormalities in chronic graft-versus-host disease in humans. Gastroenterology. 1981;80:914–921.
48. Vogelsang GB, Pavletic SZ. Chronic Graft Versus Host Disease: Interdisciplinary Management. New York: Cambridge University Press, 2009.
49. Filipovich AH, Weisdorf D, Pavletic S et al. National Institutes of Health consensus development project on criteria for clinical trials in chronic graft-versus-host disease: I. Diagnosis and staging working group report, Biol Bone Marrow Transplant. 2005;11:945–956.
50. Akpek G, Valladares JL, Lee L, et al. Pancreatic insufficiency in patients with chronic graft-versus-host disease. Bone Marrow Transplant. 2001;27:163–166.
51. Levine JE, Logan BR, Wu J, et al. Acute graft-versus-host disease biomarkers measured during therapy can predict treatment outcomes: a Blood and Marrow Transplant Clinical Trials Network study. Blood. 2012;119:3854–3860.
52. Harris AC, Ferrara JL, Braun TM, et al. Plasma biomarkers of lower gastrointestinal and liver acute GVHD. Blood. 2012;119:2960–2963.
53. Bojarski C, Gunther U, Rieger K, et al. *In vivo* diagnosis of acute intestinal graft-versus-host disease by confocal endomicroscopy. Endoscopy. 2009;41:433–438.
54. Stelljes M, Hermann S, Albring J, et al. Clinical molecular imaging in intestinal graft-versus-host disease: mapping of disease activity, prediction, and monitoring of treatment efficiency by positron emission tomography. Blood. 2008; 111:2909–2918.
55. National Cancer Institute. Cancer Therapy Evaluation Program, Common Terminology Criteria for Adverse Events v3.0, 2006.
56. Glucksberg H, Storb R, Fefer A, et al. Clinical manifestations of graft-versus-host disease in human recipients of marrow from HL-A-matched sibling donors. Transplantation. 1974; 18:295–304.
57. Volc-Platzer B. Graft versus host disease. Hautarzt. 1992; 43:669–677 (in German).
58. Przepiorka D, Weisdorf D, Martin P, et al. 1994 Consensus Conference on Acute GVHD Grading. Bone Marrow Transplant. 1995;15:825–828.

28

CHAPTER 28

Hepatic complications of hematopoietic stem cell transplantation

Niharika Samala[1], *Preet Bagi*[2], *Theo Heller*[1], *and Steven Pavletic*[3]

[1]Liver Disease Branch, The National Institute of Diabetes and Digestive and Kidney Diseases (NIDDK), National Institutes of Health, Bethesda, MD, USA

[2]The National Institute of Diabetes and Digestive and Kidney Diseases (NIDDK), National Institutes of Health, Bethesda, MD, USA

[3]Graft-versus-Host and Autoimmunity Unit, Center for Cancer Research, National Cancer Institute, Bethesda, MD, USA

Introduction

Hematopoietic stem cell transplantion (HSCT) poses a unique therapeutic challenge: balancing the benefit of the graft-versus-tumor effect against the risk of graft-versus-host complications. Liver abnormalities in this population can be a diagnostic challenge as their differential is broad. Furthermore, liver chemistries often fluctuate and clinical symptoms can be subtle to absent. Possible hepatic complications in this cohort include graft-versus-host disease (GVHD), iron overload, sinusoidal obstruction syndrome (SOS), viral hepatitis, and drug-induced liver injury (DILI). Furthermore, HSCT patients are at risk of the same liver diseases that can affect the general population, and these must be not be neglected.

Initial evaluation

When an HSCT recipient is assessed for liver disease, the most important aspect of evaluation is a thorough history and physical examination. The history should include evaluation for preexisting liver disease prior to initiation of preconditioning. Patients who have undergone multiple transfusions must be screened for iron overload and treated with chelation and serial phlelbotomy. Date(s) of HSCT and any donor lymphocyte infusions are important when considering GVHD, as is evaluation for preexisting GVHD in other organs. Other relevant historical information includes history of other organ transplantation and presence of cardiovascular, pulmonary, or renal disease. Current therapy and timing of recent changes in immunosuppressive therapy should also be noted. Examination should include evaluation for scleral icterus, jaundice, hepatosplenomegaly, caput medusae, and ascites.

Beyond a good history, laboratory assessment is helpful in supporting the presence of liver disease and narrowing the differential diagnosis. Almost all markers of liver disease are nonspecific, and many can originate from sources other than the liver (Table 28.1). AST and ALT can originate from skeletal or cardiac muscle. ALP may originate from osteocytes, malignant cells, or placental cells. GGT is an enzyme present in the cells lining the

Blood and Marrow Transplantation Long-Term Management: Prevention and Complications, First Edition. Edited by Bipin N Savani.

Table 28.1 Indicators of liver disease

Markers of liver injury	Signs of liver synthetic dysfunction	Indicators of portal hypertension
↑ transaminases (ALT/AST)	Low albumin	Low platelet count
↑ ALP	Elevated coagulation studies (PT, PTT, INR)	Imaging findings (hepatomegaly, splenomegaly, vessel collaterals)
↑ GGT[a]	Low platelet count	Clinical features (ascites, edema, anasarca)
↑ total and direct bilirubin		Endoscopic findings (esophageal/gastric/rectal varices, portal hypertensive gastropathy)
↑ LDH		

AST: aspartate aminotransferase; ALT: alanine aminotransferase; ALP: alkaline phosphatase (ALP); GGT: gamma-glutamyl transpeptidase; LDH: lactate dehydrogenase; PT: prothrombin time; PTT: partial thromboplastin time; INR: international normalized ratio.
[a]Marker specific to the liver.

biliary tract and is useful in assessing whether the ALP elevation is of liver origin. Liver synthetic function is assessed by albumin, bilirubin, platelet count, and coagulation factors (PT, PTT, and INR). As an acute-phase reactant, albumin may be low due to chronic inflammation or from protein-losing enteropathy, significant burns, nephrotic syndrome, malabsorption, malnutrition, and malignancy. Clinical features of hypoalbuminemia may include ascites, peripheral edema, or anasarca. Total bilirubin has long been noted to correlate with mortality and is an important marker of hepatic injury and dysfunction. Bilirubin is also affected by hemolysis and renal function. Thrombocytopenia may occur due to bone marrow suppression from preconditioning, immunosuppression side effect, or delayed transplant engraftment. Elevated indirect bilirubin may be a marker of excess hemolysis. Elevated LDH is seen in acute hepatitis, hepatocellular necrosis, and hematological diseases. Once the presence of liver injury is confirmed, the pattern of liver injury is an important distinction. In general,

Table 28.2 Patterns of liver injury

Hepatocellular	↑ ALT ± AST
Cholestatic	↑ ALP ± bilirubin
Mixed	↑ ALT, AST, ALP ± bilirubin

there are three patterns of liver injury: hepatocellular injury, cholestatic injury, or a mixed injury pattern (Table 28.2).

Hepatic complications after HSCT

Acute

Acute liver GVHD

Background

Liver GVHD is a significant complication of HSCT. Studies performed in HSCT patients indicate that nearly 60% may develop liver abnormalities [1]. Early liver involvement has been shown to be associated with steroid-refractory GVHD and increased nonrelapse mortality [2].

Diagnosis

Although there is a lack of specificity of liver enzyme elevation for GVHD, some conclusions can be made based on the pattern of abnormal liver chemistries. With acute liver GVHD, primarily there is a cholestatic pattern of liver injury and transaminases rarely rise to greater than 10 times the upper limit of normal (ULN), but there is an acute hepatic variant where transaminases can reach over 10 times the ULN. Making a definite diagnosis of acute liver GVHD may require liver biopsy for a histopathologic assessment. Biopsy is often indicated when multiple other confounding factors are present that may contribute to liver chemistry abnormalities. If skin or gastrointestinal (GI) acute GVHD can be diagnosed upon less invasive skin or GI biopsy, then liver biopsy may be deferred. If required, the transjugular approach is preferred to the percutaneous liver biopsy, given less risk of bleeding, especially during thrombocytopenia. If there are no other cofounding variables, then acute liver GVHD may be presumed and treated according to stage, especially if skin and/or GI acute GVHD is suspected [3]. Acute liver GVHD pathology may include dysmorphic or destroyed small bile ducts and cholestasis with lobular and/or portal inflammation. Confounding variables that can alter histology findings include decreased inflammation from concomitant immunosuppression, mimicry from infection or medications, sampling error, or biopsy too early prior to engraftment at day 15. Biomarkers as surrogate indicators of liver GVHD have been studied and include regenerating islet derived $\alpha 3$ (REGα3), hepatocyte growth factor (HGF), and cytokeratin fragment 18 (KRT18); however, these have been largely unsuccessful in correlating levels with histopathologic evidence of liver GVHD [4].

Treatment

Acute liver GVHD increases mortality, and early diagnosis after HSCT improves nonrelapse mortality rates as well as decreases the risk of liver fibrosis and cirrhosis. First-line treatment includes high-dose steroids (prednisone 1 mg/kg daily with ultimate taper or methylprednisolone 1–2 mg/kg per day), usually with calcineurin inhibitor-based systemic immunosuppression. Additionally, ursodiol can be given as 300 mg orally twice to three times daily. Ursodiol has been shown to decrease liver chemistries in those with acute liver GVHD but has questionable efficacy as a preventative measure against acute GVHD in the immediate post-HSCT phase [5, 6].

Sinusoidal obstruction syndrome

Background

SOS, also known as hepatic veno-occlusive disease, typically occurs after HSCT. It can occur to a lesser extent in nontransplant subjects after chemotherapy, radiotherapy, liver transplant, or alkaloid consumption [7]. SOS was noted initially after bone marrow transplant as a constellation of symptoms of jaundice, ascites, and painful hepatomegaly with histopathology changes involving hepatocytes, hepatic venules, and sinusoids [8]. The prevalence of SOS after transplant has been reported to varying degrees with documentation as low as 5% to as high as 54% [9–11]. The initiating mechanism is suspected to be injury to the endothelium of the hepatic venules. Risk factors for SOS that have been identified include total body irritation, drugs (cyclophosphamide, busulfan, gemtuzumab, or cytarabine), underlying liver disease, such as hepatitis B or C, and female gender [9, 12]. With the initiation of reduced-intensity conditioning regimens, the prevalence of SOS has been declining.

Diagnosis

There is no gold standard diagnostic test for SOS. This syndrome is characterized by ascites, rapid onset weight gain, jaundice, and painful hepatomegaly and is classified as mild, moderate, or severe. The severe form can progress to multiorgan failure, which carries a high risk of mortality, potentially as high as 84% [13]. The diagnosis of SOS may be made based upon clinical parameters alone. One set of criteria used for diagnosis are the Seattle criteria, which requires two of the following: painful hepatomegaly, bilirubin ≥2 mg/dL, and ascites with or without unexplained weight gain greater than 2% of baseline within 30 days of transplantation [14]. The modified Seattle criteria require symptoms to occur within 20 days after HSCT [10]. Another set of diagnostic criteria are the Baltimore criteria, which includes a bilirubin ≥2 mg/dL plus two of the following within 21 days after HSCT: hepatomegaly (typically with pain), ascites, and weight gain 5% over baseline [15]. In circumstances where clinical findings are inadequate in reaching a diagnosis, percutaneous liver biopsy can be useful. However, biopsy should be performed with caution as coexisting thrombocytopenia and coagulopathy may increase the overall bleeding risk and in these individuals the transjugular approach is safer. Additionally, a hepatic venous pressure gradient >10 mmHg is common in SOS [16]. In addition, portal pressures can be measured at the same time as the transjugular liver biopsy if needed. There is no pathognomonic imaging finding or laboratory marker that is used to diagnosis SOS.

Treatment

The treatment of SOS is primarily supportive as, at present, there is no effective and established therapy. Given the lack of treatment options once SOS develops, particularly in the severe form, it is essential to take appropriate preventative measures. Individuals at high risk of developing SOS should begin ursodeoxycholic acid prior to induction therapy [17]. Hepatic insults must be minimized and fluid overload should be prevented with use of diuretics if needed [17]. Once SOS develops, supportive care to maintain intravascular volume status without promoting fluid overload is crucial. Transjugular intrahepatic portosystemic shunt and orthotopic liver transplantation have been attempted but carry high morbidity and mortality and are not routinely recommended [18, 19]. Future potential therapy may involve defibrotide, an oligonucleotide with anti-thrombotic properties within small vessels, whose exact mechanism of action in SOS is unknown [12].

Drug-induced liver injury

Background

DILI is a common problem that can manifest as various degrees of hepatotoxicity ranging from asymptomatic mild liver chemistry elevation to histologic abnormalities to acute liver failure. In fact, acute DILI is thought to be a very common cause of acute liver failure in the USA [20]. Prognosis declines once transaminases rise to greater than three times the upper limit of normal along with a bilirubin ≥2 mg/dL, also known as Hy's law [21]. Drugs commonly used in HSCT patients that can lead to DILI include calcineurin inhibitors, cyclophosphamide, busulfan, and azole antifungal agents amongst others. In addition total parenteral nutrition can also cause cholestasis.

Diagnosis

DILI may mimic other causes of liver injury and is often a diagnosis of exclusion.

A thorough history and timeline of medication use is required. Underlying liver disease must be excluded as well. The pattern of liver chemistry elevation can represent a hepatotoxic, cholestatic, or mixed picture of injury (Table 28.2). There is no gold standard laboratory marker or histologic finding that can be used to confidently diagnose DILI. Histology can mimic many other findings and often reveals plasma cells, portal inflammation, fibrosis, intracellular cholestasis, and portal neutrophils. These findings can mimic autoimmune hepatitis; however, the presence of intracellular cholestasis and portal neutrophils appear to be more common in DILI and less common in autoimmune hepatitis [22].

Treatment

Removal of the offending agent is the treatment for DILI, and hepatic injury often improves once the drug is discontinued. Recovery may take days to weeks depending upon the degree of initial injury, particularly in cases of liver failure. In cases of suspected severe drug-induced toxicity related to acetaminophen, the use of *N*-acetylcysteine is recommended [23]. If multiple medications are suspected, then after all have been discontinued they may be restarted one at a time with close monitoring for any recurrent injury in order to determine the exact offending drug(s).

Cholangitis lenta

Background

Cholangitis lenta, or subacute non-supprative cholangitis, is a rare yet important condition that can occur after transplantation. The distinct histological features of cholangitis lenta help distinguish it from other causes of posttransplant cholestasis. The presence of cholangitis lenta suggests an underlying severe local or systemic infection, such as sepsis.

Diagnosis

No specific laboratory marker exists to diagnose cholangitis. It is typically characterized by a mild to moderate elevation of bilirubin, typically without a rise in alkaline phosphatase, in patients who have fever with or without sepsis [24]. This condition can exacerbate any preexisting liver condition and confound the diagnosis. Cholangitis lenta may be difficult to differentiate from acute GVHD, yet it appears that the GGT level may be high in GVHD while not in cholangitis lenta [25], mirroring the alkaline phosphatase. Histologic changes include proliferation of bile ducts at the edges of portal tracts, inspissated bile within bile ducts that are dilated, lack of acute inflammation within ducts, and normal interlobular bile ducts [26].

Treatment

Treatment of the underlying cause of fever and/or sepsis ultimately leads to resolution of the cholangitis lenta.

Other

Certain underlying malignancies, such as the lymphomas and leukemias, can manifest as recurrence with direct liver infiltration from the tumor itself. These can lead to any of the patterns of liver injury, and infiltration of malignant cells can be seen upon liver biopsy. Hepatic congestion as a result of cardiac failure or ischemic injury may also occur in the acute post-HSCT phase. Infectious complications post-HSCT that can involve the liver include fungal abscess or acute hepatitis from hepatitis B virus (HBV), hepatitis C virus (HCV), herpes simplex virus (HSV), varicella zoster virus (VZV), or adenovirus [3, 27].

Chronic complications

Chronic liver GVHD

Diagnosis

Per National Institutes of Health criteria, there are no diagnostic signs of chronic GVHD in the liver. In the absence of chronic GVHD in other organs, elevated liver function tests and biopsy cannot distinguish such clinical presentation from acute GVHD. Laboratory tests in chronic liver GVHD may follow a variety of patterns: (a) chronic asymptomatic elevation of transaminases alone; (b) slowly progressive cholestatic disease, usually with a primary elevation of alkaline phosphatase, thought to be a result of chronic bile duct damage, and is seen more commonly after acute liver GVHD that has progressed to chronic liver GVHD; or (c) acute hepatocellular injury as a mixed pattern of liver injury, usually associated with immunosuppressive taper or donor lymphocyte infusions. If advanced fibrosis or cirrhosis has developed, markers of liver synthetic function will likely be abnormal as well, including coagulation factors, albumin, and platelet count. Multiple other factors can contribute to elevated liver chemistries, and a liver biopsy is required to diagnose liver involvement from GVHD. Chronic liver GVHD histology may reveal complete loss of small bile ducts, chronic cholestasis, and portal fibrosis. None of these pathologic findings are specific enough to make a definite diagnosis of chronic GVHD. Therefore, the diagnosis of chronic GVHD relies on either one diagnostic clinical finding (chronic skin, oral, genital, pulmonary (bronchiolitis obliterans), muscular/articular findings) or a suggestive clinical finding plus pertinent biopsy or test results and must be used in conjunction with other diagnostic criteria for chronic GVHD [28].

Treatment

The treatment of chronic liver GVHD is similar to acute liver GVHD using corticosteroids and/or immunosuppression.

Viral hepatitis

Chronic viral hepatitis affects approximately 500 million individuals worldwide [29]. Up to 75% of these people may be unaware of their diagnosis [15]. Our immune system attempts to suppress the viral activity of chronic hepatitis, and HSCT is a risk for worsening of chronic viral hepatitis or reactivation of a chronically inactive virus. Viral hepatitis may be caused by hepatitis A, HBV (with potential hepatitis D co-infection), HCV, hepatitis E, adenovirus, HSV-1 or -2, VZV, Epstein–Barr virus, and cytomegalovirus.

Hepatitis B virus

Diagnosis

HBV serologies must be checked pretransplant (Table 28.3). Reactivation of hepatitis B is defined as a sudden increase in hepatitis B viral replication in a patient with inactive or resolved hepatitis B [30]. The latter is also known as reverse seroconversion, as hepatitis B surface antigen (HBsAg) becomes detectable in an individual who has recovered from hepatitis B. The presence of hepatitis B surface antibody (HBsAb) is actually protective against reactivation or infection however in this setting is lost and HBsAg reappears. Hepatitis B core antibody (HBcAb) indicates recovery from past HBV infection. Isolated HBcAb without HBsAb suggests prior exposure and is associated with high rate of HBsAg recurrence, with a risk up of to 8% [31]. HBcAb should be

Table 28.3 Interpretation of HBV serology tests

HBsAg	HBcAb IgG	HBcAb IgM	Anti-HBs	Interpretation
+	−	+	−	Acute HBV infection
+	+	−	−	Chronic HBV
−	+	−	−	Previous or current infection/false positive
−	+	−	+	Recovered infection
−	−	−	+	Immune after vaccination
−	−	−	−	No exposure to HBV

screened for carefully as it can develop after blood transfusion or after intravenous immunoglobulin therapy.

Treatment

Positive HBsAg individuals, including chronic inactive HBV carriers, should begin treatment with an oral nucleos(t)ide prior to induction chemotherapy. Without this antiviral prophylaxis, there is a risk of fulminant hepatitis which can be fatal. After transplant, HBV viral load should be monitored. Antiviral treatment should be considered in those with isolated HBcAb positivity, particularly if B-cell cytotoxic agents are used.

Hepatitis C virus

Diagnosis

Transplant recipients must be screened for HCV with HCV antibody testing. If positive with a detectable viral load, these individuals should be treated if possible prior to HSCT.

Treatment

Standard of care HCV treatment currently uses interferon-alpha plus ribavirin. Interferon-based regimens must be discontinued prior to immunosuppression and ribavirin alone continued in the setting of immunosuppression. The treatment of HCV is changing rapidly and it is likely that the new oral directly acting antiviral therapies will revolutionize treatment of patients with HCV. The presence of HCV pre-HSCT appears to lead to a greater risk of cirrhosis and hepatocellular carcinoma post-HSCT and must be screened with biannual liver ultrasound and serum alpha fetoprotein [3].

Iron overload

Background

Multiple factors can contribute to hepatic iron overload in transplanted patients, including transfusion dependency and marrow dysfunction.

Diagnosis

Iron studies will reveal elevated serum iron, ferritin (typically >1000 μg/dL), and elevated percentage saturation [32]. In those with elevated iron stores, *HFE* gene testing should be performed. Of note, ferritin may be falsely elevated in the setting of other inflammatory states. Liver biopsy or hepatic magnetic resonance imaging can detect iron overload.

Treatment

If the hepatic iron content is low (<7000 μg/g dry weight), treatment is only indicated if liver involvement is present. If iron content is between 7000 and 15 000 μg/g dry weight then serial phlebotomy is required. If greater than 15 000 μg/g dry weight is present, then chelation and phlebotomy are indicated [33].

Non-alcoholic fatty liver disease

Background

Non-alcoholic fatty liver disease (NAFLD) can be seen in transplant recipients due to medications such as corticosteroids or methotrexate. Non-alcoholic steatohepatitis is a more extreme form of NAFLD and can progress to cirrhosis.

Diagnosis

Liver imaging tests may reveal steatosis but will not always be detected. Liver biopsy is the gold standard of diagnosis and will reveal steatosis in the perivenular regions and possibly periportal regions. Ballooning of the hepatocytes with neutrophil-predominant inflammation can be seen as well [34].

Treatment

Weight loss is the mainstay of therapy for NAFLD. A goal of 3–5% body weight loss will improve steatosis and an up to 10% body weight loss is needed to decrease necroinflammation [35].

Nodular regenerative hyperplasia

Background

Nodular regenerative hyperplasia (NRH) was first described as clinical and laboratory findings suggestive of cirrhosis without histologic evidence of cirrhosis [14]. NRH is thought to be a complication of the underlying disease, preconditioning chemotherapy, or HSCT.

Diagnosis

Clinical findings can include hepatomegaly and ascites, but often no clinical abnormalities are found. Variceal bleeding is a less common complication in this setting however, patients are predisposed to infection. Laboratory tests primarily show a cholestatic picture of liver chemistry elevation. Pathology findings reveal hepatic hyperplasia in the absence of fibrous tissue proliferation with the presence of nodules [36, 37].

Treatment

Treatment is primarily supportive with monitoring and treatment of portal.

Conclusion

The physician caring for the HSCT patient must be cognizant of hepatologic complications that can arise as a direct result of the HSCT process and also not forget the potential for developing underlying liver diseases that the general population is at risk for as well. In addition, patients are at risk for recurrence of the original reason for HSCT as well, and this may often affect the liver. Preexisting liver disease leads to a more challenging post-HSCT course, and expert hepatology consultation should be sought in these cases on an as-needed basis.

References

1. Pidala J, Vogelsang G, Martin P, et al. Overlap subtype of chronic graft-versus-host disease is associated with an adverse prognosis, functional impairment, and inferior patient-reported outcomes: a Chronic Graft-versus-Host Disease Consortium study. Haematologica. 2012;97:451–458.
2. Robin M, Porcher R, de Castro R, et al. Initial liver involvement in acute GVHD is predictive for nonrelapse mortality. Transplantation. 2009;88:1131–1136.
3. Tuncer HH, Rana N, Milani C, et al. Gastrointestinal and hepatic complications of hematopoietic stem cell transplantation. World J Gastroenterol. 2012;18:1851–1860.
4. Harris AC, Ferrara JL, Braun TM, et al. Plasma biomarkers of lower gastrointestinal and liver acute GVHD. Blood. 2012;119:2960–2963.
5. Arat M, Idilman R, Soydan EA, et al. Ursodeoxycholic acid treatment in isolated chronic graft-vs.-host disease of the liver. Clin Transplant. 2005;19:798–803.
6. Ruutu T, Eriksson B, Remes K, et al. Ursodeoxycholic acid for the prevention of hepatic complications in allogeneic stem cell transplantation. Blood. 2002;100:1977–1983.
7. Wadleigh M, Ho V, Momtaz P, Richardson P. Hepatic veno-occlusive disease: pathogenesis, diagnosis and treatment. Curr Opin Hematol. 2003;10:451–462.
8. Shulman HM, Hinterberger W. Hepatic veno-occlusive disease – liver toxicity syndrome after bone marrow transplantation. Bone Marrow Transplant. 1992;10:197–214.
9. Carreras E, Bertz H, Arcese W, et al. Incidence and outcome of hepatic veno-occlusive disease after blood or marrow transplantation: a prospective cohort study of the European Group for Blood and Marrow Transplantation. European Group for Blood and Marrow Transplantation Chronic Leukemia Working Party. Blood. 1998;92:3599–3604.
10. McDonald GB, Hinds MS, Fisher LD, et al. Veno-occlusive disease of the liver and multiorgan failure after bone marrow transplantation: a cohort study of 355 patients. Ann Intern Med. 1993;118:255–267.
11. Shulman HM, McDonald GB, Matthews D, et al. An analysis of hepatic venocclusive disease and centrilobular hepatic degeneration following bone marrow transplantation. Gastroenterology. 1980;79:1178–1191.
12. Richardson PG, Soiffer RJ, Antin JH, et al. Defibrotide for the treatment of severe hepatic veno-occlusive disease and multiorgan failure after stem cell transplantation: a multicenter, randomized, dose-finding trial. Biol Blood Marrow Transplant. 2010;16:1005–1017.
13. Coppell JA, Richardson PG, Soiffer R, et al. Hepatic veno-occlusive disease following stem cell transplantation: incidence, clinical course, and outcome. Biol Blood Marrow Transplant. 2010;16:157–168.
14. McDonald GB, Sharma P, Matthews DE, et al. Venocclusive disease of the liver after bone marrow transplantation: diagnosis, incidence, and predisposing factors. Hepatology. 1984;4:116–122.
15. Jones RJ, Lee KS, Beschorner WE, et al. Venoocclusive disease of the liver following bone marrow transplantation. Transplantation. 1987;44:778–783.
16. Shulman HM, Gooley T, Dudley MD, et al. Utility of transvenous liver biopsies and wedged hepatic venous pressure measurements in sixty marrow transplant recipients. Transplantation. 1995;59:1015–1022.
17. Johnson DB, Savani BN. How can we reduce hepatic veno-occlusive disease-related deaths after allogeneic stem cell transplantation? Exp Hematol. 2012;40:513–517.
18. Fried MW, Connaghan DG, Sharma S, et al. Transjugular intrahepatic portosystemic shunt for the management of severe venoocclusive disease following bone marrow transplantation. Hepatology. 1996;24:588–591.
19. Rosen HR, Martin P, Schiller GJ, et al. Orthotopic liver transplantation for bone-marrow transplant-associated veno-occlusive disease and graft-versus-host disease of the liver. Liver Transpl Surg. 1996;2:225–232.
20. Ostapowicz G, Fontana RJ, Schiodt FV, et al. Results of a prospective study of acute liver failure at 17 tertiary care centers in the United States. Ann Intern Med. 2002;137:947–954.
21. Reuben A. Hy's law. Hepatology. 2004;39:574–578.
22. Suzuki A, Brunt EM, Kleiner DE, et al. The use of liver biopsy evaluation in discrimination of idiopathic autoimmune hepatitis versus drug-induced liver injury. Hepatology. 2011;54:931–939.

23. Polson J, Lee WM. AASLD position paper: the management of acute liver failure. Hepatology. 2005;41:1179–1197.
24. Strasser SI, Shulman HM, McDonald GB. Cholestasis after hematopoietic cell transplantation. Clin Liver Dis. 1999;3:651–668, x.
25. McDonald GB. Hepatobiliary complications of hematopoietic cell transplantation, 40 years on. Hepatology. 2010;51: 1450–1460.
26. Lin CC, Sundaram SS, Hart J, Whitington PF. Subacute nonsuppurative cholangitis (cholangitis lenta) in pediatric liver transplant patients. J Pediatr Gastroenterol Nutr. 2007; 45:228–233.
27. DeLeve LD, Valla DC, Garcia-Tsao G. Vascular disorders of the liver. Hepatology. 2009;49:1729–1764.
28. Filipovich AH, Weisdorf D, Pavletic S, et al. National Institutes of Health consensus development project on criteria for clinical trials in chronic graft-versus-host disease: I. Diagnosis and Staging Working Group Report. Biol Blood Marrow Transplant. 2005;11:945–956.
29. Perz JF, Armstrong GL, Farrington LA, et al. The contributions of hepatitis B virus and hepatitis C virus infections to cirrhosis and primary liver cancer worldwide. J Hepatol. 2006;45:529–538.
30. Hoofnagle JH. Reactivation of hepatitis B. Hepatology. 2009;49:S156–S165.
31. Teh BW, Slavin MA, Szer J, Sasadeusz JJ. Hepatitis B serological changes following allogeneic bone marrow transplantation. Transpl Infect Dis. 2013;15:98–103.
32. Jensen PD, Jensen FT, Christensen T, et al. Relationship between hepatocellular injury and transfusional iron overload prior to and during iron chelation with desferrioxamine: a study in adult patients with acquired anemias. Blood. 2003;101:91–96.
33. Angelucci E, Muretto P, Lucarelli G, et al. Phlebotomy to reduce iron overload in patients cured of thalassemia by bone marrow transplantation. Italian Cooperative Group for Phlebotomy Treatment of Transplanted Thalassemia Patients. Blood. 1997;90:994–998.
34. Hubscher SG. Histological assessment of non-alcoholic fatty liver disease. Histopathology. 2006;49:450–465.
35. Chalasani N, Younossi Z, Lavine JE, et al. The diagnosis and management of non-alcoholic fatty liver disease: practice Guideline by the American Association for the Study of Liver Diseases, American College of Gastroenterology, and the American Gastroenterological Association. Hepatology. 2012;55:2005–2023.
36. Steiner PE. Nodular regenerative hyperplasia of the liver. Am J Pathol. 1959;35:943–953.
37. Kida A, McDonald GB. Gastrointestinal, hepatobiliary, pancreatic, and iron-related diseases in long-term survivors of allogeneic hematopoietic cell transplantation. Semin Hematol. 2012;49:43–58.

29

CHAPTER 29

Monitoring and management of hepatitis B, hepatitis C, and HIV infection before and after transplantation

Keith Luckett and Stephen Dummer

Division of Infectious Diseases, Department of Medicine, Vanderbilt University School of Medicine, Nashville TN, USA

Introduction

Infections are one of the main causes of morbidity and mortality after stem cell transplantation (SCT). In general, the incidence of severe infections is highest in the first 6 months after SCT. In the past, many patients succumbed in this period to severe acute viral, bacterial, and fungal infections. Today, the availability of an enlarging anti-infective armamentarium and the vigorous implementation of modern approaches to supportive care have resulted in most patients being shepherded through this early period with relative safety. The great effort expended to control these early infections is feasible because it is focused on a relatively narrow time interval. The chronic viral infections discussed in this chapter represent a somewhat different infectious challenge that often has implications for patients' outcomes many years after transplantation and requires a commitment to long-term monitoring. The transplanting physician needs to understand the biology of these viruses, their potential for long-term harm, the necessary laboratory monitoring for their identification and characterization, and the pharmacological interventions for their control. The complexity of these viral infections and the ever-expanding list of drugs available for their treatment means that the transplant team usually needs to consult and collaborate with experts familiar with managing these infections, both during their early encounters with the patient and in follow-up.

Hepatitis B infection

Background

Over 350 million people worldwide are chronically infected with hepatitis B virus (HBV); it is the leading global cause of chronic hepatitis, cirrhosis, and hepatocellular carcinoma (HCC) and is thought to be responsible for 1 million deaths yearly [1]. The burden of HBV in the USA is much lower, but it is still estimated to cause over a million cases of chronic infection and 4000–5500 deaths annually from the sequelae of liver disease [2].

Hepatitis B is a small, partially double-stranded, non-enveloped DNA virus. It matures to a covalently closed circular DNA in the nucleus and can persist in a latent state after resolution of viremia [2]. The likelihood of developing a chronic infection after initial infection is high in neonates and immunocompromised individuals

Blood and Marrow Transplantation Long-Term Management: Prevention and Complications, First Edition. Edited by Bipin N Savani.

but is 5% or less in immuncompetent adults. The intensity of acute liver injury from the viral infection relates to the strength of the immune response. Thus, a healthy adult with a robust immune response to the virus may die of fulminant hepatitis after initial infection while demonstrating low viral titers in the blood. An immuncompromised individual, by contrast, may have little laboratory evidence of liver injury, despite displaying high titers of virus in liver and blood. Patients with serological markers showing cleared hepatitis B infection are at risk of reactivation of the virus when they are immunosuppressed. This phenomenon has been most frequently described after SCT and the use of certain cancer chemotherapeutic agents.

Pre-transplant evaluation

The prevalence of HBV surface antigen (HBsAg) positivity in various regions of the world ranges from <1% to 25%, with the highest prevalence in Asia and Africa and the lowest in northern Europe and the USA [1, 2]. The number of persons with antibodies to hepatitis core antigen, reflecting any past HBV infection, is 2 to 10 times higher. Because of the risk of reactivation and donor-derived infection after SCT, all candidates for SCT and their donors should be screened for HBV. A minimal screening panel should include tests for HBsAg, HBV core antibody (anti-HBc), and the HBV surface antibody (anti-HBs). All patients with a positive HBsAg or anti-HBc should undergo further screening with an HBV DNA assay to detect viremia.

Transplantation from a donor who is positive for HBsAg carries a high risk of transmission of the viral infection to the recipient, and outcomes are worse if the recipient is HBV naive [3]. If the only available donor is HBsAg positive, HBV antiviral therapy should be initiated in the donor prior to stem cell harvest to decrease the viral load and thus minimize the likelihood of transmission. Transplant candidates who are HBV-seronegative and who are being transplanted with cells from an HBsAg positive donor should receive HBV immunization before transplantation. After transplantation these recipients should be carefully monitored for *de novo* infection and managed either with antiviral prophylaxis or preemptive antiviral therapy if emergent HBV infection is detected.

Stem cell donors who have developed natural immunity to hepatitis B may adoptively transfer this immunity to actively infected recipients, who may then clear that infection more easily after transplantation [4]. Hui et al. demonstrated sustained clearance of HBsAg and seroconversion to anti-HBs positivity in 64.5% of recipients who received stem cells from donors with natural immunity [5]. All of these stem cell recipients also received antiviral therapy against HBV – usually lamivudine. None of the HBV-infected recipients who received stem cells from donors who were anti-HBc negative cleared the infection after transplantation. This experience demonstrates that one should always attempt to find a hepatitis B immune donor for any recipient who is actively infected with the virus. This may be quite difficult, however, in regions of the world such as the USA, where the prevalence of hepatitis B infection is low.

Immunizing HBV-naive patients

If feasible, HBV-naive patients should be vaccinated before transplantation. The traditional vaccination schedule includes three doses of vaccine at 0, 1, and 6 months. Every attempt should be made to immunize with at least two doses prior to SCT, given at least 3–4 weeks apart. The final dose can be given after SCT. Delaying the third dose up to 1 year after the first dose may actually lead to an increase in the anti-HBs levels as significant immune recovery will have occurred by then in most patients [1]. Anti-HBs levels should be checked 1 month after completion of the series. If no seroconversion has occurred, repeat vaccination should be attempted, but not until at least 1 year after transplantation.

Complications from hepatitis B virus infection following SCT

The risk for adverse outcomes from hepatitis B infection is most marked in patients going into transplantation with active infection as denoted by positive tests for HBsAg. Prior to the availability of antiviral therapy, hepatitis occurred in >50% of such patients. Effective antiviral prophylaxis has decreased this risk to 0–9% [1, 6]. The mean time to HBV reactivation (defined as a greater than twofold rise in alanine aminotransferase) is 4 months in patients who do not receive prophylaxis, and the associated mortality rate has varied from 5 to 40% in different case series [1, 6, 7].

Reverse seroconversion, with reappearance of HbsAg in patients with evidence of prior healed hepatitis B infection can also be problematic. These patients are negative for HBsAg before transplantation but have anti-HBc. Most, but not all, patients also have anti-HBs. The reported incidence of reverse seroconversion varies widely from 9 to 50% in patients followed from 12 to 48 months posttransplantation [8–13]. This reactivation occurs later after transplantation than in patients who are HBsAg positive going into transplantation and may be first detected many years after transplantation. In patients who have anti-HBs antibody and are followed with serial serological tests, one first sees a fall in anti-HBs titers to undetectable levels before HBsAg appears and viremia is detectable. Identified risk factors for reverse seroconversion include extensive chronic graft-versus-host disease (GVHD), low pre-transplant anti-HBs titers, a history of multiple rounds of chemotherapy, and a diagnosis of chronic hematological disease [1, 11, 13]. Biochemical or clinical hepatitis is reported in the majority of patients with reverse seroconversion [11, 13]. Fulminant hepatitis and death from liver failure can occur when the patients' recovering immune systems recognize the reappearing viral antigens. Fortunately, the occurrence of severe hepatitis has become uncommon since the availability of antiviral therapy.

No evidence links chronic HBV infection to an increased risk of veno-occlusive disease in the absence of underlying cirrhosis. One study performed prior to widespread use of prophylactic or preemptive antiviral therapy showed that patients who were HBsAg positive before transplantation had an increased incidence of acute GVHD [6]. Not surprisingly, these patients were also significantly more likely to develop cirrhosis (8/82) than stem cell transplant controls (0/721) without hepatitis B infection [5].

Management of HBV-infected transplant recipients based on pre-transplant status

Patients with active infection (HBsAg positive)

Historically, patients who were HBsAg positive before transplantation had a high risk of posttransplant liver disease. In a long-term follow-up of 82 HBsAg positive stem cell recipients from one institution, 19.5% had developed hepatitis and 10% had progressed to cirrhosis [5]. None of the 20 patients who cleared their virus went on to develop cirrhosis. Viral reactivation and hepatitis occurred as late as 10 years after transplantation.

The armamentarium of drugs with proven efficacy against HBV has expanded in recent years. Current guidelines from the American Association for the Study of Liver Diseases recommend treatment for at least 6 months after completion of chemotherapy or immunosuppressive therapy, but no specific guidelines exist for SCT. Owing to the degree of immunosuppression and the possible delay of immune recovery in these SCT recipients, a duration of antiviral therapy of at least 12 months after cessation of immunosuppression is preferred [7]. Current antiviral options are shown in Table 29.1. Lamivudine (100 mg/day) is well tolerated and has been the antiviral compound most used in stem cell recipients. However, resistance to lamivudine occurs in 15–30% of patients who take it for a year. Patients being treated with lamivudine need to be carefully monitored for viral breakthrough [2]. The two newer antiviral agents that are

Table 29.1 HBV antiviral treatment options

Drug	Dose (mg/day)	Resistance at 1 year	Side effects
Lamivudine	100	15–30%	Lactic acidosis, hepatic steatosis, pancreatitis, lipodystrophy
Telbivudine	600	6%	Lactic acidosis, hepatic steatosis, myopathy, peripheral neuropathy
Entecavir	0.5 (treatment naive) 1 (lamivudine-resistant virus)	None for treatment naive; 7% if virus is lamivudine-resistant	Lactic acidosis, hepatic steatosis, edema
Adefovir	10	Minimal	Lactic acidosis, hepatic steatosis, weakness
Tenofovir	300	None	Lactic acidosis, hepatic steatosis, renal toxicity, decreased bone mineral density

most often recommended are entecavir (0.5 mg/day) and tenofovir (300 mg/day). Both are associated with a very low rate of resistance development, but are more expensive. Entecavir has few side-effects. Tenofovir carries a low risk of renal toxicity. All of the antiviral agents active against hepatitis B are cleared by the kidney and, therefore, dose reduction may be necessary in patients with renal dysfunction.

The optimal timing for initiation of antiviral treatment in patients with active HBV receiving chemotherapy was studied by Lau et al. [14]. Thirty HBsAg-positive patients were randomized to either start lamivudine 1 week before initiating chemotherapy or delay it until the earliest signs of HBV reactivation. Eight cases of viral reactivation and seven cases of HBV-related hepatitis occurred in the deferred group versus none in the prophylactic group, showing that beginning HBV treatment prior to chemotherapy is more efficacious.

All patients should have baseline HBV viral loads determined before chemotherapy begins. The optimal frequency of laboratory monitoring after transplantation has not been standardized, but should probably be no less than every 3–4 months, even after discontinuation of antiviral therapy. Any increase in viral load while the patient is on an antiviral therapy should prompt resistance testing and consideration of an alternative agent.

Patients with resolved infection (HBsAg negative, anti-HBc positive, anti-HBs positive)

These patients have resolved their hepatitis B infection and have serological evidence of natural immunity to the virus but are at risk for reactivation, which increases steadily over time. In one study, the cumulative risk of HBsAg reactivation was 9% at 1 year, 21.7% at 2 years, and 42.9% at 4 years after transplantation [13]. There does not appear to be any date beyond which one can be sure that reactivation will not occur. These recipients should be followed with assays for HBsAG, viral DNA, and liver function testing every 2–3 months. Patients who develop a detectable viral load should be initiated on antiviral treatment with continuation of monitoring as with the HBsAg-positive group.

Patients with indeterminate infection: anti-HBc positive but negative for HBsAg and anti-HBs

This serological profile can represent one of three states: occult infection, past resolution of infection with a waning antibody titer to HBsAg, or a false positive anti-HBc with no prior or current infection. Some authorities recommend repeating the serological tests after giving a booster dose of the HBV vaccine as a brisk rise in anti-HBs in response to the vaccine usually indicates that the patient has true past infection with underlying natural immunity [1]. An HBV DNA assay should be obtained in all patients with this profile. If the DNA assay is positive for circulating HBV, then prophylactic antivirals should be administered with serial monitoring of the antiviral response. If the viral DNA assay is negative, one may manage the patient prophylactically with antiviral medications, but the most cost-effective practice is to withhold antiviral therapy and monitor the patient at 2–3-month intervals for re-emergent viral infection.

Hepatitis C infection

Background

Approximately 150 million people worldwide are infected with hepatitis C virus (HCV) and the prevalence in most countries ranges between 1 and 5% [15]. In the USA it is the most common cause of blood-borne infection and chronic liver disease [16]. Universal screening of blood products for HCV in 1992 led to a dramatic drop in new infections. However, the burden of infection remains high as HCV continues to be transmitted through intravenous drug use, non-sterile tattoo equipment, and high-risk sexual behavior.

Hepatitis C is an enveloped, positive strand RNA virus with tropism for hepatocytes, in which it replicates prolifically, producing up to 10^{12} viral particles per day. Typically, acute hepatitis C infection is asymptomatic and the subsequent course is also indolent with symptoms only appearing later in the course. Roughly 20% of people clear HCV after initial infection The remainder progress to chronic infection, which entails a 20% risk of cirrhosis over the next 20 years [15]. A substantial proportion of these patients will die from liver failure or develop HCC.

Pre-transplant evaluation for HCV

All transplant candidates and their donors require screening for HCV. Donors, who have a normal immune system, can be screened initially by checking for circulating antibodies to HCV, but if they are seropositive they should also be checked for HCV RNA. Owing to their weakened immune systems, SCT recipients may not mount an effective antibody response; thus, they should be screened with tests both for anti-HCV antibodies and HCV RNA. Unlike HBV, HCV does not have a protected reservoir in cells. Patients who previously cleared the virus (HCV antibody positive and polymerase chain reaction negative) are not at risk to transmit the virus or reactivate it in the posttransplant period.

Transmission of HCV from stem cell donors to recipients is very efficient (50–100%) [17]. Transplantation from an HCV-positive donor can be considered if no other suitable donor is available. If the HCV-infected donor fulfills standard criteria for treatment and the SCT can be postponed, treatment of the donor should be initiated to eliminate or reduce viremia [18]. In these instances, stem cell harvest should not be attempted until the donor has been off treatment for at least 2 weeks, as interferon (IFN) may affect the quality of the stem cell preparation [19].

Short-term complications

Patients infected with HCV before transplantation are at risk of early exacerbations of hepatitis. The early impact of HCV on liver function after SCT has been best documented in a large Seattle cohort of patients transplanted before any HCV screening tests were available [20]. In that study, HCV-positive patients with pre-transplant elevations in aspartate transaminase had an increased likelihood of developing severe veno-occlusive disease in the first 20 days after transplantation with a relative risk of 9.6. However, two other studies could not duplicate this finding, although there were much smaller numbers of HCV-infected patients under study [21, 22]. HCV-infected recipients in the Seattle study also had higher transaminase levels compared with uninfected controls at various times from early to very late after transplantation. For example, 31% of HCV-positive patients experienced aspartate transaminase elevations greater than 10 times the upper limit of normal between 61 and 365 days after transplantation, compared with only 5% of uninfected patients. These elevations of transaminases in the HCV-positive recipients coincided with cessation or tapering of immunosuppressve medications and were thought to be due to unmasking of the immune response. Thus, if transaminase elevations occur posttransplant and coincide with discontinuation of immunosuppressive medications, a reasonable tactic would be to re-initiate a tapering course of corticosteroids in an effort to prevent progression to severe hepatic failure. Most studies of HCV infection in SCT focus primarily on allogeneic transplantation, which has been shown in one study to carry a much higher risk of posttransplant hepatitis (100%) than autologous transplantation (16%) does [23].

Long-term complications

Early studies of HCV-positive patients undergoing SCT showed no excess mortality up to 10 years posttransplantation [20, 21]. Subsequent studies of long-term complications have focused primarily on progression to cirrhosis and HCC. De Latour et al. followed a cohort of 96 stem cell recipients infected with HCV for a median of 15.8 years [24]. Fifteen patients developed biopsy-proven cirrhosis. The cumulative incidence of cirrhosis was 11% at 15 years and 24% at 20 years. Three patients developed HCC, and HCV-related complications were the third leading cause (behind infection and GVHD) of late deaths in this population. The calculated median time to cirrhosis in this cohort was found to be 18 years compared with 40 years in a control population of patients with HCV infection who had not received transplants [24]. In a separate pan-European study, the frequency of severe long-term liver complications in 195 HCV-infected SCT recipients (134 allogeneic, 61 autologous) was 6.9% at 15 years and 11.7% at 20 years [16]. Surprisingly, no patient in the European study developed HCC.

While HCV does not appear to affect short-term survival in SCT recipients, the frequent progression to cirrhosis in the second decade after transplantation mandates close follow-up in long-term survivors.

Treatment of HCV post SCT

The evidence that HCV-positive patients have an accelerated progression to severe liver disease late after SCT has generated interest in treatment options. In 2005, de Latour et al. reported on 22 HCV-positive SCT recipients who met clinical and pathological treatment criteria and did not have any contraindications to treatment [25]. Those patients underwent 41 treatment courses. A sustained viral response was observed in 10% of those treated with IFN monotherapy and in 20% receiving ribavirin with either IFN or pegylated IFN. Hematologic side-effects were more common in patients receiving ribavirin and three patients treated with IFN had a flare of GVHD. Ljungman et al. described 99 treatment courses for HCV in 85 SCT recipients [16]. These included 38 courses of IFN monotherapy, 47 courses of IFN and ribavirin, and 14 courses of pegylated-IFN and ribavirin. In all, 41 patients (48%) became HCV RNA negative after treatment. The sustained viral response was 31% for IFN monotherapy and 59% for combinations of IFN with ribavirin. The side-effects of the medications were comparable to those seen in a nontransplant population and no GVHD recurrence was seen. There was a strong trend (OR = 0.33; $p = 0.058$) towards decreased risk of severe liver complications in the treated group.

No studies have been done in stem cell recipients with the two new FDA-approved direct-acting antiviral agents boceprevir and telaprevir, but if results from nontransplant studies hold true then these agents should represent an important advance in treating transplant recipients. Table 29.2 lists currently available treatment options for hepatitis C with information on drug dosing, clearance, and side effects [26]. Care is required in using these drugs in transplant recipients. IFN requires some dose adjustment for renal dysfunction, and all of the available drugs have hematological side effects. Both bocepravir and telapravir are cleared by the CYP450 system and have numerous drug interactions with agents such as immunosuppressive drugs and azole antifungal drugs that are often used in transplant recipients. Despite these issues, the future of HCV therapy appears bright as there are almost 20 new compounds for the treatment HCV in various stages of investigation [27].

Although no firm guidelines regarding management of hepatitis C infection after SCT have been promulgated, the available data suggest that clinicians should be aggressive in identifying, characterizing, and, when appropriate, treating HCV in stem cell populations according to current guidelines [26].

Human immunodeficiency virus (HIV) infection

Historical experience with SCT in HIV-infected patients

In the early days of the HIV epidemic, no effective treatment was available and the diagnosis of AIDS was essentially a death sentence. The favorable experience with allogeneic SCT in children with severe combined immunodeficiency led to allogeneic SCT being carried out in patients with AIDS. These early efforts have been summarized by Hütter and Zaia [28]. These attempts at SCT showed that the patients were not able to clear their viral infection or reestablish adequate immune function; as a consequence, most died in the first few months after transplantation.

Table 29.2 HCV antiviral treatment options

Drug	Dose	Metabolism	Side effects
Pegylated INF alfa-2a	180 µg subcutaneously weekly	Renal	Flu-like syndrome, marrow suppression, colitis, hypersensitivity, neuropsychiatric disorders pancreatitis, ocular changes
Pegylated INF alfa-2b	1.5 µg/kg subcutaneously weekly	Renal	
Ribavirin	Varies based on weight, genotype, coinfection with HIV, and type of interferon used	Hepatic to active metabolites, then primarily renal excretion	Hemolytic anemia, teratogenicity
Boceprevir	800 mg TID	CYP3A4 inhibitor; hepatic metabolism to inactive metabolites	Anemia, neutropenia
Telaprevir	750 mg TID	CYP3A4 inhibitor; hepatic metabolism to less active and inactive metabolites	Anemia, rash (including drug reaction with eosinophilia and systemic symptoms and Stevens–Johnson syndrome)

TID: three times a day.

Holland et al. reported the first allogeneic SCT in a patient on antiretroviral therapy (ART) [29]. A 41-year-old man with HIV and non-Hodgkin's lymphoma (NHL) received a myeloablative transplant from his HLA-identical sister. His ART was monotherapy with zidovudine begun 2 weeks before the transplantation. He engrafted on day 17 with complete donor chimerism, but soon relapsed and died on day 47. His HIV culture from blood and HIV polymerase chain reaction from blood and bone marrow were negative at autopsy. The authors postulated that the HIV reservoir had been ablated by his chemotherapy and radiation and that zidovudine had prevented reinfection of the donor cells. Several further allogeneic SCTs were performed with patients on zidovudine, however, without any effect on the course of infection [28].

Despite these unpropitious beginnings, the introduction of highly active ART for HIV infection in the mid 1990s provided superior virologic suppression and allowed for further experience with allogeneic SCT in HIV-infected patients. In a retrospective analysis in 2011 of 28 HIV-positive patients undergoing SCT on ART, the median time to engraftment was found to be 19.7 days, and there was a trend towards increasing CD4 cell numbers during follow-up [29]. Infectious complications during neutropenia were similar to those seen in HIV-negative patients. An improvement in survival was demonstrated in patients who had received ongoing ART (~50% at 3 years) versus historical controls who had not (~25% at 3 years). A similar study by Gupta et al. demonstrated that the introduction of ART had led to increased survival in patients with HIV infection after allogeneic SCT (44% versus 14% at 59 months follow-up) [30]. Other advances in supportive therapy over the same time period may, of course, have contributed to the improved outcomes.

The most interesting advance in the use of allogeneic SCT for HIV-infected patients was the experience of the so-called "Berlin patient" [35]. This 40-year-old man with HIV infection and acute myeloid leukemia underwent allogeneic SCT from a donor who was homozygous for the CCR5-Δ32 allele. CCR5 is one of the co-receptors (along with CXCR4) that HIV uses to gain entry into host cells. Homozygosity of the CCR5-Δ32 allele (a 32-base-pair deletion), which occurs in about 1% of Caucasians, leads to an inactive receptor and high resistance to infection with HIV. After transplantation and engraftment, the patient's ART was discontinued and his viral load remained undetectable in both peripheral blood and bone marrow after greater than 3 years of follow-up. Currently, other sites are investigating this therapy to see if the results can be duplicated.

Autologous SCT in HIV-positive patients

Advances in ART have enabled HIV patients to better tolerate intensive chemotherapy regimens for HIV-associated Hodgkin's lymphoma and NHL. This has led to an increased rate of complete remissions. Relapsed or refractory lymphoma still has poor survival and necessitates autologous SCT as either rescue or consolidative therapy. A retrospective comparison was performed of 53 HIV-positive patients and a matched cohort of HIV-negative patients undergoing autologous SCT for lymphoma [31]. At the time of transplantation, the HIV-positive cohort had a median CD4 count of 163 cells/μL and 93% were on ART. Both cohorts had similar neutrophil engraftment, but the HIV-positive cohort had a lower cumulative incidence of platelet engraftment (92% versus 98%). The overall and progression-free survival as well as relapse rates were not statistically different between the two groups at a median follow-up of 30 months.

In a similar study, Krishnan et al. compared the long-term outcomes of autologous SCT in 59 HIV-positive patients with NHL with a matched HIV-negative cohort [32]. Despite the HIV-positive arm having a higher proportion of patients with high-grade disease (59% versus 7%), the 2-year disease-free survival and overall survival were similar between the two groups.

The results of these two cited studies provide strong support that autologous transplantation is a reasonable option for HIV-positive patients who require it for refractory or relapsed lymphoma.

Practical considerations for HIV-positive patients undergoing SCT

Transplantation should only be considered for patients in whom HIV infection can be controlled. Baseline CD4 counts, HIV viral loads, and resistance genotypes are useful in making these decisions. In a patient naive to ART, a typical response would be an increase in CD4 count of 50–150 cells/mm^3 per year and a decrease in viral load to <50 copies/mL by 24 weeks. Patients failing their current regimen of ART should not be excluded until resistance testing is obtained to verify whether an alternate regimen might achieve virologic suppression.

Many antiretroviral medications have significant drug–drug interactions with chemotherapeutic agents used in the conditioning regimen. Mounier et al. performed a comprehensive analysis of drug interactions between ART and antineoplastic agents [33]. Nucleoside reverse transcriptase inhibitors generally have no interactions as most are cleared by the kidney and they do not induce or inhibit the CYP450 system. The non-nucleoside reverse transcriptase inhibitors (NNRTIs) induce metabolism of alkylating agents (cyclophosphamide and ifosfamide), while protease inhibitors (PIs) block their metabolism. Two small clinical studies cited in Mounier et al.'s review suggest that marrow toxicity may be greater when alkylating agents are combined with PIs. The metabolism of vinca alkaloids (vincristine), taxanes (paclitaxel), epipodophyllotoxins (etoposide), and kinase inhibitors (imatinib) is inhibited by PIs and induced by NNRTIs. However, guidance from clinical data on whether dose changes are need when these drugs are used concomitantly with ART is limited.

NNRTIs and PIs also have significant drug–drug interactions with commonly used immunosuppressive agents posttransplant. The NNRTIs have been shown to decrease the levels of glucocorticoids, calcineurin inhibitors (CNIs), and mTor inhibitors through induction of cytochrome enzymes; however, the clinical relevance of this effect is uncertain [34]. These combinations need not be avoided, but immunosuppressant drug level monitoring is advisable. The NNRTIs also cause transaminase elevation more frequently than other classes of ART and, thus, could demonstrate synergistic hepatotoxicity with CNIs. The most problematic class of ART is the PIs. PIs are strong inhibitors of the CYP450 system and can lead to significantly higher serum levels of glucocorticoids, CNIs, and mTor inhibitors. All patients on PIs require immunosuppressant dose reductions, but those on ritonavir-boosted PIs often require a 10- to 100-fold reduction of the dosage of CNIs and mTor inhibitors. For instance, doses as low as 0.5–1 mg of tacrolimus weekly suffice to achieve therapeutic levels when administered concomitantly with PIs.

The most recently released antiretrovirals include integrase inhibitors, CCR5-antagonists, and fusion inhibitors. These medications offer potential advantages in the transplant setting, because they have few drug interactions and do not require dose modifications when combined with commonly used transplant medications.

Keeping patients on ART during the early posttransplant period is often a challenge, as mucositis and GVHD may interfere with administration or absorption of oral medications. Most antiretrovirals are not available in intravenous formulations. Abrupt cessation of ART, for whatever reason, can lead to the patient being essentially on monotherapy for some time as the half-life of antiretrovirals often differs markedly. Development of antiviral resistance is more likely when patients are on monotherapy, especially with the NNRTIs. Anticipating this risk before transplantation may enable the transplanting physician to confer with an HIV practitioner and provide an ART regimen in which the component drugs have similar half-lives.

The role of SCT in patients with HIV infection seems likely to expand in upcoming years. Autologous SCT is now widely accepted as a treatment modality for patients with Hodgkin's lymphoma and NHL, regardless of HIV status. Continued experience with allogeneic SCT in these patients will undoubtedly further solidify its role as a therapeutic option. Further forays will also likely be taken into using transplantation as a means to curing HIV infection.

References

1. Lalazar G, Rund D, Shouval D. Screening, prevention and treatment of viral hepatitis B reactivation in patients with hematological malignancies. Br J Haematol. 2007;136: 699–712.
2. Dienstag JL. Hepatitis B virus infection. N Engl J Med. 2008;359:1486–1500.
3. Lau GK, Lie AK, Kwong YL, et al. A case-controlled study on the use of HBsAg positive donors for allogeneic hematopoietic stem cell transplantation. Blood. 2000;96:452–458.
4. Lau GKK, Liang R, Lee CK, et al. Clearance of persistent hepatitis B virus infection in Chinese bone marrow transplant recipients whose donors were anti-hepatitis B core- and anti-hepatitis B surface antibody-positive. J Infect Dis. 1998;178:1585–1591.
5. Hui C-K, Lie A, Au W-Y, et al. A long-term follow-up study on hepatitis B surface antigen-positive patients undergoing allogeneic hematopoietic stem cell transplantation. Blood. 2005;106:464–469.

6. Lau GKK, Liang R, Chiu EKW, et al. Hepatic events after bone marrow transplantation in patients with hepatitis B infection: a case controlled study. Bone Marrow Transplant. 1997;19:795–799.
7. Liang R. How I treat and monitor viral hepatitis B infection in patients receiving intensive immunosuppressive therapies or undergoing hematopoietic stem cell transplantation. Blood. 2009;113:3147–3153.
8. Dhédin N, Douvin C, Kuentz M, et al. Reverse seroconversion of hepatitis B after allogeneic bone marrow transplantation: a retrospective study of 37 patients with pretransplant anti-HBs and anti-HBc. Transplantation. 1998;66:616–619.
9. Onozawa M, Hashino S, Izumiyama K, et al. Progressive disappearance of anti-hepatitis B surface antigen antibody and reverse seroconversion after allogeneic hematopoietic stem cell transplantation in patients with previous hepatitis B virus infection. Transplantation. 2005;79:616–619.
10. Borentain P, Colson P, Coso D, et al. Clinical and virological factors associated with hepatitis B virus reactivation in HBsAg-negative and anti-HBc antibodies-positive patients undergoing chemotherapy and/or autologous stem cell transplantation for cancer. J Viral Hepat. 2010;17:807–815.
11. Vigano M, Vener C, Lampertico P, et al. Risk of hepatitis B surface antigen seroreversion after allogeneic hematopoietic SCT. Bone Marrow Transplant. 2011;46:125–131.
12. Knöll A, Boehm S, Hahn J, et al. Reactivation of resolved hepatitis B virus infection after allogeneic hematopoietic stem cell transplantation. Bone Marrow Transplant. 2004;33:925–929.
13. Hammond SP, Borchelt AM, Ukomadu C, et al. Hepatitis B virus reactivation following allogeneic hematopoietic stem cell transplantation. Biol Blood Marrow Transplant. 2009;15:1049–1059.
14. Lau GKK, Yiu HHY, Fong DYT, et al. Early is superior to deferred preemptive lamivudine therapy for hepatitis B patients undergoing chemotherapy. Gastroenterology. 2003;125:1742–1749.
15. WHO. Hepatitis C, Fact Sheet No. 164, 2012. Available at: http://www.who.int/mediacentre/factsheets/fs164/en/index.html (accessed 25 May 2013).
16. Ljungman P, Locasciulli A, de Soria VG, et al. Long-term follow-up of HCV-infected hematopoietic SCT patients and effects of antiviral therapy. Bone Marrow Transplant. 2012;47:1217–1221.
17. Shuhart MC, Myerson D, Childs BH, et al. Marrow transplantation from hepatitis C virus seropositive donors: transmission rates and clinical course. Blood. 1994;84:3229–3235.
18. Vance EA, Soiffer RJ, McDonald GB, et al. Prevention of transmission of hepatitis C virus in bone marrow transplantation by treating the donor with alpha-interferon. Transplantation. 1996;62:1358–1360.
19. Drapeau CM, Remotti D, Noto P, et al. Bone marrow toxicity in HCV genotype 5a-infected patient after peg-IFN alpha-2a and ribavirin therapy. J Chemother. 2008;20:648–651.
20. Strasser SI, Myerson D, Spurgeon CL, et al. Hepatitis C virus infection and bone marrow transplantation: a cohort study with 10 year follow up. Hepatology. 1999;29:1893–1899.
21. Ljungman P, Johansson J, Aschan H, et al. Long term effects of hepatitis C virus infection in allogeneic bone marrow transplant recipients. Blood. 1995;86:1614–1618.
22. Locasciulli A, Bacigalupo A, VanLint MT, et al. Hepatitis C virus infection and liver failure in patients undergoing allogeneic bone marrow transplantation. Bone Marrow Transplant. 1995;16:407–411.
23. Locasciulli A, Bruno B, Alessandrino EP, et al. Hepatitis reactivation and liver failure in hematopoietic stem cell transplants for hepatitis B virus (HBV)/hepatitis C virus (HCV) positive recipients. Bone Marrow Transplant. 2003;31:295–300.
24. de Latour RP, Lévy V, Asselah T, et al. Long-term outcome of hepatitis C infection after bone marrow transplantation. Blood. 2004;103:1618–1624.
25. de Latour RP, Asselah T, Lévy V, et al. Treatment of chronic hepatitis C virus in allogeneic bone marrow transplant recipients. Bone Marrow Transplant. 2005;36:709–713.
26. Yee HS, Chang MF, Pocha C, et al. Update on the management and treatment of hepatitis C virus infection: recommendations from the Department of Veterans Affairs Hepatitis C Resource Center Program and the National Hepatitis C Program Office. Am J Gastroenterol. 2012;107:669–689.
27. Cooper C, Hepatitis C. Treatment highlights from the 2011 American Association for the study of liver disease meeting. Clin Infect Dis. 2012;55:418–425.
28. Hütter G, Zaia JA. Allogeneic haematopoietic stem cell transplantation in patients with human immunodeficiency virus: the experiences of more than 25 years. Clin Exp Immunol. 2011;163:284–295.
29. Holland HK, Saral R, Rossi JJ, et al. Allogeneic bone marrow transplantation, zidovudine, and human immunodeficiency virus type 1 infection. Studies in a patient with non-Hodgkin lymphoma. Ann Intern Med. 1989;111:973–981.
30. Gupta V, Tomblyn M, Pedersen TL, et al. Allogeneic hematopoietic cell transplantation in human immunodeficiency virus-positive patients with hematologic disorders: a report from the Center for International Blood and Marrow Transplant Research. Biol Blood Marrow Transplant. 2009;15:864–871.
31. Diez-Martin J, Balsalobre P, Re A, et al. Comparable survival between HIV+ and HIV− non-Hodgkin and Hodgkin

lymphoma patients undergoing autologous peripheral blood stem cell transplantation. Blood. 2009;113:6011–6014.

32. Krishnan A, Palmer JM, Zaia JA, et al. HIV status does not affect the outcome of autologous stem cell transplantation (ASCT) for non-Hodgkin lymphoma. Biol Blood Marrow Transplant. 2010;16:1302–1308.
33. Mounier N, Katlama C, Costagliola D, et al. Drug interactions between antineoplastic and antiretroviral therapies: implications and management for clinical practice. Crit Rev Oncol Hematol. 2009;72:10–20.
34. van Maarseveen EM, Rogers CC, Trofe-Clark J, et al. Drug–drug interactions between antiretroviral and immunosuppressive agents in HIV-infected patients after solid organ transplantation. AIDS Patient Care STDS. 2012; 26:568–581.
35. Hütter G, Nowak D, Mossner M, et al. Long-term control of HIV by *CCR5* delta32/delta32 stem cell transplantation. N Engl J Med. 2009;360:692–698.

30

CHAPTER 30

Prevention and management of renal complications in long-term survivors

Michael Dickenmann[1] *and Joerg P Halter*[2]

[1]Clinic for Transplantation Immunology and Nephrology, University Hospital Basel, Basel, Switzerland
[2]Clinic for Hematology, University Hospital Basel, Basel, Switzerland

Introduction

Acute kidney disease (AKD) and chronic kidney disease (CKD) are important complications of both autologous and allogeneic hematopoietic stem cell transplantation (HSCT). This can be due to structural or functional abnormalities of the kidneys and manifested by reduced glomerular filtration rate (GFR), proteinuria, or other pathologic findings in urine sediment. Impaired kidney function ranges from a clinically irrelevant decrease in kidney function to end-stage renal disease (ESRD) requiring dialysis or kidney transplantation. Usually, CKD posttransplantation is the result of multiple insults associated with the transplantation, including adverse drug effects. In contrast, renal graft-versus-host disease (GVHD) is a rather rare posttransplant complication.

Epidemiology of CKD after HSCT

The number of patients at risk for posttransplant kidney dysfunction is steadily increasing for several reasons: (a) the numbers of HSCTs are continuously growing every year [1, 2], (b) long-term survival rate has improved, leading to more patients who experience sequelae from this procedure, (c) the increasing use of reduced-intensity conditioning regimens allows patients with comorbidities, including preexisting impaired renal function, to undergo HSCT who would not have previously qualified for intensive conditioning, and (d) an increasing prevalence of patients with chronic GVHD on long term-immunosuppression – frequently including calcineurin inhibitors.

The reported incidence of CKD after HSCT varies widely owing to different study populations and different definitions of CKD [3–6]. A recent systematic review addressed this topic in detail [7]. According to that analysis, which included 28 cohorts with more than 5000 patients who survived more than 100 days, the overall incidence of CKD was approximately 16%. The post-transplant decline of kidney function over 24 months was more pronounced in patients undergoing allogeneic HSCT (ΔeGFR −40 mL/min per 1.73 m^2 – eGFR: estimated GFR) as compared with autologous HSCT (ΔeGFR −18.6 mL/min per 1.73 m^2). This fall is more than expected in the general population, where an average annual decline of 0.25 mL/min per 1.73 m^2 is observed. ESRD occurred in 0.8% in this analysis. The 10-year cumulative incidence rate of CKD after myeloablative allogeneic HSCT, defined as a GFR of <60 mL/min per 1.73 m^2, has been reported to be 27%. Severe [8, 9] kidney disease (GFR of <30 mL/min per 1.73 m^2) [2] developed in 3% of patients in this analysis. Different risk factors for the development of CKD were reported; for

Blood and Marrow Transplantation Long-Term Management: Prevention and Complications, First Edition. Edited by Bipin N Savani.

example, recipient's age at transplantation, previous HSCT, preexisting kidney damage in the recipient, the type of transplantation (e.g., autologous, allogeneic, non-myeloablative), therapeutic regimens (e.g., chemotherapy, radiation, immunosuppressive agents), posttransplant infectious complications, acute kidney injury (AKI) within 100 days posttransplant, and the extent of GVHD [4, 9]. However, there is substantial heterogeneity among the studies that makes a real estimate very difficult [7], and incidence may change with the time after transplantation [10]. Most probably, the etiology is multifactorial. Renal biopsy and autopsy specimens from hematopoietic cell transplant recipients with signs of renal dysfunction reveal multiple pathologic findings in many cases [3, 11]. Membranous glomerulonephritis is the most common diagnosis (47%) [3, 11, 12]. Other glomerular pathology includes focal segmental glomerulosclerosis [3, 11], tubulointerstitial nephropathy, and minimal change disease. IgA nephropathy has also been described [11, 13]. Thrombotic microangiopathy (TMA) [3, 14], isolated or combined with other pathology, is frequently observed. Also polyoma BK virus nephropathy is increasingly recognized as a cause of CKD in patients after HSCT [9, 15, 16].

Etiology of CKD after HSCT

Basically, patients after HSCT are prone to the same risk factors and causes that lead to CKD in the general population. In addition, some specific conditions in association with the initial disease and HSCT predispose further to CKD. A significant number of patients develop AKI during the peritransplant period, and this has recently been reviewed in detail [17, 18]. Even if AKI is reversible, it represents an independent risk factor for late CKD [19].

Transplantation-associated TMA

Transplantation-associated TMA (TA-TMA) in HSCT is the result of endothelium damage with thrombosis and fibrin deposition of the renal microcirculation, caused by multiple factors, that are: calcineurin inhibitors, chemotherapy, total body irradiation, infection, and/or GVHD [20]. The incidence varies widely in different studies [21–24]. Whereas mortality rates are high in the most severe forms, chronic TMA may be a more common cause of CKD. In contrast to the classic TA-TMA manifesting early after transplantation and often associated with severe acute GVHD, this subacute or chronic type of TA-TMA typically occurs late (i.e. months after HSCT) [21–27]. Current clinical diagnostic criteria for TA-TMA [20] are unsatisfactory with only a weak correlation with autopsy studies, most probably because patients who have received a transplant frequently have multiple other reasons for the laboratory abnormalities currently used to diagnose TA-TMA. Affected patients present with microangiopathic hemolytic anemia, thrombocytopenia, and a gradual rise of serum creatinine. Urinalysis is often normal or shows only mild proteinuria and hematuria (i.e., hemoglobinuria). Arterial hypertension is frequently present. The kidneys seem to be the primary site of microangiopathy, since systemic clinical signs with the exception of hypertension are typically absent and autopsy studies have not identified systemic thrombi [14, 25, 27]. Acute infection may contribute to TMA, as has been shown in an autopsy study [27]. The hematologic abnormalities eventually resolve, although hypertension and CKD can persist. In contrast to other forms of hemolytic uremic syndrome/thrombotic thrombocytopenic purpura, plasma exchange has usually no benefit in patients with TA-TMA after HSCT [23, 27, 28]. Potential exceptions are rare patients where an antibody-mediated endothelial injury is suspected [20].

TA-TMA is typically associated with calcineurin inhibitor toxicity. Hence, a change of the immunosuppression with discontinuation of cyclosporine A or tacrolimus is advisable in patients with TA-TMA, whereas a beneficial effect of dose reduction is less clear. Treatment of arterial hypertension (and proteinuria) in TA-TMA patients with angiotensin-converting-enzyme (ACE) inhibitors may be effective, but there are no controlled studies in HSCT recipients yet.

Role of calcineurin inhibitors and other immunosuppressants

Since the number of patients with chronic GVHD is steadily increasing, long-term treatment with calcineurin inhibitors or other immunosuppressive drugs is now more frequently needed. Chronic calcineurin inhibitor therapy (cyclosporine or tacrolimus) as well as treatment with mTOR inhibitors (sirolimus or everolimus) can cause acute and chronic nephrotoxicity, as it is observed in solid organ transplantation [29–31]. The characteristic vascular and interstitial changes of chronic calcineurin inhibitor-induced nephrotoxicity can occur with prolonged therapy for GVHD. Typically, there is a slow but continuous rise in serum creatinine and a decline in eGFR associated with the onset of tubular or glomerular proteinuria. Treatment with sirolimus/everolimus in non-renal organ transplantation may be associated with acute tubular toxicity and chronic glomerular damage leading to tubular or glomerular proteinuria [32–34]. Therefore, a switch from calcineurin inhibitors to mTOR inhibitors to avoid nephrotoxicity has to be carefully evaluated. Reported effects in the literature on renal function are controversial. Both stabilization and improvement and a further decline have been observed in patients after solid organ transplantation. Data for HSCT recipients are largely lacking. If a switch is performed, careful monitoring and treatment of hyperlipidemia and proteinuria are recommended.

Nephrotic range proteinuria

The onset of nephrotic proteinuria or nephrotic syndrome after HSCT has been reported in several case series [35–38]. The most common findings in kidney biopsies are membranous nephropathy followed by minimal change disease [37–39]. For many patients, there is a temporal relationship between the development of nephrotic syndrome – predominantly membranous nephropathy – with decreased or discontinued immunosuppression and with the diagnosis of chronic GVHD. Glomerular lesions after hematopoietic cell transplantation may therefore represent a renal manifestation of GVHD. Nephrotic syndrome is usually diagnosed several months posttransplant, and usually manifests after the diagnosis of chronic GVHD [38]. Rarely, nephrotic syndrome is reported without concomitant chronic GVHD. Reintroduction or increase of immunosuppressive therapy is required to achieve remission, with better prognosis for minimal change disease than membranous nephropathy. Treatment regimens are basically the same as applied in idiopathic membranous nephropathy; that is, high-dose steroids, calcineurin inhibitors, mycophenolic acid, or rituximab. ACE-inhibitors or angiotensin II receptor blockers are recommended to lower proteinuria and blood pressure. Lipids need to be monitored and treated if indicated, and anticoagulation should be considered.

The discovery of a major podocyte antigen, the M-type phospholipase A2 receptor 1 (PLA2R1), has significantly changed the understanding of the pathogenesis of idiopathic membranous nephropathy [38, 40–42]. Anti-PLA2R antibodies appear to predict activity of the disease as well as response to therapy. But preliminary results do not confirm an association of circulating Anti-PLA2R antibodies with the onset of membranous nephropathy after HSCT [41], which does not rule out that other antibodies or cellular alloimmune mechanisms may play an important role in the pathogenesis.

Polyoma BK virus-associated nephropathy after HSCT

Polyoma BK virus-associated nephropathy (PVAN) is a cause of graft loss in kidney transplant recipients in the setting of more intensive immunosuppression [43, 44]. Reports of PVAN in native kidneys following allogeneic hematopoietic cell transplantation are rare [9, 15, 16], but some cases have been reported that occurred even later than 2 years posttransplantation [45]. Hence, PVAN should be considered in the differential diagnosis for decreasing renal function in patients with impaired immune reconstitution and/or prolonged and intensive immunosuppression after HSCT. Typically, there is initially a slow decrease of kidney function without significant proteinuria. Micro- or macrohematuria, which is often present in BK virus replication early after HSCT, is not regularly seen. Screening for PVAN comprises the examination of the urine for the presence of decoy cells and for the polyoma BK polymerase chain reaction (PCR) in the blood [43, 44]. Testing BK PCR in the urine in patients after renal transplantation has a high negative predictive value to rule out PVAN, but the predictive value of a positive BK PCR in the urine for presence of PVAN is low. The same may be true for recipients of HSCT. Renal biopsy is the gold standard in the diagnosis of PVAN. Treatment mainly consists of the reduction of immunosuppression. Antiviral therapy with cidofovir or leflunamide is controversially discussed in patients after solid organ transplantation and has not been validated after HSCT. BK-virus-specific cytotoxic T cells may present an alternative therapeutic approach in the future.

Initial evaluation and long-term follow-up of kidney function

Patients who are evaluated for HSCT should be carefully screened for CKD before specific HSCT therapy starts. The assessment of baseline data is crucial for the planning of HSCT and the comparison with follow-up data. CKD is defined as the presence of kidney damage, usually detected as pathologic urinary protein or albumin excretion or a pathologic urine sediment, *or* decreased kidney function, defined as a GFR less than 60 mL/min per 1.73 m^2 [2] for three or more months, irrespective of the cause [46]. Screening for kidney disease should include the following points: (i) assessment of kidney function, (ii) screening for and quantification of proteinuria, (iii) urinalysis, and (iv) ultrasonography of the urinary tract. Kidney function should be assessed by the eGFR, since a serum creatinine in the normal range does not exclude a significant impairment of the renal function, and even less so in patients with decreased muscle mass.

Estimation of GFR should be done with a formula based on the serum creatinine. eGFR should be preferably estimated by the CKD-EPI formula [47] as this estimation is validated in Caucasians and Afro-Americans for normal and impaired kidney function, whereas the MDRD formula [48] and the estimated creatinine clearance by Cockcroft–Gault [49] are not validated for normal kidney function. A 24-h urine collection to calculate the creatinine clearance is not necessary in the usual clinical setting. The estimation of serum cystatin C has not been validated in HSCT patients and seems not to provide additional benefit. Proteinuria is screened for by urine dipstick. In the case of a positive dipstick a quantitative analysis is mandatory. Nowadays, the quantification of proteinuria is performed by the measurement of the protein-to-creatinine or the albumin-to-creatinine ratio in the spot urine. This analysis is easy to perform, independent from patient's compliance, and excludes misleading collection failures. If the protein-to-creatinine ratio in the urine is pathologically elevated, then a detailed analysis of the proteins in the urine can help to differentiate the origin of injury (i.e., glomerular or tubular damage). Elevated albumin, transferrin, and immunoglobulin G ratios in the urine, so-called glomerular proteinuria, are markers of glomerular damage with pathological loss of big proteins usually retained by an intact glomerular barrier. Glomerular proteinuria indicates any kind of glomerular damage; for example, acute or chronic glomerulonephritis, focal segmental glomerulosclerosis, hypertensive or atherosclerotic glomerular injury. As the amount of protein loss is quantified, the ratio can be used to document the course of kidney damage and the effect of a therapeutic intervention. Figure 30.1a gives an example of glomerular proteinuria. The presence of small, freely glomerular-filtered proteins in the urine (e.g., retinol-binding protein, α-1 microglobulin, or β-2 microglobulins, so-called tubular proteins) is an indicator of tubular damage in the kidney, typically associated with drug toxicity by different substances. Acute toxicity by aminoglycoside antibiotics or vancomycin can lead to tubular toxicity. The presence of tubular proteins in the urine is also a marker of tubular damage by calcineurin inhibitors (tacrolimus, cyclosporine) and m-Tor inhibitor (sirolimus, everolimus) [30]. Therefore, the appearance of tubular proteins in the urine in patients with long-term immunosuppression can be an indicator of calcineurin-inhibitor-induced toxicity and makes a critical reevaluation of the therapeutic regimen necessary. Figure 30.1b gives an example of tubular proteinuria.

If urine dipstick analysis reveals the presence of blood or leucocytes in the urine a further diagnostic step with urine sediment examination is indicated as positive dipstick results are rather unspecific and often false positive. In case of a positive dipstick result for blood the urine sediment helps to distinguish between erythrocytes of glomerular and non-glomerular origin. The former suggests acute glomerulonephritis or glomerular damage especially if also glomerular proteinuria (see above) is present. A diagnosis of non-glomerular erythrocytes in the urine is suggestive for bleeding in the ureter, bladder or urethra (e.g. hemorrhagic cystitis). If urine dipstick is positive for blood but erythrocytes in the urine sediment are absent myoglobinuria or hemoglobinuria may be the reason and should be looked for if there is clinical suspicion.

Imaging of the urinary tract, preferably by ultrasound, before HSCT treatment starts is advisable to exclude preexisting pathology like postrenal obstruction, unilateral renal agenesis or signs of CKD.

The onset of AKD or CKD in the follow-up after HSCT that cannot be explained by clinical or non-invasive

(a)

Parameter	Value	Class	Norm
a-2-macrogl.	0.00	n.d.	<0.23 mg/mmol Krea
Immungl. G.	0.55	norm	<1.13 mg/mmol Krea
Transferrin	0.44	+	<0.19 mg/mmol Krea
Albumin	14.29	++	<2.26 mg/mmol Krea
a-1-microgl.	1.33	norm	<1.58 mg/mmol Krea
Retinolb. protein.	<0.05	<sen	<0.08 mg/mmol Krea
ß-2-microglob.	0.00	n.d.	<0.00 mg/mmol Krea
Total Protein	21.86	+	<11.31 mg/mmol Krea
Crea	12.81	+	11.31 mmol/l

Chart: Multiple of the Upper Reference Range

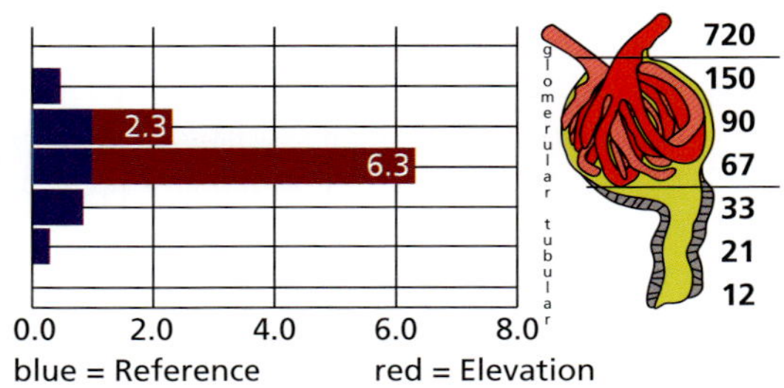

(b)

Parameter	Value	Class	Norm
a-2-macrogl.	n.d.	n.d.	<0.23 mg/mmol Krea
Immungl. G.	3.39	+	<1.13 mg/mmol Krea
Transferrin	0.38	+	<0.19 mg/mmol Krea
Albumin	7.34	+	<2.26 mg/mmol Krea
a-1-microgl.	35.78	++++	<1.58 mg/mmol Krea
Retinolb. protein.	2.82	+++	<0.08 mg/mmol Krea
ß-2-microglob.	n.d.	n.d.	<0.00 mg/mmol Krea
Total Protein	26.37	+	<11.31 mg/mmol Krea
Crea	5.31	norm	11.31 mmol/l

Chart: Multiple of the Upper Reference Range

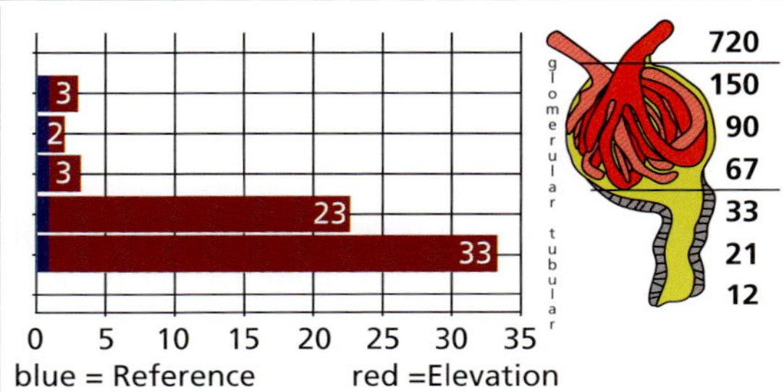

Figure 30.1 Quantification of proteinuria in the spot urine. (a) An example of glomerular proteinuria with elevated albumin and transferrin in the urine, (b) Mainly tubular proteinuria in the urine as α-1 microglobulin and retinol binding protein are pathologically increased.

diagnostic methods strongly suggests a kidney biopsy. Their findings can help to guide further therapy; for example, reduction or change of calcineurin inhibitor therapy in the case of chronic toxicity to avoid or at least slow progression of CKD. In the case of thrombocytopenia or an impaired coagulation state, a transjugular instead of a percutaneous kidney biopsy might be considered. However, diagnostic information might be less conclusive because samples collected by this approach tend to contain mainly tissue from the medulla than from the renal cortex.

Renal function should be evaluated annually after HSCT with serum creatinine, calculation of eGFR, urinalysis, and urine protein-to-creatinine ratio. Presenting signs of chronic renal injury include reductions in the GFR, proteinuria, and pathologic urine sediment.

Management of patients with CKD after HSCT

The management of patients with CKD after HSCT basically does not differ from other patient populations with CKD. It is directed by the stage of impaired kidney function. Table 30.1 shows the classification of CKD according to the GFR. Every stage demands specific diagnostic and therapeutic procedures (see Table 30.1). Independent of the stage, it is crucial to obtain a specific diagnosis of the underlying kidney disease. A kidney biopsy should be considered in all cases in which a diagnosis cannot be made by the medical history and/or noninvasive analyses. A prognosis of the decline in renal function in CKD can be made with a graph of the reciprocal of the serum creatinine concentration or with the eGFR calculated by the MDRD formula [48, 50]. eGFR can be used instead of reciprocal serum creatinine since the GFR varies inversely with the reciprocal of the serum creatinine concentration. The graph helps to roughly predict the estimated time for need of a renal replacement therapy. Figure 30.2 denotes an example using the eGFR.

Table 30.1 Classification of CKD and screening scheme for complications of CKD [46, 65]

GFR stage	GFR (mL/min per 1.73 m²)	Screen for and treat if necessary
G1	≥90	Cause of kidney disease (all stages) presence of renal abnormalities (e.g., proteinuria, pathologic urine sediment)
G2	60–89	Hypertension (all stages)
G3a	45–59	Renal anemia
G3b	30–44	Renal bone disease
G4	15–29	Metabolic acidosis
G5	<15	Nausea, neuropathy, pericarditis, itching, central nervous abnormalities

Choice of renal replacement therapy

Once it is determined that renal replacement therapy will eventually be required, the patient should be counseled to consider the advantages and disadvantages of hemodialysis (in-center or at home), peritoneal dialysis (continuous or intermittent modalities), and renal transplantation (living or deceased donor). The 2006 K/DOQI guidelines recommend that patients with a GFR less than 30 mL/min per 1.73 m² [2] should be educated concerning these issues [51]. The following key questions should be answered: (i) Is the patient suitable for any kind of renal replacement therapy? (ii) Is kidney transplantation an option? (iii) If transplantation is no option, does the patient qualify for or do they want a dialysis treatment?

Kidney transplantation

Kidney transplantation is the treatment of choice for patients with ESRD and should also be considered in patients after HSCT [52]. A successful kidney transplant reduces the mortality risk compared with maintenance dialysis in all age groups. In contrast to dialysis treatment, it offers a normal professional life in many cases and has a beneficial impact on costs [53–55]. There are only a few generally accepted contraindications to transplantation

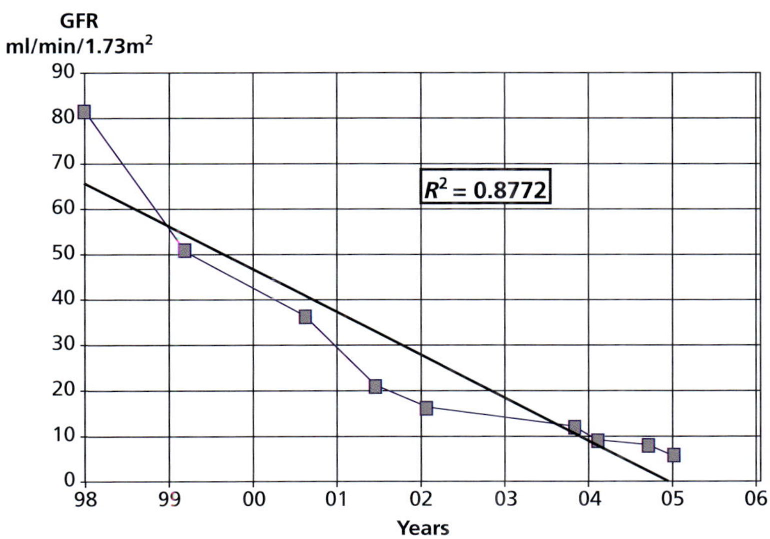

Figure 30.2 A patient's example of a graph with the eGFR plotted against time. The intersection of the line with a GFR of 10 mL/min per 1.73 m² [2] roughly denotes the time for need of a renal replacement therapy.

[56]: untreated infection, active malignancy life expectancy less than 2 years (this also includes a careful assessment of the prognosis for disease-free survival after transplantation and the prognosis of chronic GVHD if present), chronic illness with short life expectancy, poorly controlled psychosis, and active substance abuse. Relative contraindications include: active infection, untreated or untreatable coronary heart disease, and symptomatic peripheral vascular disease, especially in the pelvis axis. Advanced age, prior transplantation, and renal diagnosis are *a priori* no contraindications to transplantation. Long-term immunosuppressive therapy contributes to an increased risk for malignancy in organ transplant recipients. It is not known yet if the risk is even higher after HSCT and solid organ transplantation. Skin is the most common site for the development of malignancy; in particular, cutaneous squamous cell carcinomas and basal cell carcinomas are frequently detected [57]. Poor drug adherence, especially in young patients, is also a substantial problem [58].

Living donor kidney transplantation

Preemptive kidney transplantation in the case of ESRD after HSCT from the same donor who provided cells for the preceding hematopoietic cell transplantation would be a preferred option as specific immunosuppression may be obviated due to immunologic tolerance [59, 60]. However, it is important to emphasize that both hematopoietic stem cell and kidney donation are volunteer acts, and every pressure from health-care providers to the donor to donate a kidney shall be avoided. Hence, mechanisms need to be in place to enable the donor a free decision. Combined hematopoietic cell and kidney transplant has also resulted in the development of tolerance to the transplanted kidney and withdrawal of immunosuppressive medications [61]. Beside the superior graft survival, the preemptive approach offers the possibility to transplant at the best time (i.e., recipient has best medical and social conditions) and to minimize the risk of delayed graft function. Avoiding a time on dialysis is also a cost saving as a dialysis treatment is more expensive than a patient with a kidney transplant [54, 55], and transplanted patients have a greater opportunity to avoid unemployment or dependence from welfare. In recent years the barrier of blood group incompatibility has been successfully overcome [62, 63]. Today, blood-group-incompatible living donor kidney transplantation offers equal short- and long-term results to blood-group-compatible transplantation and is performed in up to 20% of living donor transplantations. Kidney paired donation between two donor–recipient pairs with blood group incompatibility or presence of donor-specific antibodies against the own donor is another promising new strategy to further increase the number of living donor kidney transplantations [64]. Living donor kidney transplantation offers the best solution for a patient with ESRD and has an acceptable risk for the donor. It should therefore be the treatment of choice, and its possibility should be evaluated in every patient with ESRD. Patients with no opportunity for a living donated kidney should be listed on the national kidney waiting lists.

General considerations

Radio-contrast media and gadolinium

The application of radio-contrast media enhances the risk of AKI, especially in patients with CKD. The rise in serum creatinine usually starts 1–3 days after the application. The risk is further increased by a low circulating volume, ACE inhibitor therapy, known diabetic nephropathy, or plasma cell myeloma. AKI is reversible in many, but not all, cases but it can lead to end-stage renal failure in patients with previous severe CKD [65]. The indication for radio imaging with contrast media should be very restrictive for patients with eGFR below 30 mL/min. Patients should be appropriately hydrated, preferable with sodium chloride 0.9%, and therapy with ACE inhibitors, angiotensin receptor antagonists, or non-steroidal anti-inflammatory drugs should be paused. On the other side, radio-contrast imaging should not be avoided due to the risk of AKI if the examination is crucial and decisive for the patient management.

Nephrogenic systemic fibrosis is a rare but deleterious fibrosing disorder after gadolinium application seen in patients with impaired kidney function. About 400 cases have been reported so far [66, 67]. Most cases are associated with the use of gadolamide, whereas the association with other gadolinium preparations is less certain. Among patients with an eGFR <30 mL/min or those on dialysis, gadolinium-containing contrast agents are contraindicated, unless clinical conditions make gadolinium-based imaging absolutely necessary. If inevitable, an immediate dialysis treatment should follow the gadolinium application.

Drug administration in CKD

Drug administration in CKD should be carefully evaluated, and potentially nephrotoxic drugs should be avoided. This might be feasible for non-steroidal anti-inflammatory drugs and other drugs that are not regularly used or for which alternatives exist, but it might be more difficult for other drugs for which there is no adequate substitute. Many drugs and/or their metabolites are renal eliminated. Dose adaptation has to be checked prior to the application according to the calculated eGFR (see earlier). In general, drug dose adaptation is necessary if the eGFR falls below 30 mL/min. Calculation of eGFR needs to be repeated at regular intervals. For many drugs, serum or whole blood levels can be measured, which is helpful to define the correct dose.

Various drugs, including opiates, antihypertensive drugs, or antidepressants, may lead to urinary retention, especially in elderly men, and contribute to CKD by postrenal outflow obstruction.

Need for integral patient care

Occurrence and progression of CKD is often associated with concomitant diseases, including arterial hypertension, diabetes mellitus, metabolic syndrome, or infections. These might be amplified from preexisting diseases or triggered by posttransplant complications or its treatment, including steroids and calcineurin inhibitors. Hence, a broad scope is mandatory for both prevention and treatment of CKD and its complications.

References

1. Passweg JR, Baldomero H, Gratwohl A, et al. European Group for Blood and Marrow Transplantation (EBMT). The EBMT activity survey: 1990–2010. Bone Marrow Transplant. 2012;47(7):906–923.
2. Pasquini MC, Wang Z. Current use and outcome of hematopoietic stem cell transplantation: CIBMTR summary slides, 2011. Available at: http://www.cibmtr.org/ReferenceCenter/SlidesReports/SummarySlides/pages/index.aspx (accessed 9 May 2013).
3. Troxell ML, Pilapil M, Miklos DB, et al. Renal pathology in hematopoietic cell transplantation recipients. Mod Pathol. 2008;21(4):396–406.
4. Touzot M, Elie C, van Massenhove J, et al. Long-term renal function after allogenic haematopoietic stem cell transplantation in adult patients: a single-centre study. Nephrol Dial Transplant. 2010;25(2):624–627.
5. Saddadi F, Hakemi M, Najafi I, et al. Chronic kidney disease after hematopoietic cell transplantation: frequency, risk factors, and outcomes. Transplant Proc. 2009;41(7):2895–2897.
6. Hingorani S, Guthrie KA, Schoch G, et al. Chronic kidney disease in long-term survivors of hematopoietic cell transplant. Bone Marrow Transplant. 2007;39(4):223–229.
7. Ellis MJ, Parikh CR, Inrig JK, et al. Chronic kidney disease after hematopoietic cell transplantation: a systematic review. Am J Transplant. 2008;8(11):2378–2390.
8. Kersting S, Hene RJ, Koomans HA, Verdonck LF. Chronic kidney disease after myeloablative allogeneic hematopoietic stem cell transplantation. Biol Blood Marrow Transplant. 2007;13(10):1169–1175.
9. Weiss AS, Sandmaier BM, Storer B, et al. Chronic kidney disease following non-myeloablative hematopoietic cell transplantation. Am J Transplant. 2006;6(1):89–94.
10. Abboud I, Porcher R, Robin M, et al. Chronic kidney dysfunction in patients alive without relapse 2 years after allogeneic hematopoietic stem cell transplantation. Biol Blood Marrow Transplant. 2009;15(10):1251–1257.
11. Chan GS, Lam MF, Au WY, et al. Clinicopathologic analysis of renal biopsies after haematopoietic stem cell transplantation. Nephrology (Carlton). 2008;13(4):322–330.
12. Hu SL. The role of graft-versus-host disease in haematopoietic cell transplantation-associated glomerular disease. Nephrol Dial Transplant. 2011;26(6):2025–2031.
13. Hu SL, Colvin GA, Rifai A, et al. Glomerulonephritis after hematopoietic cell transplantation: IgA nephropathy with increased excretion of galactose-deficient IgA1. Nephrol Dial Transplant. 2010;25(5):1708–1713
14. Siami K, Kojouri K, Swisher KK, et al. Thrombotic microangiopathy after allogeneic hematopoietic stem cell transplantation: an autopsy study. Transplantation. 2008;85(1):22–28.
15. Raval M, Gulbis A, Bollard C, et al. Evaluation and management of BK virus-associated nephropathy following allogeneic hematopoietic cell transplantation. Biol Blood Marrow Transplant. 2011;17(11):1589–1593.
16. Lekakis LJ, Macrinici V, Baraboutis IG, et al. BK virus nephropathy after allogeneic stem cell transplantation: a case report and literature review. Am J Hematol. 2009;84(4):243–246.
17. Lopes JA, Jorge S. Acute kidney injury following HCT: incidence, risk factors and outcome. Bone Marrow Transplant. 2011;46(11):1399–1408.

18. Kogon A, Hingorani S. Acute kidney injury in hematopoietic cell transplantation. Semin Nephrol. 2010;30(6): 615–626.
19. Coca SG, Singanamala S, Parikh CR. Chronic kidney disease after acute kidney injury: a systematic review and meta-analysis. Kidney Int. 2012;81(5):442–448.
20. Laskin BL, Goebel J, Davies SM, Jodele S. Small vessels, big trouble in the kidneys and beyond: hematopoietic stem cell transplantation-associated thrombotic microangiopathy. Blood. 2011;118(6):1452–1462.
21. Changsirikulchai S, Myerson D, Guthrie KA, et al. Renal thrombotic microangiopathy after hematopoietic cell transplant: role of GVHD in pathogenesis. Clin J Am Soc Nephrol. 2009;4(2):345–353.
22. Loomis LJ, Aronson AJ, Rudinsky R, Spargo BH. Hemolytic uremic syndrome following bone marrow transplantation: a case report and review of the literature. Am J Kidney Dis. 1989;14(4):324–328.
23. Fuge R, Bird JM, Fraser A, et al. The clinical features, risk factors and outcome of thrombotic thrombocytopenic purpura occurring after bone marrow transplantation. Br J Haematol. 2001;113(1):58–64.
24. Imai H, Oyama Y, Miura AB, et al. Hematopoietic cell transplantation-related nephropathy in Japan. Am J Kidney Dis. 2000;36(3):474–480.
25. Parikh CR, Coca SG. Acute renal failure in hematopoietic cell transplantation. Kidney Int. 2006;69(3):430–435.
26. Ruutu T, Hermans J, Niederwieser D, et al. Thrombotic thrombocytopenic purpura after allogeneic stem cell transplantation: a survey of the European Group for Blood and Marrow Transplantation (EBMT). Br J Haematol. 2002; 118(4):1112–1119.
27. George JN, Li X, McMinn JR, et al. Thrombotic thrombocytopenic purpura–hemolytic uremic syndrome following allogeneic HPC transplantation: a diagnostic dilemma. Transfusion. 2004;44(2):294–304.
28. Zager RA. Acute renal failure in the setting of bone marrow transplantation. Kidney Int. 1994;46(5):1443–1458.
29. Dieterle A, Gratwohl A, Nizze H, et al. Chronic cyclosporine-associated nephrotoxicity in bone marrow transplant patients. Transplantation. 1990;49(6):1093–1100.
30. Franz S, Regeniter A, Hopfer H, et al. Tubular toxicity in sirolimus- and cyclosporine-based transplant immunosuppression strategies: an ancillary study from a randomized controlled trial. Am J Kidney Dis. 2010;55(2):335–343.
31. Fioretto P, Najafian B, Sutherland DE, Mauer M. Tacrolimus and cyclosporine nephrotoxicity in native kidneys of pancreas transplant recipients. Clin.J Am Soc Nephrol. 2011; 6(1):101–106.
32. Wadei HM, Zaky ZS, Keaveny AP, et al. Proteinuria following sirolimus conversion is associated with deterioration of kidney function in liver transplant recipients. Transplantation. 2012;93(10):1006–1012.
33. Uhlmann D, Weber T, Ludwig S, et al. Long-term outcome of conversion to sirolimus monotherapy after liver transplant. Exp Clin Transplant. 2012;10(1):30–38.
34. Aliabadi AZ, Pohanka E, Seebacher G, et al. Development of proteinuria after switch to sirolimus-based immunosuppression in long-term cardiac transplant patients. Am J Transplant. 2008;8(4):854–861.
35. Reddy P, Johnson K, Uberti JP, et al. Nephrotic syndrome associated with chronic graft-versus-host disease after allogeneic hematopoietic stem cell transplantation. Bone Marrow Transplant. 2006;38(5):351–357.
36. Hingorani S. Chronic kidney disease in long-term survivors of hematopoietic cell transplantation: epidemiology, pathogenesis, and treatment. J Am Soc Nephrol. 2006;17(7): 1995–2005.
37. Srinivasan R, Balow JE, Sabnis S, et al. Nephrotic syndrome: an under-recognised immune-mediated complication of non-myeloablative allogeneic haematopoietic cell transplantation. Br J Haematol. 2005;131(1):74–79.
38. Brukamp K, Doyle AM, Bloom RD, et al. Nephrotic syndrome after hematopoietic cell transplantation: do glomerular lesions represent renal graft-versus-host disease? Clin.J Am Soc Nephrol. 2006;1(4):685–694.
39. Terrier B, Delmas Y, Hummel A, et al. Post-allogeneic haematopoietic stem cell transplantation membranous nephropathy: clinical presentation, outcome and pathogenic aspects. Nephrol Dial Transplant. 2007;22(5):1369–1376.
40. Beck LH Jr, Bonegio RG, Lambeau G, et al. M-type phospholipase A2 receptor as target antigen in idiopathic membranous nephropathy. N Engl J Med. 2009;361(1):11–21.
41. Huang X, Qin W, Zhang M, et al. Detection of anti-PLA2R autoantibodies and IgG subclasses in post-allogeneic hematopoietic stem cell transplantation membranous nephropathy. Am J Med Sci. 2013;346(1):32–37.
42. Beck LH Jr. Monoclonal anti-PLA2R and recurrent membranous nephropathy: another piece of the puzzle. J Am Soc Nephrol. 2012;23(12):1911–1913.
43. Ramos E, Drachenberg CB, Wali R, Hirsch HH. The decade of polyomavirus BK-associated nephropathy: state of affairs. Transplantation. 2009;87(5):621–630.
44. Hirsch HH, Knowles W, Dickenmann M, et al. Prospective study of polyomavirus type BK replication and nephropathy in renal-transplant recipients. N Engl J Med. 2002;347(7): 488–496.
45. O'Donnell PH, Swanson K, Josephson MA, et al. BK virus infection is associated with hematuria and renal impairment in recipients of allogeneic hematopoetic stem cell transplants. Biol Blood Marrow Transplant. 2009;15(9): 1038–1048.

46. Levey AS, Coresh J. Chronic kidney disease. Lancet. 2012;379(9811):165–180.
47. Levey AS, Stevens LA, Schmid CH, et al. A new equation to estimate glomerular filtration rate. Ann Intern Med. 2009;150(9):604–612.
48. Levey AS, Bosch JP, Lewis JB, et al. A more accurate method to estimate glomerular filtration rate from serum creatinine: a new prediction equation. Modification of Diet in Renal Disease Study Group. Ann Intern Med. 1999;130(6): 461–470.
49. Cockcroft DW, Gault MH. Prediction of creatinine clearance from serum creatinine. Nephron. 1976;16(1):31–41.
50. Mitch WE, Walser M, Buffington GA, Lemann J Jr. A simple method of estimating progression of chronic renal failure. Lancet. 1976;2(7999):1326–1328.
51. Hemodialysis Adequacy 2006 Work Group. Clinical practice guidelines for hemodialysis adequacy, update 2006. Am J Kidney Dis. 2006;48(Suppl 1):S2–S90.
52. Koenecke C, Hertenstein B, Schetelig J, et al. Solid organ transplantation after allogeneic hematopoietic stem cell transplantation: a retrospective, multicenter study of the EBMT. Am J Transplant. 2010;10(8):1897–1906.
53. US Renal Data System, USRDS 2010 Annual Data Report: Atlas of Chronic Kidney Disease and End-Stage Renal Disease in the United States. National Institutes of Health, National Institute of Diabetes and Digestive and Kidney Diseases, Bethesda, MD, 2010.
54. Salonen T, Reina T, Oksa H, et al. Cost analysis of renal replacement therapies in Finland. Am J Kidney Dis. 2003; 42(6):1228–1238.
55. Villa G, Rodriguez-Carmona A, Fernandez-Ortiz L, et al. Cost analysis of the Spanish renal replacement therapy programme. Nephrol Dial Transplant. 2011;26(11):3709–3714.
56. Siddqi N, Hariharan S, Danovitch M. Evaluation and preparation of renal transplant candidates. In: Danovitch GM (ed.). Handbook of Kidney Transplantation, 4th edition. Philadelphia: Lippincott Williams and Wilkins, 2005; pp. 169–172.
57. Vajdic CM, van Leeuwen MT. Cancer incidence and risk factors after solid organ transplantation. Int J Cancer. 2009;125(8):1747–1754.
58. Nevins TE, Thomas W. Quantitative patterns of azathioprine adherence after renal transplantation. Transplantation. 2009;87(5):711–718.
59. Butcher JA, Hariharan S, Adams MB, et al. Renal transplantation for end-stage renal disease following bone marrow transplantation: a report of six cases, with and without immunosuppression. Clin Transplant. 1999;13(4):330–335.
60. Sayegh MH, Fine NA, Smith JL, et al. Immunologic tolerance to renal allografts after bone marrow transplants from the same donors. Ann Intern Med. 1991;114(11): 954–955.
61. Scandling JD, Busque S, Dejbakhsh-Jones S, et al. Tolerance and chimerism after renal and hematopoietic-cell transplantation. N Engl J Med. 2008;358(4):362–363.
62. Oettl T, Halter J, Bachmann A, et al. ABO blood group-incompatible living donor kidney transplantation: a prospective, single-centre analysis including serial protocol biopsies. Nephrol Dial Transplant. 2009;24(1):298–303.
63. Oettl T, Zuliani E, Gaspert A, et al. Late steroid withdrawal after ABO blood group-incompatible living donor kidney transplantation: high rate of mild cellular rejection. Transplantation. 2010;89(6):702–706.
64. Gentry SE, Montgomery RA, Segev DL. Kidney paired donation: fundamentals, limitations, and expansions. Am J Kidney Dis. 2011;57(1):144–151.
65. National Kidney Foundation. K/DOQI clinical practice guidelines for chronic kidney disease: evaluation, classification, and stratification. Am J Kidney Dis. 2002;39(2): S1–S266.
66. Cowper SE. Nephrogenic Systemic Fibrosis. 2001–2009. Available at: http://www.icnfdr.org (accessed 13 May 2013).
67. Bongartz G. Imaging in the time of NFD/NSF: do we have to change our routines concerning renal insufficiency? MAGMA. 2007;20(2):57–62.

31

CHAPTER 31

Immunosuppressive agents and monitoring in long-term survivors

Paul Shaughnessy[1] *and Helen Leather*[2]

[1]Texas Transplant Physician Group, San Antonio, TX, USA
[2]Department of Medicine, University of Florida, FL, USA

Introduction

The goal of this chapter is to review the management of immunosuppressive agents in the care of long-term survivors after hematopoietic stem cell transplant (HSCT). Progress has been made in improving survival after both autologous and allogeneic HSCT, predominately by advances in supportive care [1–3]. In recent years more attention has been given to not just survival of patients after HSCT, but also to the quality of life (QoL) and symptom management of HSCT survivors [4]. Use of immunosuppressive agents after HSCT can be an important part of supportive care of these patients, but also may lead to its own set of complications to manage and negatively impact a patient's QoL.

This chapter is not meant to recommend agents to treat graft-versus-host disease (GVHD) or be an exhaustive list of all drugs used for immunosuppression, but rather to review monitoring and common toxicities of agents that may affect the long-term health of patients after HSCT.

General recommendations for monitoring

Recommendations for routine health maintenance and screening for long-term survivors of HSCT have been well described [5]. This chapter is not meant to supplant these recommendations, but add to them for specific complications or monitoring that may be needed for particular immunosuppressive agents. For example, 1-year postallogeneic HSCT routine health screening for asymptomatic patients may include evaluating thyroid function, iron levels, pulmonary function testing, and cataract screening, among other tests; but if that same patient has new-onset chronic GVHD (cGHVD) and receives rituximab or anti-thymocyte globulin (ATG) therapy, then additional testing for viral reactivation (cytomegalovirus (CMV) and/or Epstein–Barr virus (EBV)) may be warranted. Also, signs and symptoms of infection, changes in vital signs, or evidence of end organ damage may point to different etiologies in patients on different immunosuppressive agents. Unexplained decreases in platelet counts may herald viral reactivations in patients, especially if they recently received agents such as ATG, campath, or rituximab. Laboratory results changes, such as increased lactate dehydrogenase (LDH) and decreased platelets with hypertension, may warrant closer evaluations or changes for those patients on both a calcineurin inhibitor and mammalian target of rapamycin (mTOR) inhibitor. There are limited randomized controlled studies on the recommendations for monitoring or the schedule for evaluations. The most important guide to monitoring is for health-care providers to be aware of potential toxicities and drug interactions, and evaluate

Blood and Marrow Transplantation Long-Term Management: Prevention and Complications, First Edition. Edited by Bipin N Savani.

changes in the patient's clinical symptoms or laboratory parameters associated with the use of immunosuppressive therapy.

Need for long-term immunosuppressive agents

The use of any immunosuppressive therapy needs to always weigh the possible risks and side effects against any possible benefit. Immunosuppressive agents are used less often in recipients of autologous HSCT, although several possible uses are briefly described herein. The use of maintenance therapy with lenalidomide or bortezomib in patients with multiple myeloma, or rituximab in patients with diffuse large B-cell non-Hodgkin lymphoma (NHL) after autologous HSCT, needs to weigh carefully the risks of therapy with any proven survival advantage in the particular patient population.

cGVHD in allogeneic recipients of HSCT can take on many different forms, and not all manifestations of cGVHD require systemic immunosuppressive therapy. Some patients with cGVHD may have limited symptoms that do not impede their functionality or QoL and, therefore, may just be followed carefully for progression without any specific therapy. Other patients with cGVHD may have manifestations of disease amenable to local therapy and also avoid systemic use of immunosuppressive therapy. Several reviews on the medical management of cGVHD have been published, and providers who care for patients with cGVHD should be familiar with local therapy options [6, 7].

After immunosuppressive therapy is tapered, patients may still require 2 years to recover baseline immunologic function [8]. Long-term survivors of allogeneic HSCT who demonstrate recurrent viral or bacterial infections, even if systemic immunosuppressive therapy is stopped, may require ongoing monitoring of viral reactivation and immunoglobulin G (IgG) levels. Also, cGVHD is in itself an immunosuppressive state, and patients with low-level cGVHD on no systemic immunosuppressive therapy may still need monitoring. Hypogamaglobulinemia is often seen after allogeneic HSCT and in patients with cGVHD. Several studies have assessed the use of prophylactic intravenous immunoglobulin (IVIG) after allogeneic HSCT, outside of the use with CMV infection, and did not demonstrate an advantage for patients in the prophylactic setting [9]. However, some centers may treat long-term survivors of allogeneic HSCT with recurrent infections and hypogamaglobulinemia with IVIG infusions of 0.5 g/kg monthly or as needed based on serum IgG levels.

Autologous HSCT and immunosuppressive monitoring

The use of immunosuppressive agents in long-term survivors of autologous HSCT is not routinely used but may be encountered in select circumstances. The immunomodulatory class of drugs, including thalidomide and lenalidomide, are most commonly used as maintenance therapy after autologous HSCT [10, 11]. The exact mechanism by which these agents mediate their antimyeloma effect is not clear, but it is believed they may have an immune modulating effect. The risk of thrombosis and its management is well described in the literature, but no increased risk of infection or need for antimicrobial prophylaxis has been described. The possible association of secondary malignancies in patients exposed to lenalidomide may be a consequence of the immunosuppressive state of myeloma itself, a direct effect of the drug, or unknown etiologies [12]. Pomalidomide is now approved by the US Food and Drug Administration for relapsed or refractory myeloma, and further studies will clarify the monitoring and risks of long-term use. Bortezomib has also been used for long-term maintenance in some patients with multiple myeloma, and this agent has been associated with an increased risk for varicella zoster, and routine antiviral prophylaxis should be employed in these patients. Carfilzomib, a second-generation proteasome inhibitor, was recently approved by the US Food and Drug Administration for treatment of relapsed and refractory multiple myeloma. Most patients enrolled in the clinical trials with carfilzomib received prophylactic antiviral medication; and as such, routine antiviral prophylaxis should be considered with this agent [13].

Several studies have described a long-term maintenance schedule with rituximab in some patients with NHL, and even when used as a single agent after autologous HSCT rituximab has been associated with cytopenias [14] and viral infections such as hepatitis B reactivation [15]. Although rare, any patient who receives rituximab is at risk for progressive multifocal leukoencephalopathy secondary to JC virus infections, which may occur up to a year after rituximab has been discontinued [16].

Immunosuppressive agents: long-term complications and monitoring

Corticosteroids

The most common class of immunosuppressive agents used in long-term survivors of HSCTs are corticosteroids [17–22]. This very important class of agents may be the most effective single agent with the quickest clinical effect in cGVHD, but also is associated with the most devastating and wide-ranging list of side effects [17–22].

Long-term cGVHD usually does not require doses of corticosteroids above 1 mg/kg methylprednisolone, or equivalent [17, 20]. Corticosteroids should always be tapered to the lowest possible dose necessary to control manifestations of disease. Long-term use of corticosteroids requires monitoring and management of hyperglycemia, hypertension, hyperlipidemia, osteoporosis, and renal impairment. Yearly bone mineral density screening may be warranted to screen for osteoporosis. Joint pain should warrant radiologic evaluation for avascular necrosis. Adrenal insufficiency may occur as steroids are tapered or if the patient should become acutely ill, and stress-dose steroids may be needed for acute illnesses or if elective surgery is planned. Employing an every other day dosing of corticosteroids may help alleviate some of the risk of adrenal insufficiency yet maintain treatment [17, 22].

Calcineurin inhibitors (tacrolimus, cyclosporine)

Tacrolimus and cyclosporine are commonly employed in long-term survivors of allogeneic HSCT to control symptoms and to allow for steroid-sparing effects. There are limited randomized controlled data on the effectiveness of calcineurin inhibitors in long-standing or refractory cGVHD, so their use should always be weighed against possible side effects. One randomized study comparing the use of cyclosporine and daily prednisone with prednisone alone showed no difference in transplant-related mortality or secondary therapy for cGVHD, but there was significantly less avascular necrosis in the cyclosporine arm, indicating a possible steroid-sparing effect [23].

Regular monitoring of drug levels is warranted whenever calcineurin inhibitors are used to assess for toxicity. Levels may be needed once or twice a week during loading phases or when doses are changed, but patients on stable doses with no other major changes in medical management may have levels monitored less frequently. Good communication and education are necessary with the patient, pharmacy, and other medical providers because of the long list of medicine interactions with calcineurin inhibitors. Medicines that inhibit the cytochrome p450 system may increase calcineurin levels and interactions that promote the cytochrome p450 system may decrease levels. A list of medicines that interact with calcineurin inhibitors is provided in Appendix 3.

Drug levels for calcineurin inhibitors are used to monitor dosing and therapy, but toxicities of these drugs can occur even in the presence of normal therapeutic levels. Therefore, patients on long-term use of calcineurin inhibitors should be screened for toxicities even if calcineurin levels are in the therapeutic range. Patients should have serum electrolytes and renal function monitored for the development of renal insufficiency. If patients present with new neurologic symptoms, the presence of thrombotic thrombocytopenic purpura can be screened for with a blood smear, serum creatinine, and LDH. Global neurological changes, seizures, and encephalopathy with white matter changes evident on brain magnetic resonance imaging and posterior reversible encephalopathy syndrome (PRES) may also be related to calcineurin inhibitors. Toxicities that are associated with high serum calcineurin inhibitor levels may resolve with holding of the drug and then reinstituting at lower doses with close monitoring. Some toxicity, such as PRES, seizures, or encephalopathy related to white matter changes that occur despite nontoxic levels of calcineurin inhibitor, may make reusing any calcineurin inhibitor difficult. Switching from tacrolimus to cyclosporine or vice versa because of toxicities may be tried, but close monitoring for the same toxicity will be needed. Physical findings such as tremor and hypertension may not warrant stopping of the calcineurin inhibitor, but may require closer monitoring and medical management of the side effect.

Generic versions of both tacrolimus and cyclosporine now exist, and patients, physicians, and pharmacists need to communicate if the drug is being switched from brand name to generic because some variations in serum levels, and therefore in effectiveness and toxicities, may occur.

Mycophenolate mofetil

Mycophenolate mofetil (MMF) is the prodrug of mycophenolic acid (MPA) and is often used in long-term survivors of allogeneic HSCT to treat refractory cGVHD and to taper and spare corticosteroids based on small retrospective reviews [24, 25]. A randomized prospective study by Martin et al. comparing MMF with placebo for initial treatment of cGVHD was closed early because an interim analysis revealed a low probability of finding a positive result. That study also demonstrated a hazard ratio of death of 1.99 (95% confidence interval 0.9–4.3) for patients who received MMF, with the majority of deaths due to infection or relapse [26].

If patients have severe renal insufficiency (glomerular filtration rate, <25 ml/min per 1.73 m^2), plasma MPA area under the curve may be 75% higher than in patients with normal renal function and use of the drug should be avoided or appropriately reduced in this patient population, whereas no dose adjustments for hepatic impairment are described [27]. A common toxicity of MMF is myelosuppression, and patients who are first started on the drug and/or develop renal insufficiency may have blood counts monitored weekly for the first month, twice weekly for the second and third months, and then monthly while they continue on therapy.

MMF can lead to a variety of gastrointestinal (GI) mucosal injuries, including ulcerative stomatitis, esophagitis, gastropathy, and GVHD-like features on intestinal biopsies [28]. GI hemorrhage or perforation may occur, and patients with active GI inflammation, infection, or other disorders should use MMF with caution and be monitored closely for worsening of these disorders. Patients with acute GVHD or cGVHD with GI symptoms or mucosal disease treated with MMF should be monitored for possible worsening of these symptoms.

Important drug interactions exist with MMF [29]. Antacids containing magnesium and proton pump inhibitors may increase gastric pH and, therefore, decrease absorption of MMF and so should not be taken concomitantly. Oral dosing of MMF involves some entero-hepatic recirculation; therefore, agents such as cholestyramine that interfere with entero-hepatic recirculation should not be used together. Antibiotics that effect bowel flora (norfloxacin, metronidazole, ciprofloxacin, amoxicillin plus clavulanic acid) may reduce glucuronidase-possessing enteric organisms, leading to a decrease in entero-hepatic recirculation of MPA [29]. Trough serum levels of MPA can be monitored but no data exist for monitoring levels in long-term survivors of HSCT.

Sirolimus

Sirolimus is a macrolide antibiotic that inhibits T-lymphocyte activation and proliferation by a mechanism that is distinct from calcineurin inhibitors, blocking progression of cells from the G1 phase to the S phase via mTOR blockade. Sirolimus, therefore, is an intriguing agent to use for long-term survivors of HSCT to afford steroid-sparing benefits and also provide immunosuppression to patients who may not be able to tolerate calcineurin inhibitors. Thrombotic thrombocytopenic purpura is a well-described complication that may occur in patients using both calcineurin inhibitors and mTOR inhibitors [30]. Patients using these agents together should have levels monitored closely once or twice weekly during loading and dosing increases. Clinical indicators such as petechiae or neurologic changes or hypertension, as well as laboratory indicators of increasing LDH, renal insufficiency, and dropping platelets should also be clues to impending toxicity.

Sirolimus has a long half-life and may be affected by many drug interactions and hepatic impairment; therefore, drug level monitoring is needed. The maintenance dose of sirolimus should be reduced by approximately one-third in patients with mild to moderate hepatic impairment and by one-half in patients with severe hepatic impairment [31]. Renal impairment does not necessarily affect dosing of sirolimus, but renal toxicity can occur from the drug, which may warrant dose adjustments or holding the agent.

Sirolimus is known to be a substrate for both cytochrome CYP3A4 and P-gp, and many drug interactions involving this metabolic pathway have been described. Sirolimus can be taken with or without food, but it is important to remember that grapefruit juice reduces the CYP3A4-mediated drug metabolism.

Serum levels of sirolimus should be monitored at least weekly during initial use until steady-state levels are documented. Renal function and electrolytes should also be monitored for toxicity. Increased serum cholesterol and triglycerides may occur with sirolimus, and these parameters should be monitored [31]. In patients who have received a solid organ transplant and received sirolimus, poor wound healing or the development of a lymphocele has been described [31]. Long-term HSCT patients with cGVHD may already be at risk for poor wound healing or chronic ulcerations and should use sirolimus cautiously.

Rituximab

Common side effects such as infusional reactions, especially after the first dose, and risk of infection are well described. Cytopenias can occur, especially after HSCT, and complete blood counts should be checked before each course. During treatment, blood counts should be monitored at weekly intervals and then monthly or more frequently in those who do develop cytopenias. The duration of cytopenias can last for months after treatment when rituximab is discontinued. Viral reactivation with the hepatitis viruses and JC virus are described above.

Antithymocyte globulins

There are several different antithymocyte globulin formulations, and protein composition and concentrations vary depending on the source of the ATG used (rabbit/horse). During infusion and immediately afterward, infusion-related effects on renal, hepatic, and possibly lung function due to capillary leak or hypoperfusion may occur. Several studies have reported high rates of CMV reactivation and infection, as well as other viral infections and EBV-related posttransplant lymphoproliferative disease (PTLD) [32]. No standard recommendation for frequency and timing of viral monitoring exists, but viral monitoring should be done at least weekly early in the transplant course or after use of ATG. Early detection of EBV may allow prophylactic use of rituximab in some patients to prevent the development of PTLD [33, 34]. Continued viral monitoring is maintained beyond the first 3 months in most allogeneic HSCT recipients for the first year posttransplant, or for as long as the patient requires systemic immunosuppression, or if patients present with clinical symptoms of infection. No specific monitoring schedule exists long term, but viral testing may be done at each clinic visit for routine visits or if symptoms or changes in the patient's clinical condition warrant evaluation.

Deniluekin diftitox

Denileukin diftitox has been used to treat steroid refractory acute GVHD, and infusional reactions are described as well as third spacing, especially with a low serum albumin [35, 36]. Severe liver toxicities were also seen in some patients, especially those patients with underlying liver disease [36]. Cytopenias, especially lymphopenia, may occur after use, and atypical or viral infections should be considered if patients develop signs or symptoms of infection.

Alemtuzumab

Alemtuzumab has been used in multiple studies as part of the transplant regimen for prophylaxis of acute GVHD, and more rarely as treatment for steroid refractory acute GVHD or cGVHD [37, 38]. There are no specific long-term monitoring requirements, but the immunosuppressive effects of alemtuzumab may be very long lasting for a year or more after use. Viral reactivation is described after use of alemtuzumab, and routine viral monitoring for CMV and EBV may be necessary at least weekly initially after use. No specific schedule for long-term viral monitoring is described, but clinical symptoms of infection may warrant screening for common viral etiologies.

Tumor necrosis factor inhibitors

Etanercept is a given as a subcutaneous injection that binds to tumor necrosis factor (TNF) and blocks its interaction with cell surface TNF receptors, while infliximab is given as an intravenous infusion and is a monoclonal antibody that binds to TNF and inhibits binding of TNF with its receptors. Use in cGVHD is limited [39, 40] and no standard requirements for monitoring, besides the standard clinical screening for active infections, tuberculosis, or other fungal infections (histoplasmosis, coccidiomycosis, blastomycosis) exists.

Cytotoxic agents

Treatment of cGVHD in long-term survivors of HSCT may include the use of cytotoxic agents such methotrexate, cyclophosphamide, and pentostatin. Monitoring for myelosuppression by evaluating complete blood counts prior to each dose and weekly during initial dosing may be needed. Methotrexate may cause liver and renal toxicity, and these laboratory values should be monitored initially before each dose; but for patients who are stable on long-term weekly use, less frequent monthly evaluations may be adequate. Pentostatin may cause a profound lymphopenia with less effect on other cell lines; therefore, monitoring the differential on the blood counts may be warranted.

Conclusion

Monitoring of immunosuppressive agents in long-term survivors of HSCT is primarily based on close clinical care of patients and knowledge of the toxicities and interactions of medications used in these patients. In the future, as more prospective studies are done to better treat long-term survivors of HSCT, developing specific guidelines for monitoring and use of immunosuppressive agents will help all providers care for these patients.

References

1. Gooley TA, Chien JW, Pergam SA, et al. Reduced mortality after allogeneic hematopoietic cell transplantation. N Engl J Med. 2010;363:2091–2101.
2. Gyurkocza B, Rezvani A, Storb R. Allogeneic hematopoietic cell transplantation: the state of the art. Expert Rev Hematol. 2010;3:285–299.
3. Pasquini MC, Wang Z, Horowitz MM, et al. Report from the Center for International Blood and Marrow Transplant Research (CIMBTR): current uses and outcomes of hematopoietic cell transplants for blood and bone marrow disorders. Clin Transpl. 2010;2010:87–105.
4. Syrjala KL, Martin PJ, Lee SJ. Delivering care to long-term adult survivors of hematopoietic cell transplantation. J Clin Oncol. 2012;30:3746–3751.
5. Majhail NS, Rizzo DJ, Lee S, et al. Recommended screening and preventative fractices for long term survivors after hematopoietic cell transplantation. Biol Blood Marrow Transplant. 2012;18:348–371.
6. Couriel D, Carpenter P, Cutler C, et al. Ancillary therapy and supportive care of chronic graft-versus-host disease: national institutes of health consensus development project on criteria for clinical trials in chronic Graft-versus-host disease: V. Ancillary Therapy and Supportive Care Working Group Report. Biol Blood Marrow Transplant. 2012;12: 375–376.
7. Blazar A, Murphy WJ, Abedi M. Advances in graft-versus-host disease biology and therapy. Nat Rev Immunol. 2012;12(6):443–458.
8. Bosch M, Khan FM, Storek J. Immune reconstitution after hematopoietic cell transplantation. Curr Opin Hematol. 2012;19(4):324–335.
9. Sokos DR, Berger M, Lazarus HM. Intravenous immunoglobulin: appropriate indications and uses in hematopoietic stem cell transplantation. Biol Blood Marrow Transplant. 2002;8(3):117–130.
10. Spencer A, Prince HM, Roberts AW, et al. Consolidation therapy with low dose thalidomide and prednisolone prolongs the survival of multiple myeloma patients undergoing a single autologous stem cell transplantation procedure. J Clin Oncol. 2009;27(11):1788–1793.
11. Dimopoulos MA, Chen C, Spencer A, et al. Long-term follow up on overall survival from the MM-009 and MM-010 phase III trials of lenalidomide plus dexamethasone in patients with relapsed or refractory multiple myeloma. Leukemia. 2009;23(11):2147–2152.
12. Scott E, Reece D. What is the benefit of maintenance therapy with lenalidomide or bortezomib after autologous stem cell transplantation in multiple myeloma and what is the risk of developing secondary primary malignancy? Hematology Am Soc Hematol Educ Program. 2011; 2011:205–207.
13. Siegel DS, Martin T, Wang M, et al. A phase 2 study of single agent carfizomib in patients with relapsed and refractory multiple myeloma. Blood. 2012;120(14):2817–2825.
14. Cattaneo C, Spendini P, Casari S, et al. Delayed onset peripheral blood cytopenia after rituximab: frequency and risk factor assessment in a consecutive series of 77 treatments. Leuk Lymphoma. 2006;47(6):1013–1017.
15. Carson KR, Evens AM, Richey EA, et al. Progressive multifocal leukoencephalopathy after rituximab therapy in HIV negative patients: a report of 57 cases from the Research on Adverse Drug Events and Reports project. Blood. 2009; 113(20):4834–4840.
16. Aksoy S, Harputluoglu H, Kilickap S, et al. Rituximab related viral infections in lymphoma patients. Leuk Lymphoma. 2007;48(7):1307–1312.
17. Syrjala K, Martin P, Lee S. Delivering care to long-term adult survivors of hematopoietic cell transplantation. J Clin Oncol. 2012;30:3745–3751.
18. Sun C, Francisco L, Kawashima T, et al. Prevalence and predictors of chronic health conditions after hematopoietic cell transplantation: a report from the bone marrow transplant survivor study. Blood. 2010;116:3129–3139.
19. Fraser C, Bhatia S, Ness K, et al. Impact of chronic graft-versus-host disease on the health status of hematopoietic cell transplantation survivors: a report from the Bone Marrow Transplant Survivor Study. Blood 2006;108: 2867–2873.
20. Mohty B, Mohty M. Long-term complications and side effects after allogeneic hematopoietic stem cell transplantation: an update. Blood Cancer J. 2011;1:e16. doi: 10.1038/bcj.2011.14 (accessed 21 May 2013). [Internet]

21. Bhatia S, Francisco L, Carter A, et al. Late mortality after allogeneic hematopoietic cell transplant and functional status of long-term survivors: report from the Bone Marrow Transplant Survivor Study. Blood. 2007;110:3784–3792.
22. Majhail NS, Rizzo JD. Surviving the cure: long term follow up of hematopoietic cell transplant recipients. Bone Marrow Transplant. 2013. doi: 10.1038/bmt.2012.258 [Epub ahead of print].
23. Koc S, Leisenring W, Flowers ME, et al. Therapy for chronic graft versus host disease: a randomized trial comparing cyclosporine plus prednisone versus prednisone alone. Blood. 2002;100:48–51.
24. Mookerjee B, Altomonte V, Vogelsang G. Salvage therapy for refractory chronic graft versus host disease with mycophenolate mofetil and tacrolimus. Bone Marrow Transplant. 1999;24:517–520.
25. Baudard M, Vincent A, Moreau P, et al. Mycophenolate mofetil for the treatment of acute and chronic GVHD is effective and well tolerated but induces a high risk of infectious complications: a series of 21 BMT or PBSC transplant patients. Bone Marrow Transplant. 2002;5:287–295.
26. Martin PJ, Storer BE, Rowley SD, et al. Evaluation of myclophenolate mofetil for initial treatment of chronic graft versus host disease. Blood. 2009;113:5074–5082.
27. Van Hest RM, Doorduign JK, de Winter BC, et al. Pharmacokinetics of mycophenolate mofetil in hematopoietic stem cell transplant recipients. Ther Drug Monit. 2007;29: 353–360.
28. Parfitt JR, Jaayakumar S, Driman DK. Mycophenolate mofetil related gastrointestinal mucosal injury: variable injury patterns, including gaft versus host disease like changes. Am J Surg Pathol. 2008;32:1367–1372.
29. Genentech Mycophenolate mofetil package insert. Genentech USA Inc South San Francisco, CA. 2012. Available from: http://www.gene.com/download/pdf/cellcept_prescribing.pdf (accessed 23 May 2013).
30. Couriel DR, Saliba R, Escalon MP, et al. Sirolimus in combination with tacrolimus and corticosteroids for the treatment of resistant chronic graft versus host disease. Br J Haematol. 2005;130:409–417.
31. Wyeth Pharmaceuticals Inc. Sirolimus package insert. Philadelphia, PA: Pfizer Inc, 2012. Available from: http://labeling.pfizer.com/showlabeling.aspx?id=139 (accessed 23 May 2013).
32. Schonberger S, Meisel R, Adams O, et al. Prospective, comprehensive, and effective viral monitoring in children undergoing allogeneic hematopoietic stem cell transplantation. Biol Blood Marrow Transplant. 2010;16:1428–1435.
33. Blaes AH, Cao Q, Wagner JE, et al. Monitoring and preemptive rituximab therapy for Epstein Barr virus reactivation after antithymothyte globulin containing nonmyeloablative conditioning for umbilical cord blood transplantation. Biol Blood Marrow Transplant. 2010;16:287–291.
34. Peres E, Savasan S, Klein J, et al. High fatality rate of Epstein Barr Virus associated lymphproliferative disorder occurring after bone marrow transplantation with rabbit antithymothyte globulin conditioning regimens. J Clin Microbiol. 2005;43:3540–3543.
35. Ho VT, Zahrieh D, Hochber E, et al. Safety and efficacy of denileukin diftitox in patients with steroid refractory acute graft versus host disease after allogeneic hematopoietic stem cell transplantation. Blood. 2004;104:1224–1226.
36. Shaughnessy P, Bachier C, Grimley M, et al. Denileukin diftitox for the treatment of steroid resistant acute graft versus host disease. Biol Blood Marrow Transplant. 2005;11: 188–193.
37. Giralt S. The role of alemtuzumab in non-myeloablative hematopoietic transplantation. Semin Oncol. 2006;33: S36–S43.
38. Ruiz-Arguelles GJ, Gil-Beristain J, Magana M, Ruiz Delgado GJ. Alemtuzumab induced resolution of refractory cutaneous chronic graft versus host disease. Biol Blood Marrow Transplant. 2008;14:7–9.
39. Sleight BS, Chan KW, Braun TM, et al. Infliximab for GVHD therapy in children. Bone Marrow Transplant. 2007;40: 473–480.
40. Chiang KY, Abhyankar S, Bridges K, et al. Recombinant human tumor necrosis factor receptor fusion protein as complementary treatment for chronic graft versus host disease. Transplantation. 2002;73:665–667.

3

SECTION 3

Supportive care for long-term survivors after HSCT

CHAPTER 32

Nutritional assessments and nutritional supplementation for long-term transplant survivors: multivitamins, vitamin D, calcium, antioxidants, and minerals

Lauren Zatarain[1], *LaQuisa Hill*[2], *Daniel R Thomas*[3], *and Stacey A Goodman*[4]

[1]Division of Hematology/Oncology, Vanderbilt University, Nashville, TN, USA
[2]Department of Medicine, Vanderbilt University, Nashville, TN, USA
[3]Vanderbilt University Medical Center, Nashville, TN, USA
[4]Hematology and Stem Cell Transplant, Vanderbilt University, Nashville, TN, USA

Introduction

Much of the traditional focus of nutrition in hematopoietic cell transplantation (HCT) lies in the acute peritransplant period. During this period, there is increased risk for malnutrition due to gastrointestinal (GI) toxicity from preparative regimens, as well as increased metabolic requirements while awaiting engraftment. However, it is important to recognize that engraftment does not end the necessity for monitoring nutritional problems in HCT patients. Reduced dietary intake, weight loss, and body composition alterations occur throughout the posttransplant period, although the trajectory improves over time.

Prevalence of nutritional problems

Reductions in dietary intake occur for a variety of reasons, including anorexia, taste alterations, nausea, and xerostomia [1]. Poor appetite was reported in two-thirds of patients 50 days posttransplant in a prospective longitudinal study of 58 patients [2]. At 1 year, nearly one-quarter of patients still report eating difficulties. Xerostomia is reported with similar frequencies early posttransplant and at the 1 year mark. Separate reports reveal a strong negative correlation between anorexia and quality of life in long-term HCT survivors [3]. Taste sensation remains altered after HCT, with a raised threshold for salt lasting for more than 1 year [4]. Diet tolerance varies widely and may be limited by oral complaints or fungal infections (refer to Chapter 17). Lactose intake may not be tolerated during the first year after HCT. Despite nutritionist recommendations for energy, protein, and micronutrient enrichments, compliance with dietary advice is poor and decreases over time [2].

Weight changes are cited as the most frequent nutritional problem, with 28% of patients experiencing weight loss in a study of 192 long-term survivors of allogeneic

Blood and Marrow Transplantation Long-Term Management: Prevention and Complications, First Edition. Edited by Bipin N Savani.

transplant [1]. In fact, 17% of patients were 10% or more below their ideal body weight at 1 year posttransplant, with the most significant body composition alterations noted in patients with extensive graft-versus-host disease (GVHD). Similar results are described with only half of patients regaining at least 95% of their pretreatment body weight, 1 year after transplant, with greater rates of growth retardation in the total-body irradiation-treated cohort [2]. Up to 1 year after unrelated donor bone marrow transplant, nearly one-quarter of patients still reported weight loss [3].

Body composition alterations

Body composition alterations are prevalent in long-term transplant survivors. Anthropometry (height, weight, body mass index (BMI), upper arm measurements), dual-energy X-ray absorptiometry (DEXA) total body scans, and bioelectrical impedance analysis are tools employed for the assessment of total body composition. Total body weight is composed of fat mass (20–50%), lean mass (47–75%), and bone mineral (5%) [5]. Body composition alterations manifest as weight redistribution of lean and fat mass with muscle mass loss and adipose tissue gain. Loss of body weight after discharge from the transplant unit preferentially consists of muscle mass loss [5]. There is universal muscle mass loss and adipose tissue gain in all posttransplant groups studied, with more extensive alterations noted in patients with extensive chronic GVHD [1]. Chronic GVHD is known to be a highly inflammatory, catabolic state resulting in wasting with negative calorie and nitrogen balances, likely accounting for these findings. However, even apparently healthy patients do not appear to return to their baseline, as evidenced by an increased frequency of depleted muscle reserves at 1 year posttransplant [1]. In a separate 6-year longitudinal study, 38% of HCT patients did not regain their pretransplant lean body mass [6]. Similarly, low performance status is associated with decreased lean body mass. Decrements in grip strength are also noted in long-term transplant survivors, reflecting their depleted physical functioning within 1 year of transplant [5]. These anthropometric changes may be attributable to activity restrictions in the posttransplant period. Unfortunately, only a minority of allogeneic transplant patients regain their pretransplant physical condition and nutrition status by 1 year, thus requiring continued monitoring.

Extensive pediatric transplant literature demonstrates similar body composition alterations with effects on growth (refer to Chapter 20). Low BMI remains an important predictor of morbidity and mortality and is associated with physiologic, immunologic, and psychologic changes [7]. Chronic GVHD is a risk factor for low BMI and depressed lean muscle mass [8]. The association of low BMI is also seen in T-cell-depleted grafts, possibly due to complications with delayed immune reconstitution [8]. Total-body irradiation consistently results in low BMI values in the pediatric population [9]. However, BMI values in long-term transplant survivors remained unchanged from initiation of HCT to long-term follow-up in a cohort of 151 adult patients [10].

There are shortcomings in BMI assessments that should be noted. It is difficult to distinguish lean mass and fat mass alterations with BMI measurements alone. This is particularly problematic in patients with inflammatory conditions, such as chronic GVHD, as excess fat mass may conceal lean mass deficits [11]. In addition, fluid retention with third spacing stabilizes overall weight, leading to potentially normal BMI values, which obscures potential nutritional deficits [12]. Several studies reveal discrepancies between BMI and lean mass percentages in allogeneic transplant patients; thus, multiple assessment tools are necessary for monitoring body composition changes [6, 8, 11, 13]. Therefore, even patients with normal BMI values should undergo assessments of lean mass to ensure appropriate and timely intervention by nutritionists and physical therapists. Assessments with DEXA, bioelectrical impedance analysis, and anthropometric measures assist in accurately measuring both lean and fat mass.

Chronic GVHD is a hypercatabolic state with increased circulating pro-inflammatory cytokines [14], contributing to extensive lean muscle mass loss. There are significant associations between low lean body mass and chronic GVHD, suggesting that the complications and treatment of GVHD increase rates of muscle mass depletion [6]. Glucocorticoids are known to increase protein oxidation and decrease fat oxidation, leading to altered body composition [15]. Thus, long-term survivors of transplant with chronic GVHD require intensive nutritional surveillance throughout the follow-up period.

Nutrition assessments

Nutrition screening questionnaires

There are several validated patient questionnaires used to assess nutritional status. The Subjective Global Assessment (SGA) [16] and the Patient-Generated Subjective Global Assessment (PG-SGA) [17], which was specifically designed for patients with cancer, are useful tools to identify malnutrition. The SGA uses information from the history, such as weight change, dietary intake change, GI symptoms, functional capacity, and metabolic demands. Physical examination findings such as muscle wasting and loss of subcutaneous fat from triceps and chest measurements are included in the assessment. The SGA places patients into one of three categories: (1) well nourished, (2) moderately malnourished, and (3) severe malnutrition. The SGA has proven effectiveness in correlating nutritional status to biochemical complications, anthropometric changes, immunologic parameters, infections, and length of hospital stay [18]. The PG-SGA incorporates more nutritional symptoms and weight loss questions, allowing for the patient to provide the majority of the history. A potential advantage of the PG-SGA over the SGA includes the generation of a numerical score. This score correlates to the degree of malnutrition with higher assessed numbers indicating increased risk for malnutrition. A numerical score allows for a more sensitive triage for intervening on malnutrition. The PG-SGA also provides more objective data, demonstrating subtle changes in nutritional status that may not be garnered from the SGA. In addition, there is high sensitivity (98%) and specificity (82%) for correlation of the PG-SGA and SGA questionnaires, appropriately identifying patients at risk for malnutrition [19].

Laboratory assessments

Biochemical laboratory values, such as albumin, prealbumin, transferrin, and retinol-binding protein, are used as adjunctive tests in nutritional assessments. Rapid turnover proteins are more sensitive markers owing to shorter half-lives when compared with albumin, which tends to reflect chronic nutritional changes [20]. However, protein levels are variable and may be affected by infections, hyper-hydration, or liver and renal insufficiency [21]. Transferrin levels serve as a negative prognostic marker in patients undergoing HCT, as lower levels correlate with increased death [5]. Similarly, depressed albumin levels predict for in-patient death, nosocomial infections, and length of hospitalization.

Prevalence of supplement use

Use of vitamin and mineral supplementation occurs more frequently in the cancer population as compared with the general US population. A systematic summary of studies demonstrates that long-term cancer survivors report supplement use rates of 64–81% as compared with 50% in the general population [22]. In addition, 30–50% of patients initiate supplement use after their initial cancer diagnosis [23]. Increased supplementation after diagnosis and through survivorship occurs for a multitude of reasons, including healthy lifestyle behavioral changes, following the advice of health care providers or others, treating symptoms, ensuring adequate nutritional intake, strengthening immune systems, or preventing cancer recurrence [24]. Daily multivitamins in amounts equivalent to 100% of the US Department of Agriculture recommended daily value are generally considered safe and recommend by the National Cancer Institute and the American Cancer Society. However, the associated risks and benefits of vitamin and mineral supplementation in long-term cancer survivors and their effects on cancer treatment toxicity, cancer recurrence, and overall survival warrant further investigation.

Over 75% of patients taking supplements consume more than one; however, nearly half of patients do not communicate usage to their physicians. The underreporting may be due to patients' perceptions of physician indifference or opposition, poor medical documentation, or underrecognition of its medical implications by both patients and their physicians [25]. This lack of communication is not attributable to patient education, as higher levels of education are consistently associated with higher supplement use [22]. This highlights the importance of an open dialogue between healthcare providers and their patients regarding vitamin and mineral supplementation.

Multivitamins

Multivitamins are the most prevalent supplement utilized among cancer survivors, with reported rates of 26–77% [22]. Following HCT, daily iron-free multivitamin supplementation is recommended for a minimum of 1 year. Seventy percent of allogeneic transplant patients report continuing their multivitamins, with higher compliance rates among patients with more extensive GVHD [1]. Lower rates of folate, calcium, and magnesium supplementation were reported in 39%, 11%, and 4% of all transplant patients, respectively.

Vitamin D

Vitamin D exerts hormonal effects regulating calcium homeostasis (refer to Chapter 15), modulating inflammatory pathways [26], and regulating cellular pathways involved in cancer [27]. Vitamin D, 25(OH)D_3, requires hydroxylation in the kidneys to form the biologically active form of vitamin D, 1,25(OH_2)D_3. Several studies reveal that low serum 25-hydroxyvitamin D_3 (25(OH)D_3) concentrations may be associated with poorer overall survival in both solid and hematologic malignancies [28], although long-term outcome data in the transplant population are lacking.

Sunlight exposure, dietary intake, and supplementation are the primary routes through which humans attain vitamin D. Deficiencies may result from reduced endogenous skin synthesis of vitamin D_3 (cholecalciferol) due to decreased UV sunlight exposure. Thus, it is important to take into account the time of year that a patient's vitamin D level is measured. In addition, there may be reduced absorption of vitamin D_2 (ergocalciferol) and vitamin D_3 in the GI tract as a result of GI GVHD, biliary salt deficiency, pancreatic enzyme insufficiency, or bacterial overgrowth. Organ injury, including hepatic and renal insufficiency, may contribute to decreased synthesis of vitamin D. Specific medications, including glucocorticoids and antirejection medications, increase catabolism of vitamin D.

Vitamin D deficiency is defined as a 25(OH)D_3 level less than 20–30 ng/mL (50–75 nmol/L) [29]. Baseline serum vitamin D (25(OH)D_3) concentrations in patients presenting for HCT are frequently below recommended levels of at least 30 ng/mL. There is growing consensus that serum 25(OH)D_3 concentrations of at least 75–80 nmol/L are needed for optimal bone health. Vitamin D deficiency (15–29 ng/mL) is present in 39–89% of allogeneic transplant patients [30, 31], with 25% of patients exhibiting extremely low levels (≤10 ng/mL) prior to HCT [32]. Both exogenous and endogenous vitamin D supply are low in HCT patients at baseline. Direct sunlight exposure of less than 3 h is reported in 68% of patients, accounting for low endogenous synthesis [32]. In addition, few patients report high consumption of vitamin D-rich foods or use of vitamin D_3 supplements prior to HCT.

Patients with grades 3–4 GVHD experience more profound reductions in vitamin D levels [33]. Drops of up to 23% from baseline vitamin D levels are reported by day 100 [32]. There is impaired absorption of lipid-soluble vitamins via the intestinal tract in patients with GVHD. In addition, treatment of GVHD with corticosteroids increases vitamin D catabolism. It remains unclear whether vitamin D deficiency increases risk for the development of GVHD, given its role in T-lymphocyte regulation [34]. Thus, future studies are needed to address whether vitamin D supplementation prior to HCT affects GVHD incidence and severity.

Routine vitamin D testing is performed in a minority of long-term HCT survivors. In a cohort of 289 patients, only 20% underwent vitamin D testing [35]. Female and older patients were more likely to be offered testing, most often occurring in the metabolic disease clinic. Interestingly, 90% of the patients tested still had low levels of vitamin D approximately 1 year after transplant, with 58% of patients tested exhibiting extremely low levels (≤10 ng/mL). In addition, 95% of patients had coexisting chronic GVHD with steroid requirements, both known to increase the incidence of vitamin D deficiency. Instructions to avoid sun exposure and use of sunscreen are routinely given to HCT patients, which may contribute to vitamin D deficiency in this population. One-fifth of patients were taking vitamin D supplements when diagnosed with vitamin D deficiency. Despite supplementation, clinically apparent osteopenia and osteoporosis were present in 65% of patients tested. Thus, HCT providers should consider evaluation of vitamin D levels intermittently in long-term survivors.

Both pediatric and adult HCT long-term survivors are at risk for continued vitamin D deficiency, even after accounting for seasonal variation. A cohort study of 78 pediatric and adolescent acute lymphoblastic leukemia patients found that 53% were insufficient and 12% were deficient in vitamin D [36]. Although 35% of patients reported taking 400 IU/day vitamin D supplementation, only 8% of HCT patients met the recommended dietary allowance (RDA) for dietary vitamin D intake. A separate cohort of 95 long-term survivors, including children, adolescents, and adults, revealed that 64% were vitamin

D replete [37]. Supplemental vitamin D use was prevalent in over 50% of patients in this cohort, likely accounting for the lower incidence of vitamin D deficiency. Of the deficient patients, 80% were not taking any vitamin D supplementation. Routine supplementation of 400–1000 IU vitamin D per day should be considered for long-term HCT survivors.

Treatment with either vitamin D_2 (ergocalciferol) or D_3 (cholecalciferol) is preferred [29], although some studies suggest vitamin D_3 may be more potent [38]. Recommended intake of vitamin D in healthy adults aged 19–70 is at least 600 IU/day and in healthy adults aged >71 is 800 IU/day in order to maximize bone health and muscle function [29, 39]. Obese adults or adults on medications known to decrease vitamin D levels should be treated with two to three times more vitamin D for their age group [29]. Thus, routine supplementation of 400–1000 IU vitamin D per day should be considered for long-term HCT survivors for prevention of vitamin D deficiency. All adults who are found to be vitamin D deficient should be treated with 50 000 IU/week of vitamin D_2 or D_3 (equivalent to 6000 IU/day) to achieve serum levels greater than 30 ng/mL. This should be followed by maintenance therapy of 1500–2000 IU/day [29]. If the 25(OH)D_3 concentration does not increase by 25% with treatment dosing, malabsorption or poor compliance should be considered as the etiology of persistently low levels [40].

Calcium

Calcium is the most abundant macroelement in the human body and can be found in a variety of foods and drugs (e.g., antacids). Calcium is involved in a number of important biological functions, including contraction of muscles and blood vessels, secretion of hormones and enzymes, and transmission of impulses in the nervous system. Most of the calcium in the body is stored in bones and teeth. Similar to vitamin D, most Americans do not achieve adequate calcium intake from their daily diets. Vitamin D must be replete, as it is responsible for stimulating intestinal enterocytes, leading to appropriate calcium absorption. In fact, only 10–15% of dietary calcium is absorbed without vitamin D [29]. Calcium absorption is affected by several other factors, including age, low estrogen levels, hypochlorhydria, and a high-fiber diet [41].

Calcium supplements are widely available in the USA, although reported use in allogeneic transplant patients is only 11% [1]. Calcium supplementation should be considered in all individuals who fail to meet adequate dietary intake, persons at risk of calcium and/or vitamin D deficiency, osteoporosis patients on antiresorptive or anabolic medications, and persons receiving glucocorticoids. Benefits of calcium supplementation are most apparent when complemented with vitamin D supplementation. Calcium citrate and calcium carbonate are the most common forms of calcium supplementation. Calcium carbonate must be taken with a meal to ensure optimal absorption. Calcium citrate can be taken without food and is the supplement of choice for individuals with achlorhydria or those taking H2 blockers or proton pump inhibitors [41]. Thus, calcium citrate is the preferred supplement for transplant patients and should be prescribed in divided doses. Each dose should not exceed 500 mg, as this is the maximum amount that can be absorbed.

Current recommended allowances of calcium in healthy men and women between the ages of 19 and 50 years are 1000 mg/day. Recommendations for calcium supplementation increase to 1200 mg/day in women over the age of 50 years and men over the age of 71 years [39, 41]. However, higher doses of 1500 mg/day are traditionally recommended in allogeneic transplant patients over the age of 18 years. Intake in excess of 2500 mg/day may interfere with the absorption of other minerals, including zinc, magnesium, and phosphorus [41]. Dietary calcium intake should be considered in calculating the need for additional supplementation, especially in light of recent concerns raised regarding calcium supplementation and cardiovascular risk [15].

There has been recent controversy regarding the safety of calcium supplementation owing to a possibility of increased cardiovascular risk. One meta-analysis demonstrated an increase in the incidence of myocardial infarction of approximately 30% in individuals on calcium supplements in excess of 500 mg/day compared with those taking placebo [42]. However, no significant increase was observed in the incidence of a number of related vascular endpoints, including stroke and death. In addition, the studies included in the analysis were designed to assess the effects of calcium only (without vitamin D) on bone density and fracture risk, and none of the included trials had cardiovascular outcomes as primary or secondary endpoints. Subsequent randomized, placebo-controlled studies did not demonstrate increased risk of death or first-time hospitalization from atherosclerotic vascular disease in healthy patients taking calcium supplementation [43]. Thus, further studies regarding the appropriate dosage of calcium supplementation in transplant patients who already have premature atherosclerotic risks are warranted.

Antioxidants

Concentrations of vitamin C, vitamin E (α-tocopherol), and β-carotene decline following high-dose chemotherapy and radiation in patients undergoing HCT [44]. Glutathione, an endogenous antioxidant, also declines in response to chemotherapy, but may also be decreased as a result of depleted vitamin C and E levels [45]. Total parenteral nutrition administration during HCT does not prevent antioxidant depletion. In fact, α-tocopherol depletion occurred with nadir at day 14 despite intravenous supplementation at twice the recommended dose [46]. Prolonged periods of reduced α-tocopherol concentrations appear to increase risk for organ toxicity. However, α-tocopherol may reduce the immunosuppressive effects of cyclosporine, potentially heightening GVHD risk [47].

Approximately two-thirds of HCT patients report taking antioxidants prior to HCT, with rates of 31% vitamin C use, 19% vitamin E use, 8% β-carotene use, and 6% vitamin A (retinol) use [47]. A cohort of approximately 350 patients with acute leukemia demonstrated that nonrelapse mortality was increased at 2 years in those patients taking ≥500 mg/day of vitamin C prior to HCT. Similarly, patients taking ≥400 IU/day of vitamin E had increased risk of mortality or relapse.

Antioxidant supplementation raises a particular concern given their protective effects on oxidative damage to cancer cells, potentially rendering chemotherapeutic and radiation therapies less effective [48]. Future studies in the HCT population are warranted to determine whether the antioxidant benefits of organ protection do not come at the expense of disease-free survival. Thus, high-dose supplementation is discouraged in the general oncology and HCT populations.

Minerals

Trace elements, particularly zinc and copper, are not adequately preserved in severely stressed patients. Micronutrient shifts of potassium, phosphorus, magnesium, and zinc occur in chronic malnutrition, although serum levels may be initially normal [49]. As patients increase their calorie intake, utilization of these stored elements leads to precipitous drops in serum concentrations. Thus, chronically ill long-term transplant survivors with increased nutrition requirements should undergo weekly serum trace element monitoring, in order to avoid excess chromium, manganese, and copper supplementation.

Zinc deficiency following HCT transplant is observed in the immediate post-HCT period, but recovers over time [50]. This occurs despite daily supplementation with zinc via a commercial trace element concentration within the first 30 days of transplant. Decreased zinc stores are reflected clinically as low levels of serum alkaline phosphatase. Zinc deficiency is the result of hypoalbuminemia and impaired absorption with excess GI losses. In general, long-term HCT survivors do not need additional zinc repletion in excess of amounts contained in a multivitamin.

Iron overload due to transfusions occurs in 30–60% of long-term allogeneic HCT survivors [51] and may increase risk for hepatic and cardiac toxicity (refer to Chapter 27). Hyperferritinemia (ferritin >1000 ng/mL) is used as a screening test for iron overload; however, this may not accurately reflect total body iron stores. Hyperferritinemia is associated with increased risk for early nonrelapse mortality and overall survival [52, 53]. In addition, vitamin C supplementation may intensify oxidative damage in patients with high iron stores owing to the strong pro-oxidant nature of the iron–ascorbate complex. Vitamin C promotes the conversion of the ferric form of iron to the ferrous form, increasing reactive oxygen species generation. Therefore, most HCT patients should avoid supplements containing iron, unless proven to be iron deficient.

Hypomagnesemia may result in hypocalcemia, peripheral vitamin D resistance, and resistance to parathyroid hormone. Maintenance of serum magnesium levels in the normal range may prevent osteopenia and bone fragility. Symptoms of magnesium deficiency include symptomatic hypocalcemia, muscle cramps, latent tetany, carpal-pedal spasms, and seizures. Patients on cyclosporine or tacrolimus should receive adequate magnesium supplementation in order to maintain normal concentrations and undergo monthly magnesium testing. It should be noted that assessments of magnesium are problematic owing to the distribution of magnesium in the body [54]. About half of the total body magnesium (1 mol) is located in the bone and the other half is in the soft tissues. Extracellular magnesium accounts for approximately 1% of total body magnesium. Therefore, the measurement of serum magnesium does not exactly reflect its intracellular level. The magnesium requirements range from 200 to 2500 mg/day, and some patients require intravenous supplementation with magnesium sulfate owing to significant diarrhea which may occur with oral administration (refer to Chapter 30).

Herbal preparations

All medications, including over-the-counter supplements and alternative treatments such as herbal preparations, must be reported to HCT providers. Potent drug interactions may occur with necessary posttransplantation medications; thus, an open dialogue between patients and their physicians is necessary to avoid potentially deleterious effects.

Conclusions

It is clear that HCT recipients require long-term monitoring and management of nutritional problems. Dietitians specializing in the care of transplant patients are integral components to the HCT team. Patients should undergo monthly weight evaluations in the first year after transplant, allowing for timely intervention. Patients identified with inappropriate weight loss or eating problems should be referred to nutrition services. Patients with chronic GVHD may require more comprehensive nutrition evaluations given their highly catabolic state.

Supplement use in long-term transplant survivors should be carefully monitored by the HCT team (refer to Table 32.1). An iron-free daily multivitamin is recommended for a minimum of 1 year following HCT. Calcium and vitamin D supplementation is also recommended for bone health maintenance. There should be cautious use of antioxidants, minerals, and herbal preparations in excess of RDA values. The associated risks and benefits of vitamin and mineral supplementation in long-term survivors and their potential effects on cancer treatment toxicity, cancer recurrence, and overall survival must be weighed.

Table 32.1 Recommended vitamin supplementation in long-term transplant survivors

Multivitamin	Daily for minimum of 1 year (iron-free preparations)
Vitamin D	400–1000 IU/day for prevention of vitamin D deficiency 50 000 IU/week until replete for treatment of vitamin D deficiency
Calcium	1500 mg/day
Antioxidants	Not to exceed 100% RDA values *Avoid high-dose supplementation
Minerals	Not to exceed 100% RDA values *As clinically indicated (e.g. magnesium with calcineurin-inhibitor associated renal wasting)

References

1. Lenssen P, Sherry ME, Cheney CL, et al. Prevalence of nutrition-related problems among long-term survivors of allogeneic marrow transplantation. J Am Diet Assoc. 1990;90:835–842.
2. Iestra JA, Fibbe WE, Zwinderman AH, et al. Body weight recovery, eating difficulties and compliance with dietary advice in the first year after stem cell transplantation: a prospective study. Bone Marrow Transplant. 2002; 29(5):417–424.
3. Molassiotis A. Anorexia and weight loss in long-term survivors of haematological malignancies. J Clin Nurs 2003;12:925–927.
4. Mattsson T, Arvidson K, Heimdahl A, et al. Alterations in taste acuity associated with allogeneic bone marrow transplantation. J Oral Pathol Med. 1992;21:33–37.
5. Schulte C, Reinhardt W, Beelen D, et al. Low T3-syndrome and nutritional status as prognostic factors in patients undergoing bone marrow transplantation. Bone Marrow Transplant. 1998;22(12):1171–1178.
6. Kyle UG, Chalandon Y, Miralbell R, et al. Longitudinal follow-up of body compositionin hematopoietic stem cell transplant patients. Bone Marrow Transplant. 2005;35(12): 1171–1177.
7. Deeg HJ, Seidel K, Bruemmer B, et al. Impact of patient weight on non-relapse mortality after marrow transplantation. Bone Marrow Transplant. 1995;15(3):461–468.
8. Inaba H, Yang J, Kaste SC, et al. Longitudinal changes in body mass and composition in survivors of childhood hematologic malignancies after allogeneic hematopoietic

stem-cell transplantation. J Clin Oncol. 2012;30:3991–3997. Epub 2012 Oct 1.

9. Couto-Silva AC, Trivin C, Esperou H, et al. Changes in height, weight and plasma leptin after bone marrow transplantation. Bone Marrow Transplant. 2000;26(11):1205–1210.
10. Cohen A, Duell T, Socié G, et al. Nutritional status and growth after bone marrow transplantation (BMT) during childhood: EBMT Late-Effects Working Party retrospective data. European Group for Blood and Marrow Transplantation. Bone Marrow Transplant. 1999;23(10): 1043–1047.
11. Mostoufi-Moab S, Ginsberg JP, Bunin N, et al. Body composition abnormalities in long-term survivors of pediatric hematopoietic stem cell transplantation. J Pediatr. 2012;160(1):122–128. Epub 2011 Aug 11.
12. Cheney CL, Abson KG, Aker SN, et al. Body composition changes in marrow transplant recipients receiving total parenteral nutrition. Cancer. 1987;59(8):1515–1519.
13. Urbain P, Birlinger J, Lambert C, et al. Longitudinal follow-up of nutritional status and its influencing factors in adults undergoing allogeneic hematopoietic cell transplantation. Bone Marrow Transplant. 2013;48:446–451. Epub 2012 Aug 27.
14. Zatarain L, Savani BN. The role of nutrition and effects on the cytokine milieu in allogeneic hematopoietic stem cell transplantation. Cell Immunol. 2012;276(1–2):6–9. Epub 2012 May 17.
15. Horber FF, Marsh HM, Haymond MW. Differential effects of prednisone and growth hormone on fuel metabolism and insulin antagonism in humans. Diabetes. 1991;40(1): 141–149.
16. Detsky AS, McLaughlin JR, Baker JP, et al. What is subjective global assessment of nutritional status? JPEN J Parenter Enteral Nutr. 1987;11(1):8–13.
17. Ottery F. Definition of standardized nutritional assessment and interventional pathways in oncology. Nutrition. 1996;12(1 Suppl):S15–S19.
18. Makhija S, Baker J. The Subjective Global Assessment: a review of its use in clinical practice. Nutr Clin Pract. 2008;23(4):405–409.
19. Bauer J, Capra S, Ferguson M. Use of the scored Patient-Generated Subjective Global Assessment (PG-SGA) as a nutrition assessment tool in patients with cancer. Eur J Clin Nutr. 2002;56(8):779–785.
20. Inoue Y, Nezu R, Matsuda H, et al. Rapid turnover proteins as a prognostic indicator in cancer patients. Surg Today. 1995;25(6):498–506.
21. Rzepecki P, Barzal J, Sarosiek T, Szczylik C. Biochemical indices for the assessment of nutritional status during hematopoietic stem cell transplantation: are they worth using? A single center experience. Bone Marrow Transplant. 2007;40(6):567–572.
22. Velicer CM, Ulrich CM. Vitamin and mineral supplement use among US adults after cancer diagnosis: a systematic review. J Clin Oncol. 2008;26(4):665–673.
23. Miller PE, Vasey JJ, Short PF, Hartman TJ. Dietary supplement use in adult cancer survivors. Oncol Nurs Forum. 2009;36(1):61–68.
24. Rock CL, Doyle C, Demark-Wahnefried W, et al. Nutrition and physical activity guidelines for cancer survivors. CA Cancer J Clin. 2012;62:242–274.
25. Lee MM, Lin SS, Wrensch MR, et al. Alternative therapies used by women with breast cancer in four ethnic populations. J Natl Cancer Inst. 2000;92(1):42–47.
26. Cantorna MT, Zhu Y, Froicu M, Wittke A. Vitamin D status, 1,25-dihydroxyvitamin D_3, and the immune system. Am J Clin Nutr. 2004;80(6 Suppl):1717S–1720S.
27. Perkins SL, Kling SJ, Ross FP, Teitelbaum SL. 1,25 Dihydroxyvitamin D_3 stimulates differentiation of committed murine bone marrow-derived macrophage precursor cells. Endocrinology. 1995;136(12):5643–5650.
28. Shanafelt TD, Drake MT, Maurer MJ, et al. Vitamin D insufficiency and prognosis in chronic lymphocytic leukemia. Blood. 2011;117(5):1492–1498. Epub 2010 Nov 3.
29. Holick MF, Binkley NC, Bischoff-Ferrari HA, et al. Evaluation, treatment, and prevention of vitamin D deficiency: an Endocrine Society clinical practice guideline. J Clin Endocrinol Metab. 2011;96(7):1911–1930. Epub 2011 Jun 6.
30. Massenkeil G, Fiene C, Rosen O, et al. Loss of bone mass and vitamin D deficiency after hematopoietic stem cell transplantation: standard prophylactic measures fail to prevent osteoporosis. Leukemia. 2001;15(11):1701–1705.
31. Schulte C, Beelen DW, Schaefer UW, Mann K. Bone loss in long-term survivors after transplantation of hematopoietic stem cells: a prospective study. Osteoporos Int. 2000;11(4): 344–353.
32. Urbain P, Ihorst G, Biesalski H-K, Bertz H. Course of serum 25-hydroxyvitamin D_3 status and its influencing factors in adults undergoing allogeneic hematopoietic cell transplantation. Ann Hematol. 2012;91(5):759–766.
33. Kreutz M, Eissner G, Hahn J, et al. Variations in 1α,25-dihydroxyvitamin D_3 and 25-hydroxyvitamin D_3 serum levels during allogeneic bone marrow transplantation. Bone Marrow Transplant. 2004;33:871–873.
34. Benrashid M, Moyers K, Mohty M, Savani BN. Vitamin D deficiency, autoimmunity, and graft-versus-host-disease risk: implication for preventive therapy. Exp Hematol. 2012;40(4):263–267. Epub 2012 Jan 17.
35. Sproat L, Bolwell B, Rybicki L, et al. Vitamin D level after allogeneic hematopoietic stem cell transplant. Biol Blood

Marrow Transplant. 2011;17(7):1079–1083. Epub 2010 Dec 27.

36. Simmons JH, Chow EJ, Koehler E, et al. Significant 25-hydroxyvitamin D deficiency in child and adolescent survivors of acute lymphoblastic leukemia: treatment with chemotherapy compared with allogeneic stem cell transplant. Pediatr Blood Cancer. 2011;56(7):1114–1119.
37. Robien K, Strayer L, Majhail N, et al. Vitamin D status among long-term survivors of hematopoietic cell transplantation. Bone Marrow Transplant. 2011;46(11):1472–1479. Epub 2011 Jan 17.
38. Dawson-Hughes B, Mithal A, Bonjour JP, et al. IOF position statement: vitamin D recommendations for older adults. Osteoporos Int. 2010;21(7):1151–1154.
39. Ross AC, Manson JE, Abrams SA, et al. The 2011 report on dietary reference intakes for calcium and vitamin D from the Institute of Medicine: what clinicians need to know. J Clin Endocrinol Metab. 2011;96(1):53–58.
40. Holick M. Vitamin D: importance in the prevention of cancers, type 1 diabetes, heart disease, and osteoporosis. Am J Clin Nutr. 2004;79(3):362–371.
41. Onakpoya IJ, Perry R, Zhang J, Ernst E. Efficacy of calcium supplementation for management of overweight and obesity: systematic review of randomized clinical trials. Nutr Rev. 2011;69(6):335–343.
42. Bolland MJ, Grey A, Avenell A, et al. Calcium supplements with or without vitamin D and risk of cardiovascular events: reanalysis of the Women's Health Initiative limited access dataset and meta-analysis. BMJ. 2011;342:d2040.
43. Lewis JR, Calver J, Zhu K, et al. Calcium supplementation and the risks of atherosclerotic vascular disease in older women: results of a 5-year RCT and a 4.5-year follow-up. J Bone Miner Res. 2011;26(1):35–41.
44. Clemens MR, Ladner C, Ehninger G, et al. Plasma vitamin E and beta-carotene concentrations during radiochemotherapy preceding bone marrow transplantation. Am J Clin Nutr. 1990;51(2):216–219.
45. Bhuvarahamurthy V, Balasubramanian N, Govindasamy S. Effect of radiotherapy and chemoradiotherapy on circulating antioxidant system of human uterine cervical carcinoma. Mol Cell Biochem. 1996;158:17–23.
46. Jonas CR, Puckett AB, Jones DP, et al. Plasma antioxidant status after high-dose chemotherapy: a randomized trial of parenteral nutrition in bone marrow transplantation patients. Am J Clin Nutr. 2000;72:181–189.
47. Breummer B, Patterson RE, Cheney C, et al. The association between vitamin C and vitamin E supplement use before hematopoietic stem cell transplant and outcomes to two years. J Am Diet Assoc. 2003;103:982–990.
48. Lawenda BD, Kelly KM, Ladas EJ, et al. Should supplemental antioxidant administration be avoided during chemotherapy and radiation therapy? J Natl Cancer Inst. 2008; 100(11):773–783. Epub 2008 May 27.
49. Weisdorf-Schindele S, Schwarzenberg SJ. Nutritional support of hematopoietic cell recipients. In: Blume KG, Forman SJ, Appelbaum FR (eds). Thomas' Hematopoietic Cell Transplantation. Malden, MA: Wiley-Blackwell Publishing Ltd, 2007; pp. 883–893.
50. Antila HM, Salo MS, Kirvelä O, et al. Serum trace element concentrations and iron metabolism in allogeneic bone marrow transplant recipients. Ann Med. 1992;24(1):55–59.
51. Majhail NS, Lazarus HM, Burns LJ. A prospective study of iron overload management in allogeneic hematopoietic cell transplantation survivors. Biol Blood Marrow Transplant. 2010;16(6):832–837.
52. Armand P, Kim HT, Cutler CS, et al. Prognostic impact of elevated pretransplantation serum ferritin in patients undergoing myeloablative stem cell transplantation. Blood. 2007;109(10):4586–4588.
53. Pullarkat V, Blanchard S, Tegtmeier B, et al. Iron overload adversely affects outcome of allogeneic hematopoietic cell transplantation. Bone Marrow Transplant. 2008;42(12): 799–805.
54. Witkowski M, Hubert J, Mazur A. Methods of assessment of magnesium status in humans: a systematic review. Magnes Res. 2011;24(4):163–180.

CHAPTER 33
Daily routines and guidelines: driving, infection isolation, masks, food/diet, activities, exercise, pets, sun exposures, and others

Angela M Woods
National VA Transplant Program, Bone Marrow/ Stem Cell Transplant Service, Veterans Affairs Medical Center, Nashville, TN, USA

Introduction

If multiple transplant centers were questioned, you may receive various answers to questions regarding transplant precautionary routines and guidelines. Many worry about the first 100 days, but as transplant and infectious disease medicine improves, that time period can be smoother and uneventful as patients are kept close to the transplant center and observed carefully. Sometimes the complications appear for the first time after they go home, which is usually after day 90–100 for an allogeneic transplant patient and day 30 for an autologous transplant patient. As the centers try to help manage these new or continued problems such as graft-versus-host disease (GVHD), infection, or their cancer/disease, many issues are being discussed and managed by their local team or primary care providers. Repetitive instruction and education are attempted prior to leaving the transplant centers to ensure they are more prepared once they go home. But many times these topics become more important once they have less frequent visits with their transplant center. Often, questions regarding their daily living are forgotten before the transplant because the worries are focused on their chances of survival, disease, chemotherapy, and the unknown of the transplant procedure itself. Some are thinking they are going to have just another round of chemotherapy and plan to lose their hair yet again. While others have never had the chemotherapy experience of gastrointestinal distress, fevers, and bleeding and cannot imagine losing their hair. Some know all about the neutropenic precautions from having myelodysplastic syndrome or from their acute leukemia treatments, while others have never experienced such treatments or complications having chronic myeloid leukemia or myelofibrosis. So some patients focus on different aspects before and after transplant. Education, even if repetitive, is crucial.

Posttransplant follow-up

Autologous stem cell transplant patients (received their own stem cells as a rescue from high-dose chemotherapy) who are not on maintenance therapy (drugs to treat their disease or trying to prevent it from returning) or any therapy for relapsed (disease that has returned) or

Blood and Marrow Transplantation Long-Term Management: Prevention and Complications, First Edition. Edited by Bipin N Savani.

progressive (growing) disease are generally instructed and educated to follow the same guidelines from engraftment (when bone marrow stem cells start producing new blood cells) to day 100 posttransplant, which are discussed below. Allogeneic transplant patients (received stem cells from another person) have lower immune systems for longer. This high-risk timeframe is usually 6 months or longer. It is also recommended to check all patients' white blood cells with differential, immunoglobulins, and T and B cell subsets at day 100 to obtain a partial glimpse at their immune system, as some autologous patients may also have an extended immunosuppression (decreased immune system) for various reasons. But in general, autologous patients are not on immunosuppressive therapy, such as cyclosporine or tacrolimus, as the allogeneics continue, which decreases their immune system and makes them more susceptible to infections. Depending on the allogeneic patient's disease and GVHD status, the weaning of these drugs may start at day 100–180, or the drugs may continue indefinitely if they have experienced significant GVHD. Allogeneic patients are also more likely to be treated with drugs such as thymoglobulin that have extensive, longer term immunosuppression. Even though autologous patients continue to have an impaired immune system, they are not as immunocompromised as the post-allogeneic transplant patients, whom sometimes have almost no immune system to help fight infections. This is why allogeneic patients continue preventative medications for bacterial, fungal, and viral infections for a longer period of time. (If a post-autologous patient is on any kind of active treatment/chemotherapy, infection precautions should be taken for bacterial, fungal, and viral infections, as their active disease places their immune system at risk along with their risk of the previous and current treatment/therapy.) Any allogeneic patient still taking immunosuppressive therapy, such as cyclosporine or tacrolimus, still has a low immune system even if it is years after the transplant, so precautions should be taken. If a patient is on steroids, they are very high risk for many complications, including rare infections, so maintain high alert for all precautions, and transplant centers should be called for any questions. High-risk patients also include neutropenic and thrombocytopenic patients. Posttransplant blood counts can be affected by many factors, such as infections and GVHD. Continue strict precautions for infection if a patient is neutropenic (absolute neutrophil count less than 1000 cells/mm^3) such as frequent hand washing, wearing masks, avoiding crowds, no suppositories or rectal manipulation, avoiding frequent acetaminophen, which can hide a fever, and continue a neutropenic diet. If thrombocytopenic, remember to use only electric razors, use gentle dental care, avoid blowing nose, prevent falls/injuries, and avoid using ibuprofen or aspirin.

Infection prevention

Posttransplant patients need to avoid sick people and wash their hands frequently. Hand sanitizers should be used when soap and water are not available. Both autologous and allogeneic patients do not start their repeat vaccines until usually 1 year posttransplant (the influenza vaccine is usually started earlier, at approximately 6 months and especially if it is influenza season, then continued yearly) when it is believed that their immune system is recovered enough to make antibodies from immunizations/vaccines and redevelop that protection. These can be given by any clinician's office or hospital, and a list/schedule should be available from the patient's transplant center. Until they achieve immunity again, these patients need to remember that they may not have the protection of their previous immunizations/vaccines as those antibodies are affected from the high-dose chemotherapy they received as their conditioning/preparative regimen for their transplant/stem cell rescue. They can acquire these illnesses as usually contracted, but they can also become infected with these diseases from people (usually children) that have received live vaccines. As someone with a low immune system that has lost their antibodies, they can actually become infected with the illness within the live vaccine. So it is always best to avoid these people/children for 2–3 weeks after they receive a live vaccine (this is recommended until the transplant patient achieves immunity from their own repeat vaccines). Parents, of any children that will be exposed to a low immune system patient, should discuss with their pediatrician if vaccines are live. In general, these patients should wear any surgical-type mask (N95 masks are not necessary for daily, routine use) in public places (especially the hospital). They are taught to keep these masks on unless they are in a private room with known staff, family, or friends (or outside in open air away from strangers, like when walking for exercise). A mask is not proven to prevent all infections, but this does act as a barrier and more importantly keeps others distanced from the patient. The mask guideline is loosened as patients are further out from transplant as their immune systems recover and their medications are discontinued. When in doubt, wear the mask. Autologous patients, whom have no active disease/cancer and are not on any treatment that can affect their immune system, should wear the mask for 100 days. If it is still the cold/flu season, they should still wear it to places such as church and to hospital/medical appointments. Allogeneic patients should wear it for at least 6 months or until off all immunosuppressive medications; again, blood work can be assessed to see whether their immune system is strengthening.

Routines after transplantation

After transplant, there needs to be a daily goal of planning ahead. Go out in public at less popular times. Complete errands such as grocery shopping when stores are least busy, so do not shop at a mall on a weekend. Go out to eat for late lunches and early dinners. Ask if you can be seated in the most private area, if you are wearing your mask, they will most likely not question your request. Of course, you will need to remove your mask when eating. Do not go to the movies on Friday night or weekends, but feel free to attend when less crowded, such as weekday matinees. Anywhere you go, if you arrive and there is a visible crowd of people or a full parking lot, please change your plans or stay in the car while your family/friends go inside. Try to avoid cruise ships as long as possible, and preferably until after vaccines. Large concerts and athletic events should also be cautioned against for at least 6 months or until off immunosuppressive medications. Vigilance should be used for places such as church. Many patients choose to avoid church for approximately 6 months as they feel that their church is too crowded or that they would have difficulty avoiding kisses, especially during influenza season. Others feel comfortable sitting in the back of the church or up in a balcony, while wearing their mask to remind their fellow church members to be cautious. Either way, it is always recommended to wash hands frequently and use hand sanitizer for when a sink is unavailable.

How family and friends help prevent infectious complications

These patients are always encouraged to visit with family and friends, unless family/friends are currently ill or have been in close contact with an ill person (such as caring for their ill child or grandchild). A good plan is to speak with family and friends via phone and discuss this topic before their arrival, and that should prevent surprises. When going to public places, you do not have the benefit of speaking to all those people before your exposure, as they may have a contagious virus. A good custom is to have all friends/family wash their hands on arrival, and then visit as you normally would (and wash hands as you and they normally would; that is, after using the bathroom or blowing nose and before eating). If someone is ill or caring for an ill person, such as their child with a virus, they should postpone their visit for at least 1 week. More caution should be taken with young children, as they spread germs more easily. So pay close attention to any new symptom; then, when discussing their illness with a healthcare provider, always ask if the illness is contagious and for how long. If a patient's family member within the household becomes ill, sometimes there may not be somewhere else for them to stay during this illness to prevent transmission. So they need to be as cautious as they are able. Sleep in different beds if possible, use disinfectants/antibacterial cleaners/sanitizers, frequent hand washing for all, and avoid kissing, and so on. As always, check temperature for any new symptoms which could be related to infection, such as chills, feeling feverish or hot, headache, sore throat, cough, sinus drainage or congestion, runny nose, sneezing, nausea, vomiting, diarrhea, burning with urination. Bathing daily can help prevent bacterial infections, as we have bacteria that live on our skin. Family and friends want a good outcome and want to know what they can do to help, so please educate and train them on how to prevent infections.

It is recommended that friends/family of posttransplant patients receive the (non-live injection/shot is preferred) influenza vaccine (unless contraindicated). No one can develop influenza from the flu shot. Some develop symptoms as their body reacts to the vaccine, making antibodies. If someone truly develops influenza after the flu shot, it was a strain not covered by the vaccine, as the vaccine does not protect from all strains of the virus.

Home environment

Patients with low immune systems are more at risk to contract viral and bacterial infections, and most patients are aware of these. Also, patients have heard of yeast infections, but they are not usually familiar with infections such as aspergillus and mucor, which can be very difficult to treat. Normal people with normal immune systems come in contact with these organisms frequently and no infection is developed. When the immune system is impaired, exposure to fungus can cause an infection. So the higher risk behaviors that can place you in contact with these infections are avoided, such as dusting, vacuuming, construction (tearing down walls, etc.), grass cutting, digging in the dirt, baling hay, planting flowers, and chopping wood. Tell patients to avoid fungus, mold, and mildew. So you should not strip down old wallpaper in your basement or repair that water damage in the ceiling. Now sometimes there are circumstances such as someone living alone and not having someone to help them dust/vacuum/clean; just ask them to wear a mask and gloves, but it is always best if someone could deep clean the house before they come home from the transplant. People ask if they need to get their air ducts or carpets cleaned, but this is not necessary unless you feel they are overly dirty or there has been a known problem. Sometimes an allogeneic patient has not been able to cut the grass for years because they have been on immunosuppressive medications for GVHD. In circumstances like this, sometimes these patients beg to participate in these tasks because it makes them feel normal again. This should be discussed with their transplant team and sometimes in these circumstances they may be allowed with a mask, if they are on low-dose immunosuppression. Smoking of tobacco, cigarettes, cigars, and marijuana is prohibited indefinitely due to the fungal pneumonia risk, as those leaves may contain fungus that can infect a person with a low immune system. Fungal pneumonia is difficult to treat and can be fatal. Patients are usually prescribed medications to prevent bacterial, viral, and fungal infections when infection risk is highest. Patients should try to follow all infection precautions for 6 months or until off immunosuppressive medications, unless discussed with their transplant team first.

Issues such as living arrangements and conditions of a home should be discussed and addressed pretransplant. Issues include living alone and clarifying who is available to help cook, clean, transport to appointments, and so on. How far away does the patient live from a willing caregiver and how far is the nearest clinician and hospital? Frequently, people live in close proximity to a clinic, lab, infusion clinic, and emergency room but at a much farther distance from their transplant center or metro hospital. This scenario can be successful as long as there is open communication with their transplant center and hematologist/oncologist. It should also be addressed pretransplant whether the patient has electricity/gas for cooking, heat/air conditioning, plus clean water with working plumbing. There should also be discussions about who lives in the house with them (any children or pets), along with potential physical hurdles such as living on the fourth floor with no elevator. Children place them at higher risks for infection, so greater care needs to be taken, along with future planning for family/friends to help out when children are sick in the hope of preventing spreading to the patient with a low immune system. Pets are allowed, but some need more caution than others; see below.

Exercise and activities

Exercise is somewhat limited while an external catheter, such as a Hickman or Groshong, is still in place. Guidelines given at placement should still be followed, such as with heavy lifting. Once the catheter is out, exercise is mostly based on how the patient feels (energy level) and it is best to proceed slow and steady. Start out slower and with less weight, even if they were previously very active. Pulled muscles and injuries can happen. Even fatigue and sore muscles can set them back and discourage them. Walking is the best exercise to start and continue, which can be done even if a catheter is still present. This is recommended pre-, peri-, and posttransplant. Walking is great exercise. It strengthens lungs and muscles. This can help prevent pneumonia and muscle weakness, which can be very important with prolonged admissions or steroid use for GVHD. Walking is also good for improving sleep and blood sugar. Patients should walk twice every day, then increase distance every few days. This may start in the hospital hallway or as one block in the city. Always encourage stopping for a break if needed; watch for benches to sit on for rest. Getting mildly winded is expected, and walking should resume after a rest. Plus with time, their stamina and energy will improve and so will their breathing/lungs. If the patient has trouble breathing, shortness of breath, or chest pain, this should be reported to their medical team immediately. Any new breathing symptom at rest (not induced by activity such as walking) should also be reported. Most patients find that they cannot walk as far as they previously did comfortably, so they must start at a shorter distance and slowly increase back to their prior level. This happens as the activity level decreases during chemotherapy and hospitalizations, infections, and complications. Many also find climbing stairs more difficult, so this is avoided until their energy, stamina, and muscle strength increases. This can be a proud moment for them, when they can take the stairs again. The thigh muscles tend to weaken first and more often when patients have taken steroids as part of their treatment. These muscles are important when climbing stairs and standing up from a chair. Treadmills can be used instead of outdoor walking, especially if weather and sun exposure are concerns. Elliptical machines are a popular next step for many people. Then patients can add light free weights. Sexual activity is allowed once energy permits, barring platelets are greater than 50 000/μL. A condom is recommended to prevent bacterial or yeast infection exposure from their partner for 6 months or until off of immunosuppressive medications. Swimming is not recommended when they have an external catheter such as a Hickman, Groshong, or a peripherally inserted central catheter, as infection is a risk. Later, when swimming is allowed, a well-maintained pool owned by a family or friend is recommended over a public pool. A public pool along with swimming in a river, lake, or ocean should wait until 6 months after transplant or off immunosuppressive medications. Do not drink water or swim with open wounds. Of course, remember sun limitations (covered below). Other common activity questions include hunting and fishing. Both are acceptable. The patient should avoid touching the bait, such as worms, along with handling the animal or fish itself. Friends and family should assist the patient. Gloves should be used along with using a hand sanitizer frequently. Again, follow sun exposure recommendations.

Sun exposure

Sun exposure is a concern for all allogeneic patients (no limitations specific to autologous). Patients are instructed that sun exposure can cause or trigger GVHD, so precautions should be taken. They do not have to get burned for this to happen. This applies for all patients, all ethnicities, and skin colors. After transplant, this continues indefinitely, as there is no definite date that GVHD risk disappears. Many of these posttransplant precautions are not exact, and this is another one. We know exposure can cause changes in the skin which can trigger GVHD, but there is no definite amount of time of sun exposure, as we are all different. This is still a concern for dark complexion patients, as again you do not have to experience sunburn for these changes to occur. Outdoor walks are still encouraged, as are other short amounts of time outside, as long as sun protection is enforced. Outdoor activities are better in early and late daylight hours, as during midday the sun's rays are strongest. Sunscreen must be applied every day, even on cloudy days (not needed on skin covered by SPF (sun protection factor) clothing if worn). Snow also reflects the sun's rays just as water and sand. Patients are taught to make daily habits to prevent complications related to sun exposure. After bathing daily, apply moisturizing lotion (dry skin can also cause complications), and then apply sunscreen. According to the American Academy of Dermatology, sunscreen should be at least 30 SPF, protect against UVA and UVB rays, and be water resistant. It should also be *para*-aminobenzoic acid free. Sunscreen should be applied generously to all exposed areas and under thin clothing such as a T-shirt. A hat is encouraged to help protect their head, but sunscreen is still recommended for their face/neck and their ears, especially if it is a baseball cap. Remember to apply to hands also. Many also chose to wear long sleeves and pants to protect their skin and decrease the amount of sunscreen needed daily. In addition, many are increasing their coverage confidence by purchasing SPF clothing. This is not mandatory because of the cost, just convenient. These patients cannot sunbathe. They must be aware of their location to the equator, as those patients must be extra careful.

Depending on climate and time of year, many patients must time their activities to be early morning or evening, such as with outdoor walking. Exposure should be limited to 30–60 min per block, with sunscreen. Otherwise they should not be participating in outdoor activities where they are not completely protected in the shade (along with sunscreen). Reapplying sunscreen is recommended after 2 h or excessive sweating or swimming. Be aware that patients have experienced too much sun exposure riding in a car or covered by an umbrella. As you would guess because the sun provides vitamin D, most of these patients require a vitamin D supplement owing to the lack of sun exposure and use of sunscreen.

Driving after transplantation

Driving is part of our daily life that many of us take for granted. We drive to work, for errands, and wherever we choose. Once you have cancer and have to face your own mortality, the little things in life become more appreciated. Many of these patients have not driven for months because of treatment-related symptoms, side effects, and complications. The leukemia patients have spent months in the hospital before their transplant. So after transplant, some are more eager than others. They want to know, when can I drive? They want to go shopping or maybe just take a ride to explore. They could do this at the transplant center, but they were always the passenger. They commonly feel that they have lost their independence because their medical team and caregivers have made most of their decisions for an extended period. As a general rule, there is no driving for the first 100 days for the allogeneic patients. That gives time to see how they tolerate medications such as cyclosporine and tacrolimus, which can cause tremors. This also gives them time to regain energy from fatigue, which can be from chemotherapy or complications such as infections and GVHD. Sometimes patients forget that driving requires energy, strength, coordination, and quick responses. They must be able to check their blind spots quickly and make fast decisions. One of the best judges to help decide if they are ready is their caregiver. They have been with them for 3 months and seen their strength, coordination, and cognition throughout the day, every day. Usually they know if they are ready or if it should be postponed a little longer. Autologous patients could be ready at 30–60 days. But there are some that will not have the physical strength for several months, and this should be decided by a healthcare professional as with any other medical or elderly patient. Remember that patients can also have weak muscles from steroids and neuropathy from previous chemotherapy or diabetes mellitus. If medication levels, such as cyclosporine or tacrolimus, are followed and patients take these drugs consistently on a tight schedule as they are instructed, then these levels should remain stable. Always remember that new medications can alter these levels, which can affect their tremor and other side effects, especially starting antifungals. So levels should be checked more often in these circumstances, along with any change in kidney function which also affects levels. Also, if immunosuppressive drugs are changed, such as cyclosporine to tacrolimus or vice versa, seizures can happen rarely, so they should not drive for at least 2 weeks after this change or until levels are stabilized. When someone is on high-dose steroids, it is most likely causing some side effects such as blurred vision, insomnia, fluid retention, rapid weight gain, muscle weakness, and possibly high blood sugar or blood pressure. Most likely driving should be postponed until the steroid dose is low and better tolerated. If there is any doubt, do not drive. Remind patients that they should assess how they feel every time they get behind the wheel. Do I feel tired? Do I feel shaky? Once driving is deemed safe by your medical team to attempt, remember that safety is important for you, plus other people out on the streets. So please take a practice drive in a parking lot with someone else in your car first.

Pets after transplantation

Pets are our best friends and considered family members for countless patients, so it is usually encouraged to keep pets and maintain these relationships. Remember that any pet can potentially transmit an infection just as a human, especially if precautions are not taken. So a general recommendation is that pets are taken to a veterinarian for yearly, comprehensive visits and receive recommended immunizations. People can contract some of their illnesses, such as parvovirus. Patients' low immune systems should be explained to the veterinarians. Always remember to wash hands frequently and avoid animal kisses on the face. In general, it is best to avoid contact with any feces, but especially cats' and birds' feces as these can cause serious infections. Patients should not clean litter boxes or bird cages, and these boxes/cages should be kept away from the patient, such as in a room that the patient does not frequently visit. If possible, birds should be cared for by a friend/family member at another location owing to higher infection risks. Avoid close exposure to hay and barns or petting zoos. Horses can be rode and touched, but someone else should clean barns and work with hay.

Cooking and food habits

For some, cooking is a hobby. They enjoy going out to eat and experimenting with new foods. Most people with normal immune systems can eat risky foods frequently, and they may only experience diarrhea, if anything. Patients after transplant with lowered immune systems must be more careful as they could get very ill and require hospitalization or even die if they ingest certain bacteria. When patients are neutropenic (low neutrophils/white blood cells important for fighting infection), neutropenic (sometimes called low microbial) diets are followed. A neutropenic diet prohibits raw fruits and vegetables that are unprotected by a tough, thick skin, in addition to high-risk foods discussed below. This is to avoid bacteria (and also pesticides). So oranges, bananas, and melons (washed and peeled by caregiver) are allowed, in addition to canned/jarred fruits/vegetables. It is safe to eat cooked fruits and vegetables and pasteurized juice. Even if not neutropenic, all fresh fruits and vegetables should be washed well under running water with a brush before cutting or peeling (cleaners and detergents are not necessary). This prevents the spread of bacteria while cutting and peeling. Transplant patients should try to avoid food-borne illnesses by taking precautions such as heating up leftovers well to kill any bacteria (to at least 165 °F). Now some may choose not to eat leftovers at all, but it is always best to throw them out once >24 h old. After reheating leftovers, throw away food that still has not been eaten; so do not reheat twice. It is best to avoid buffets as germs can spread with coughing and sneezing and unwashed hands, but there is also a concern that the food may not be kept cold or hot enough, which can cause an illness. Transplant patients should avoid ingesting high-risk foods, which are more likely to cause illness/food poisoning. High-risk foods include raw or undercooked eggs and meat. Many patients worry this means they have to eat their meat dry and burnt, but some meats are still pink even though they have been cooked to the minimum temperature. So cook by temperature not color. Now ground meat can be more likely to contain bacteria, so it should always be cooked well; for example, ground beef should be gray. Always remember to wash the thermometer with hot water and soap after use. So if eating out in public, it is safest to order all meat well done, as you cannot be sure that they are using a thermometer. Also remember that some foods have raw eggs as a standard ingredient; for instance, raw cookie dough, aioli, mousse, hollandaise sauce, and homemade Caesar dressing. Raw fish, sushi, or ceviche is considered a high-risk food, so it should be avoided. Great care should be taken by those that are cooking and preparing food for these patients. Hands should be washed well before cooking. Contamination from raw meat, poultry, seafood, or uncooked eggs should be prevented by cleaning hands, utensils, and surfaces after contact with these foods. Cleaning requires soap and water or an antibacterial cleaner. There is a web site managed by the US Department of Health and Human Services at www.foodsafety.gov which can teach people how to safely cook at home. Their basics include washing hands frequently, always for at least 20 s with soap and running water. Always wash hands after contact with raw meat, poultry, seafood, or uncooked eggs and before touching anything else. These foods should also be separated from other foods while shopping and transporting home from the store, along with storage in the refrigerator. Packages can leak. Use two bags, supplied at the store in the meat section, to keep meats separate from other food in your cart and refrigerator. Do not store dairy products on the doors of refrigerators, as they may not stay cool enough. Follow expiration dates. Never thaw or marinate food at room temperature. Label foods with dates. Do not eat food left out for more than 2 h at room temperature. Well water needs to be boiled. Avoid unpasteurized dairy products (this may include cheese queso or moldy cheeses) or honey. Deli meats and hot dogs are safe if cooked until steaming. Certain nuts (factory/commercial nuts are safe) and soft-serve ice cream, along with fountain drinks, uncooked spices, tea made with cold water, and raw mushrooms, can also be higher risk foods. Many patients avoid fast food, but always eat at restaurants that look and feel clean. You can

Table 33.1 Posttransplant routines and guidelines

	Autologous	Allogeneic
Driving	Discouraged for 30 days posttransplant or until strength has returned	Discouraged for 100 days posttransplant or until strength has returned
Sun exposure	No definitive limitations Sunscreen suggested to prevent skin cancer	Must limit sun exposure daily Must use sunscreen daily All ethnicities
Masks Surgical-type masks (N95 masks are not necessary for daily, routine use)	At least 100 days	At least 6 months or until off all immunosuppressive medications
Vaccines Follow chart provided by transplant center	Influenza at 6 months posttransplant if flu season Rest of vaccines start at 1 year post transplant	Influenza at 6 months posttransplant if flu season Rest of vaccines start at 1 year post transplant

read their health department score, which should always be posted. No herbal supplements. Because there are so many factors and variants that affect a situation, it is hard to discuss every situation. High-risk situations and foods may harm one person and not the next; so when in doubt, just avoid it. The risk may be small or rare, but the patient's safety and health is the ultimate goal.

Summary

Given that there are no published guidelines and protocols on this subject, therefore, this chapter offers practical advice and outlines our personal approaches in posttransplant routines for long-term survivors after transplantation. This is summarized in Table 33.1.

CHAPTER 34
Caregivers of long-term survivors

Elizabeth Wulff-Burchfield

Division of Hematology/Oncology, Department of Medicine, Vanderbilt University Hospital, Nashville, TN, USA

Introduction

By the time that a patient crosses the threshold of a transplant center, he and his caregiver have undoubtedly already endured numerous challenges concerning his presenting disease process. Not only have they suffered the sadness, fear, and anger of his initial diagnosis, but they have also endured treatment for this condition. Treatment for the presenting condition is followed by a lengthy and anxiety-provoking hematopoietic stem cell transplant (HSCT) evaluation, only to enter a new phase of high-stakes treatments with no guarantee of cure. The relief of having a matched stem cell donor is coupled with the fear of the consequences of transplant, both short- and long-term. A significant portion of the pretransplant evaluation revolves around potential candidates' social and caregiver support, a valid initiative given that there is data demonstrating that patients with better informal caregiver support have improved survival and progression-free survival [1]. Furthermore, patients and caregivers are frequently required to move to temporary housing near the transplant center, far from any other social support. In short, even the uncomplicated HSCT course places significant demands upon caregivers, frequently resulting in adverse mental and physical health consequences. In spite of this, a majority of HSCT patient caregivers still regard that their role as a caregiver is rewarding and meaningful [2].

HSCT caregivers are unique among all caregivers

HSCT recipients have a unique set of challenges and mandate having a primary caregiver to provide support throughout the course of their illness and transplant. Unlike caregivers for patients with chronic or progressive illnesses such as dementia, amyotrophic lateral sclerosis, or mental illness, allogeneic HSCT patients maintain a chance for cure and, thus, they and their caregivers experience an unpredictable course over time. Patients undergoing HSCT have a lengthy treatment course characterized by periods of critical illness and periods of relative health. To some extent, this is shared by all cancer patients, who frequently have periods of worsened physical and mental health during cancer therapy. Caregiver distress is generally associated with worse physical or mental health on the part of the patient [3], so caregivers of all cancer patients, including HSCT patients, likely experience waxing and waning symptoms and levels of distress. All cancer patients can, at times, experience the stresses of determining eligibility for various treatments, although this process is typically not formalized for non-HSCT cancer patients and often retains some degree of flexibility. However, one notable difference between cancer patients not treated with HSCT is that they do not necessarily undergo the stresses associated with relocation to a transplant center and lengthy inpatient hospitalizations required to complete a transplant.

Blood and Marrow Transplantation Long-Term Management: Prevention and Complications, First Edition. Edited by Bipin N Savani.

Another group of caregivers with comparable hardships to HSCT caregivers is caregivers for solid organ transplant recipients. This patient population shares some key attributes with the HSCT population, in that patients have been treated for life-threatening illnesses for months or years prior to transplant, they have undergone a rigorous pretransplant workup, and transplant is typically the only chance for cure of their illness. Caregivers for both HSCT [4] and solid organ transplant [5, 6] recipients have been demonstrated to have the highest levels of distress in the pretransplant period with slow improvement after transplant. However, one major difference between HSCT and solid organ transplant recipients is that solid organ transplant patients typically experience the peak of adverse symptoms and poor health immediately prior to transplantation; thus, transplantation itself typically results in significant relief of symptoms. In contrast, HSCT candidates are usually not experiencing the most severe period of illness immediately prior to transplantation, so their HSCT typically brings about new and more severe symptoms than that which they experienced preceding their transplant. Thus, the transplant process itself typically brings about a new wave of caregiving tasks and responsibilities. Data demonstrate that the more personal the caregiving tasks are, the greater are the levels of caregiver distress [7], so new health problems such as graft-versus-host disease (GVHD) likely result in more intense degrees of caregiver burden. Caregivers for HSCT recipients are an essential part of the transplant process and have proven themselves to be unique among all groups of caregivers, so it is fitting that transplant centers have begun to attend to the issues of this population.

Informal caregivers of HSCT patients frequently experience distress

Informal or family caregivers of HSCT patients frequently experience burnout, distress, and self-reported diminished quality of life. In fact, the prevalence of caregiver distress in this population has been demonstrated to be as high as 88% [8], although most estimates are that approximately one-third of caregivers experience significant distress [9]. This reported rate has been demonstrated in multiple studies to be comparable to, if not higher than, that of the HCST patients themselves [2, 9]. Among the psychological sequelae, HSCT caregivers have been shown to experience anxiety, depression, and decreased motivation. Some portion of their anxiety appears to be related to living a life characterized by uncertainty. One descriptive study by Eilers et al. characterized the HSCT caregiving experience as "riding a roller coaster in the dark" [10]. Despite this, levels of anxiety tend to peak prior to transplantation and improve during the posttransplant period, although there is little data exploring prevalence of anxiety later that 1 year posttransplantation [4, 11, 12].

Depression appears to be an even more widespread problem with some evidence of persistence into the posttransplant period. Multiple studies have demonstrated that caregivers of HSCT patients frequently develop depressive symptoms or major depressive disorder [2, 8, 9, 12–14]. One study demonstrated that the proportion of caregivers with depression is not significantly different from the proportion of survivors with depression, but that both are significantly greater than age- and gender-matched controls [9]. Despite the high proportion of caregivers with depression and the higher proportion of caregivers with depressive symptoms, caregivers do not appear to transfer their depression to patients [8]. It appears that caregiver depression is greatest pretransplantation and improves slowly over time, beginning in the immediate posttransplant period [8, 12]. There is growing recognition of the risk of depression amongst all caregivers, but, despite the fact that caregivers for HSCT patients have similar rates of depression, they not appear to seek care for their depression with the same frequency as patients do [9].

Caregivers of HSCT recipients also experience multiple physical symptoms and adverse health outcomes. Fatigue appears to be the most commonly reported symptom, and this has been shown to persist until after the acute phase of stem cell transplantation [12, 15]. Sleep disturbance is another commonly reported symptom, as are pain, loss of appetite, and unintentional weight loss [14]. HSCT caregivers have often left their homes to live nearer to transplant centers, which likely means that they are geographically separated from their own healthcare providers and unlikely to seek care for these pervasive symptoms. There is evidence in the literature from caregivers of solid organ transplant recipients that they not only experience the bothersome symptoms outlined above, but also that their health is adversely affected [16]. While there are not yet data to support this assertion, caregivers for HSCT patients likely suffer adverse health outcomes in much the same way.

Reasons for caregiver distress

Just as HSCT patients have many reasons to experience psychosocial distress, there are numerous factors that predispose their caregivers to suffer similar consequences. First, one seemingly ubiquitous trend among multiple groups of caregivers is a positive association between caregiver distress and worse patient health or outcomes. This association has been seen among cancer caregivers, including caregivers for HSCT patients and solid-organ transplant recipients [5, 6, 11, 17]. Recent literature suggests that as many as 40–60% of HSCT recipients may suffer from chronic GVHD, which carries with it significant morbidity [18–20]. By all logic, the high propensity for chronic GVHD in the allogeneic HSCT patient population likely predisposes their caregivers to significant distress related to the health outcomes of patients.

An international trend toward the delivery of more transplant-related care in the outpatient setting places a greater burden of caregiving onto these informal caregivers. In fact, during the outpatient phase of the HSCT, informal caregivers are typically the sole providers of physical and emotional support for the HSCT patients [14, 21]. Despite the myriad of resources available to HSCT patients, one study by Laizner et al. demonstrated that up to one-third of HSCT caregivers report having no assistance [21]. Isolation is a frequently cited contributor to the distress of HSCT caregivers. Despite the fact that multiple studies have demonstrated that social isolation and increasing proportion of outpatient care contribute to the burden of HSCT caregivers, two studies have paradoxically demonstrated that levels of caregiver distress often decline when care is transitioned to the outpatient setting [11, 22].

Two additional causes of caregiver distress are changing family roles associated with assumption of the caregiving role and financial strain associated with the transplant process. These are frequently intertwined, since the majority of allogeneic HSCT patients are male and transplantation often results in these patients' withdrawal from the workforce. This change frequently requires caregivers to take on new involvement with family finances in addition to their new caregiving roles. Family dynamics have been shown to become altered even prior to transplant, as demonstrated by Siston et al. [15]. This change in family dynamics frequently proves challenging for caregivers, who have been shown to make maintenance of typical family dynamics a central priority in addition to their caregiving responsibilities [23]. Unfortunately, a high proportion of caregivers of HSCT patients report marital dissatisfaction beginning in the early transplant period and often extending even into survivorship [24, 25]. To add to the strain, the same caregiving responsibilities that result in shifts in family roles or decreased marital satisfaction often result in an inability for caregivers to work, resulting in significant loss of income throughout the transplant process [26].

Gender-based differences in caregiving experiences

Male and female caregivers have demonstrated to have notably different caregiving experiences and, thus, different degrees and manifestations of distress. Currently, a majority of patients receiving HSCT are male. Given that a majority of caregivers for HSCT patients are spouses or partners, a majority of HSCT caregivers are, consequently, female [11]. Review of the relevant literature reveals that female caregivers report more severe symptoms, both psychological and physical. Specifically, female caregivers report higher levels of stress than male caregivers, more depressive symptoms, and more anxiety [9, 25]. Female HSCT caregivers also report lower marital satisfaction, more sexual problems, and poorer social functioning [9]. The cause for these discrepancies remains unclear. There have been several explanations for this phenomenon proposed by Fife et al. [11]: the first is that if the primary caregiver is male, he typically recruits assistance from outside the family, whereas female primary caregivers are more likely to care for the patient alone. Another theory is that female caregivers may be more empathetic, resulting in more internalization of the patient's own anxiety. In addition to studies in the HSCT literature regarding gender differences and caregiver distress, the non-HSCT cancer literature has also shown that female informal caregivers report higher levels of psychological distress [27, 28].

Assessment of caregiver distress

Numerous tools have been used in the medical literature in the evaluation of HSCT caregiver distress. These tools can be categorized by way of the primary aims of the assessment tool and the targeted audience. The first type of assessment is diagnostic screening tools for mental health problems such as anxiety or depression. These tools are validated for their use in the clinical setting and can amount to diagnosing the condition for which they screen. Examples of this include the State Trait Anxiety Index, and the Beck Depression and Anxiety Inventories. A second type of assessment strives to characterize the mental state of the person taking the survey; examples include the Profile of Mood States, Distress Thermometer, and Life Orientation Test. The final type of assessment is designed to characterize the caregiving experience. This type of assessment focuses on issues specific to the caregiver role, such as psychosocial stress, relationships and roles, and related issues. Examples of this type of assessment tool include the Caregiver Distress Scale, Bakas Caregiving Outcomes Scale, and Zarit Burden Interview. At least 20 different assessment tools have been used in the medical literature to evaluate caregivers of HSCT patients. Most have not been validated for use with this population of caregivers, but they nonetheless provide valuable insight into the functional status and mental state of caregivers for HSCT patients.

Impact of caregiver distress

To date, caregiver distress and burnout have not been proven to affect the outcomes of HSCT patients. However, there are data in other caregiver populations that suggest increased levels of distress are associated with worse patient outcomes. Specifically, increased levels of distress in caregivers for patients with dementia are associated with increased frequency of institutionalization and increased all-cause mortality [29], increased levels of distress in caregivers of patients with bipolar disorder are associated with increased frequency of affective episodes [30], and the overall health and health-related quality of life of caregivers are positively associated with mortality of cardiothoracic transplant recipients [16]. Further study is required in order to determine the impact of caregiver quality of life and distress upon the health outcomes of HSCT recipients.

Conclusions

HSCT is a unique and demanding process with substantial morbidity for both the transplant recipient and their caregiver. Numbers of HSCTs increase every year, as do the number of caregivers available to help these patients. As HSCT becomes a less morbid and mortal process, more effort can and should be expended on determining and attending to the needs of the HSCT caregiver. Although it has not been demonstrated to date, it is highly likely HSCT caregiver distress or burnout impacts HSCT patient outcomes and may represent a useful point of intervention through which we can further improve transplant outcomes.

References

1. Foster LW, McLellan L, Rybicki L, et al. Validating the positive impact of in-hospital lay care-partner support on patient survival in allogeneic BMT: a prospective study. Bone Marrow Transplant. 2013;48(5):671–677.
2. Bishop MM. Psychosocial sequelae of hematopoietic cell transplantation in survivors and caregivers. Biol Blood Marrow Transplant. 2009;15(1 Suppl):29–32.
3. Bevans M, Sternberg EM. Caregiving burden, stress, and health effects. J Am Med Assoc. 2012;307(4):398–403.
4. Beattie S, Lebel S. The experience of caregivers of hematological cancer patients undergoing a hematopoietic stem cell transplant: a comprehensive literature review. Psychooncology. 2011;20(11):1137–1150.
5. Rodrigue JR, Dimitri N, Reed A, et al. Spouse caregivers of kidney transplant patients: quality of life and psychosocial outcomes. Prog Transplant. 2010;20(4):335–342, quiz 343.
6. Rodrigue JR, Dimitri N, Reed A, et al. Quality of life and psychosocial functioning of spouse/partner caregivers before and after liver transplantation. Clin Transplant. 2011;25(2):239–247.
7. Nijboer C, Tempelaar R, Sanderman R, et al. Cancer and caregiving: the impact on the caregiver's health. Psychooncology. 1998;13:3–13.
8. Keogh F, O'Riordan J, McNamara C, et al. Psychosocial adaptation of patients and families following bone marrow transplantation: a prospective, longitudinal study. Bone Marrow Transplant. 1998;22(9):905–911.

9. Bishop MM, Beaumont JL, Hahn EA, et al. Late effects of cancer and hematopoietic stem-cell transplantation on spouses or partners compared with survivors and survivor-matched controls. J Clin Oncol. 2007;25(11):1403–1411.
10. Eilers J, Heermann JA, Wilson ME, Million R. The experience of spouses as informal caregivers for recipients of hematopoietic stem cell transplants. Support Care Cancer. 2009;32(3):15–23.
11. Fife BL, Monahan PO, Abonour R, et al. Adaptation of family caregivers during the acute phase of adult BMT. Bone Marrow Transplant. 2008;43(12):959–966.
12. Foxall MJ, Gaston-Johansson F. Burden and health outcomes of family caregivers of hospitalized bone marrow transplant patients. J Adv Nurs. 1996;24:915–923.
13. Rexilius SJ, Mundt CA, Megel ME, Agrawal S. Therapeutic effects of massage therapy and healing touch on caregivers of patients undergoing autologous hematopoietic stem cell transplant. Depression. 2002;29(3):35–44.
14. Stenberg U, Ruland CM, Miaskowski C. Review of the literature on the effects of caring for a patient with cancer. Psychooncology. 2010;19(10):1013–1025.
15. Siston AK, List MA, Daugherty CK, et al. Psychosocial considerations Psychosocial adjustment of patients and caregivers prior to allogeneic bone marrow transplantation. Bone Marrow Transplant. 2001;27:1181–1188.
16. Myaskovsky L, Posluszny DM, Schulz R, et al. Predictors and outcomes of health-related quality of life in caregivers of cardiothoracic transplant recipients. Am J Transplant. 2012;12(12):3387–3397.
17. Bevans M, Sternberg EM. Caregiving burden, stress, and health effects among family caregivers of adult cancer patients. J Am Med Assoc. 2012;307(4):398–403.
18. Jagasia M, Giglia J, Chinratanalab W, et al. Incidence and outcome of chronic graft-versus-host disease using National Institutes of Health concensus criteria. Biol Blood Marrow Transplant. 2007;1215:1207–1215.
19. Mohty M, Apperley JF. Long-term physiological side effects after allogeneic bone marrow transplantation. Hematology Am Soc Hematol Educ Program. 2010;2010:229–236.
20. Inamoto Y, Flowers MED. Treatment of chronic graft-versus-host disease in 2011. Curr Opin Hematol. 2011; 18(6):414–420.
21. Laizner AM, Yost LMS, Barg FK, McCorkle R. Needs of family caregivers of persons with cancer. Semin Oncol. 1993;9(2):114–120.
22. Grimm PM, Zawacki KL, Mock V, et al. Caregiver responses and needs. an ambulatory bone marrow transplant model. Cancer Pract. 2000;8(3):120–128.
23. Mayer DK, Tighiouart H, Terrin N. A brief report of caregiver needs and resource utilization during pediatric hematopoietic stem cell transplantation. J Pediatr. 2011; 26(4):223–229.
24. Langer SL, Yi JC, Storer BE, Syrjala KL. Marital adjustment, satisfaction and dissolution among hematopoietic stem cell transplant patients and spouses: a prospective, five-year longitudinal investigation. Psychooncology. 2010;19(2): 190–200.
25. Langer SL, Abrams J, Syrjala K. Caregiver and patient marital satisfaction and affect following hematopoietic stem cell transplantation: a prospective, longitudinal investigation. Psychooncology. 2003;12(3):239–253.
26. Meehan KR, Fitzmaurice T, Root L, et al. The financial requirements and time autologous stem cell transplant recipients. J Support Oncol. 2006;4(4):187–190.
27. Kim Y, Loscalzo MJ, Wellisch DK, Spillers RL. Gender differences in caregiving stress among caregivers of cancer survivors. Psychooncology. 2006;15(12):1086–1092.
28. Kim Y, Baker F, Spillers RL. Cancer caregivers' quality of life: effects of gender, relationship, and appraisal. J Pain Symptom Manage. 2007;34(3):294–304.
29. Kuzuya M, Enoki H, Hasegawa J, et al. Impact of caregiver burden on adverse health outcomes in community-dwelling dependent older care recipients. Am J Geriatr Psychiatry. 2011;19:382–91.
30. Perlick DA, Rosenheck RR, Clarkin JF, et al. Impact of family burden and patient symptom status on clinical outcome in bipolar affective disorder e. J Nerv Ment Dis. 2001; 189(1):31–37.

35

CHAPTER 35

Health-related quality of life in adult and pediatric survivors of hematopoietic stem cell transplantation

Margaret Bevans[1] *and Lori Wiener*[2]

[1]LCDR, United States Public Health Service, National Institutes of Health, Clinical Center, Bethesda, MD, USA

[2]Psychosocial Support and Research Program, Center for Cancer Research, Pediatric Oncology Branch, NIH, Bethesda, MD, USA

Introduction

In 2007, the number of cancer survivors in the USA was estimated at 11.7 million, with one of the contributing factors being improved treatments [1]. Hematopoietic stem cell transplantation (HSCT) is one treatment that has seen considerable progress in the past 50 years [2] as a potentially curative treatment for a variety of malignant and nonmalignant conditions. As the number of survivors continues to grow, heath-related quality of life (HRQL), including psychosocial effects, has become a priority in this population. In adults, HRQL outcomes have been well reviewed [3, 4], while in children there remains a considerable gap [5]. Despite the clinical and moral imperative to inform patients and their families of potential late effects, the decision to undergo this potentially curative treatment is seldom affected [6]. Therefore, attentive oncology programs recognize that supportive interventions to manage HRQL and psychosocial effects should begin at the time a decision to undergo HSCT is made, continue through the donor search, and extend throughout long-term follow-up care [7]. This chapter defines HRQL and highlights areas of potential impact for the patient and family throughout the course of treatment and beyond for both pediatric and adult patients and their family members. As some specific differences have been found in factors affecting HRQL in adult and pediatric patients, the chapter will address the age groups separately for purposes of clarity. Positive outcomes along with ongoing challenges are discussed. Suggested screening, assessment, and interventions to improve care are offered.

Quality of life

Quality of life (QOL) is a phrase often used to describe an overall perception by the patient of their recovery and return to a meaningful way of living. The World Health Organization has defined QOL as "an individual's perceptions of their position in life in the context of the culture and value systems in which they live and in relation to their goals, expectations, standards, and concerns." [8] HRQL considers QOL in the context of one's health. HRQL incorporates biologic and physiologic variables, symptom status, functional status (physical, psychological, social/family), general health perception, and overall quality of life [9]. Quality health care, especially

Blood and Marrow Transplantation Long-Term Management: Prevention and Complications, First Edition. Edited by Bipin N Savani.

relative to cancer treatment, requires a comprehensive assessment of the patient, including the HRQL and psychosocial outcomes [10, 11].

HSCT process and procedure

HSCT is an intense and arduous treatment with HRQL effects that vary based on a variety of factors related to the process and procedure itself. Individual and disease-specific factors such as age, co-morbidities, disease, disease stage, and donor availability are embedded in the transplant-specific decision, including additional factors such as HSCT type (autologous or allogeneic), conditioning (myeloablative or reduced intensity), and stem cell source (bone marrow, peripheral blood stem cells, cord blood). These elements of the HSCT process define the transplant experience and influence the patient's HRQL and psychosocial outcomes. For example, despite some similarities between the conditioning regimens of an autologous and allogeneic HSCT, the allogeneic HSCT recipients have a higher level of treatment-related morbidity and mortality and an increased incidence of late-effects (e.g., chronic graft-versus-host disease (c-GVHD)) from long-term immunosuppressive medications and a new donor immune system. In addition, the intensity of the conditioning regimen may vary for allogeneic HSCT recipients. Patients receiving reduced-intensity conditioning will likely have lower levels of physical functioning pre-HSCT; and although their recovery pattern may be similar to those receiving myeloablative conditioning, their absolute level of recovery may differ [12].

Moreover, stem cell source can contribute to the speed of recovery posttransplant with neutrophil recovery 2–4 weeks after HSCT [13]. Overall, engraftment time is shortest with peripheral blood stem cells compared with both bone marrow and cord blood, a factor that can impact treatment-related morbidity and length of hospitalization. In children (<20 years), bone marrow is the leading source of stem cells, with peripheral and cord blood accounting for 27% and 23%, respectively, of allogeneic transplants. In adult patients (≥20 years) peripheral blood is the predominate source, with cord blood use increasing, although still quite low (estimated 5%) [14].

The "phase" of HSCT offers another layer of context that should be considered when trying to understand the factors that affect HRQL in survivors. The pre-HSCT phase includes stressors that (1) surround the decision-making process to consent to a potentially life-threatening procedure, (2) disrupt and often relocate the patient and at least one family member as caregiver, and (3) reveal preexisting psychosocial challenges. For example, if non-compliance exists prior to HSCT, it will warrant consistent assessment during survivorship to prevent serious consequences, including elevated rates of morbidity and mortality, increased use of resources, and inadequate management following HSCT [15]. Post-HSCT management consists of providing interventions aimed at decreasing or managing preexisting psychosocial risk factors. Assessing and addressing potential negative effects on medical outcome are critical prior to transplant [16].

The infusion of hematopoietic stem cells often creates a sense of anxiety for the patient and family although the procedure is generally clinical unremarkable. During the acute phase of the HSCT procedure, the focus is primarily on minimizing toxicities and survival. Therefore, the conditioning regimen and its associated side effects often define the early experience. The symptom experience during the first 100 days is quite extensive [17, 18] and requires complex and specialized management, especially for allogeneic HSCT patients who face the additional complication of acute GVHD. The acute toxicity of the high-dose chemotherapy and/or radiotherapy used in conditioning regimens, along with aversive daily routines and medications administered post cell infusion, require adherence and professional support to limit and manage the treatment-related morbidity, particularly while waiting for count recovery [19].

In the later phases, usually after day 100, there is a focus on reintegration and the "new normal." The resumption of roles in the family and beyond (e.g., student or work) becomes a major focus in this phase. Depending on the course of treatment following HSCT (such as continued treatment with immunosuppressive medications), patients of all ages may have additional limitations related to their resumption of activities. It is also common for patients to transition from the transplant center and specialists to their local hematologist or oncologist provider, which may affect quality of care and subsequently HRQL. Providing a comprehensive summary of the HSCT experience and a suggested plan of follow-up prior to discharge from the transplant center is an important component of quality care [20].

Global heath-related quality of life

Adults

The multidimensional concept of HRQL is a composite measure often including physical, social, role, and psychological or emotional function. Long-term HRQL is an essential component of comprehensive quality care, but understanding the recipient's status prior to HSCT is essential; baseline HRQL can be a strong predictor of HRQL following HSCT [21]. For example, an individual who received less treatment prior to HSCT will likely report better HRQL compared with those who have received more treatment prior to HSCT, specifically those preparing for an autologous HSCT [4].

The pattern of HRQL recovery following HSCT has been well documented in adult recipients [3, 4]. For the majority of recipients, HRQL impairments are greatest during the first 10–30 days [12, 22, 23], with survivors returning to baseline as early as 3 months following HSCT [12, 22, 24, 25]. Recipients who have not yet returned to baseline will likely have gradual improvements over months and even years following HSCT [26, 27], although the trajectory is not likely to be linear. Residual impairment along with "bumps" in recovery, primarily due to c-GVHD [28, 29] and multiple symptoms [30], negatively affect HRQL [31]. Overall, however, survivors often report positive HRQL, which may be a result of a "response shift" in their perspective where HRQL is reframed by their standards or values in the context of their HSCT experience [32, 33]. Optimism (positive attitude) and quality social support are often factors that also predict better global HRQL [32, 34].

Pediatrics

As with adults, there is evidence of a nonlinear recovery of HRQL post-HSCT. However, the significant advances in HSCT pertaining to pharmacologic symptom management may play a role in less emotional trauma and more positive reported HRQL outcomes. Several variables have been shown to positively affect HRQL scores in pediatric HCST survivors, many of which have been described in critical reviews of the literature [35–40]. These include high family cohesion, child's adaptive functioning [41], and lower parental distress prior to transplant [42–46]. Other factors associated with more positive HRQL outcomes include donor versus unrelated donor (for the first year only) [43, 47], low worry, good communication during the acute recovery period [47], younger age [45, 48, 49], male gender [48, 49], African-America race [48], and father raters [50].

Few studies have examined HRQL outcomes longitudinally or beyond 12 months following HSCT in pediatric survivors. The few that have looked at pediatric survivors 5 years posttransplant report reasonably good HRQL, with variables such as psychological distress, cognitive problems, and long-term physical problems negatively affecting HRQL [49, 51]. Yet the final samples in several of these studies were considerably smaller than those at baseline due to either being lost to follow-up or disease-related factors (e.g., relapse) [47], all of which could alter accurate estimates of HRQL. Older age at transplant and female gender have been reported as significant predictors of improved global HRQL at baseline and over time in both self and parent reports [48].

Specific disease factors also play a role in HRQL outcomes. An association has been found between those who have endured high-risk medical interventions prior to transplant (e.g., leukemia, neuroblastoma) with poorer physical and emotional HRQL outcomes years post-SCT [48, 49]. Similar to the adult survivors, moderate to severe GVHD has been consistently associated with worsening HRQL at both early and later time points posttransplant [43, 52, 53].

Physical function

Adults

As with overall HRQL, an awareness of any limitation in physical function that existed prior to HSCT is essential to the assessment and management plan during survivorship. The greatest impact of HSCT on physical function is during the acute phase, specifically through day 100, without regard to the type of transplant or conditioning regimen intensity [4, 12]. Physical functioning following autologous HSCT follows a similar pattern as that following allogeneic HSCT, with a more rapid recovery to baseline beginning at 3 months [4]. Generally, as recipients move beyond day 100 and through the first year, symptoms become less prevalent and physical function returns to baseline [4]. Assuming the absence of persistent late effects, survivors often report a return to baseline prior to 1 year posttransplant [54]. This level of physical function is often similar to that reported by survivors who have received conventional-dose chemotherapy only [55], but below that of the population norm [56, 57].

Symptoms are a significant factor contributing to limitations in physical function [30, 31, 57]. In the presence of late effects such as c-GVHD, symptoms will once again become a major contributing factor to physical function [58, 59]. More specifically, the most prevalent and bothersome symptoms during the survivorship phase are associated with impairments in sexual function and intimacy, fatigue, sleep disturbance, and mood symptoms [30, 31, 54, 57, 60–62]. Other symptoms that can persist years following HSCT, that are often, but not exclusively associated with c-GVHD, include eye problems, musculoskeletal dysfunction, pain, and difficulties with memory and attention [31].

Pediatrics

In children, the largest improvements in overall functioning occur between the 4 and 6 months assessment with continued improvement from 6 to 12 months [43, 63]. Physical function and late effects in pediatric survivors is often documented with different measures compared with adults. The studies that are available in pediatric cohorts have found physical disability rates that range from 7% to 40% depending on whether the outcome was based on clinician report, self-report, or an objective measure of physical performance [37]. Not surprisingly, children who did not survive the first year posttransplant exhibited deterioration in HRQL in the months prior to their death. These trajectories were strikingly different than for survivors [43].

As with adults, symptoms are an important component of physical function and are often generated by late treatment effects years following allogeneic HSCT. Those whose HRQL was already compromised prior to transplant were further impaired immediately following conditioning but improved 4–12 months posttransplant. Chronic GVHD was the most significant factor associated with lower HRQL scores following HSCT [64–66]. One study reported female gender significantly predicted lowered self-reported physical HRQL over time [48]. Nausea and pain during the acute phase of treatment have not been associated with HRQL [47], while psychological distress (i.e., depression and anxiety) has been identified as a strong predictor of functional status [67]. Relapse of disease, which often results in symptoms as well as co-morbidities from intense treatments such as osteopenias, may impact overall physical function.

Psychological function

Adult

Both persistent psychological symptoms and tremendous resiliency in HSCT survivors have been reported [3, 4]. Psychological distress and negative mood states, such as anxiety and depression, have been evaluated most often in HSCT survivors and continue to be of concern 3–5 years following HSCT [54]. High levels of emotional distress before HSCT [68] often continue during HSCT, with slight improvements reported by 3 months [12, 24, 58]. Although negative psychological effects may wane over time, survivors more than 10 years from HSCT report levels of psychological function comparable to controls and cancer survivors who received chemotherapy only [56, 57].

Posttraumatic stress disorder (PTSD) has also been identified in a subset of HSCT survivors. A review reports its presence in both autologous and allogeneic HSCT survivors ranging from 5 to 19% [3]. This diagnosis can include symptom clusters defined as re-experiencing, avoidance, numbing, and arousal that are not commonly assessed during routine HSCT follow-up [69]. However, these reports suggest the presence of PTSD is possible in HSCT survivors and can serve to validate the significant impact of HSCT on the psychological health of survivors.

Additional effects of HSCT on the emotional health of survivors include impaired self-concept [70], self-esteem [71], and self-image [72]. These "nonclinical" concerns are less seldom discussed but may present challenges to survivors during the reintegration into roles within their family or work. Additional factors that place adult HSCT survivors at risk for poor long-term psychological outcomes vary across studies but often include problems involving physical function or symptoms [3]. In addition, more psychological distress has been found in females [34], those who report negative psychological effects during transplantation, individuals with preexisting family conflict [58], those who are not married [58], and those with c-GVHD [58, 73].

Pediatric

Research has tried to identify time points throughout the transplant that may pose greatest psychological distress to pediatric patients. Distress during the acute phase of HSCT has been noted as a possible factor in poor outcomes post-HSCT. A 5-year longitudinal study examining the HRQL of pediatric survivors reported compromised emotional functioning, a high level of worry, and reduced communication during the acute phase of treatment result in a negative impact on HRQL at 1 year posttransplant [47].

Several studies in the pediatric literature have also examined psychological impact post-HSCT and varying results have been reported. Early reports found clinical challenges associated with prolonged engraftment and medically required isolation. These include regressive behavior and an overall sense that the reduction in normal interactions and emotional supports enhances the stress associated with transplant [74, 75]. In these studies, the intensity of symptoms was noted to increase the child's dependence on their parents and other adults and to decrease participation in peer and school-based activities. Dependency and social withdrawal could pose a threat to the accomplishment of developmental milestones. Some later studies have documented symptoms of psychological stress, problems with social adaptation, anxiety, depression, PTSD, and disruptive behavior [41, 43, 47, 76–79], with females and those with more treatment to be at highest risk of depression [49]. In a small qualitative report with adolescent children who survived bone marrow transplant (BMT), youth reported descriptions of their life having been permeated by insecurity, changed body image, and physical and emotional problems [80]. Another qualitative study found that survivors remain affected by feeling different, continued loss of contact with friends, and dependence on parents [81].

In contrast, other data illustrate favorable adjustment, low distress, and tremendous resilience following HSCT [82–84]. A prospective longitudinal study of 153 pediatric and adolescent HSCT patients found a low prevalence of behavioral and social problems and stable functioning over time [85]. In a study of young adults approximately 14 years post-BMT, patients scored significantly higher on the "emotional well-being" subscale of the FACT-BMT [86]. More recently, Phipps et al. found significant improvements on all HRQL outcomes from admission to week 24; patients who had reported low levels of adjustment difficulties at admission improved to normative or better than average levels of adjustment and HRQL at week 24 [84]. These studies support earlier reports that pre-HSCT emotional functioning and ability to cope with stress appear to be strongly predictive of later functioning.

The literature points to a few key psychological factors that appear to place HSCT survivors at highest risk of poor long-term psychosocial outcomes. In younger recipients these include low family cohesion and expressiveness and poor childhood adaptive functioning prior to transplant [41, 48, 87]. Certain demographic factors have been identified as well. Early studies found children undergoing matched unrelated donor transplants experiencing the highest levels of distress, followed by those undergoing matched-sibling BMT, while those undergoing autologous transplant experienced the lowest levels of distress [88], though these findings have not been substantiated over time. However, in 2011, Brice et al. [48] identified specific ethnic differences with African-American children reporting highest HRQL and those of Asian descent with the worst decline in psychosocial HRQL post-HSCT. Families of lower socioeconomic status have demonstrated greater distress and disturbance in HRQL throughout the first 6 months post-BMT [88].

The pediatric literature has used a framework of traumatic stress to describe psychological outcomes in children who have experienced a chronic illness, including transplant survivors and their family members. Ingerski et al. compared traumatic stress symptoms of youth being considered for solid organ and bone marrow transplantation and other chronic conditions and found 10% of youth by self-report, 18% of youth by parent-proxy report, and 13% of caregivers described symptoms suggestive of PTSD [92]. Phipps et al. [84] found significant reduction in PTSD symptoms from admission for HSCT to week 24. Moreover, parents of pediatric transplant patients self-reported greater symptoms than caregivers of youth with other conditions and those with higher traumatic stress symptoms reported greater symptoms in their children.

Parental psychological function

The traumatic stress model has also been used to investigate the role of posttraumatic stress symptoms and PTSD among parents of children undergoing HSCT.

Manne et al. [183] assessed emotional distress, BMT-related fears, and negative responses of family and friends in 90 mothers at the time of the BMT infusion and 3 and 6 months post-BMT. PTSD symptoms were measured 6 months post-BMT by both paper-and-pencil and structured interview methods. Emotional distress, BMT-related fears, and negative responses of family and friends assessed at the time of BMT hospitalization were predictive of later PTSD symptoms. None of these variables prospectively predicted a PTSD diagnosis as measured by the structured interview. Other studies in parents of children who survived HSCT have identified PTSD 18 months posttransplant [89, 90], with mothers reporting significantly worse mental well-being compared with population norms [91]. Each of these findings suggest that traumatic stress symptoms may be especially salient for families of pediatric transplant candidates [92]. In fact, data supporting the negative psychological impact on parents both during and after HSCT have been much less contradictory than the data on mental health outcomes in pediatric transplant survivors.

While most parents return to healthy levels of psychosocial functioning at evaluations following HSCT (including PTSD), a subset report persistent symptoms years later, particularly when there are clinical complications [93] and in parents who perceive their child to be much more vulnerable compared with parents of healthy children [46]. Qualitative findings have provided insight into the stresses incurred during transplant and post-transplant and have described parents' paradoxical existence within an "abnormal normality," a sense of isolation, coping differences between mothers and fathers, as well as the experience of "positive growth" [94]. These findings speak to the potential ongoing toll of parents' well-being and the need for screening and comprehensive assessment of family coping and adaptation in the standard of care provided to all families. Intervening at critical junctures throughout and following HSCT could mitigate potential negative consequences for parents and their children [93].

Social and role functioning

Adults

Throughout the transplant experience, effects on social and role function can be quite profound, with the greatest impact occurring during the acute phase of HSCT. Beginning with the selection of a transplant center, a patient and at least one family member will likely travel great distances for care, often separating them from family and community support. The relocation close to the transplant center, often an out-of-pocket cost [95], creates a variety of additional challenges with roles and support within their family, the community, employment, and school. Although significant adjustments are required, there is an attitude of "acceptance" during the transplant phase because of the potentially curative nature of the HSCT and focus on the treatment-related toxicities.

However, as the initial hurdles of treatment-related effects become manageable, the effect on social function and roles becomes more relevant. This often begins with the return home when the resumption of work or school becomes a focus in recovery. Although the social effects associated with hospitalization and frequent hospital visits reduce with time, diminished social relationships and social function continue into the survivorship phase [96–98]. The return to work is quite variable, with reports ranging from 50 to 84% [54, 56, 99], although there is evidence that the majority of survivors 5 years or more from HSCT without relapse have an employment rate that does not differ from that of controls without cancer [57]. A significant factor that may delay return to work or school is c-GVHD [100].

The HSCT patient also reports that the impact of HSCT on their family is a factor that impacts their degree of stress [101]. The patient's concern for their family members or caregiver has been validated across multiple studies [102]. Although there are documented benefits to helping a family member undergoing HSCT, caregivers often have significant psychological, social, and physical problems [102] that might be having invisible effects on their health [103]. Challenges for the patient and caregiver often overlap with issues of sexual dysfunction, which has been well reviewed and documented as one of the most significant concerns for HSCT survivors [104] and is further described in Chapter 18. In addition, patients and spouses report poor dyadic adjustment [96], with female spouses (male patient) reporting an increased risk of relationship difficulties [105].

Pediatrics

Generally, owing to risk of infection, children do not participate in group activities with other children for up to a year posttransplant. While nonattendance at school can result in lower educational achievement levels, the social impact on pediatric HSCT survivors is also greatly impacted by the child being separated from their peers and age-appropriate activities. In fact, the enforced isolation both during and subsequent to hospitalization is a serious stressor for youth [106]. The perceived isolation associated with wearing a mask in public is particularly difficult in adolescence, when identity achievement is so crucial. Encouraging the child to continue with their academics via hospital school programs or homebound tutoring reduces academic lag and the possibility of having to repeat a grade upon return to the classroom. While an early study of HSCT survivors suggested a pattern of difficulties with peers and the potential to disrupt normal social and emotional development [107], this has not been substantiated in later studies.

Social and romantic outcomes of survivors of non-central nervous system (CNS) cancer have been found to be similar when compared with peers during the transition from adolescence to emerging adulthood [108]. Similarly, a recent case-matched study examining life satisfaction with long-term survivors of HSCT for childhood malignant and nonmalignant disease found no significant social or role impairment compared with healthy controls [109]. Survivors with CNS disease have not fared as well. Some studies have documented declines in cognitive function up to 3 years posttransplant [110, 111], particularly those whose sample included patients under the age of 5 at the time of transplant, those who had cranial irradiation or total body irradiation as part of their preparatory regimen [112, 113], and female survivors showing more cognitive symptoms than male survivors [49]. Another study that followed HSCT patients for 5 years posttransplant reported no significant changes in global intelligence quotient and academic achievement [114]. Socioeconomic status was a significant determinant of all cognitive and academic outcomes, including diagnosis, type of transplant, total body irradiation, and c-GVHD [87, 114, 115]. These are described in Chapter 20.

Survivors with CNS disease have also shown future problems in the areas of cognitive, social, and romantic functioning [116]. As social acceptance and friendships are powerful predictors of future success or failure, any observation of social isolation or rejection should prompt a psychological evaluation [117]. Owing to differences between peer, teacher, and self-reports, the need for multiple informants is always helpful, particularly when examining cognitive, peer, and social outcomes.

Benefit-finding and posttrauma growth

As noted throughout this chapter, HSCT can be a traumatic experience with data supporting long-lasting psychological challenges in a subset of patients and family members. Fortunately, there is a growing body of research that supports that the experience might also include highly meaningful and positive outcomes [118] in both pediatric and adult survivors, including a greater appreciation of life and changed priorities, better relationships with family and others, and deeper spirituality [84, 119–124]. In fact, recent trauma literature has supported a philosophical shift from examining pathogenic features to a paradigm in which the focus is on positive as well as negative posttraumatic changes. However, empirical knowledge exploring the different domains of positive change or posttraumatic growth (PTG) is scarce.

Survivors have now reported similar levels of positive growth compared with controls [96], with a greater meaning in life positively related to psychological adjustment [125], increased personal strengths, and enhanced interpersonal relationships [84, 119–124]. Woman and older survivors are more likely to report growth in one or more dimensions, as are HSCT survivors with dispositional optimism and more social support [124]. This personal growth is also found in terms of limited regret, as survivors often report that they would make the same decision again to undergo an HSCT [126, 127].

Specific to children HSCT survivors, empirical knowledge exploring the different domains of positive change or PTG is scarce. This area of research has important implications for redefining the "victims" of transplant-related trauma as individuals capable of positive change rather than merely surviving. In a study of childhood cancer survivors and their parents, a majority of adolescent survivors and their mothers and fathers reported at least one of the following positive changes in their lives: (1) how they think about their lives, (2) how they treat other people, and (3) how careful they are [119]. In that study, PTG was positively correlated with age at diagnosis, posttraumatic symptomatology, greater treatment intensity, and greater perceived life threat [119]. The authors suggest that PTG outcomes in these survivors may be consistent with developmental tasks and challenges of adolescence; that is, with cognitive and emotional development the youth begin to understand and appreciate the support and encouragement they received during their treatment and the strength they were able to exhibit in the face of a life-threatening experience. In another study, Phipps et al. examined perceived benefits prior to and following transplant: HSCT children survivors reported significantly higher benefit finding at week 24 posttransplant [84]. Perceptions of benefit following pediatric HSCT have also been studied in parents of pediatric HSCT survivors. Predictors of benefit include optimism and reduced medical risk [128]. From the limited research available with pediatric cohorts, the impact of benefit-finding with adaptive outcomes is not straightforward. Further research examining variables such as family cohesion, developmental understanding, disease severity, and individual personality characteristics will bring greater light to this promising area of investigation [129].

General health and health-promoting behaviors

HSCT survivors are living longer and are at an increased risk for late effects such as cardiovascular disease and secondary cancers, yet little is known about their health behaviors to manage this increased risk [130]. Health behavior related to illness prevention includes *health-promoting behaviors* such as healthy eating, *health-risk behaviors* such as tobacco and alcohol use, and *health-responsibility behaviors* such as routine screening. The utilization of health care during HSCT survivorship is more likely to include a general physical exam compared with a cancer or transplant-specific visit [131]. Although the attention to overall health by HSCT survivors is comparable to other cancer survivors, and may be adequate in some cases, the intensity of an allogeneic HSCT suggests greater attention to illness prevention and cancer screening [132]. The findings from one study of HSCT survivors suggest that some cancer screening practices may be better compared with their unaffected siblings, although survivors who were younger, without health insurance, and less education were more likely to participate in unhealthy behaviors such as alcohol use and smoking [133]. This has also been seen in pediatric survivors, where the risk for late effects is significantly increased by behavior, including obesity, physical inactivity, smoking, and unprotected sun exposure [134–136]. Behavioral interventions to successfully promote health behaviors in HSCT survivors is not well studied [137].

Application to practice

Adults

Assessing the HRQL status of an HSCT patient is not without its challenges. During the more acute phases of HSCT, the transplant center is likely to have an expert interdisciplinary team to assess the impact of the procedure on HRQL and psychosocial outcomes. Once the survivors have returned to their primary residence and often the care of their nontransplant provider, assessment may be more difficult to complete, although guidelines have been established suggesting that, at a minimum, all HSCT survivors should have HRQL and psychosocial outcomes assessed 6 and 12 months following HSCT and then annually [95].

Overestimating function and HRQL has been documented in the HSCT settings [138] and could be addressed by collecting information directly from the patient. The use of self-report measures is likely to increase the accuracy and completeness of the assessment [139], and improve physician–patient communication [140] and patient outcomes [139]. However, selecting a measure to use in practice can seem overwhelming. Pencil-and-paper questionnaires are the traditional method for including patient-reported outcomes (PROs) such as HRQL into an assessment, but electronic methods are becoming increasingly more available. To ensure the patient's valid perspective, the inclusion of PROs for HRQL and psychosocial outcomes should be guided by individuals with expertise in the field. Published guidance exists relative to the use of PROs [141] as well as resources that describe the various measures available [142]. Table 35.1 offers a summary of the most commonly administered HRQL measures in HSCT.

The process of incorporating questionnaires in practice is quite different from their use for research. Pencil-

Table 35.1 Common measures for HRQL outcomes in HSCT patients

Measure	Ages	# items	Time to complete	Details
Adults				
EORTC Quality of Life Questionnaire – Core Questionnaire (EORTC QLQ-C30) [162]	Adult	30	10 min	*Population:* Cancer *Scales:* Physical, role, cognitive, emotional, social, fatigue, pain, nausea and vomiting, and global health *Response frame:* Past 7 days
Functional Assessment of Chronic Illness Therapy Measurement System (FACIT) [163] Functional Assessment of Cancer Therapy – General (FACT-G) Functional Assessment of Cancer Therapy –BMT (FACT-BMT) [163]	Adult	Variable	5–10 min	*Population:* Cancer and chronic illnesses *Scales:* Physical, social/family, emotional, function and BMT specific scale *Response frame:* Past 7 days
Rotterdam Symptom Checklist (RSCL) [164]	Adult	39	8 min	*Population:* Cancer *Scales:* Physical symptom distress, psychological distress, activity level and overall global life quality *Response frame:* Past 7 days
SF-36® Health Survey and SF-36v2™ Health Survey (SF-36®/ SF-36v2™) [165]	14 years old	36	5–10 min	*Population:* Generic, all diseases *Scales:* Physical functioning, physical role, bodily pain, general health, vitality (energy/fatigue), social, emotional role, and mental health *Response frame:* Past 4 weeks or past 7 days
SF-12® Health Survey and SF-12v2® Health Survey (SF-12®/SF-12v2®) [166]		12		
Sickness Impact Profile (SIP) [167]	Adult	136	20–30 min	*Population:* Generic, all diseases *Scales:* Sleep and rest, emotional behavior, body care and movement, home management, mobility, social interaction, ambulation, alertness behavior, communication, work, recreation and pastimes and eating *Response frame:* Today
City of Hope Quality of Life (COH-QOL) [168] City of Hope Quality of Life Bone Marrow Transplant Survivors [168]	Adult	41 84	10–20 min	*Population:* Cancer *Scales:* Physical well-being, psychological well-being, social well-being, and spiritual well-being; BMT scale *Response frame:* Today
Patient-Reported Outcomes Measurement Information System (PROMIS) [169]	Adult & Pediatric	Variable	Variable	*Population:* Generic, all diseases *Scales:* Concepts common to BMT population include, but not limited to: anxiety, depression, pain, physical function, and sleep disturbance *Response frame:* Past 7 days *Comment:* Electronic administration and scoring
Satisfaction with Life Domains Scale for Bone Marrow Transplantation (SLDS-BMT) [170]	Adult	18	<10 min	Population: BMT specific Scales: Health, spouse, other relatives, friends, body, daily activities, job, leisure time, appearance, strength overall comfort, BMT, sex, eating, control, quality of life, future, and life as a whole Response frame: Past 4 weeks

(*Continued*)

Table 35.1 (*Continued*)

Measure	Ages	# items	Time to complete	Details
Symptoms of Chronic Graft-versus-Host Disease (cGVHD scale) [171]	Adult	30	5–10 min	*Population:* c-GVHD *Scales:* Skin, vitality, lung, nutritional status, psychological functioning, eye and mouth *Response frame:* Past 4 weeks
Pediatric				
Child Health and Illness Profile (CHIP) [172]	6–17	45–108		*Population:* Generic *Scales:* Well-being, symptoms, behaviors, and illnesses
Child report (CHIP-CE)			15 min	*Response frame:* Past 4 weeks(well-being, symptoms and behaviors); past year (illnesses)
Adolescent-report (CHIP-AE)			25 min	
Parent-report on adolescents (CHIP-PRF) Parent-report on children (CHIP-CPRF)				*Comment:* Proxy and self-administered options
Child Health Questionnaire (CHQ) [173]	5–18	87–98		*Population:* Generic *Scales:* Child health, well-being, and impact of illness on life function
Child-report (CHQ-CF)			16–25 min	
Parent-report (CHQ-PF)			5–15 min	*Response frame:* Past 4 weeks *Comment:* Proxy and self-administered options
Pediatric Quality of Life Inventory (PedsQL) [174] PedsQL 28 item Cancer Module (5–18) PedsQL short form: 15 items	2–25	15–23	<4 min	*Population:* Pediatric cancer *Scales:* Pain, hurt, nausea, procedural anxiety, treatment anxiety, worry, cognitive problems, perceived physical appearance and communication *Response frame:* Past 4 weeks and past 7 days
Youth Quality of Life (YQOL) [175] Child-report Surveillance (YQOL-S): 13 items Child-report Research & Program Evaluation (YQOL-R): 41 items	12–18	13–41	~10 min	*Population:* Generic *Scales:* Self, relationships, environment, and general quality of life *Response frame:* Today
Miami Pediatric Quality of Life Questionnaire (MPQLQ) [176]	1–18	39		*Population:* Pediatric cancer *Scales:* Social competence, emotional stability, self-competence, and total quality of life *Response frame:* Today *Comment:* Proxy and self-administered options
Pediatric Oncology Quality of Life Scale (POQOL) [177]	2–19	23		*Population:* Pediatric cancer *Scales:* Physical functioning, emotional distress and role restriction and total QOL score *Response frame:* Past 2 weeks *Comment:* Proxy and self-administered options

Table 35.1 (*Continued*)

Measure	Ages	# items	Time to complete	Details
Play Performance Scale for Children (PPSC) [178]	6 months–16 years	1		*Population:* Pediatric cancer *Scales:* Physical functioning, emotional distress and role restriction and total QOL score *Response frame:* Past 2 weeks *Comment:* Proxy and self-administered options. Parent-report: observational domains vary by age. Differentiates between inpatient, outpatient, and healthy children
Functional Disability				
Child Activity Limitations Interview (CALI) [179]	8–16	21	5–7 min	*Population:* Generic *Scales:* Pain-related activity limitation, functional impairment, age-appropriate activities of daily life *Response frame:* Past 4 weeks *Comment:* Proxy and self-administered options
Functional Disability Inventory (FDI) [180]	8–17	15	5–10 min	*Population:* Generic *Scales:* Global measure of functional disability, with somatic complaints, depression, anxiety, bed days, and medication use *Response frame:* The last few days *Comment:* Proxy and self-administered options
Transplant Specific				
Behavioral, Affective and Somatic Experiences Scale (BASES) [181] BASES-C	1–20	38 14		*Population:* Pediatric transplant *Scales:* Somatic distress, compliance, mood/behavior (anxious, depressive), quality of interactions, and activity *Response frame:* Over the last day *Comment:* Proxy and self-administered options
Child Health Ratings Inventory (CHRIs) [182] Accompanying measure: Disease Impairment Inventories-Bone Marrow Transplant (DSII-BMT(DSII) – HSCT module	5–20	20 10	3–4 min	*Population:* Pediatric transplant *Scales:* Physical functioning, role functioning, emotional functioning, and energy *Response frame:* Past 4 weeks *Comment:* Proxy and self-administered options

and-paper questionnaires can be resource intensive and involve the administration, scoring, interpretation, and communication to the provider for each individual patient. However, electronic methods for collection have grown over the last decade. Web-based programs for routine collection of HRQL outcomes are being considered in HSCT patients [99], with more widely used systems such as Patient-Reported Outcomes Measurement Information System (PROMIS) providing an efficient, psychometrically robust assessment in a wide range of chronic diseases, across outcomes [143]. Advances in collection methods will allow for providers to screen survivors for possible effects that linger from the HSCT experience or current late effects.

Pediatrics

An important consideration in interpreting HRQL findings in children is the question of who is rating the child's functioning. Parent proxy reports are almost always used when assessing a child's HRQL. In addition, discrepant outcomes related to ability to function socially based on physical limitation and self-esteem have been noted [52], with parental reports of child's HRQL tending to be worse than self-reports [53, 144–146]. The association between maternal distress and the child's HRQL has also been found to reflect the parents' own distress [45, 52].

The questionable reliability of reporting by children under the age of 5 has resulted in few measures that rely solely on self-report for this age group. Even for older children, most questionnaires that assess HRQL collect proxy ratings from parents or other adults (teachers, nurses, physicians). Assessment of the validity and reliability of parent proxy ratings suggests that these may be satisfactory in the case of some questionnaires (e.g., the PedsQLTM) [147]. However, parents tend to underrate children's HRQL. They may also be poor judges of which consequences of illness matter most to their children, be influenced by their own response to their child's illness, and may use different reference points than their children against which to judge HRQL [148]. These problems are confounded by the fact that children's behavior – which necessarily forms the basis for proxy reports – varies depending on the situation and whether they are at home versus school versus the hospital [149]. For teenagers and young adults, a parent may be aware of acting out behavior that has been brought to their attention, but feelings of sadness, loneliness, and fear may not have been shared, resulting in richer data obtained from using multiple informants.

Interventions

Adults

Interventions to improve the HRQL outcomes of an HSCT survivor tend to focus on the individual dimension(s) most affected. As mentioned earlier, an awareness of the baseline status of the patient is important to their continued management following HSCT. When an individual patient, family member, or caregiver is determined to have a problem that could potentially impact the transplant experience (e.g., previous trauma) it is important to refer them to an expert for a more in-depth assessment and treatment plan. Quality health care can be improved with the collaboration across disciplines [150]. For example, if physical function is determined to be impaired in a clinically stable patient, then an exercise regimen is likely to provide improvement [151]. An exercise program might be best guided by a specialist in rehabilitation medicine, although on account of the intensity of treatment and the time burden a formal program may be difficult to attend [152]. Similarly, benefit might be found through cognitive–behavioral techniques guided by a mental health specialist for those survivors with persistent psychological or treatment-related symptoms [153–155].

Although mental health services are often available at transplant centers, there is evidence that HSCT survivors are underutilizing this service to aid with their adjustment during recovery [72]. Reported barriers include scheduling, finances, limited knowledge of HSCT by mental health providers, specific illness-related factors, and hesitancy of survivors to "rehash" their transplant experience with others. Survivors who are male, with a lower income, and those who are unemployed as well as those with c-GVHD or those with greater physical and functional limitations are also more likely not to obtain mental health services. It is suggested that education and tailoring the mental health services to the individual and their identified barriers may improve the use of services [72].

Access to accurate information for patients and their family is a critical component of effective care. Both patients and caregivers have indicated that lack of information results in more distress. Despite the need for information to address unmet concern, it is essential to assess the specific needs of the patient and develop an individualized plan of education [156]. This plan might consist of both center-specific materials and those available online. Online resources are especially valuable to survivors who are not linked to a direct transplant center (Table 35.2). Self-care and return to a normal lifestyle is a priority area for cancer patient [156].

Pediatrics

Although HSCT has become standard therapy for many life-threatening disorders of childhood, there is little

Table 35.2 Common online patient resources

Resource	Website address	Description
American Cancer Society	http://www.cancer.org/treatment/treatmentsandsideeffects/treatmenttypes/bonemarrowandperipheralbloodstemcelltransplant/bone-marrow-and-peripheral-blood-stem-cell-transplant-toc	• Treatment specific topics • Links to support and treatment topics
Be The Match® by The National Marrow Donor Program	http://marrow.org/Patient/Patients_and_Families.aspx	• Disease, treatment, transplant donor search information and resources • Support resources for patients, families and caregivers throughout the transplant continuum (pretransplant through survivorship)
Blood & Marrow Transplant Information Network	http://bmtinfonet.org/	• Emotional support, information and education for patients and families before, during, and after blood and marrow transplant
Cancer*care*	http://www.cancercare.org/patients_and_survivors	• Support groups, education, workshops, counseling services, financial assistance
CarePages.com	www.carepages.com/	• Site to create video/website blog to connect with family and others going through similar situations
CARING BRIDGE	www.CARINGBRIDGE.org	• Site to connect with friends and family
ExploreBMT™	http://www.explorebmt.org/	• One-stop site for transplant-related resources
Health Resources and Services Administration	http://bloodcell.transplant.hrsa.gov/	• Transplant education, donor and cord blood information • Research, data, and outcomes reports
Mayo Clinic	http://www.mayoclinic.com/health/stem-cell-transplant/MY00089	• Stem cell transplant and educational materials
The Leukemia & Lymphoma Society	www.lls.org/diseaseinformation	• Disease and treatment information
NIH Medline Plus	http://www.nlm.nih.gov/medlineplus/bonemarrowtransplantation.html	• Disease and treatment information • Links to research studies
National Bone Marrow Transplant Link	http://nbmtlink.org/resources_support/resources.htm	• Transplant resources, guides, and support • Links to disease-specific and symptom support groups, financial resources, and local support organizations
National Cancer Institute	http://www.cancer.gov/cancertopics/factsheet/Therapy/bone-marrow-transplant	• Education resources for patients and donors • Links to clinical trials
National Heart, Lung, and Blood Institute	http://www.nhlbi.nih.gov/health/health-topics/topics/bmsct/	• Disease and treatment information • Links to clinical trials

research on interventions aimed at decreasing distress and improving long-term emotional and psychosocial functioning. Guidelines for the medical and psychosocial care of pediatric cancer survivors, including survivors of HSCT are available through the Children's Oncology Group (www.survivorshipguidelines.org/pdf/ltfuguidelines.pdf). These guidelines address management of late effects that may potentially arise as a result of therapeutic exposures used during treatment and are intended to increase awareness of potential late effects and to standardize and enhance follow-up care provided to survivors of pediatric malignancies throughout their lifespan.

Early evidence on effective interventions provides some direction for practice. One study identified acceptance, humor, and positive cognitive appraisal during the active phase of HSCT as protective factors [90]. An early pilot study designed to evaluate a technique to help parents manage stress associated with their child's illness and transplant found parents are interested in such interventions particularly during the preadmission phase, a time point when they experience considerable stress [157]. In a recent study of 171 patients and parents who were randomized to receive a child-based intervention (massage and humor therapy), a parent intervention (massage and relaxation/imagery) or standard care, Phipps et al. found no benefit from the complementary interventions over standard care; the authors discuss the remarkable resilience and overall positive adjustment seen in their sample as well as the improvements in medical and psychosocial supportive care during transplant [84].

Well-established approaches for caring for children living with chronic and acute illness, including cognitive–behavioral interventions, show great promise in improving procedural distress, compliance with treatment, and behavioral problems associated with HSCT [158]. Familial interventions that aim to enhance protective factors, improve communication, and decrease parental anxiety and depression are crucial, and cancer-specific interventions may serve as a template for the development of HSCT-specific interventions [158]. Social media can allow hospitalized youth to remain connected with their peers. Other creative interventions may also play an important role, such as bibliotherapy [7], therapeutic board games [159], therapeutic music videos [160], and those using Web-based technology that are easily accessible from the hospital or home posttransplant and reflect changing needs over time [67].

A health-related website for parents of children receiving hematopoietic stem cell transplant (HSCT-CHESS) has been created and it is currently being tested in a randomized control trial [161]. Similar e-health interventions might prove quite effective in educating pediatric survivors about ways to enhance their quality of life.

Summary

As future progress in the field of transplantation unfolds, shorter courses of treatment, more outpatient care, better supportive care, and less severe GVHD will lead to improvements in HRQL outcomes. Nevertheless, HSCT remains one of the most intense and life-threatening procedures for hematological malignancies and nonmalignant hematological diseases, and survivors, and their family, often experience impairments and symptoms for many years following HSCT. Although the evidence on the HRQL effects in adults is quite extensive, the translation of this knowledge into practice remains limited. Notably, the research examining HRQL in pediatric HSCT recipients has lagged behind [37] that of its adult counterparts. From the available studies, overall conclusions regarding psychological, cognitive, academic, and social outcomes of HCT survivors have been constrained by methodological issues, including different measures and inconsistent raters, modest sample sizes, narrow measurement strategies (i.e., self-report versus direct observation), wide age range of participants, lack of qualitative data, and limited long-term follow-up. While the results suggest risk of developing long-term emotional problems in a subset of young patients who underwent HSCT, most studies are limited by a retrospective or cross-sectional design and longitudinal studies with considerably small sample sizes at long-term evaluations.

To ensure the provision of quality care to HSCT survivors, an approach to assessing HRQL outcomes and incorporating the findings in "real time" needs to become a universal practice. This imperative in practice will be the key to success for survivors and will likely be dependent on an electronic health record that has a patient portal for outcome assessment. The evidence base for interventions continues to be developed, but HSCT providers can benefit from the cancer literature more broadly where intervention recommendations are more extensive (Table 35.3).The overall goal is to ensure a well-informed

Table 35.3 Common HRQL and psychosocial impairments and matched interventions

HRQL dimension	Behavior or outcome	Risk factor	Intervention
Adults			
Physical function	Limitations in ADLs	Persistent symptoms: Pain Musculoskeletal Fatigue Depression c-GVHD	• Comprehensive assessment • Symptom management
Psychological function	Anxiety Depression Worry Low self-esteem	Females Single Family conflict Poor social support Impaired physical health	• Comprehensive psychological assessment • Cognitive behavioral techniques • Couples counseling
Social–family function	Isolation Intimacy Employment Poor dyadic adjustment Infertility	Female spouses (poor dyadic adjustment)	• Comprehensive assessment by mental health professional including spouse and family as indicated • Cognitive behavioral techniques • Encourage strong support networks • Sexual counseling and function assessment by specialist
Symptoms	Fatigue Sleep disturbance	Pretransplant medical or psychological symptoms	• Exercise program • Relaxation interventions
General health	Preventive health screening Risky behaviors	Prior history of nonadherence	• Education
Pediatrics			
Physical function	Withdrawal from friends/social activities/ school Depression Anger	Limited mobility Pain c-GVHD	• Comprehensive assessment • Symptom management • Physical activity – consider rehabilitation medicine referral • Camp programs
Psychological function	Anxiety Destructive outbursts Regression	Preexisting mental health problems (e.g., anxiety disorder, mood dysregulation) Lack of trust in the medical system or family members Slow to recover: poor resiliency Difficulty coping with change	• Comprehensive psychological assessment • Cognitive behavioral techniques (e.g., problem solving) • Individual counseling • Expressive therapies • Specialized camping programs

(Continued)

Table 35.3 (*Continued*)

HRQL dimension	Behavior or outcome	Risk factor	Intervention
Social–family function	Poor academic performance Family conflict Isolation/withdrawal	Parental conflict Significant sibling rivalry Poor peer relationships Limited support	• Comprehensive assessment by mental health professional including siblings and extended family as indicated • Cognitive behavioral techniques/remediation • School intervention • Peer support groups • Encourage support networks • Family/marital counseling, as indicated
Symptoms	Sleep disturbance Fatigue Excessive use of narcotics (pain)	Previous medical problems exacerbated by HSCT Separation anxiety cGVHD	• Education • Cognitive behavioral techniques • Sleep specialist • Pain specialist • Medications, as indicated
General health	Alcohol or substance abuse Adherence	Previous medical problems exacerbated by HSCT cGVHD	• Individual counseling • Education • Close follow-up

HSCT survivor and family and to encourage the appropriate use of services both online or within the healthcare system to manage the HRQL effects.

Acknowledgments

The authors thank the following individuals for their support and thoughtful review of this chapter: Leslie Wehrlen, Stephen D. Klagholz, and Adrienne Viola.

References

1. CDC. Cancer survivors – United States, 2007: Centers for Disease Control and Prevention 2011, 2011 Mar 11, Contract No.: 9.
2. Thomas ED, Blume KG. Historical markers in the development of allogeneic hematopoietic cell transplantation. Biol Blood Marrow Transplant. 1999;5(6):341–346.
3. Mosher CE, Redd WH, Rini CM, et al. Physical, psychological, and social sequelae following hematopoietic stem cell transplantation: a review of the literature. Psychooncology. 2009;18(2):113–127.
4. Pidala J, Anasetti C, Jim H. Quality of life after allogeneic hematopoietic cell transplantation. Blood. 2009;114(1): 7–19.
5. Tanzi EM. Health-related quality of life of hematopoietic stem cell transplant childhood survivors: state of the science. J Pediatr Oncol Nurs. 2011;28(4):191–202.
6. Lee SJ, Joffe S, Kim HT, et al. Physicians' attitudes about quality-of-life issues in hematopoietic stem cell transplantation. Blood. 2004;104(7):2194–2200.
7. Wiener L, Pao M. Comprehensive and family-centered psychosocial care in pediatric oncology: integration of clinical practice and research. In: Kreitler S, Ben-Arush M, Martin A (eds). Pediatric Psycho-Oncology: Psychosocial Aspects and Clinical Interventions, 2nd edition. Chichester, UK: John Wiley & Sons, Ltd, 2012; pp. 7–17.
8. Harper A, Power M, Orley J, et al. Development of the World Health Organization WHOQOL-BREF quality of life assessment. Psychol Med. 1998;28(3):551–558.
9. Wilson IB, Cleary PD. Linking clinical variables with health-related quality of life: a conceptual model of patient outcomes. J Am Med Assoc. 1995;273(1):59–65.
10. IOM. Cancer Care for the Whole Patient: Meeting Psychosocial Health Needs. Washington, DC, 2008.
11. Johnson J, Temple R. Food and Drug Administration requirement for approval of new anti-cancer drugs. Cancer Treat Rep. 1985;69(10):1155–1157.

12. Bevans MF, Marden S, Leidy NK, et al. Health-related quality of life in patients receiving reduced-intensity conditioning allogeneic hematopoietic stem cell transplantation. Bone Marrow Transplant. 2006;38(2):101–109.
13. Bosch M, Khan FM, Storek J. Immune reconstitution after hematopoietic cell transplantation. Curr Opin Hematol. 2012;19(4):324–335.
14. Pasquini MC, Wang Z. Current use and outcome of hematopoietic stem cell transplantation: CIBMTR Summary Slides, 2011. Available at: http://www.cibmtr.org/ReferenceCenter/SlidesReports/SummarySlides/pages/index.aspx (accessed 22 May 2013).
15. Bishop MM, Rodrigue JR, Wingard JR. Mismanaging the gift of life: noncompliance in the context of adult stem cell transplantation. Bone Marrow Transplant. 2002;29(11): 875–880.
16. Foster LW, McLellan L, Rybicki L, et al. Ethical reasoning about patient eligibility in allogeneic BMT based on psychosocial criteria. Bone Marrow Transplant. 2009;44(9): 607–612.
17. Bevans MF, Mitchell SA, Marden S. The symptom experience in the first 100 days following allogeneic hematopoietic stem cell transplantation (HSCT). Support Care Cancer. 2008;16(11):1243–1254.
18. Cohen MZ, Rozmus CL, Mendoza TR, et al. Symptoms and quality of life in diverse patients undergoing hematopoietic stem cell transplantation. J Pain Symptom Manage. 2012; 44(2):168–180.
19. Patenaude AF. Psychological impact of bone-marrow transplantation – current perspectives. Yale J Biol Med. 1990;63(5):515–519.
20. IOM. Implementing Cancer Survivorship Care Planning: Workshop Summary: Institue of Medicine, 2006
21. Andorsky DJ, Loberiza FR Jr, Lee SJ. Pre-transplantation physical and mental functioning is strongly associated with self-reported recovery from stem cell transplantation. Bone Marrow Transplant. 2006;37(9):889–895.
22. McQuellon RP, Russell GB, Rambo TD, et al. Quality of life and psychological distress of bone marrow transplant recipients: the "time trajectory" to recovery over the first year 16. Bone Marrow Transplant. 1998;21(5): 477–486.
23. Sherman AC, Simonton S, Latif U, et al. Changes in quality-of-life and psychosocial adjustment among multiple myeloma patients treated with high-dose melphalan and autologous stem cell transplantation Biol Blood Marrow Transplant. 2009;15(1):12–20.
24. Schulz-Kindermann F, Mehnert A, Scherwath A, et al. Cognitive function in the acute course of allogeneic hematopoietic stem cell transplantation for hematological malignancies. Bone Marrow Transplant. 2007;39(12):789–799.
25. van Agthoven M, Vellenga E, Fibbe WE, et al. Cost analysis and quality of life assessment comparing patients undergoing autologous peripheral blood stem cell transplantation or autologous bone marrow transplantation for refractory or relapsed non-Hodgkin's lymphoma or Hodgkin's disease. A prospective randomised trial. Eur J Cancer. 2001;37(14):1781–1789.
26. Molassiotis A, van den Akker OB, Milligan DW, et al. Quality of life in long-term survivors of marrow transplantation: comparison with a matched group receiving maintenance chemotherapy. Bone Marrow Transplant. 1996; 17(2):249–258.
27. Redaelli A, Stephens JM, Brandt S, et al. Short- and long-term effects of acute myeloid leukemia on patient health-related quality of life. Cancer Treat Rev. 2004;30(1): 103–117.
28. Lee SJ, Kim HT, Ho VT, et al. Quality of life associated with acute and chronic graft-versus-host disease. Bone Marrow Transplant. 2006;38(4):305–310.
29. Prieto JM, Saez R, Carreras E, et al. Physical and psychosocial functioning of 117 survivors of bone marrow transplantation. Bone Marrow Transplant. 1996;17(6): 1133–1142.
30. Syrjala KL, Martin PJ, Lee SJ. Delivering care to long-term adult survivors of hematopoietic cell transplantation. J Clin Oncol. 2012;30(30):3746–3751.
31. Le RQ, Bevans M, Savani BN, et al. Favorable outcomes in patients surviving 5 or more years after allogeneic hematopoietic stem cell transplantation for hematologic malignancies. Biol Blood Marrow Transplant. 2010;16(8): 1162–1170.
32. Beeken RJ, Eiser C, Dalley C. Health-related quality of life in haematopoietic stem cell transplant survivors: a qualitative study on the role of psychosocial variables and response shifts. Qual Life Res. 2011;20(2):153–160.
33. Tierney DKPRN, Facione NPRN, Padilla GP, Dodd MPRN. Response shift: a theoretical exploration of quality of life following hematopoietic cell transplantation. Cancer Nurs. 2007;30(2):125–138.
34. Heinonen H, Volin L, Uutela A, et al. Quality of life and factors related to perceived satisfaction with quality of life after allogeneic bone marrow transplantation. Ann Hematol. 2001;80(3):137–143.
35. Baker KS, Bresters D, Sande JE. The burden of cure: long-term side effects following hematopoietic stem cell transplantation (HSCT) in children. Pediatr Clin North Am. 2010;57(1):323.
36. Clarke SA, Eiser C, Skinner R. Health-related quality of life in survivors of BMT for paediatric malignancy: a systematic review of the literature. Bone Marrow Transplant. 2008;42(2):73–82.

37. Parsons SK, Phipps S, Sung L, et al. NCI, NHLBI/PBMTC First International Conference on Late Effects after Pediatric Hematopoietic Cell Transplantation: health-related quality of life, functional, and neurocognitive outcomes. Biol Blood Marrow Transplant. 2012;18(2):162–171.
38. Tremolada M, Bonichini S, Pillon M, et al. Quality of life and psychosocial sequelae in children undergoing hematopoietic stem-cell transplantation: a review. Pediatr Transplant. 2009;13(8):955–970.
39. Tsimicalis A, Stinson J, Stevens B. Quality of life of children following bone marrow transplantation: critical review of the research literature. Eur J Oncol Nurs. 2005;9(3): 218–238.
40. Schmidt D, Anderson L, Bingen K, et al. Late effects in adult survivors of childhood cancer: considerations for the general practitioner. WMJ. 2010;109(2):98–107.
41. Barrera M, Boyd-Pringle LA, Sumbler K, Saunders F. Quality of life and behavioral adjustment after pediatric bone marrow transplantation. Bone Marrow Transplant. 2000;26(4):427–435.
42. Jobe-Shields L, Alderfer MA, Barrera M, et al. Parental depression and family environment predict distress in children before stem cell transplantation. J Dev Behav Pediatr. 2009;30(2):140–146.
43. Parsons SK, Shih MC, Duhamel KN, et al. Maternal perspectives on children's health-related quality of life during the first year after pediatric hematopoietic stem cell transplant. J Pediatr Psychol. 2006;31(10):1100–1115.
44. Alderfer MA, Navsaria N, Kazak AE. Family functioning and posttraumatic stress disorder in adolescent survivors of childhood cancer. J Fam Psychol. 2009;23(5):717–725.
45. Barrera M, Atenafu E, Hancock K. Longitudinal health-related quality of life outcomes and related factors after pediatric SCT. Bone Marrow Transplant. 2009;44(4):249–256.
46. Vrijmoet-Wiersma CMJ, Egeler RM, Koopman HM, et al. Parental stress and perceived vulnerability at 5 and 10 years after pediatric SCT. Bone Marrow Transplant. 2010;45(6): 1102–1108.
47. Felder-Puig R, di Gallo A, Waldenmair M, et al. Health-related quality of life of pediatric patients receiving allogeneic stem cell or bone marrow transplantation: results of a longitudinal, multi-center study. Bone Marrow Transplant. 2006;38(2):119–126.
48. Brice L, Weiss R, Wei Y, et al. Health-related quality of life (HRQoL): the impact of medical and demographic variables upon pediatric recipients of hematopoietic stem cell transplantation. Pediatr Blood Cancer. 2011;57(7):1179–1185.
49. Sanders JE, Hoffmeister PA, Storer BE, et al. The quality of life of adult survivors of childhood hematopoietic cell transplant. Bone Marrow Transplant. 2010;45(4):746–754.
50. Barrera M, Atenafu E, Doyle J, et al. Differences in mothers' and fathers' health-related quality of life after pediatric SCT: a longitudinal study. Bone Marrow Transplant. 2012;47(6):855–859.
51. Lof CM, Winiarski J, Giesecke A, et al. Health-related quality of life in adult survivors after paediatric allo-SCT. Bone Marrow Transplant. 2009;43(6):461–468.
52. Forinder U, Lof C, Winiarski J. Quality of life following allogeneic stem cell transplantation, comparing parents' and children's perspective. Pediatr Transplant. 2006;10(4): 491–496.
53. Parsons SK, Barlow SE, Levy SL, et al. Health-related quality of life in pediatric bone marrow transplant survivors: according to whom? Int J Cancer Suppl. 1999; 12:46–51.
54. Syrjala KL, Langer SL, Abrams JR, et al. Recovery and long-term function after hematopoietic cell transplantation for leukemia or lymphoma. JAMA. 2004;291(19):2335–2343.
55. Messerer D, Engel J, Hasford J, et al. Impact of different post-remission strategies on quality of life in patients with acute myeloid leukemia. Haematologica. 2008;93(6): 826–833.
56. Kiss TL, Abdolell M, Jamal N, et al. Long-term medical outcomes and quality-of-life assessment of patients with chronic myeloid leukemia followed at least 10 years after allogeneic bone marrow transplantation. J Clin Oncol. 2002;20(9):2334–2343.
57. Syrjala KL, Langer SL, Abrams JR, et al. Late effects of hematopoietic cell transplantation among 10-year adult survivors compared with case-matched controls. J Clin Oncol. 2005;23(27):6596–6606.
58. Syrjala KL, Chapko MK, Vitaliano PP, et al. Recovery after allogeneic marrow transplantation: prospective study of predictors of long-term physical and psychosocial functioning. Bone Marrow Transplant. 1993;11(4):319–327.
59. Worel N, Biener D, Kalhs P, et al. Long-term outcome and quality of life of patients who are alive and in complete remission more than two years after allogeneic and syngeneic stem cell transplantation. Bone Marrow Transplant. 2002;30(9):619–626.
60. Bush NE, Haberman M, Donaldson G, Sullivan KM. Quality of life of 125 adults surviving 6–18 years after bone marrow transplantation. Soc Sci Med. 1995;40(4):479–490.
61. Mosher CE, DuHamel KN, Rini C, et al. Quality of life concerns and depression among hematopoietic stem cell transplant survivors. Support Care Cancer. 2011;19(9): 1357–1365.

62. Wellisch DK, Schains W, Grttz ER, Wang HEJ. Psychological functioning of daughters of breast cancer patients. Part III: experiences and perceptions of daughters related to mother's breast cancer. Psychooncology. 1996;5(3):271–281.
63. Phipps S, Dunavant M, Lensing S, Rai SN. Acute health-related quality of life in children undergoing stem cell transplant: II. Medical and demographic determinants. Bone Marrow Transplant. 2002;29(5):435–442.
64. Caocci G, Efficace F, Ciotti F, et al. Prospective assessment of health-related quality of life in pediatric patients with beta-thalassemia following hematopoietic stem cell transplantation. Biol Blood Marrow Transplant. 2011; 17(6):861–866.
65. Forinder U, Lof C, Winiarski J. Quality of life and health in children following allogeneic SCT. Bone Marrow Transplant. 2005;36(2):171–176.
66. Uygun V, Tayfun F, Akcan M, et al. Quality of life assessment in hematopoietic stem cell transplantation performed on thalassemia major patients. Pediatr Hematol Oncol. 2012;29(5):461–471.
67. Braamse AM, van Meijel B, Visser O, et al. Distress and quality of life after autologous stem cell transplantation: a randomized clinical trial to evaluate the outcome of a web-based stepped care intervention. BMC Cancer. 2010;10: 361.
68. Hjermstad MJ, Evensen SA, Kvaloy SO, et al. Health-related quality of life 1 year after allogeneic or autologous stem-cell transplantation: a prospective study. J Clin Oncol. 1999;17:706–718.
69. DuHamel KN, Manne S, Nereo N, et al. Cognitive processing among mothers of children undergoing bone marrow/stem cell transplantation. Psychosom Med. 2004;66(1): 92–103.
70. Beanlands HJ, Lipton JH, McCay EA, et al. Self-concept as a "BMT patient", illness intrusiveness, and engulfment in allogeneic bone marrow transplant recipients. J Psychosom Res. 2003;55(5):419–425.
71. Wolcott DL, Wellisch DK, Fawzy FI, Landsverk J. Adaptation of adult bone marrow transplant recipient long-term survivors. Transplantation. 1986;41(4):478–484.
72. Ross S, Mosher CE, Ronis-Tobin V, et al. Psychosocial adjustment of family caregivers of head and neck cancer survivors. Support Care Cancer. 2010;18(2):171–178.
73. Broers S, Kaptein AA, Le Cessie S, et al. Psychological functioning and quality of life following bone marrow transplantation: a 3-year follow-up study 26. J Psychosom Res. 2000;48(1):11–21.
74. Kellerman J, Rigler D, Siegel SE. Psychological response of children to isolation in a protected environment. J Behav Med. 1979;2(3):263–274.
75. Kutsanellou-Meyer M, Christ GH. Factors affecting coping of adolescents and infants on a reverse isolation unit. Soc Work Health Care. 1978;4(2):125–137.
76. Barrera M, Atenafu E, Pinto J. Behavioral, social, and educational outcomes after pediatric stem cell transplantation and related factors. Cancer. 2009;115(4):880–889.
77. Vrijmoet-Wiersma CM, Kolk AM, Grootenhuis MA, et al. Child and parental adaptation to pediatric stem cell transplantation. Support Care Cancer. 2009;17(6):707–714.
78. Ferry C, Gemayel G, Rocha V, et al. Long-term outcomes after allogeneic stem cell transplantation for children with hematological malignancies. Bone Marrow Transplant. 2007;40(3):219–224.
79. Ishida Y, Honda M, Ozono S, et al. Late effects and quality of life of childhood cancer survivors: part 1. Impact of stem cell transplantation. Int J Hematol. 2010;91(5): 865–876.
80. Anders JC, Lima RA. Growing up with bone marrow transplantation: repercussions for the quality of life of children and adolescents. Rev Lat Am Enfermagem. 2004;12(6):866–874 (in Portuguese).
81. Forinder U, Posse E. "A life on hold": adolescents' experiences of stem cell transplantation in a long-term perspective. J Child Health Care. 2008;12(4):301–313.
82. Kelly MJ, Pennarola BW, Rodday AM, Parsons SK. Health-related quality of life (HRQL) in children with sickle cell disease and thalassemia following hematopoietic stem cell transplant (HSCT). Pediatr Blood Cancer. 2012;59(4): 725–731.
83. Michel G, Bordigoni P, Simeoni MC, et al. Health status and quality of life in long-term survivors of childhood leukaemia: the impact of haematopoietic stem cell transplantation. Bone Marrow Transplant. 2007;40(9):897–904.
84. Phipps S, Peasant C, Barrera M, et al. Resilience in children undergoing stem cell transplantation: results of a complementary intervention trial. Pediatrics. 2012;129(3):e762–e770.
85. Kupst MJ, Penati B, Debban B, et al. Cognitive and psychosocial functioning of pediatric hematopoietic stem cell transplant patients: a prospective longitudinal study. Bone Marrow Transplant. 2002;30(9):609–617.
86. Helder DI, Bakker B, de Heer P, et al. Quality of life in adults following bone marrow transplantation during childhood. Bone Marrow Transplant. 2004;33(3):329–336.
87. Phipps S, Mulhern RK. Family cohesion and expressiveness promote resilience to the stress of pediatric bone marrow transplant: a preliminary report. J Dev Behav Pediatr. 1995;16(4):257–263.

88. Phipps S, Dunavant M, Garvie PA, et al. Acute health-related quality of life in children undergoing stem cell transplant: I. Descriptive outcomes. Bone Marrow Transplant. 2002;29(5):425–434.
89. Manne S, DuHamel K, Ostroff J, et al. Anxiety, depressive, and posttraumatic stress disorders among mothers of pediatric survivors of hematopoietic stem cell transplantation. Pediatrics. 2004;113(6):1700–1708.
90. Vrijmoet-Wiersma CMJ, Egeler RM, Koopman HM, et al. Parental stress before, during, and after pediatric stem cell transplantation: a review article. Support Care Cancer. 2009;17(12):1435–1443.
91. Clarke SA, Skinner R, Guest J, et al. Clinical outcomes and health-related quality of life (HRQOL) following haemopoietic stem cell transplantation (HSCT) for paediatric leukaemia. Child Care Health Dev. 2011;37(4):571–580.
92. Ingerski LM, Shaw K, Gray WN, Janicke DM. A pilot study comparing traumatic stress symptoms by child and parent report across pediatric chronic illness groups. J Dev Behav Pediatr. 2010;31(9):713–719.
93. Terrin N, Rodday AM, Tighiouart H, et al. Parental emotional functioning declines with occurrence of clinical complications in pediatric hematopoietic stem cell transplant. Support Care Cancer. 2013;21:687–695.
94. McDowell E, Titman P, Davidson S. Parents' experiences one year on from their child's hematopoietic stem cell transplant for primary immunodeficiency. J Health Psychol. 2010;15(6):897–904.
95. Majhail NS, Rizzo JD, Lee SJ, et al. Recommended screening and preventive practices for long-term survivors after hematopoietic cell transplantation. Bone Marrow Transplant. 2012;47(3):337–341.
96. Andrykowski MA, Bishop MM, Hahn EA, et al. Long-term health-related quality of life, growth, and spiritual well-being after hematopoietic stem-cell transplantation. J Clin Oncol. 2005;23(3):599–608.
97. Kopp M, Holzner B, Meraner V, et al. Quality of life in adult hematopoietic cell transplant patients at least 5 yr after treatment: a comparison with healthy controls. Eur J Haematol. 2005;74(4):304–308.
98. Watson M, Buck G, Wheatley K, et al. Adverse impact of bone marrow transplantation on quality of life in acute myeloid leukaemia patients; analysis of the UK Medical Research Council AML 10 Trial. Eur J Cancer. 2004;40(7):971–978.
99. Bush N, Donaldson G, Moinpour C, et al. Development, feasibility and compliance of a web-based system for very frequent QOL and symptom home self-assessment after hematopoietic stem cell transplantation. Qual Life Res. 2005;14(1):77–93.
100. Wong FL, Francisco L, Togawa K, et al. Long-term recovery after hematopoietic cell transplantation: predictors of quality-of-life concerns. Blood. 2010;115(12):2508–2519.
101. Heinonen H, Volin L, Zevon MA, et al. Stress among allogeneic bone marrow transplantation patients. Patient Educ Couns. 2005;56(1):62–71.
102. Beattie S, Lebel S. The experience of caregivers of hematological cancer patients undergoing a hematopoietic stem cell transplant: a comprehensive literature review. Psychooncology. 2011;20(11):1137–1150.
103. Bevans M, Sternberg EM. Caregiving burden, stress, and health effects among family caregivers of adult cancer patients. JAMA. 2012;307(4):398–403.
104. Thygesen KH, Schjodt I, Jarden M. The impact of hematopoietic stem cell transplantation on sexuality: a systematic review of the literature. Bone Marrow Transplant. 2012;47(5):716–724.
105. Langer SL, Yi JC, Storer BE, Syrjala KL. Marital adjustment, satisfaction and dissolution among hematopoietic stem cell transplant patients and spouses: a prospective, five-year longitudinal investigation. Psychooncology. 2010;19(2):190–200.
106. Elhasid R, Tohami T, Moustafa-Hawash N, et al. Spontaneous remission of childhood acute marrow fibrosis and megakaryoblastic leukemia. J Pediatr Hematol Oncol. 2012;34(7):565–568.
107. Vannatta K, Zeller M, Noll RB, Koontz K. Social functioning of children surviving bone marrow transplantation. J Pediatr Psychol. 1998;23(3):169–178.
108. Gerhardt CA, Vannatta K, Valerius KS, et al. Social and romantic outcomes in emerging adulthood among survivors of childhood cancer. J Adolesc Health. 2007;40(5):462 e9–462 e15.
109. Uderzo C, Corti P, Pappalettera M, et al. Life satisfaction in young adults 10 or more years after hematopoietic stem cell transplantation for childhood malignant and nonmalignant diseases does not show significant impairment compared with healthy controls: a case-matched study. Biol Blood Marrow Transplant. 2012;18:1759–1764.
110. Kramer JH, Crittenden MR, DeSantes K, Cowan MJ. Cognitive and adaptive behavior 1 and 3 years following bone marrow transplantation. Bone Marrow Transplant. 1997;19(6):607–613.
111. Kramer JH, Crittenden MR, Halberg FE, et al. A prospective study of cognitive functioning following low-dose cranial radiation for bone marrow transplantation. Pediatrics. 1992;90(3):447–450.
112. Smedler AC, Bolme P. Neuropsychological deficits in very young bone-marrow transplant recipients. Acta Paediatr. 1995;84(4):429–433.

113. Smedler AC, Winiarski J. Neuropsychological outcome in very young hematopoietic SCT recipients in relation to pretransplant conditioning. Bone Marrow Transplant. 2008;42(8):515–522.
114. Phipps S, Rai SN, Leung WH, et al. Cognitive and academic consequences of stem-cell transplantation in children. J Clin Oncol. 2008;26(12):2027–2033.
115. Phipps S, Dunavant M, Srivastava DK, et al. Cognitive and academic functioning in survivors of pediatric bone marrow transplantation. J Clin Oncol. 2000;18(5): 1004–1011.
116. Vannatta K, Gerhardt CA, Wells RJ, Noll RB. Intensity of CNS treatment for pediatric cancer: prediction of social outcomes in survivors. Pediatr Blood Cancer. 2007; 49(5):716–722.
117. Noll RB. School and peer relationships. In: Wiener L, Pao M, Kazak AE, et al. (eds). Quick Reference for Pediatric Oncology Clinicians: The Psychiatric and Psychological Dimensions of Pediatric Cancer Symptom Management. Charlottesville, VA: IPOS Press, 2009; pp. 223–235.
118. Calhoun LG, Tedeschi RG. The foundations of post-traumatic growth: new considerations. Psychol Inq. 2004; 15(1):93–102.
119. Barakat LP, Alderfer MA, Kazak AE. Posttraumatic growth in adolescent survivors of cancer and their mothers and fathers. J Pediatr Psychol. 2006;31(4):413–419.
120. Belec RH. Quality of life: perceptions of long-term survivors of bone marrow transplantation. Oncol Nurs Forum. 1992;19(1):31–37.
121. Bishop MM, Beaumont JL, Hahn EA, et al. Late effects of cancer and hematopoietic stem-cell transplantation on spouses or partners compared with survivors and survivor-matched controls. J Clin Oncol. 2007;25(11):1403–1411.
122. Curbow B, Somerfield MR, Baker F, et al. Personal changes, dispositional optimism, and psychological adjustment to bone marrow transplantation. J Behav Med. 1993;16(5): 423–443.
123. Fromm K, Andrykowski MA, Hunt J. Positive and negative psychosocial sequelae of bone marrow transplantation: implications for quality of life assessment. J Behav Med. 1996;19(3):221–240.
124. Tallman B, Shaw K, Schultz J, Altmaier E. Well-being and posttraumatic growth in unrelated donor marrow transplant survivors: a nine-year longitudinal study. Rehabil Psychol. 2010;55(2):204–210.
125. Johnson Vickberg SM, Duhamel KN, Smith MY, et al. Global meaning and psychological adjustment among survivors of bone marrow transplant. Psychooncology. 2001;10(1):29–39.
126. Molassiotis A, Morris PJ. Quality of life in patients with chronic myeloid leukemia after unrelated donor bone marrow transplantation. Cancer Nurs. 1999;22(5): 340–349.
127. Sutherland HJ, Fyles GM, Adams G, et al. Quality of life following bone marrow transplantation: a comparison of patient reports with population norms. Bone Marrow Transplant. 1997;19(11):1129–1136.
128. Rini C, Manne S, DuHamel KN, et al. Mothers' perceptions of benefit following pediatric stem cell transplantation: a longitudinal investigation of the roles of optimism, medical risk, and sociodemographic resources. Ann Behav Med. 2004;28(2):132–141.
129. Stanton AL. Positive consequences of the experience of cancer: perceptions of growth and meaning. In: Holland J, Breitbart W, Jacobsen PB, et al. (eds). Psycho-Oncol, 2nd edition. New York, NY: Oxford University Press, 2010; pp. 547–550.
130. Bishop MM, Lee SJ, Beaumont JL, et al. The preventive health behaviors of long-term survivors of cancer and hematopoietic stem cell transplantation compared with matched controls. Biol Blood Marrow Transplant. 2010; 16(2):207–214.
131. Shankar SM, Carter A, Sun CL, et al. Health care utilization by adult long-term survivors of hematopoietic cell transplant: report from the bone marrow transplant survivor study. Cancer Epidemiol Biomarkers Prev. 2007;16(4): 834–839.
132. Rizzo JD, Wingard JR, Tichelli A, et al. Recommended screening and preventive practices for long-term survivors after hematopoietic cell transplantation: joint recommendations of the European Group for Blood and Marrow Transplantation, the Center for International Blood and Marrow Transplant Research, and the American Society of Blood and Marrow Transplantation. Biol Blood Marrow Transplant. 2006;12(2):138–151.
133. Armenian SH, Sun CL, Francisco L, et al. Health behaviors and cancer screening practices in long-term survivors of hematopoietic cell transplantation (HCT): a report from the BMT Survivor Study. Bone Marrow Transplant. 2012;47(2):283–290.
134. Hudson MM, Findlay S. Health-risk behaviors and health promotion in adolescent and young adult cancer survivors. Cancer. 2006;107(7 Suppl):1695–1701.
135. Nathan PC, Ford JS, Henderson TO, et al. Health behaviors, medical care, and interventions to promote healthy living in the Childhood Cancer Survivor Study cohort. J Clin Oncol. 2009;27(14):2363–2373.
136. Garwicz S, Anderson H, Olsen JH, et al. Late and very late mortality in 5-year survivors of childhood cancer: changing pattern over four decades – experience from the Nordic countries. Int J Cancer. 2012.131(7):1659–1666.

137. Demark-Wahnefried W, Pinto BM, Gritz ER. Promoting health and physical function among cancer survivors: potential for prevention and questions that remain. J Clin Oncol. 2006;24(32):5125–5131.
138. Hendriks MG, Schouten HC. Quality of life after stem cell transplantation: a patient, partner and physician perspective. Eur J Intern Med. 2002;13(1):52–56.
139. Guyatt GH, Ferrans CE, Halyard MY, et al. Exploration of the value of health-related quality-of-life information from clinical research and into clinical practice. Mayo Clin Proc. 2007;82(10):1229–1239.
140. Detmar SB, Muller MJ, Schornagel JH, et al. Health-related quality-of-life assessments and patient–physician communication: a randomized controlled trial. JAMA. 2002; 288(23):3027–3034.
141. FDA. Patient-reported outcome measures: use in medical product development to support labeling claims (draft guidance). 2009 Available from: http://www.fda.gov/downloads/Drugs/Guidances/UCM193282.pdf (accessed 28 May 2013).
142. PROQOLID. Patient-Reported Outcomes and Quality of Life Instruments Database. 2010. Available from: http://www.proqolid.org/ (accessed 22 May 2013).
143. Ader DN. Developing the patient-reported outcomes measurement information system (PROMIS). Med Care. 2007;45(5 Suppl 1):S3–S11.
144. Feichtl RE, Rosenfeld B, Tallamy B, et al. Concordance of quality of life assessments following pediatric hematopoietic stem cell transplantation. Psychooncology. 2010; 19(7):710–717.
145. Lof CM, Forinder U, Winiarski J. Risk factors for lower health-related QoL after allogeneic stem cell transplantation in children. Pediatr Transplant. 2007;11(2): 145–151.
146. Nuss SL, Wilson ME. Health-related quality of life following hematopoietic stem cell transplant during childhood. J Pediatr Oncol Nurs. 2007;24(2):106–115.
147. Varni JW, Limbers CA, Burwinkle TM. Parent proxy-report of their children's health-related quality of life: an analysis of 13,878 parents' reliability and validity across age subgroups using the PedsQL (TM) 4.0 Generic Core Scales. Health Qual Life Outcomes. 2007;5:2.
148. De Civita M, Regier D, Alamgir AH, et al. Evaluating health-related quality-of-life studies in paediatric populations – some conceptual, methodological and developmental considerations and recent applications. Pharmacoeconomics. 2005;23(7):659–685.
149. PoCoG. Measuring quality of life in children. Psycho-oncology Co-operative Research Group (PoCoG), 2008. Available from: http://www.pocog.org.au/content.aspx?page=QOL%20in%20children (accessed 22 May 2013).
150. Zwarenstein M, Goldman J, Reeves S. Interprofessional collaboration: effects of practice-based interventions on professional practice and healthcare outcomes. Cochrane Database Syst Rev. 2009;(3): CD000072.
151. Cramp F, Byron-Daniel J. Exercise for the management of cancer-related fatigue in adults. Cochrane Database Syst Rev. 2012;(11):CD006145.
152. Bird L, Arthur A, Niblock T, et al. Rehabilitation programme after stem cell transplantation: randomized controlled trial. J Adv Nurs. 2010;66(3):607–615.
153. Cimprich B, Janz NK, Northouse LL, et al. Taking charge: a self-management program for women following breast cancer treatment. Psychooncology. 2005;14(9):707–717.
154. Cohen M, Kuten A. Cognitive-behavior group intervention for relatives of cancer patients: a controlled study. J Psychosom Res. 2006;61(2):187–196.
155. Kurtz ME, Kurtz JC, Given C, Given B. Effects of a symptom control intervention on utilization of health care services among cancer patients. Med Sci Monit. 2006;12(7):319–324.
156. Mills ME, Sullivan K. The importance of information giving for patients newly diagnosed with cancer: a review of the literature. J Clin Nurs. 1999;8(6):631–642.
157. Streisand R, Rodrigue JR, Houck C, et al. Brief report: parents of children undergoing bone marrow transplantation: documenting stress and piloting a psychological intervention program. J Pediatr Psychol. 2000;25(5): 331–337.
158. Packman W, Weber S, Wallace J, Bugescu N. Psychological effects of hematopoietic SCT on pediatric patients, siblings and parents: a review. Bone Marrow Transplant. 2010; 45(7):1134–1146.
159. Wiener L, Battles H, Mamalian C, Zadeh S. ShopTalk: a pilot study of the feasibility and utility of a therapeutic board game for youth living with cancer. Support Care Cancer. 2011;19(7):1049–1054.
160. Burns DS, Robb SL, Haase JE. Exploring the feasibility of a therapeutic music video intervention in adolescents and young adults during stem-cell transplantation. Cancer Nurs. 2009;32(5):E8–E16.
161. Mayer DK, Ratichek S, Berhe H, et al. Development of a health-related website for parents of children receiving hematopoietic stem cell transplant: HSCT-CHESS. J Cancer Surviv. 2010;4(1):67–73.
162. EORTC. EORTC Quality of Life Questionnaire – QLQ-C30. Available from: http://groups.eortc.be/qol/eortc-qlq-c30 (accessed 22 May 2013).
163. Cella D Manual of the Functional Assessment of Chronic Illness Therapy (FACIT) measurement system, Version 4.1. Evanston, IL: Center of Outcomes, Research and Education (CORE) Evanston Northwestern Healthcare and Northwestern University; 2004.

164. De Haes JC, Olschewski M, Fayers P Measuring the quality of cancer patients with Rotterdam Symptom Checklist: a manual. Groningen: Northern Center for Health Research; 1996.

165. Ware J, Snow K, Kosinski M, Gandel B. SF-36 Health Survey. Manual and Interpretation Guide. Boston, MA: The Health Institute, New England Medical Center, 1997.

166. Ware JE. SF-36 Health Survey update. Spine. 2000; 25(24):3130–3139.

167. Bergner M, Bobbitt RA, Carter WB, Gilson BS. The Sickness Impact Profile: development and final revision of a health status measure. Med Care. 1981;19(8):787–805.

168. COH. City of Hope Pain & Palliative Care Resource Center. Duarte, CA. 2012. Available from http://prc.coh.org/qual_life.asp (accessed 22 May 2013).

169. PROMIS-NIH. Patient Reported Outcomes Measurement Information System (PROMIS). 2011. Available from: http://www.nihpromis.org/ (accessed 22 May 2013).

170. Baker F, Wingard JR, Curbow B, et al. Quality of life of bone marrow transplant long-term survivors. Bone Marrow Transplant. 1994;13:589–596.

171. Lee S, Cook EF, Soiffer R, Antin JH. Development and validation of a scale to measure symptoms of chronic graft-versus-host disease. Biol Blood Marrow Transplant. 2002;8(8):444–452.

172. Starfield B, Riley A, Ensminger M, et al. Manual Child Health and Illness Profile-Adolescent Edition (CHIP-AE). 1994.

173. Landgraf JL, Abetz L, Ware JE The CHQ User's Manual. 1996.

174. Varni JW, Burwinkle TM, Katz ER, et al. The PedsQL (TM) in pediatric cancer – reliability and validity of the Pediatric Quality of Life Inventory (TM) Generic Core Scales, Multidimensional Fatigue Scale, and Cancer Module. Cancer. 2002;94(7):2090–2106.

175. Edwards TC, Huebner CE, Connell FA, Patrick DL. Adolescent quality of life, part I: conceptual and measurement model. J Adolesc. 2002;25(3):275–286.

176. Armstrong FD, Toledano SR, Miloslavich K, et al. The Miami pediatric quality of life questionnaire: parent scale. Int J Cancer Suppl. 1999;12:11–17.

177. Goodwin D, Boggs SR, Graham-Pole J. Development and validation of the pediatric oncology quality of life scale. Psychol Assess. 1994;6(4):321–328.

178. Lansky LL, List MA, Lansky SB, et al. Toward the development of a play performance scale for children (PPSC). Cancer. 1985;56(7 Suppl):1837–1840.

179. Palermo TM, Witherspoon D, Valenzuela D, Drotar DD. Development and validation of the Child Activity Limitations Interview: a measure of pain-related functional impairment in school-age children and adolescents. Pain. 2004;109(3):461–470.

180. Claar RL, Walker LS. Functional assessment of pediatric pain patients: psychometric properties of the Functional Disability Inventory. Pain. 2006;121(1–2):77–84.

181. Phipps S, Dunavant M, Jayawardene D, Srivastiva DK. Assessment of health-related quality of life in acute in-patient settings: use of the BASES instrument in children undergoing bone marrow transplantation. Int J Cancer Suppl. 1999;12:18–24.

182. Parsons SK, Shih MC, Mayer DK, et al. Preliminary psychometric evaluation of the Child Health Ratings Inventory (CHRIs) and Disease-Specific Impairment Inventory-Hematopoietic Stem Cell Transplantation (DSII-HSCT) in parents and children. Qual Life Res. 2005; 14(6):1613–1625.

183. Manne S, DuHamel K, Nereo N, et al. Predictors of PTSD in mothers of children undergoing bone marrow transplantation: the role of cognitive and social processes. J Pediatr Psychol. 2002;27(7):607–617.

36

CHAPTER 36

Prevalent psychosocial adjustment issues and solutions: lifestyle and social challenges

Katrina M Stokes

Tennessee Valley Healthcare System, Nashville, TN, USA

Introduction

In this chapter we will look at some of the more prevalent psychosocial adjustment issues for your patients and their caregivers once they reach the long-term care setting of allogeneic stem cell transplant. Resources and options will be identified that are available for patients and caregivers to aid in addressing these issues in a positive, productive manner. First, issues affecting the patient and the caregiver will be discussed, such as changes in family dynamics, the support system and caregiver stress. Then, issues will be reviewed that affect the patient–caregiver relationship and the patient as an individual as they address their sexuality and establishing intimacy in significant relationships. In the final section, issues more prevalent in the individual patient experience will be discussed, such as returning to work, addressing possible pain control or addiction issues, stabilizing mental health, and assessing the changes to their spirituality after the life-threatening experience of transplant.

The patient and their support system: coping with stress in the long-term care setting

All of the hard work that goes into the allogeneic stem cell transplant process is not only to prolong life for your patients but to give them the opportunity to live a full and realized life. It can be difficult, as a medical team, to manage successfully all the complex treatment issues of the acute phase of transplant to find yourself facing a patient and family no longer certain how to live life.

In programs across the country the vital role of the caregiver in the allogeneic stem cell transplant setting is consistently acknowledged in program protocols requiring caregiver assistance to proceed with treatment. When our transplant program first began in the early 1990s our team knew that it was our preference that patients had the support of a caregiver through their treatment, but we were somewhat flexible on the issue. Those days are long gone. The reasons are fairly obvious. Patients run the risk of becoming critically ill, physically debilitated, cognitively impaired, or so depleted that they cannot manage medications, hygiene, hydration, or proper nutrition. Of equal significance is the fear and inner struggle the physical challenges present for the patient. The patient not only needs the caregiver for their physical assistance but also for the strength they receive from them through their love, support, and encouragement [1, 2].

Although the patient and caregiver have their own personal experiences through transplant they are both affected by the stress and uncertainty they face each day [3, 4]. As individuals grow and develop they begin to establish life goals and expectations. It is rare that one

Blood and Marrow Transplantation Long-Term Management: Prevention and Complications, First Edition. Edited by Bipin N Savani.

considers the possibility of living with illness when they are making plans for their life. After diagnosis, patients and families often feel they have to function with a whole new set of life rules. Successful adjustment to these changes requires living with shorter daily goals through the ups and downs of treatment as opposed to long-term future goals. After struggling with the roller coaster ride of emotions and physical challenges during the acute phase of treatment, they blink against the light of potential recovery and find themselves back in the old world of future goals and expectations. Understandably, some patients and families approach this new phase with caution. They know how it felt to have these comforting rules of living stripped from them in the past.

Dealing with the aftermath of all the role changes experienced by a family, during a transplant, can be a daunting task. Caregivers have to learn how to care for themselves again and patients have to gain some confidence in their ability to function independently. As the healthcare providers, it is a good opportunity to provide some validation and recognition of the enormity of what they have been through as a family.

If you see that a patient and their family are struggling during this phase it could be helpful to refer them to a local family therapist or support group. You can find resources in your community through the Cancer Support Network, which offers support groups through agencies, such as Gilda's Place, addressing cancer-related issues.

Another option is to establish a support group as part of your program. This would provide a group setting more focused on the post stem cell transplant issues as opposed to a group for more general cancer-related issues. If you decide to schedule the group on your larger clinic days this could increase participation owing to the convenience. It will require some good teamwork and communication. Your program could have the social worker invite patients into the group as opposed to them waiting in the clinic waiting area. The nurse practitioner and/or physicians could then call patients out of the group as they are needed to be seen. It is a casual approach to the group setting but can be very effective. Your program may consider providing a group for caregivers only. This provides an outlet for the caregiver and a way to connect to a temporary support system while away from their homes and support network for long periods of time. Even if your patients live in your community and have family and friends available, they may still benefit from the group experience. Although friends and family may be supportive they are not always capable of understanding the emotions wrapped up in the caregiver role.

Most patients resent the time they give to medical appointments already and would often talk themselves out of coming to the clinic or the hospital on a separate day to attend group. They often appreciate the opportunity and efficient use of their time when the support group is a part of the program. Ideally, they will also experience an increase in emotional well-being from the connections they make in the group setting.

The caregiver/patient issues discussed so far have focused more on situations where the caregiver is the patients' spouse or significant other. In a discussion of the stem cell transplant caregiver it is important to take into account the different people that can fulfill this role in a patients' life.

The role of the caregiver cannot be well served by just anyone in the patients' life. It is intimate in nature, involving issues that most consider private. Whether it is financial issues, the sharing of medical information, the exposure of personal habits, or the needed assistance in hygiene issues, there are moments during a transplant that a patient cannot just share with a casual acquaintance. However, through necessity, patients and their primary caregivers may need to involve a wider net of friends and family to meet the needs of the patient.

In transplant, as in life, there is no one perfect way that an individual's support system may come together. Some people may lack a connection with their biological families, have lived their lives separate from them by choice or circumstance, or have come from small or distant families. In these circumstances, people often develop their "family" through others that have shared their lives. As with the more traditional family support system, transplant can move these relationships to a deeper level.

One of the surprises of transplant is the time that patients have to reconnect to many of the people in their lives. During transplant, patients are often able to spend focused time with their siblings, parents, cousins, aunts, uncles, grandparents, and others. They reconnect at a time that they are also faced with their mortality. In the long-term setting they are accepting their survival and deciding how to deal with these renewed relationships.

It would be naive not to acknowledge that transplant can also be the strain that breaks some relationships, both casual and significant in nature. Often when individuals are put under the stress of facing their mortality the worst of their personality traits emerge. This does not tend to enrich relationships and may leave a patient alone with regret when survival becomes a reality and not a mere dream.

It can be easy as healthcare providers to expect a certain amount of joy in our patients and their families once they have reached the long-term care setting. We have been eye witnesses to their struggle to survive and are prepared to bask in their glow of triumph but can feel perplexed when there is no expected jubilation. Patients and caregivers can be too consumed with the stressors in their lives to respond as we might expect. Their life experiences, their history with each other and with their disease and treatment are individually processed. All of these variables affect how they cope and react. Just because they may be struggling with some of the adjustments in their lives posttransplant does not mean transplant was unsuccessful. It is a sign of success that they are getting on with living a life with all of its bumps and turns.

The patient and caregiver: facing intimacy issues

In this section of the chapter concerning patient sexuality and caregiver relationships it is important to remember that many of our caregivers never imagined that they would find themselves in this situation. They may have lived their lives avoiding all aspects of "sickness," staying healthy themselves and never entering the hospital setting. Then, out of nowhere, they find themselves immersed in prescription schedules, monitoring bowel movements, learning to give shots or flush Hickman catheters. Even if the caregiver is the patient's spouse, relationships can vary. In couples that function with a mutually agreed upon independence, this level of intimacy is not what they bargained for. It is not surprising that caregivers want to run away from this responsibility. When this happens in the acute phase it is a serious complication for the patient's care. More commonly, caregivers hang in there during the acute phase, for many reasons, often guilt driven. After they have seen the patient through the acute phase they may leave out of fear of the disease returning or the unavoidable changes they have experienced in their relationship. Caregivers have expressed during group their fear of loving the patient too much because they anticipate the pain of losing them. A caregiver may have been drawn to the patient's strength and take charge personaly but has watched these characteristics disappear through the fear and uncertainty of living with cancer.

From the patient's perspective, they are often so sick of being sick and dealing with the relentless side effects of treatment that they struggle to think outside of their own misery. They will find the strength to "put on a happy face" for their healthcare team while showing all their pain and frustration to the person that is with them around the clock, assuming forgiveness and understanding. Resentment and frustration can build. The support groups mentioned previously can be a comfortable, logical place to process some of these complex issues.

Maintaining respectful communication in the patient–caregiver relationship under such stress is complicated. However, they need to reestablish trust through the emotional connection of respectful communication to move forward in reestablishing their intimate sexual relationship. An integral part of the human experience is our sexuality, and reestablishing this is an important step for the patient in their road to a healthy life.

As your patients seek this healthy life posttransplant they will be looking at different areas of their life, the changes they have experienced in those areas, and what their new expectations might be. These changes have affected their body, their mind, their priorities, their relationships with others, and so on. They may attempt to minimize the effect these changes have had, but in the end they have to face them for what they are. It would seem logical that on a subconscious level some patients could feel betrayed by their body. They may feel that their body no longer looks or functions in a way that they can predict or control. Sharing intimacy with another person can cause some feelings of vulnerability and uncertainty. When you have lost confidence in knowing your own body, sharing it with another could be an intimidating concept [5].

Whether your patients' issues relate to lowered libido, lack of confidence, or are more functional in nature, they will look to you, their healthcare providers, for some answers. This is a subject that can often be difficult for the patient to bring up, so you want to be prepared. It may be tempting to avoid the subject and assume there are no issues if the patient does not voice concerns. I would like to suggest some alternatives that might be more comfortable for everyone involved and hopefully prevent such an important issue from being neglected.

Research what resources are available within your system and/or community. The American Cancer Society has developed a refreshingly comprehensive pamphlet addressing these issues for both male and female patients (Cancer and Sexuality). It looks at some of the more intimate aspects of this question, such as sexual positions that require less physical strength while still providing the participants a satisfying option for expressing their love and/or attraction to each other. The pamphlet also offers clothing suggestions that may improve a patient's confidence with their body postsurgery and/or treatment, among other pertinent but private details. If you are in a hospital setting you may have a significant resource through your urology department to address function/libido issues for men. Any written materials, short videos, or educational support groups available only help improve your confidence in communicating with the patient on this difficult topic and will hopefully help normalize the issue for the patient. It is a win–win for all involved.

If you have a social worker and a nurse practitioner in your program you could utilize their strengths with a team approach to address the combined psychological and physical aspects of issues surrounding sexuality. It does not have to be awkward. It is a positive step toward feeling and living like a healthy person again for your patient.

I would like to encourage you to develop this aspect of your post stem cell transplant clinic. Provide this information in a logical, user-friendly manner to all your patients. If you have a large clinic it may be more efficient to develop a couple of educational classes addressing different aspects of sexuality posttransplant. Your dynamic duo team of your nurse practitioner and licensed clinical social worker could coordinate these classes, presenting information, bringing in speakers, offering a couples support group, question and answer sessions, and so on. It could help guide your development of this program by screening your clients initially for some helpful feedback. The following is an example of a survey that could be used for such a purpose. Remember . . . user friendly.

Let's talk about sex

1. Do you have some questions about posttransplant sexual issues but are uncomfortable bringing them up in the clinic setting? If yes, what are some of these questions?
2. Are you and your partner experiencing some complications in your sexual relationship?
3. Are you having trouble talking about these issues together?
4. What would your preference be for receiving answers to your questions?(Number 1–4 in order of preference.)
   (a) Support group with other couples.
   (b) Couples counseling with an individual therapist.
   (c) Educational support group/topic presentations
   (d) Pamphlets provided in posttransplant clinic setting.
5. Do any of the following statements apply to you?
   (a) I don't know how to feel sexy in my body posttransplant.
   (b) My partner has become more like a parent than a lover.
   (c) I don't know how to start dating again postcancer.

Other quality of life issues for the stem cell transplant patient

In this final section of the chapter we will be looking at quality of life issues affecting the transplant patient as an individual. On that bumpy road back to living well, patients not only have to adjust to new roles and responsibilities and reestablishing healthy relationships, but they also face the question of what to do with this new life and how to do it.

Returning to work is a goal that becomes more of a possibility when the patient reaches this long-term care stage. Again, I remind us all to remember that our patients are individuals. Feelings about returning to work vary based on the individual and can be affected by the patient's mental health, physical strength, general coping skills, age, and gender and how this affects personal and societal expectations.

If a patient is already retirement age at the time of treatment they often do not want to return to work but to return to life and activities that they see as part of a healthy retirement. The younger patient may find it hard to find their place without the concept of their career or their role as provider. Even though women have become an integral part of the workforce, society is still more accepting of alternative roles outside of the workplace for women. The pull for female patients to return to work may be more on a personal level of job satisfaction, the intellectual stimulation of the workplace, the social connection, and so on. The male patient will have these interests also, but with the added element of seeing "earning a living" as some sign of a stronger masculine role. Post stem cell transplant is all about finding their "new normal." For both male and female patients this is a challenge and may involve special training or education to develop skills more in sync with their current physical and cognitive status.

The long-term care stem cell transplant patient may have developed several physical issues that would have to be considered when evaluating job options. There could be short-term memory loss, peripheral neuropathy, or cataracts, just to name a few. Many of these issues are here to stay and some can be improved through surgery, physical therapy/occupational therapy consults, or something as simple as utilizing a notepad in day-to-day functioning. As providers, we can support the patient in their efforts to return to work by doing a thorough assessment of their individual functional issues and making referrals to appropriate resources.

If a patient is receiving social security disability benefits they have access to a program called Ticket to Work. Either through an employment network provider or an individual's state vocational rehabilitation agency they can have access to career counseling, job placement, and other supportive services in their efforts to return to work posttransplant.

The Vanderbilt transplant program, which serves not only stem cell transplant patients but also solid organ transplants, provides on-site vocational rehabilitation services through the Vanderbilt Transplant Return to Work Program. This program is funded through a grant from the Tennessee Department of Human Services, Division of Rehabilitation. Program services include career interest and vocational aptitude testing, career counseling, help with resumés and interviewing skills, and assistance with job placement and job retention. All services are offered one-on-one and provided free of charge to the patient. The program also helps individuals access additional services available through the Tennessee Division of Rehabilitation Services, including sponsorship for education and job retraining. In a transplant program that serves solid organ and stem cell transplant patients, this is a valuable resource. The less road blocks to returning to work, the more employment becomes a real possibility for the transplant patient. If your program is significant in size you may want to investigate resources in your area. In the program mentioned above they pursued the grant, provided space for the return-to-work employee, and worked out a referral system to help patients gain maximum benefit from the service. It requires some devoted effort to get off the ground but has been a thriving part of that program for approximately 15 years.

By the time the stem cell transplant patient has reached the long-term care setting they have faced challenges beyond what any of us would anticipate dealing with in an entire lifetime. Chronic illness, chronic pain, chronic reminders of your mortality, chronic fear, chronic insecurity all pile up for our patients. Because the issues they have faced are so rare, few of our patients have had life experiences that help them develop coping skills for such intense attacks on their quality of life. Depression and anxiety can be a common complaint. The level of intensity and the duration experienced by each patient will be affected by circumstance, chemical balance, genetics, and coping skills learned through each individual's unique life experience.

Transplant clinicians are often holistic in their approach to the patient, including mental health in their review of systems. It can be tempting to address any signs of anxiety or depression immediately. Prescribing medication is a remedy at hand in the fast-moving clinical setting. Just remember that there are many issues that can affect mood that are not long term. Being sad because you were told your disease relapsed is an appropriate response to a complicated issue. As clinicians, it is important to assess patient safety in relation to their mood. If you find no evidence of irrational thoughts of harm, it is important to respect the patient's right to process information through their emotions. Emotions may cause us concern in our need to "fix" things, but sadness does not have to break someone. It can often be a cathartic process for the patient to find their balance in adjusting to difficult information.

If possible, it would be advantageous for any patient dealing with some anxiety or depression to have a thorough assessment prior to starting on medication. There are many issues that affect mood that can be managed through a nutritionist, an exercise regime, or individual or group therapy. One or all of these approaches may provide the changes needed for the patient's mood to improve.

A nutritionist can do a thorough review of a patient's diet, identifying an excess daily intake of sugar and/or caffeine that can increase anxious feelings or agitation. They can also identify any food allergies or make recommendations for diet changes that can improve energy and mood. Regular exercise can also improve mood. If the patient has some limitations, they could meet with a physical therapist for recommendations of excercise options such as yoga, swimming, stationary biking, and so on.

Individual or group therapy can also be a positive resource. Meeting with a therapist gives the patient an outlet to process some of their emotions, problem solve, and develop tools for dealing with pain, anxiety, or depression. A therapist can also help the anxious patient identify triggers to their anxiety, and give them tools to address the anxiety before developing into an anxiety or panic attack.

Some of these tools could be provided through your clinic if there are any roadblocks to individual therapy. There are several excellent progressive muscle relaxation scripts available from different resources on the internet. Progressive muscle relaxation is an excellent tool to introduce to patients in a group setting. After walking them through the process and having some discussion after, the group facilitator can provide a copy of a script for the patient to use with their caregiver or a recorded copy of the script to use on their own. Discussion should focus on how the practice of relaxation techniques is a way to be in touch with how their body feels when it is fully relaxed, the goal being to eventually know how to take their bodies to that relaxed state through remembering the relaxed state. Visual imagery is another effective tool for dealing with anxiety or depression brought on by living with pain. At www.innerhealthstudio.com there are multiple visual imagery scripts providing a wide selection of visual images that walk an individual through a peaceful place while taking note of their sensory response to the image.

The goal of a good relaxation technique is to slow the breathing and focus the thoughts enough to stop the repeat track of worried thinking. If your patient is experiencing stress or anxiety in a place where they are unable to work on progressive muscle relaxation or visual imagery, it is important to keep things simple. An easy relaxation tool for patients to use in almost any setting is deep breathing. Counting, in their mind, while breathing in . . . 1 . . . 2 . . . 3 . . . 4, holding air in 1 . . . 2 . . . 3 . . . 4, and then slowly out 1 . . . 2 . . . 3 . . . 4. The patient may have to count to only two at first until they start to calm and can take slower, deeper breaths.

If the patient has a bit of privacy the mental countdown is a great tool that does not require total solace and so could be managed in an exam room or office. The patient sits comfortably and will do a countdown of five things they see, hear, and physically feel. It is important for the patient to say these things out loud, allowing the rhythm of their voice to aid in calming their mind and body. Encourage them not to worry about repeating items on the countdown. Keeping the rhythm of their voice going seems to be most critical, letting the mind relax into auto pilot.

Survival guilt is often seen during this long-term care stage and can be connected to some of the feelings of depression or anxiety. If you see signs of this in your patient it is important to recommend short-term therapy. The patient needs to process these feelings with a therapist that will help them see that they had no control or responsibility for the other patients' loss of life. To help them move to a place of joy and appreciation that they have done well.

Although patients see us less and less as they get farther out from transplant, the hospital and clinic setting is still part of their lives and can be a source of stress. Some simple steps from an administrative perspective can improve quality of life for a chronically ill individual. It is easy to be focused on how many patients we need to see in a limited amount of time in clinic rather than the schedule for each individual patient. This is one of those areas where I would encourage each long-term care stem cell transplant program to spend some time thinking of how an individual might feel managing their care through your program.

By the time we are treating the stem cell transplant patient in the long-term care setting they have become overly sensitized to the treatment setting. Some patients have spent months in the hospital, many days each week in clinic, and suffered through countless procedures. Needing this treatment is, of course, not your fault, but you can see how the patient could resent those times when they might have to come back to repeat a test, or have two appointments in one day that are 5 hours apart.

Any small conveniences mean so much: having comfortable waiting areas, magazines, water, and so on. These things may seem unimportant in the large scheme of treatment, but your patients have been reminded of their mortality, they feel the limitation of their time here on Earth, and, as nice as we are, they would rather spend their time doing things that lift up their spirits or, at a minimum, involve their favorite recliner rather than stiff chairs in our waiting room. So, in the same way that you regularly assess the quality of the medical care you provide your patients, assess the quality of the process and how to improve patient satisfaction with their care. The following is an example of a survey that could give you some feedback on patient satisfaction:

How can we improve your care experience?

1. Were you seen on time today?
2. How long did you wait before seeing the physician after being placed in the exam room?
3. Is the waiting room comfortable?
4. Do you feel that you have privacy when being seen by your providers?
5. Do you have to repeat a lot of the same information through your check in and treatment process?
6. Would you appreciate educational materials being available in waiting area?
7. Would you like to have educational or emotional support groups during clinic time?
8. Are your appointments scheduled in a convenient manner?
9. Are you making more than one trip a week to clinic? If yes, do you feel some of these trips could be combined?
10. Do you have convenient access to restroom facilities and water?

Another issue that affects the patient's quality of life and can be complicated to assess and address is that of pain control and addiction. Pain caused by disease or treatment side effects in the posttransplant setting is a problem that cannot be ignored. The complicated aspect of posttransplant pain management is helping a patient recognize when their pain is physical and should be treated with pain medication and when their pain is psychological and should be treated with a more appropriate solution.

It is important to know your resources and to know your patient. If there are valid concerns about pain medication use and possible abuse, express these concerns to the patient in a professional manner. Assist them in meeting with a clinician trained to help them in addressing this issue. Approach the patient as you would with other issues negatively affecting their health and well-being. Approach them with respect and honesty. Clarify your limitations and guidelines that must be followed in prescribing these medications. Owing to the long-term aspect of this treatment setting it is important to address this issue quickly and foster clear communication. The concept of becoming addicted should be addressed when first beginning treatment [6, 7].

Regardless of our patients' particular spiritual belief systems, they cannot go through the ground-shaking experience of transplant without an inner response. Facing one's mortality can bring about an intense clinging to what we believe or an inability to believe in anything, since all we know has been tossed about and is no longer recognizable. This experience brings to mind a quote by Eleanor Roosevelt, "We gain strength, and courage, and confidence by each experience in which we really stop to look fear in the face . . . we must do that which we think we cannot."

The fact that this book is being published is, in itself, testament to how far "bone marrow" transplant has come. Our patients are surviving. They are looking for love, balance, and meaning to their lives. Our patients are living.

References

1. Gallant MP. The influence of social support on chronic illness self management: a review and directions for research. Health Educ Behav. 2003;30(2):170–195.
2. Wolff JL. Family matters in health care delivery. JAMA. 2012;308(15):1529–1530.
3. Nijboer C, Triemstra M, Sanderman R, van den Bos GA. Determinants of caregiving experiences and mental health of partners of cancer patients. Cancer. 1999;86(4):577–588.

4. Bevans MF, Sternberg EM. Caregiving burden, stress and health effects among family caregivers of adult cancer patients. JAMA. 2012;307(4):398–403.
5. Manne SL, Zautra AJ. Couples coping with chronic illness: women with rheumatoid arthritis and their healthy husbands. J Behav Med. 1990;13(4):327–342.
6. Zgierska A, Miller M, Rabago D. Patient satisfaction, prescription drug abuse, and potential unintended consequences. JAMA. 2012;307(13):1377–1378.
7. Nampiaparampil DE. Chronic pain: a primary care guide to practical management. JAMA. 2010;303(2):174–173.

37

CHAPTER 37

A patient's perspective: concepts of long-term survivor support groups and their roles

Michael W Brown
Private Wealth Management Group, LLC, Crossville, TN, USA

My name is Mike. I am a 66-year-old allogeneic stem cell survivor and I have had a complete recovery from non-Hodgkin's lymphoma. I refer to my self as a "recovered lymphomaniac," but then I have always confronted adversity with humor.

On a recent visit to my oncologist, Dr Bipin Savani, he asked me to write about long-term survivor support groups and the value of their role.

Following my stem cell transplant and a 4-month stay at Vanderbilt University Hospital in Nashville, Tennessee, I returned to my small community appearing healthy, alert, and ready to go back to work. Because of this outward face of energy, I was asked by the local hospital to lead its Cancer Support Group. The current leader was retiring.

It is an honor to address what I thought would be an important aspect of cancer recovery. I thought I could share, interact, and lead a special group of patients who are involved in a battle for their lives. I hoped to help them reach a recovery as I had.

I welcomed the challenge. It was a "give back" opportunity and a means of demonstrating to my fellow patient/survivors what a marvel modern medicine is. I was eager to educate about the miracle of stem cell transplantation, to offer solutions for dealing with ongoing neuropathy and muscle cramps, and to encourage attention to diet and exercise. I was psyched up about sharing solutions and remedies.

The leadership role was not what I had envisioned. The environment was needy and dark. Stories were grim. Dealing with personal disaster without humor and hope was not how my wife, Sue, and I had managed 11 years of my health issues.

I believe my outcome was directly related to how my wife, now known as The Surgeon General, and I chose to cope with the cancer diagnosis. As a married couple and soul-mates, we have always teamed up to confront life's challenges. The "You Have Cancer" is one of the greatest ones.

Non-Hodgkin's lymphoma is a slow-developing cancer and we adjusted our lives to treatment protocols laid out for us in 90-day treatment regimens. Once-a-week all-day infusions went on for a month. It became the norm. Computer axial tomography scans and positron emission tomography (PET) scans monitored the effectiveness of the drugs. There were two clinical trials. One lasted 4 months and involved a daily round-trip commute of 222 miles. We spent nearly 7 years educating ourselves on the progression of the disease, what physical maladies to expect, and how to live with them.

Patients at the clinic or the chemo sessions fell into two groups: some approached cancer as a life event

Blood and Marrow Transplantation Long-Term Management: Prevention and Complications, First Edition. Edited by Bipin N Savani.

that required adjustment of schedules; others let the cancer rule.

We chose to live with cancer, deal with it positively, and somehow find humor in what we faced.

It was our attitude for 7 years. In March 2010, I was pronounced in remission and told my port would be removed. I was officially "de-ported" the following week.

Four months later a routine PET scan showed my cancer was back and growing aggressively. My oncologist, who became a wonderful friend for all of these years, told me the drugs had run their course. In order to continue living I needed a stem cell transplant.

I entered the first stage of dealing with this news. I was never fond of "Denial", so I let Reality quickly kick in. It included months of maintenance chemo, sibling-match screening, and insurance hoop-jumping. The Medical Acceptance Board approved me for the stem cell procedure. There was ongoing blood testing, bone marrow testing doctor appointments, and my business to run.

Who was going to take care of the dog for 4 months?

My sense of Reality sharpened when, after screening my brother and two sisters, I was told my brother was the strongest candidate to be a donor. I owe a loving and great gratitude to our parents, for luckily none of us fell far from their DNA tree.

The transplant was done on St Patrick's Day 2011. I dressed in Kelly Green for the occasion of my brother literally becoming my keeper. His stem cells gave me another chance to live a normal life.

It was a 100-day episode at Vanderbilt, and when I went home and got into my own bed I was thankful for time to enjoy my wife, family, and friends.

It was at this time I was asked to lead the local Cancer Support Group in our small community. I felt it an honor to help fellow survivors navigate the road to acceptance and recovery. There were five who attended. I told them my story and they told me theirs.

One woman told a tear-filled story of congestive heart failure from chemotherapy. She added that she was the president of the Polio Survivors Group and said she owed her entire survival to herbs and alternative treatments.

Another survivor had recently moved to our small community. She came from a large metropolitan area, where she was treated for non-Hodgkin's lymphoma in a university medical setting. Her new oncologist told her she had been "overtreated", PET scans were overrated, and she no longer needed them. (The local hospital did not have a PET scanner on site at the time of her doctor's evaluation.)

I fervently believe a PET scan saved my life. My oncologist told me he was very pleased he insisted on a PET scan, otherwise he would not have detected the aggressive growth of the cancer as early as he did.

The only male in the support group was a Viet Nam vet recovering from radical surgery of his jaw and throat. He attributed his problem to Agent Orange, a defoliant used in the Viet Nam war. The Veterans Administration (VA) identified it as a carcinogen that would make him eligible for treatment. However, he was denied this treatment by the VA for reasons he did not explain. He is facing severe financial difficulties along with the ongoing discomfort associated with his cancer.

After 3 months of meetings, I researched why there was not greater participation and involvement in our chapter. I spoke with many cancer survivors I knew personally, asking why they did not attend the meetings.

The answer was the group members were complainers, who instead of supporting one another, were mostly self-indulgent.

Friends, who briefly attended a Parkinson's support group, were not enthused by that group for similar reasons.

I have had such a successful transplant. I am surrounded with positive personalities. I realize my good fortune with my outcome. However, the involvement with the local cancer support group sucked the life out of me. It left me deeply frustrated and depressed after each session.

The attitude of the members was virulent in acceptance of anything different in the format of the group meetings. It was not a "supportive" place. So, I resigned.

My negative experience with a cancer support group, I hope, is not the norm. There are organizations that are absolutely helpful.

While researching cancer support web sites, I found *CancerCare.org*, a wonderful resource for all forms of cancer. It offers the ability to participate in live lectures and to review previous presentations via podcasts. It addresses cancer on various topics, such as diet and exercise and neuropathy after chemotherapy

Meditation, relaxation techniques to reduce stress, and alternative techniques in managing cancers are other available topics. This site has several beneficial topics and presentations to educate cancer patients and caregivers. This technological age provides a world of available information.

My goal is to return to the group, but only as a member. I am far from a quitter in things I believe in. I was temporarily sidetracked by negative attitudes. I do, however, believe in helping those who seek help. It is a great way to share knowledge, and I will go back and hope we become what the names says it is supposed to be, a "Support Group."

APPENDIX 1

NMDP/Be The Match posttransplant guidelines resources

Darlene Haven

National Marrow Donor Program®/Be The Match®, Minneapolis, MN, USA

Posttransplant care guidelines resources

Advances in hematopoietic cell transplantation (HCT) technology and supportive care have led to improvements in long-term survival after HCT. Emerging indications for transplantation, introduction of newer graft sources (e,g., umbilical cord blood), and transplantation of older patients using less intense conditioning regimens have also contributed to an increase in the number of HCT survivors. These survivors are at risk for developing late complications secondary to pre-, peri-, and post-transplantation exposures and risk factors.

In support of improving planning, survival, and quality of life for these patients, the National Marrow Donor Program® (NMDP)/Be The Match® produces clinical and patient education and resources.

The need for follow-up care

As HCT recipients transition from one phase of post-transplantation care to another, transplant providers and patients both need to understand that close and ongoing monitoring are necessary to continue to improve survival. A survivorship care plan can support this follow-up to remind providers about appropriate surveillance for late complications based on an individual patient's risk factors and exposures.

Published guidelines for screening and preventative practices

To address the appropriate screening and preventative practices, guidelines for HCT survivors were published in 2006 [1]. An international group of transplantation experts was then convened in 2011 to review contemporary literature and update these recommendations while considering the changing practice of transplantation and international applicability of these guidelines. This review provided updated recommendations for screening and preventive practices for pediatric and adult survivors of autologous and allogeneic HCT [2].

NMDP/Be The Match adaptation of publication into online and mobile app resources

The NMDP/Be The Match then worked with the authors to adapt the publication into resources that can be readily used by clinicians in practice and by patients as they navigate their care after transplant. The resources provide an easy-to-follow guide that defines screening and preventative practices, based on individual risks and exposures, for specific time points of 6 months, 1 year, and every year thereafter.

The authors recommended that patients use the guidelines to set out a long-term follow-up care plan in

Blood and Marrow Transplantation Long-Term Management: Prevention and Complications, First Edition. Edited by Bipin N Savani.

consultation with their health-care providers. Likewise, the guidelines can be used by transplant clinicians to organize care once the patient transitions from the transplant center to primary treating physicians. They can also be used to educate treating physicians on appropriate monitoring and follow-up care.

The full NMDP/Be The Match guidelines resource contains:

- posttransplant care guidelines;
- graft-versus-host disease (GVHD) screening recommendations with photo atlas;
- referral timing guidelines with outcomes data [3].

Available online and via mobile app:

- Includes the list of screening and preventative practices that may be customized by the patient's risk factors (age group, gender, GVHD, steroid exposure, total body irradiation)
- Results can be e-mailed and printed by the user
- Provides links to references/outcomes data
- Provided at no charge.

How to access the resources

The NMDP/Be The Match provides the guidelines resources free online:

- online clinical version – marrow.org/HCT-guide
- online patient version – BeTheMatch.org/careguide
- mobile-friendly web – m.marrow.org/HCT.

Or free through phone marketplace – search "transplant" or NMDP:

- mobile app available on iPad®, iPhone®, Android™.[1]

[1] Apple, the Apple logo, iPhone, iPod touch, and iTunes are trademarks of Apple Inc., registered in the U.S. and other countries. iPad is a trademark of Apple Inc. App Store is a service mark of Apple Inc. Android is a trademark of Google Inc. Use of this trademark is subject to Google Permissions.

About NMDP/Be The Match

The NMDP is the global leader in providing a cure to patients with life-threatening blood cancers – like leukemia and lymphoma – or other diseases. The nonprofit organization connects patients with their donor match for a life-saving marrow or umbilical cord blood transplant, educates health-care professionals, and conducts research with the Center for International Blood and Marrow Transplant Research, the research arm of NMDP.

The NMDP also operates Be The Match, which provides patient support and operates the Be The Match Registry – the world's largest registry of potential marrow donors and donated cord blood units. Learn more at marrow.org/md.

References

1. Rizzo JD, Wingard JR, Tichelli A, et al. Recommended screening and preventive practices for long-term survivors after hematopoietic cell transplantation: joint recommendations of the European Group for Blood and Marrow Transplantation, the Center for International Blood and Marrow Transplant Research, and the American Society of Blood and Marrow Transplantation. Biol Blood Marrow Transplant. 2006;12:138–151.
2. Majhail NS, Rizzo JD, Lee SJ, et al. Recommended screening and preventive practices for long-term survivors after hematopoietic cell transplantation. Co-published in Biol Blood Marrow Transplant. 2012;18(3):348–371; Bone Marrow Transplant, 2012;47(3):337–341; and Hematol Oncol Stem Cell Ther. 2012;5(1):1–30.
3. NMDP, ASBMT. Recommended Timing for Transplant Consultation, 2011. Available from: www.marrow.org/HCT-guide (accessed 22 May 2013).

APPENDIX 2
Long-term follow-up calendar

André Tichelli, Joerg P Halter, Jakob R Passweg, and Alicia Rovó
Hematology Division, Basel University Hospital, Basel, Switzerland

Introduction

The long-term follow-up program aims to provide care for childhood and adulthood survivors after hematopoietic stem cell transplant (HSCT). Long-term care of transplanted survivors includes screening and prevention of late complications of the HSCT, education about the possible late consequences of the transplantation, and monitoring of health care needs according to risk profile of the survivor.

For transplanted patients in remission from their primary disease and without active chronic graft-versus-host disease (GVHD), annual follow-up visits are considered as a standard. More frequent controls may be needed for patients with active chronic GVHD, with recurrent infectious complications or other posttransplant complications which need close guidance from experts in post-transplant care. Because the long-term survivors often live in geographical areas away from the transplant center and have returned to work, the visit should be well prepared in advance to avoid waiting times. Health risk after HSCT is strongly associated with a number of factors, which are related to the primary disease and its previous treatment, as well as to the transplantation procedure itself. Since the magnitude of risk and the severity of the late complications for an individual patient may greatly vary, the follow-up care should be individualized on the basis of the patient's history.

In this appendix, the survivorship care plan, the organization of an annual visit, and the recommendations for screening and preventive measurements of posttransplant survivors will be discussed.

Survivorship care plan

The Institute of Medicine recommended that all patients completing primary cancer treatment are provided with a comprehensive treatment summary and a survivorship care plan, reviewed with the patient during an end-of-treatment consultation [1]. This plan is intended to improve care coordination and patient's knowledge about late effects that may occur after cancer treatment. Likewise, at transition from the transplant center to the long-term follow-up clinic or to a nontransplant health care provider a survivorship care plan has to be ready, including the treatment summary and the follow-up care plan for this patient. Such a plan should be done even when the follow-up clinic belongs to the same transplant center.

For a long time, survivorship care plan instruments that are specific for HSCT recipients were lacking; therefore, providers had to consider instruments that had been developed for cancer survivors in general (e.g., LIVESTRONG Care Plan: www.livestrongcareplan org; Passport for Care: www.txch.org/passportforcare). These instruments allowed for preparing an individualized survivorship care plan based on information that health care providers or the patient themselves provided in a brief questionnaire. This questionnaire includes demographics from the patient, as well as details on their cancer and cancer treatment received. Based in this information, a detailed individualized description of anticipated risks of late effects as well as a follow-up plan is proposed. Today, the LIVESTRONG Care Plan includes HSCT as a therapeutical option. The drugs and the possibility of total

Blood and Marrow Transplantation Long-Term Management: Prevention and Complications, First Edition. Edited by Bipin N Savani.

body irradiation (TBI) used for conditioning are integrated into the risk estimation. However, specific details such as intensity of conditioning, dose of irradiation, source of stem cells, and donor type are so far not taken into account. Recently, an internet-based survivorship care plan, Passport for Care, has been developed on the initiatives of researchers at the Texas Children's Cancer Center and Baylor College of Medicine's Center for Collaborative and Interactive Technologies in Huston. This Passport for Care should guide survivors and the health care providers, and drive algorithms to produce individualized monitoring and management recommendations for long-term follow-up [2].

Now, posttransplant care guidelines are available and include recommendations for long-term posttransplant screening and preventive practices, screening for chronic GVHD, and vaccinations. These recommendations provided by the National Marrow Donor Program (NMDP)/ Be The Match are based on Recommended Screening and Preventive Practices, developed by experts from seven international transplant professional societies [3].

The survivorship care plan is intended for the health care provider as well as the transplant survivor and their family. It is particular useful for health care providers who are not specialized in cancer treatment and in HSCT. Elements that have to be included in such a survivorship care plan are presented in Table A.2.1. From this information an individualized risk profile and a plan for follow-up care can be assessed. A patient-friendly version should be available for the survivor and their relatives. Issues to be considered when implementing a survivorship care plan concern data collection, resources needed, the way to proceed during the transition phase, and the future responsibilities of care and care planning.

Table A.2.1 Elements of a survivorship care plan for patients treated with hematopoietic stem cell transplantation, according to Ref. [4] (Section 3, delivering long-term follow-up care; p. 36)

1. *General background information*
   a. Demographics (name, sex, date of birth, contact information, insurance)
   b. Social information (matrimonial state, children, age of the children)
   c. Important medical history before primary diagnosis for which the patient is transplanted
   d. Name and address of the hemato-oncologist or primary healthcare provider
2. *Primary diagnosis (for which the patient was transplanted)*
   a. Diagnostic details (diagnosis, stage at diagnosis and at HSCT, date of diagnosis, pertinent diagnostic features, state of the disease at transition to the long-term follow-up clinic)
3. *Treatment summary*
   a. Chemotherapy (before HSCT)
      i. Drugs and route of administration
      ii. Cumulative dose (alkylators, anthracyclines, etc.)
   b. Radiation therapy
      i. Field(s) and total dose, number of fractions, radiation type
      ii. Institution/facility
   c. Surgical procedure
      i. Date of the procedures
      ii. Names and sites of the procedures
4. *Hematopoietic stem cell transplantation (HSCT)*
   a. Type(s) and date(s) of HSCT (allogeneic, syngeneic, autologous)
   b. Type of donor
   c. Source of stem cells
   d. Conditioning regimen
   e. GVHD prophylaxis and treatment in allogeneic HSCT
5. *Potential long-term effects*
   a. List of possible late effects
6. *Follow-up plan*
   a. Recommendations for screening tests (type and frequency) based on age and risk factors

Organization of the long-term follow-up visit

The annual long-term follow-up visit should last no longer than one full day; this will reduce cost for those patients coming from distant geographical areas and guarantee the attendance of long-term survivors socially integrated at school or employment. Besides the clinical visit, this follow-up visit includes a number of consultations by specialists as well as time-consuming highly specialized investigations. Furthermore, time for special questions and for counseling of the patient should be allocated. As a consequence, this visit has to be prepared carefully before the scheduled date. The long-term follow-up visit can be divided into three different phases: the preparation for the clinic visit; the structured visit itself; the post-clinic follow-up [4].

The *preparation of the follow-up visit* begins with the reviewing of all documents and medical records available. The aim of this review is to visualize the individual risk constellation of the transplant survivor, the detailed treatment schedule, and the current problems. At the first visit, all relevant information should be included in the survivorship care plan. If this plan has not been provided by the transplant clinic, the long-term follow-up clinic should take the opportunity to draw it up. In the case of a follow-up visit, recommendations provided during the previous visit should be registered for the visit. Based on this review of the documents, the structured visit with a customized screening plan can be designed. It is recommended to share the information in a team meeting held before the scheduled follow-up visit including all participants of the multidisciplinary team. After this meeting, the definitive plan is set for the visit.

The *clinic follow-up visit* includes the review of the history since last visit and the physical exam performed by the clinician. The team should decide who will address which question to the patient, in order neither to be repetitious nor to omit important questions concerning the medical, family, social, and psychological history. The physical exam should focus on organs at risk for late effects after HSCT, considering the history of the patient, their previous visits, and their new complaints. For particular examinations, the subspecialist should be involved, such as gynecologist, dermatologist, dentist, ophthalmologist, or endocrinologist. These examinations by subspecialists, as well as particular exams such as radiological exams, lung function tests, and cardiologic investigations, have to be scheduled carefully for the visit. During the follow-up visit, comment on previous recommendations, and the concrete consequences drawn from them have to be considered. Finally, adequate time has to be dedicated for a general discussion and health counseling with the survivor, and, if desired, with relatives or a person of acquaintance. A checklist of the recommendations for concrete counseling is shown in Table A.2.2.

The aim of the *post-clinic follow-up* is to summarize the patient's status and provide further recommendations for the health care provider. Therefore, all clinical and biological information obtained should be available. It is wise if a single staff member is responsible for tracking all results and information. Once all results and information are assembled, one of the clinicians is responsible for the overall summary. At a regular base, the long-term survivorship visits should be discussed in the multidisciplinary follow-up team and, if necessary, with representatives of a subspecialty. The follow-up visit will be summarized in a single, structured document. This document is a useful tool for the primary health care provider, as well as for the long-term follow-up clinic.

Depending on which model of transplant follow-up clinic is chosen, the organization of the long-term

Table A.2.2 Check-list of recommendations for counseling of the long-term survivor during the follow-up visit according to the Ref. [5]

1. *Healthy heart lifestyle recommendations*
   a. Eat healthy diet with a wide variety of foods
   b. Do not smoke (passive and active exposure), chew tobacco, or use illegal drugs. For smoker, insist on smoking cessation
   c. Use alcohol in moderation, generally <2 drinks per day
   d. Maintain a healthy weight
   e. Avoid excessive exposure and wear sunscreen protection for anticipated periods of longer exposure
   f. Follow general population age-specific guidelines for physical activity
      i. Adults aged 18 to 64 years should do 2 h 30 min a week a moderate-intensity aerobic physical activity or 1 h 15 min a week of moderate- and vigorous-intensity aerobic physical activity or an equivalent combination of moderate- and vigorous-intensity aerobic physical activity
      ii. Aerobic activity should be performed in episodes of at least 10 min
      iii. Adults should also do muscle strengthening activities that involve all major muscle groups performed on two or more days per week
2. *Other recommendations to the patient during the follow-up visit*
   a. Skin self-examination
   b. Second cancer vigilance counseling
   c. Counseling and education about preventive oral health and routine dental maintenance
   d. Avoid iron supplementation and alcohol ingestion for patients with iron overload
   e. Particular counseling for women
      i. In women with gonadal recovery, counseling contraception. Contraception is advisable if fertile or if fertility status is not known and pregnancy not desired
      ii. Counseling about preventive measures for bone loss and fractures (physical exercise; vitamin D supplementation, hormone replacement)
      iii. Self-examination of the vaginal area, general hygiene measures, and early recognition of local symptoms

follow-up visit will differ. Whatever model is chosen, however, the structured follow-up of long-term survivors will need additional personnel, time, and clinic space resources. More details are presented in Chapter 3.

Screening and preventive recommendations

Recommendations on screening and preventive practices for long-term survivors after HSCT have been published for the first time by experts from the Center for International Blood and Marrow Transplant Research, the European Group for Blood and Marrow Transplantation and the American Society for Blood and Marrow Transplantation in 2006. These guidelines were updated in 2012, expanding the working group by including participants from most of the societies of HSCT worldwide [5]. From these recommendations, the National Marrow Donor Program provided recommended posttransplant care guidelines for physicians and patients (Appendix 1) [3]. These guidelines include the most common complications, the recommended tests to be performed, and an outline of the preventive measure as well as the recommended timing, organ by organ.

References

1. Institute of Medicine. From Cancer Patient to Cancer Survivor: Lost in Transition. Washington DC: The National Academics Press, 2006.
2. Horowitz ME, Fordis M, Krause S, et al. Passport for care: implementing the survivorship care plan. J Oncol Pract. 2009;5:110–112.
3. National Marrow Donor Program/Be The Match. Recommended Post-Transplant Care: Long-Term Survival Guidelines. 2012. Physician version: http://www.marrow.org/md-guidelines; patient version: http://www.BeTheMatch.org/careguide (accessed 23 May 2013).
4. Children's Oncology Group Nursing Discipline Clinical Practice Subcommittee Survivorship in collaboration with the Late Effects Committee. Establishing and Enhancing Services for Childhood Cancer Survivors: Long-Term Follow-Up Program Resource Guide (CureSearch Children's Oncology Group edition) 2007.
5. Majhail NS, Rizzo JD, Lee SJ, et al. Recommended screening and preventive practices for long-term survivors after hematopoietic cell transplantation. Bone Marrow Transplant. 2012; 47:337–341.

APPENDIX 3
Commonly used transplant-related medications in long-term survivors

Melissa Logue
Hematology and Stem Cell Transplantation Section, Division of Hematology/Oncology, Department of Medicine, Vanderbilt University Medical Center, Nashville, TN, USA

Declaration of commercial interest

None.

Blood and Marrow Transplantation Long-Term Management: Prevention and Complications, First Edition. Edited by Bipin N Savani.

Table A.3.1 Commonly used transplant-related medications in long-term survivors (ref: Chapter 8)

Medication	Indication	Alternative
Acyclovir	Viral prophylaxis	Valacyclovir (Valtrex)
Budesonide (Entocort)	Gut graft-versus-host disease (GVHD)	
Cyclosporine (Gengraf)[a]	GVHD prophylaxis and treatment	n/a
Depo Provera	Menstrual prophylaxis	Provera, Premarin
Ergocalciferol (vitamin D_2)	Vitamin D deficiency	
Filgrastim (Neupogen; granulocyte-colony stimulating factor)	Neutropenia	
Fluconazole (Diflucan) or voriconazole (Vfend) or posaconazole or micafungin	Fungal prophylaxis and treatment- selection of drug depends on underlying condition	
Levofloxacin (Levaquin)	Bacterial prophylaxis	Cefuroxime, ciprofloxacin, moxifloxacin
Mycophenolate mofetil (Cellcept)	GVHD prophylaxis (for reduced-dose treatment regimens)	
Oxycodone	PRN pain	Morphine, Dilaudid
Prednisone	GVHD	Methylprednisolone
Prilosec (omeprazole)	Heartburn prevention	Nexium, Protonix
Prochlorperazine maleate (Compazine)	Nausea/vomiting	Ondansetron, promethazine, lorazepam
Sirolumus (rapamycin)	GVHD prophylaxis and treatment	
Sulfamethoxazole–trimethoprim (BactrimDS)	*Pneumocystis jirovecii* pneumonia prophylaxis	Dapsone, pentamidine inhalation
Tacrolimus (Prograf)[a]	GVHD prophylaxis and treatment	
Triamcinolone/hydrocortisone cream	Skin GVHD	
Ursodiol (Actigall)	Sinusoidal obstruction syndrome prophylaxis	

[a] The following increase cyclosporine (also tacrolimus) blood concentrations: diltiazem, nicardipine, verapamil, voriconazole (severe drug interactions), fluconazole, itraconazole, ketoconazole, clarithromycin, erythromycin, lansoprazole (pantoprazole and omeprazole do not change cyclosporine levels significantly), rabeprazole, cimetidine, methylprednisolone, allopurinol, bromocriptine, metoclopramide, colchicine, amiodarone, danazole, grapefruit juice. The following lower the cyclosporine (also tacrolimus) blood concentrations: nafcillin, rifabutin, rifampin, carbamazepine, phenobarbital, phenytoin, octreotide, ticlopidine, orlistat, St John's wort.

Index

Blood and Marrow Transplantation Long-Term Management: Prevention and Complications, First Edition. Edited by Bipin N Savani.